Case Studies in

Clinical Cardiac Electrophysiology

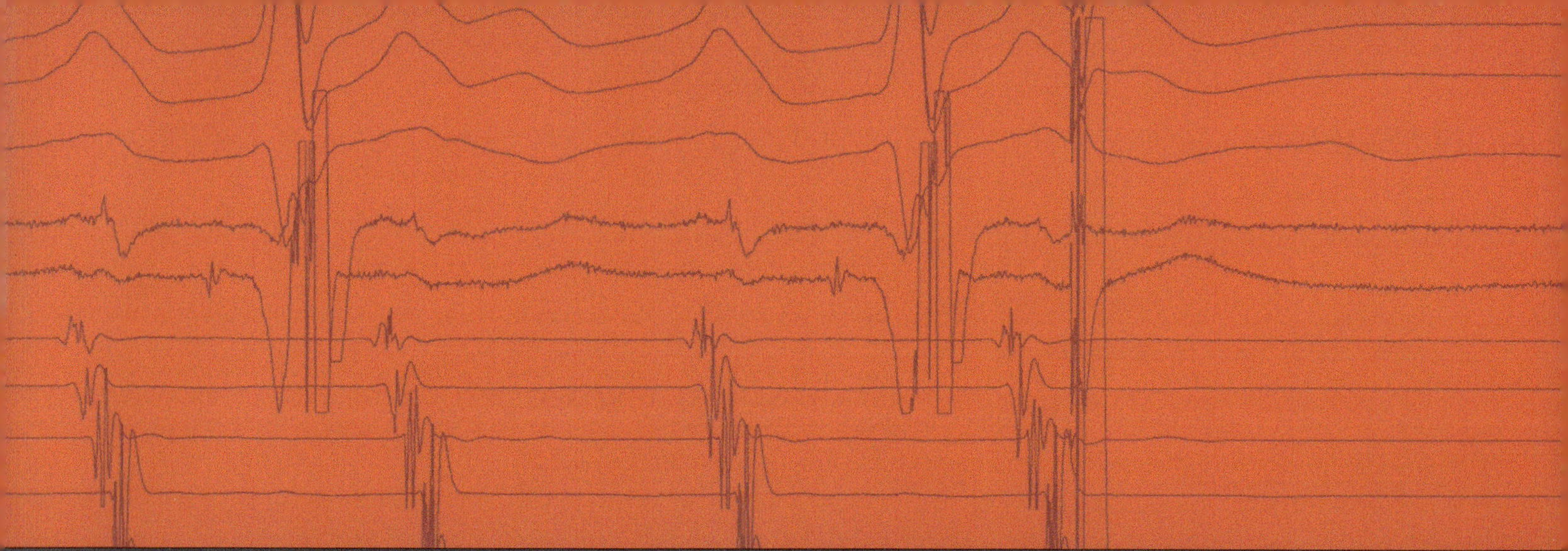

Case Studies in Clinical Cardiac Electrophysiology

John M. Miller, MD
Professor of Medicine, Indiana University School of Medicine
Director, Clinical Cardiac Electrophysiology
Indianapolis, Indiana

Mithilesh K. Das, MD
Professor of Clinical Medicine, Indiana University School of Medicine
Indianapolis, Indiana

Douglas P. Zipes, MD
Distinguished Professor Emeritus of Medicine, Pharmacology and Toxicology
Indiana University School of Medicine
Emeritus Director, Krannert Institute of Cardiology
Indianapolis, Indiana

ELSEVIER

ELSEVIER

1600 John F. Kennedy Blvd.
Ste 1800
Philadelphia, PA 19103-2899

CASE STUDIES IN CLINICAL CARDIAC ELECTROPHYSIOLOGY ISBN: 978-0-323-18772-5

Notices

Knowledge and best practice in this field are constantly changing. As new research and experience broaden our understanding, changes in research methods, professional practices, or medical treatment may become necessary.

Practitioners and researchers must always rely on their own experience and knowledge in evaluating and using any information, methods, compounds, or experiments described herein. In using such information or methods they should be mindful of their own safety and the safety of others, including parties for whom they have a professional responsibility.

With respect to any drug or pharmaceutical products identified, readers are advised to check the most current information provided (i) on procedures featured or (ii) by the manufacturer of each product to be administered, to verify the recommended dose or formula, the method and duration of administration, and contraindications. It is the responsibility of practitioners, relying on their own experience and knowledge of their patients, to make diagnoses, to determine dosages and the best treatment for each individual patient, and to take all appropriate safety precautions.

To the fullest extent of the law, neither the Publisher nor the authors, contributors, or editors, assume any liability for any injury and/or damage to persons or property as a matter of products liability, negligence or otherwise, or from any use or operation of any methods, products, instructions, or ideas contained in the material herein.

Library of Congress Cataloging-in-Publication Data

Names: Miller, John M. (John Michael), 1954- author. | Das, Mithilesh K., author. | Zipes, Douglas P., author.
Title: Case studies in clinical cardiac electrophysiology / John Miller, Mithilesh Das, Douglas Zipes.
Description: Philadelphia, PA : Elsevier, [2018] | Includes bibliographical references and index.
Identifiers: LCCN 2016053043 | ISBN 9780323187725 (hardcover : alk. paper)
Subjects: | MESH: Heart Diseases--diagnosis | Electrophysiologic Techniques,
Cardiac--methods | Case Reports
Classification: LCC RC683.5.E5 | NLM WG 141.5.F9 | DDC 616.1/2075--dc23
LC record available at https://lccn.loc.gov/2016053043

Content Strategist: Maureen Iannuzzi
Senior Content Development Specialist: Janice Galliard
Publishing Services Manager: Catherine Jackson
Project Manager: Kate Mannix
Design Direction: Brian Salisbury

Printed in the United States of America by
Sheridan Kentucky, 100 US-60, Versailles, KY 40384

Last digit is the print number: 9 8 7 6

Keenly aware of the time and energy diverted from our families that was required to perform these procedures and assemble the recordings into a form accessible by readers, we dedicate this volume to our beloved wives (Jeanne, Rekha, and Joan), who have allowed us the privilege of putting this work together. We also dedicate this work to the readers, who we hope will benefit from the lessons we have tried to convey, and finally to their patients, who we hope will in turn benefit from their learning.

Foreword

The practice of clinical cardiac electrophysiology is one of clinical exploration that starts with integration of the patient's symptoms and cardiac evaluation with electrocardiographic interpretation. One of the most gratifying experiences for patient and physician is when this process culminates in the electrophysiology laboratory with confirmation of the diagnosis and implementation of effective therapy for the arrhythmia with catheter ablation. Mastery of each component is needed, and the knowledge that is gained from each step can be applied to the previous step to refine one's diagnostic acumen. We became much better electrocardiographers by applying the knowledge gained from the pioneering work that defined cardiac activation patterns and arrhythmia mechanisms using cardiac mapping and programmed electrical stimulation. Expertise in the last step, interventional electrophysiology, is the most challenging to acquire. It requires assimilation of complex patterns of cardiac activation, interpretation of spontaneous changes in patterns, and application of maneuvers to confirm a diagnosis, and this confirmation is critical for guiding catheter ablation.

Drs. Miller, Das, and Zipes have assembled a wonderful book that captures the spirit of clinical exploration leading to effective therapy. They use cases to describe pathophysiologic concepts that start with fundamentals and proceed to complex concepts. From the electrophysiology laboratory they incorporate findings ranging from those that are classic to those that are only recently described and that require a nuanced interpretation and understanding, but that are critical to arriving at the correct diagnosis. Examples include the newest technologies that are now being applied for delineation of arrhythmia mechanisms and substrate.

The authors are renowned teachers who apply their wealth of experience in communicating complex scenarios and concepts to make the cases accessible for the complete range of students of clinical electrophysiology, from the trainee to the advanced practitioner. The cases clarify concepts and provide fundamentals for the new student, but also provide insights that will expand the knowledge of experienced clinicians. Dr Miller's hand is evident throughout in the superb graphics, for which he is widely known among teachers of cardiology.

One of the amazing aspects of biology, medicine, and certainly extending to cardiac electrophysiology, is the variability that one encounters from patient to patient. After years in the field, one still encounters new arrhythmia problems. A solid basis in understanding mapping and diagnostic maneuvers is required for solving new puzzles in the electrophysiology laboratory, and this learning is acquired from the study of cases. You can never analyze too many cases. I congratulate the authors of *Case Studies in Clinical Cardiac Electrophysiology* on a wonderful book.

William G. Stevenson, MD
Director, Cardiac Arrhythmia Program
Cardiovascular Division
Brigham and Women's Hospital
Professor of Medicine, Harvard Medical School
Boston, Massachusetts

Preface

The understanding and care of patients with heart rhythm disturbances (clinical cardiac electrophysiology [EP]) has evolved in the last three decades from simple diagnostic studies of the conduction system using a few electrodes, to complex diagnostic and therapeutic procedures involving recording and stimulation from a large number of electrodes, for the purpose of finding and ablating arrhythmogenic tissue. With this dramatic change in the character of EP studies has come the critical need for careful analysis and thorough understanding of the meaning of recordings that are made and results of stimulation in order to achieve optimal results from ablation. At the same time, EP training programs have come under increasing pressure to perform more procedures in a shorter amount of time, resulting in compromising time for careful and methodical study of and learning from these procedures that are rich with teaching material. Although many excellent texts in our field explain the principles of recording and stimulation in treatment of arrhythmias, for example, *Clinical Arrhythmology and Electrophysiology*, few are structured to show their practical application in a case-study format. In light of this, the purpose of this volume is to take the reader through a representative series of EP procedures from start to finish, evaluating results of diagnostic pacing maneuvers, sampling and comparing characteristics of electrograms, and selection of appropriate sites for ablation. It is our hope that readers will benefit from this mode of presentation, highlighting some of the limitations of techniques that are used on a daily basis, with the aim of improving the efficacy and safety of procedures they perform on their patients.

Acknowledgments

We gratefully acknowledge the role played by our nursing and technical staff with whom we performed the procedures reviewed in this work, as well as electrophysiology fellows, whose patience in keeping catheters in place during long procedures contributed greatly to the quality of the figures. We also acknowledge our patients, who provide a constant source for learning.

Contents

Sinus Node and Atrioventricular Conduction Disease

1

Case Presentation

A 56-year-old man experienced syncope while walking at work. Coworkers called emergency medical services (EMS). Upon the arrival of EMS, he was awake and feeling normal but was convinced to go to the emergency room (ER). The patient had a history of anterior wall myocardial infarction (MI), percutaneous coronary intervention (PCI), to left anterior descending coronary artery (LAD) several years before, and a negative stress test within the last 6 months. Examination results were normal except for obesity. ECG showed sinus rhythm, long PR, right bundle branch block (RBBB), left anterior fascicular block (LAFB), and anterior scar. Echocardiogram revealed ejection fraction (EF) 40% and anterior hypokinesis. The patient was referred for electrophysiology (EP) study.

Baseline ECG

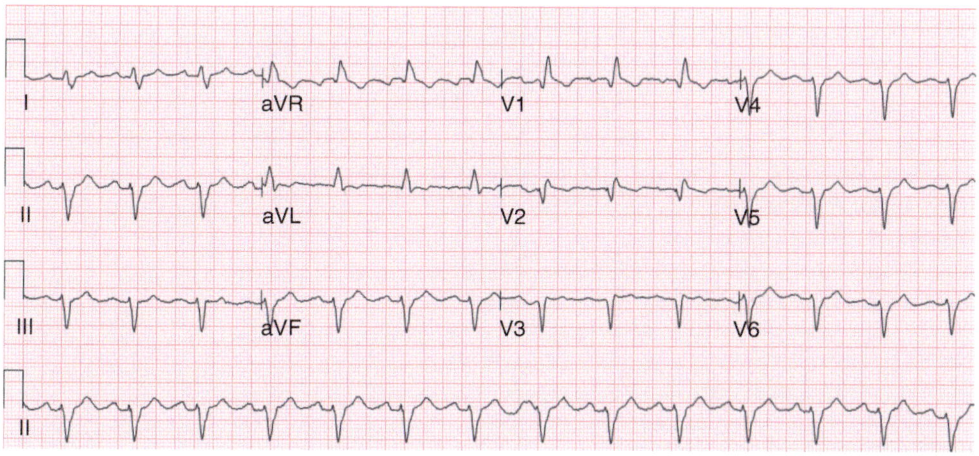

Figure 1-1

The ECG in Fig. 1-1 shows sinus rhythm with a prolonged P wave (left atrial abnormality), slightly prolonged PR interval, RBBB and left anterior fascicular block, and an extensive anterior infarction. On the basis of this, there are many possible causes of syncope—atrial arrhythmias (atrial flutter and fibrillation, other reentrant atrial tachycardias), heart block (either in AV node or His-Purkinje system), or ventricular arrhythmia (ventricular tachycardia or fibrillation). There is nothing in the ECG to favor one cause of syncope over another, and because treatment strategies are very different depending on the cause (medications or ablation for atrial arrhythmias; pacemaker for heart block; implantable defibrillator for ventricular arrhythmias), further investigation is needed.

Evaluation

Figure 1-2

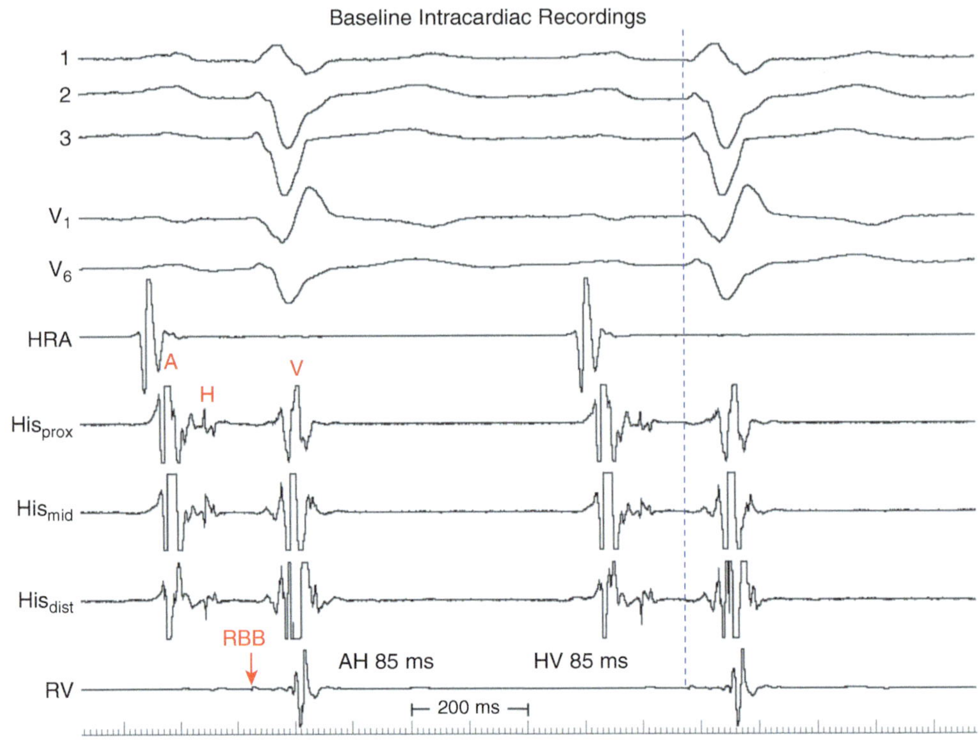

Intracardiac recordings during sinus rhythm (Fig. 1-2) show atrial (A), His (H), and ventricular (V) recordings as noted. This confirms the presence of His-Purkinje disease, with an HV interval of 85 ms—prolonged (normal, 40 to 55 ms), but not enough to implicate His-Purkinje dysfunction as a cause of heart block. Surprisingly, though the PR interval is somewhat prolonged, the AH interval is normal (85 ms [normal, 60 to 125 ms]). Usually, prolongation of the PR interval is caused by the AV nodal (AH) component, because to prolong the PR even 60 ms from His-Purkinje disease would require a lengthening of the HV to a degree (that is, from 40 ms to 100 ms) that 1:1 conduction would be unlikely. Note also that there is a delay between the distal His recording and right bundle branch (RBB)—there is usually <10 ms between these—and that the RBBB is further caused by delay or block between the RBB and RV apical electrogram, with a QRS onset *(dashed blue line)* to RV electrogram of 75 ms (normal, 10 to 35 ms).

Figure 1-3

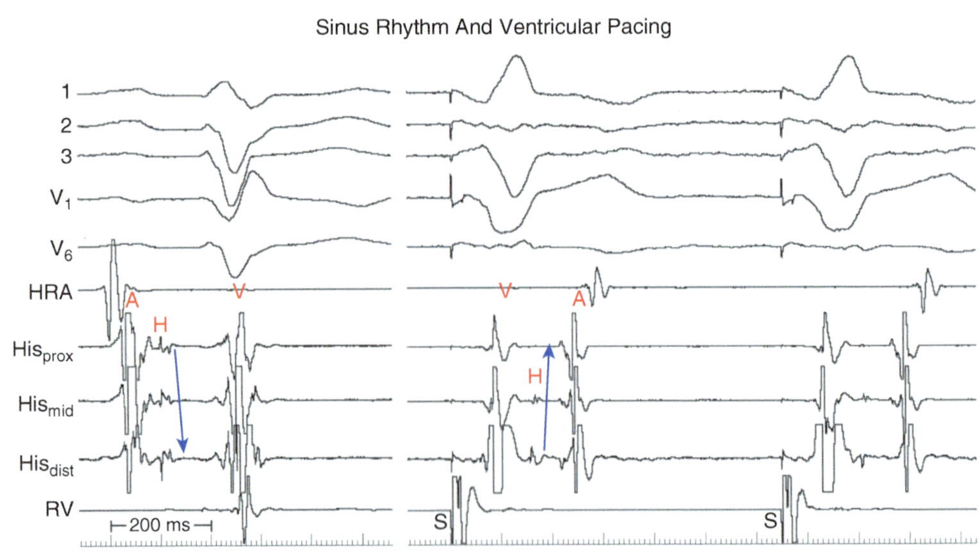

The left side of Fig. 1-3 shows a sinus rhythm complex as in the previous figure for reference, whereas the 2 complexes on the right are during pacing from the right ventricular apical region. Note that there is retrograde conduction to the atria, with the His bundle activated from distal to proximal as expected. Usually, the timing of the His potential is before the local ventricular electrogram in the His recoding, because conduction proceeds more rapidly up the RBB to the His than does muscle-to-muscle propagation from apex to base. Because there is RBBB in this case, the impulse cannot ascend the RBB as it normally would and instead must traverse the interventricular septum, enter the left bundle branch, and then activate the His retrogradely. These findings just confirm the His-Purkinje disease but give no further insight as to the cause of syncope.

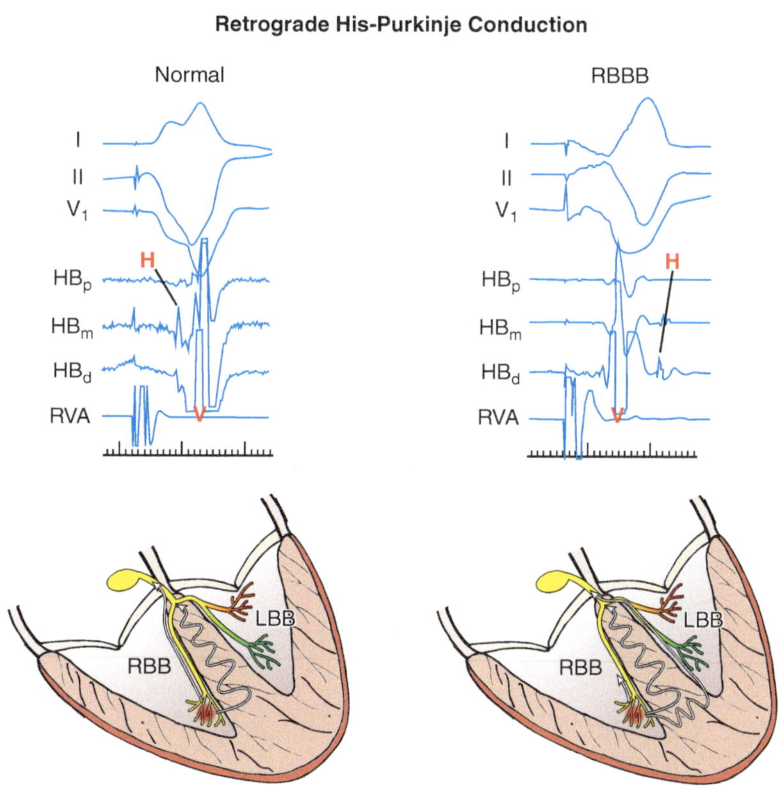

Figure 1-4

As illustrated in Fig. 1-4, in patients with normal His-Purkinje function (at *left*), pacing from the right ventricular apex *(red circle)* results in retrograde conduction over the RBB *(white line)* that is more rapid than muscle-to-muscle conduction (*wavy line* in septum), resulting in a His potential (H) inscribed before the larger local ventricular recording (V). At right, in the presence of anterograde RBBB, the paced wavefront cannot ascend the blocked right bundle and instead crosses the interventricular septum *(wavy horizontal line)* to engage the left bundle, and then proceeds rapidly to the His that now appears after the local ventricular recording (that is again generated after muscle-to-muscle spread).

Figure 1-5

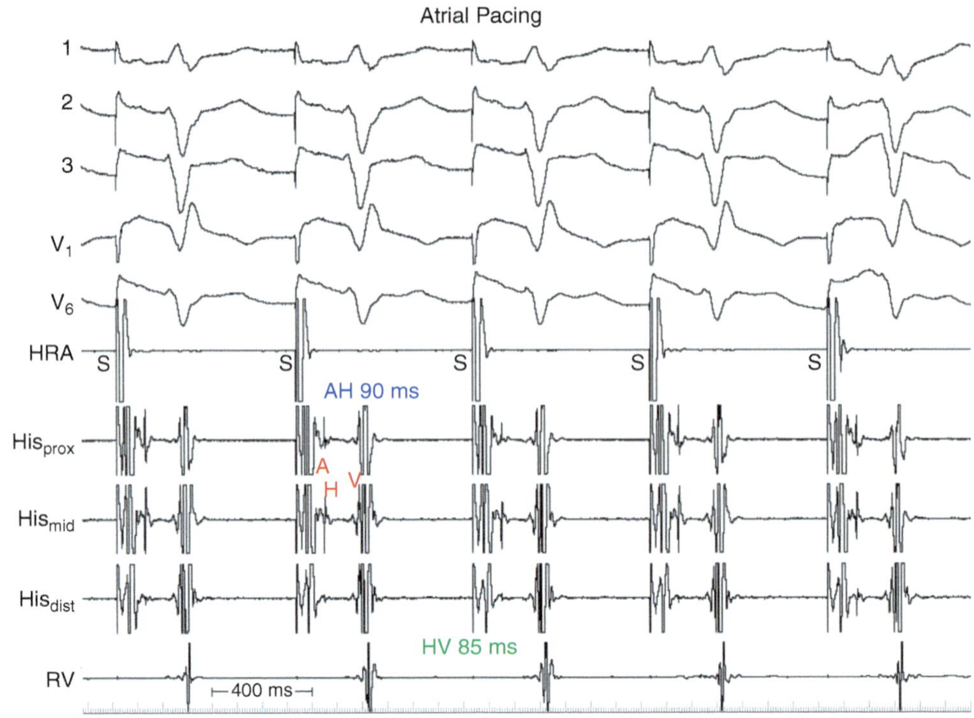

Rapid pacing can often reveal abnormalities of AV conduction that were not very evident at rest. In Fig. 1-5, pacing the atrium (S) slightly faster than the sinus rate shows minimal change in either AH (90 ms) or HV (85 ms) intervals. It is useful to display multiple electrode pairs of His recordings because the signal amplitude may vary enough between complexes that the His potential may be poorly visible or even absent in one electrode pair (His_{dist} in this case), whereas it is readily visible in other electrode pairs.

Figure 1-6

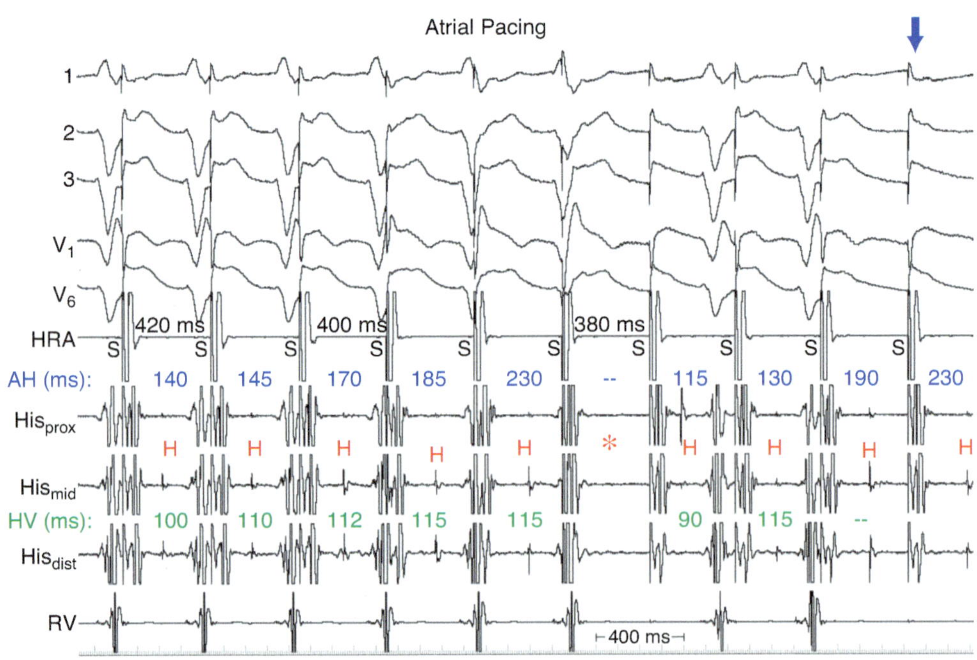

More rapid pacing starts to reveal some abnormalities. As the pacing rate increases (cycle length decreases), the AH is expected to prolong but the HV interval usually remains constant. In Fig. 1-6, the AH (in *blue*) does prolong, but so does the HV interval (in *green*). The *asterisk* denotes where AV nodal block occurs (no subsequent His potential), but three cycles after this, there is a His potential not followed by a QRS (infra-His block; *green dash*)

and the HV intervals on the prior two cycles had prolonged (thus, infra-His Wenckebach). This is distinctly abnormal and likely warrants pacemaker implantation. However, this may not be the reason that syncope had occurred (there may be other abnormalities that have not yet been uncovered during the study).

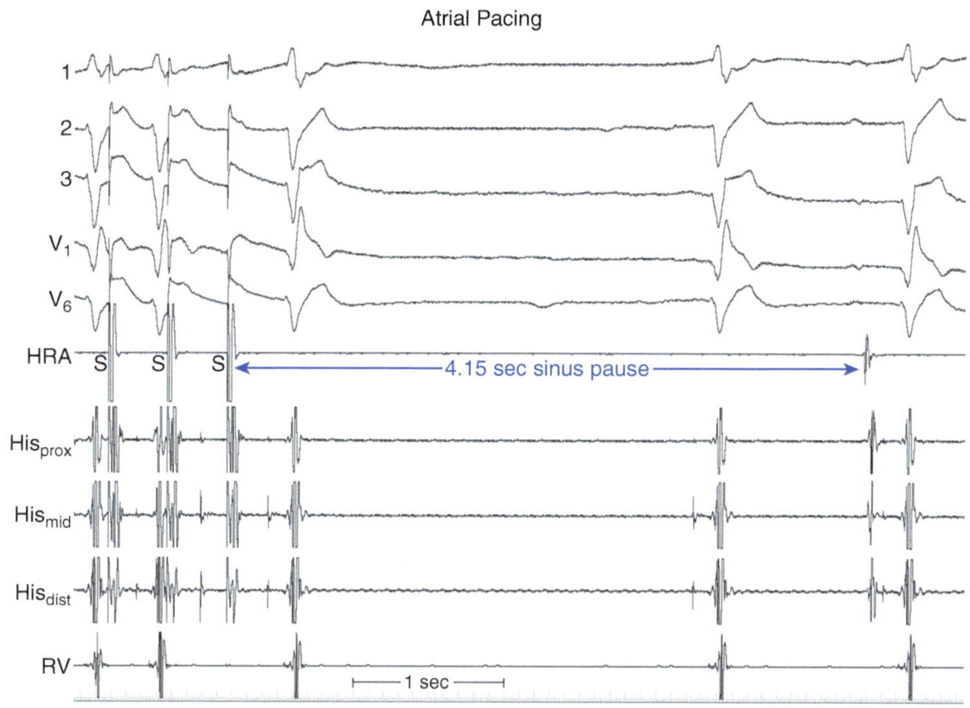

Figure 1-7

In Fig. 1-7, pacing is repeated for 1 min at the same cycle length as shown in the prior figure to stress the sinus node. Upon cessation of pacing, a prolonged sinus pause (4.15 seconds) is observed; a junctional escape complex occurs after 3 seconds. This is another potential cause of syncope (sinus node dysfunction).

Figure 1-8

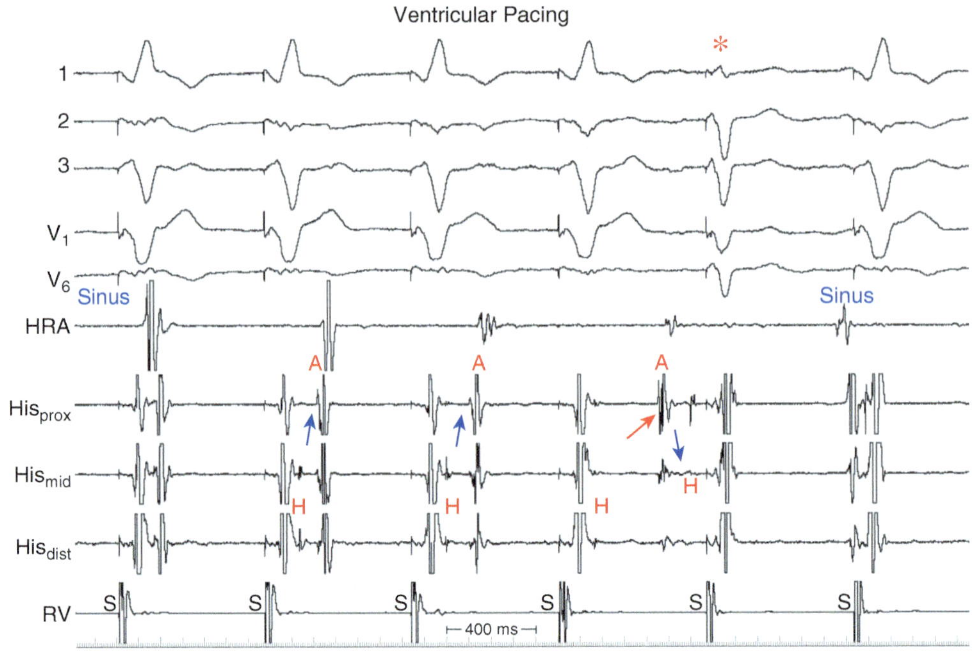

Turning to the ventricles (Fig. 1-8), slow ventricular pacing again shows that there is retrograde conduction; the first and last atrial complexes are sinus in origin (HRA before His atrial recordings) but the middle three complexes are retrogradely conducted. The first two of these *(blue arrows)* are over the fast pathway, but after the fourth ventricular stimulus, the ventriculoatrial interval suddenly increases, signifying a switch to a slow pathway *(red arrow)*. Immediately after this, there is a QRS complex that is not fully paced *(asterisk)*; this is because of fusion between the paced wavefront and one over the normal conduction system (see His potential). This is the result of an atypical AV nodal echo (retrograde slow pathway, anterograde fast—*blue arrow*). This is a common finding and, unless accompanied by sustained atypical AV nodal reentrant SVT, has no relevance for the diagnosis of syncope.

Figure 1-9

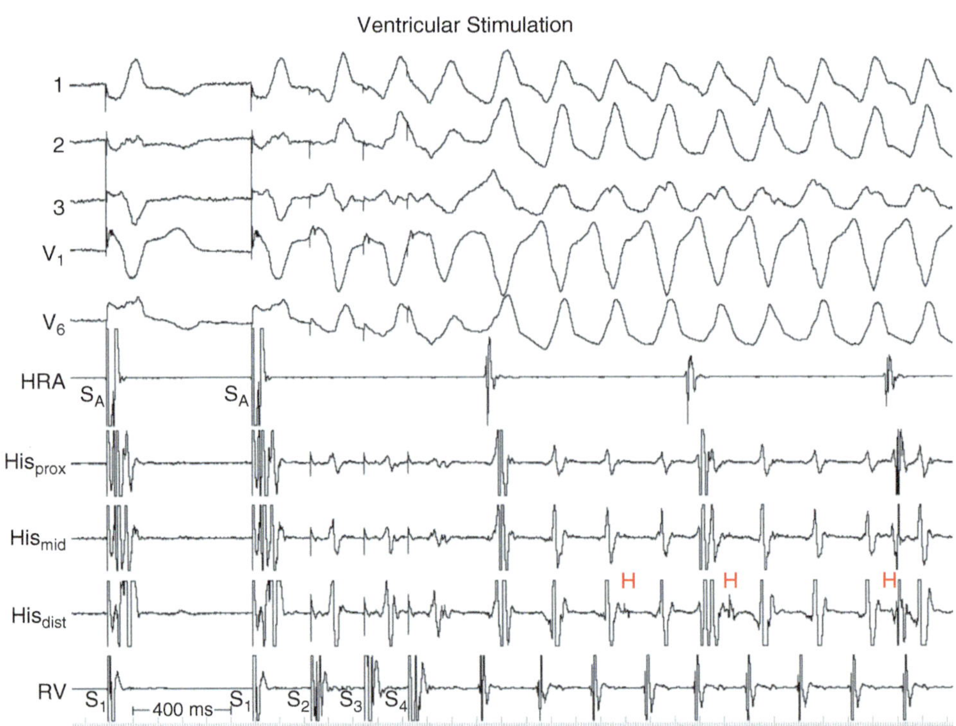

The last part of the syncope evaluation consists of programmed ventricular stimulation. As shown in Fig. 1-9, standard stimulation (here, with triple extrastimuli, S2 to S4) initiates a rapid, hemodynamically unstable ventricular tachycardia (CL 250 ms) that stopped spontaneously after 15 seconds. Given the presence of a prior MI and "serious" syncope, this arrhythmia was deemed a reasonable candidate for the cause of his syncope. He received a dual-chamber ICD later that day. Note that a His potential is seen on occasion but not with every complex—excluding bundle branch reentry as a possible cause of the tachycardia (S_A = atrial stimulus).

Summary

- This man had syncope in the presence of structural heart disease—which always needs further evaluation.
- Multiple potential causes of syncope may be present in the same patient; in this case,
  - Sinus node dysfunction
  - His-Purkinje dysfunction
  - Ventricular tachycardia
- Judgment must be used to determine which possible cause(s) of syncope should be treated and how.

Typical ("Slow-Fast") Atrioventricular Nodal Reentry 2

Case Presentation

A 48-year-old woman had a history of palpitations for ~5 years. Her episodes started and stopped suddenly, lasted 1 to 2 minutes, and were associated with lightheadedness. She came to a local emergency room with a prolonged episode: ECG showed a narrow QRS tachycardia (by report; no ECG available) that was terminated with adenosine. She was treated with oral diltiazem and metoprolol but continued to have supraventricular tachycardia (SVT) episodes. She had a normal physical exam; non-invasive evaluation showed no structural heart disease. She was referred for catheter ablation of her SVT.

Baseline ECGs and Intracardiac Recordings

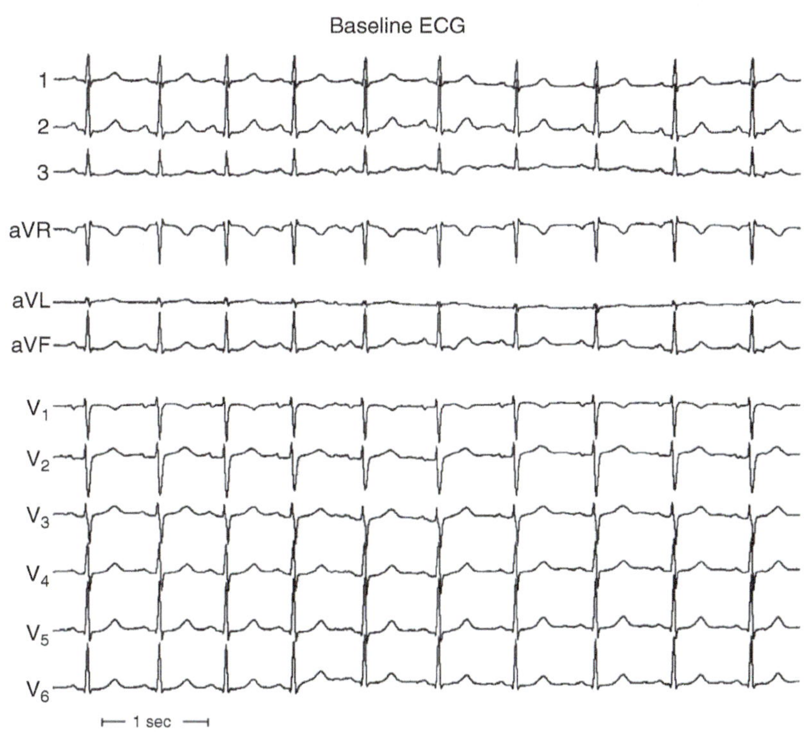

Figure 2-1

Fig. 2-1 demonstrates normal sinus rhythm without delta waves, fractionation, or prolongation of the P wave or QRS and normal QT. ECG is normal.

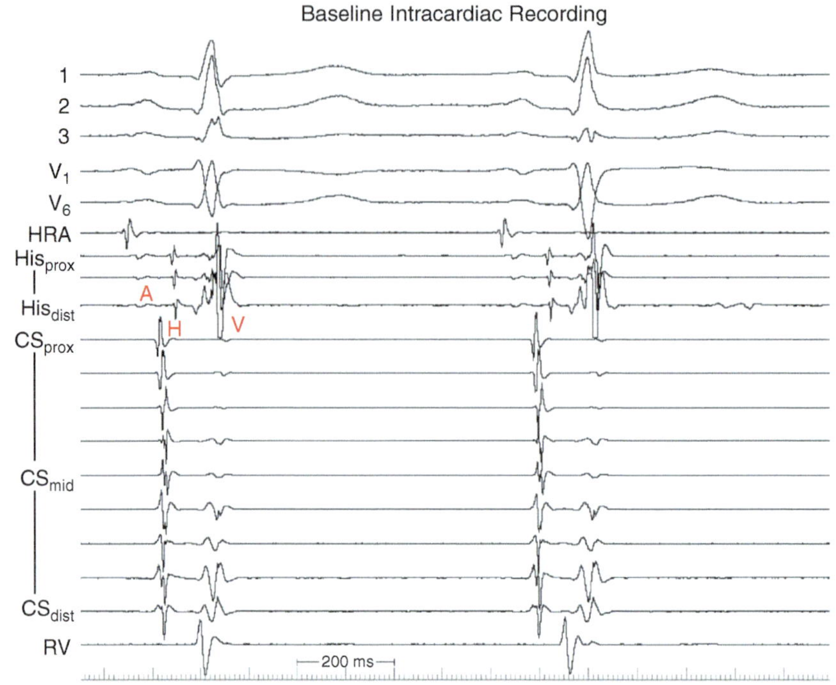

Figure 2-2

Fig. 2-2 shows normal intracardiac intervals (AH, HV); there is no evidence of preexcitation on intracardiac recordings. Normal progression of atrial activation is seen from right atrium to His to coronary sinus proximal to distal.

Ventricular Pacing

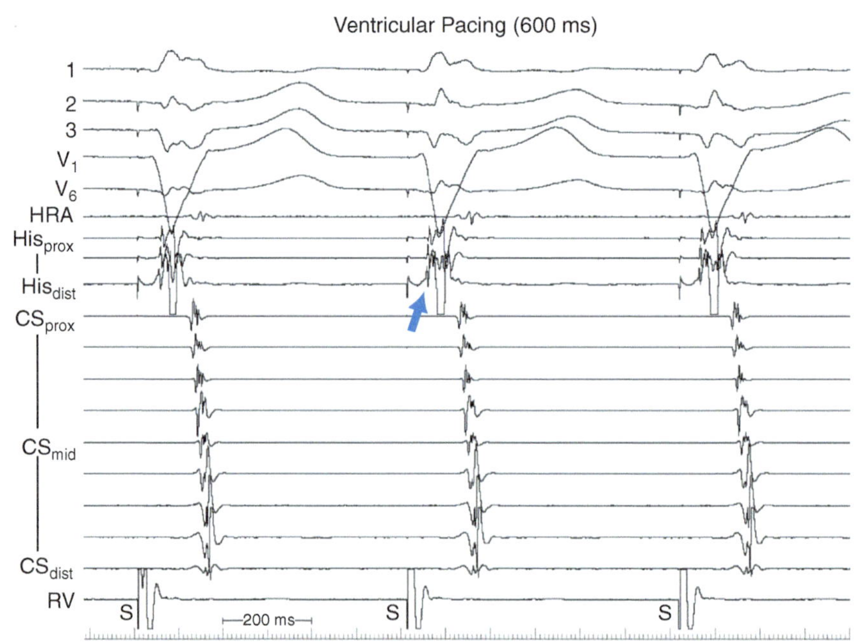

Figure 2-3

In Fig. 2-3, with ventricular pacing at 600 ms, retrograde conduction is present with a concentric activation pattern; a retrograde His potential *(arrow)* is seen between stimulus artifact and local ventricular electrogram.

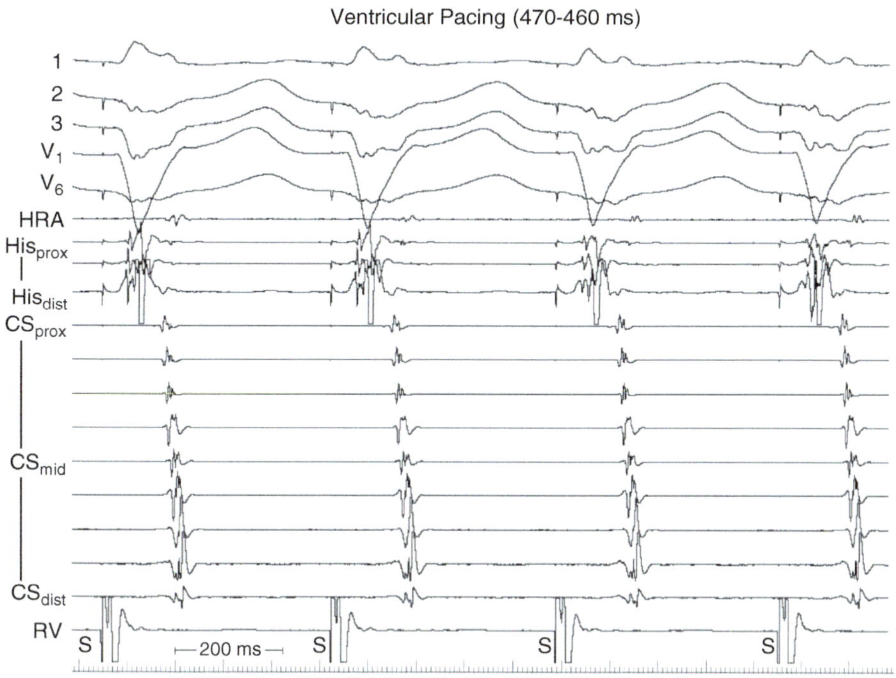

Figure 2-4

With more rapid ventricular pacing (470–460 ms) the same activation sequence is seen in Fig. 2-4, with a longer VA interval—most consistent with AV nodal conduction.

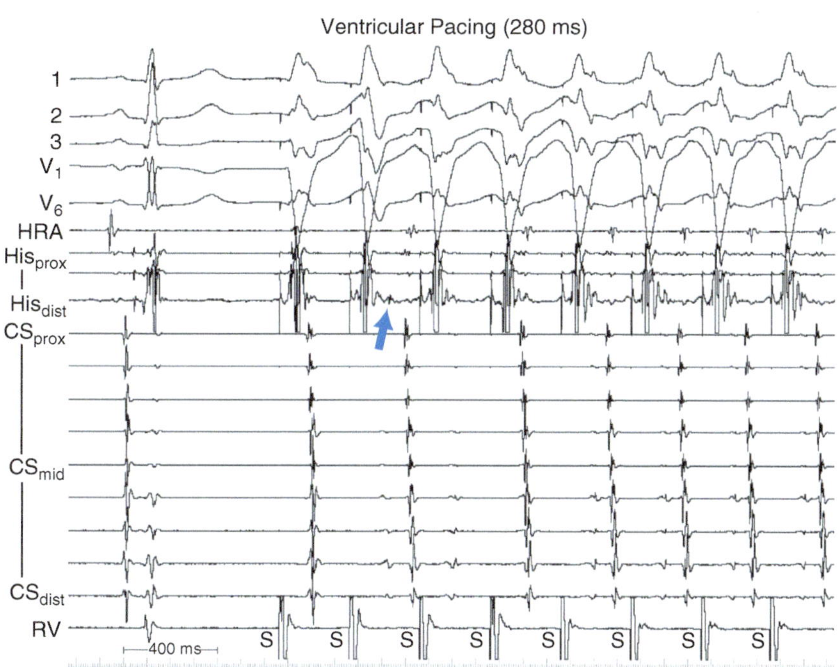

Figure 2-5

In Fig. 2-5, with the sudden onset of ventricular pacing (280 ms), a His "out the back" *(arrow)* is seen after second stimulus, with atrial activation dependent on His (ie, no bypass tract). Retrograde block occurs after the third stimulus likely because of block in the His-Purkinje system, which recovers by the fourth stimulus (after which 1:1 retrograde conduction resumes).

ECGs Compared

Figure 2-6

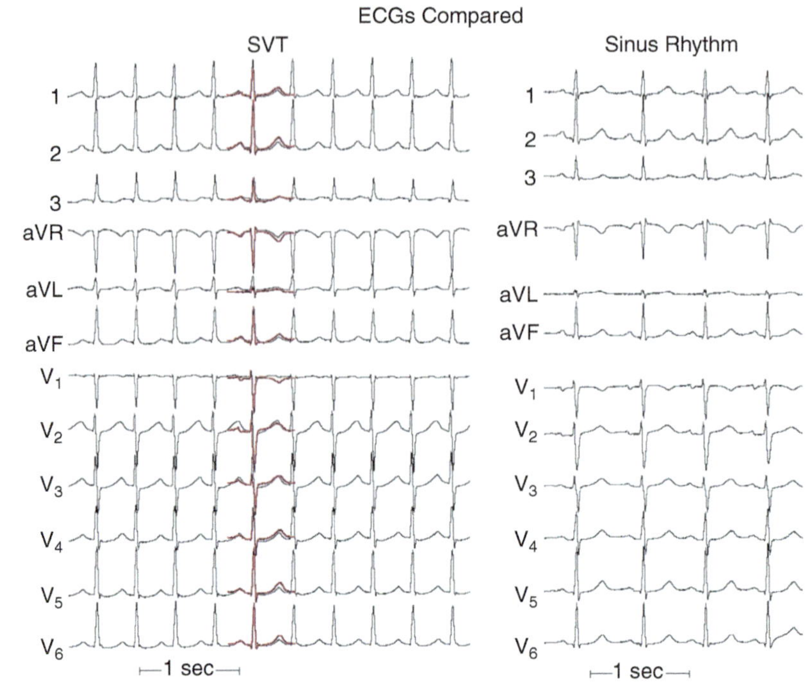

SVT was induced ((*left*); sinus rhythm is shown at right in Fig. 2-6. A superimposed sinus complex *(red)* overlaid on SVT shows no clear difference, implying that the P wave must be hidden within the QRS complex.

Ventricular Pacing in SVT

Figure 2-7

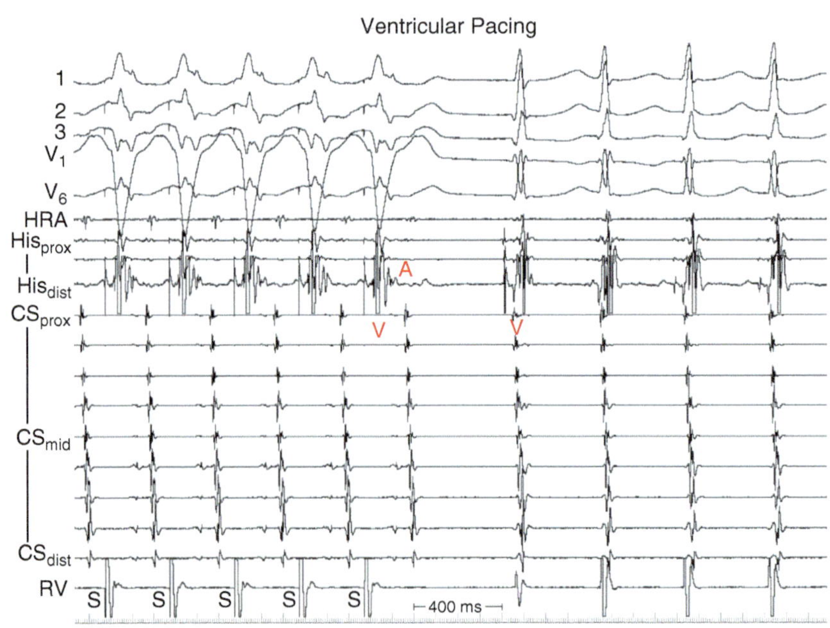

In Fig. 2-7, ventricular pacing during SVT conducts retrogradely to atrium with the same activation pattern as during SVT. During SVT that resumes on cessation of pacing, atrial activation appears concentric and within (even before) the QRS complex, excluding orthodromic SVT. The long pause after pacing suggests conduction down an AV nodal slow pathway. The "VAV" response is consistent with typical atrioventricular nodal reentry (AVNRT), not atrial tachycardia (AT).

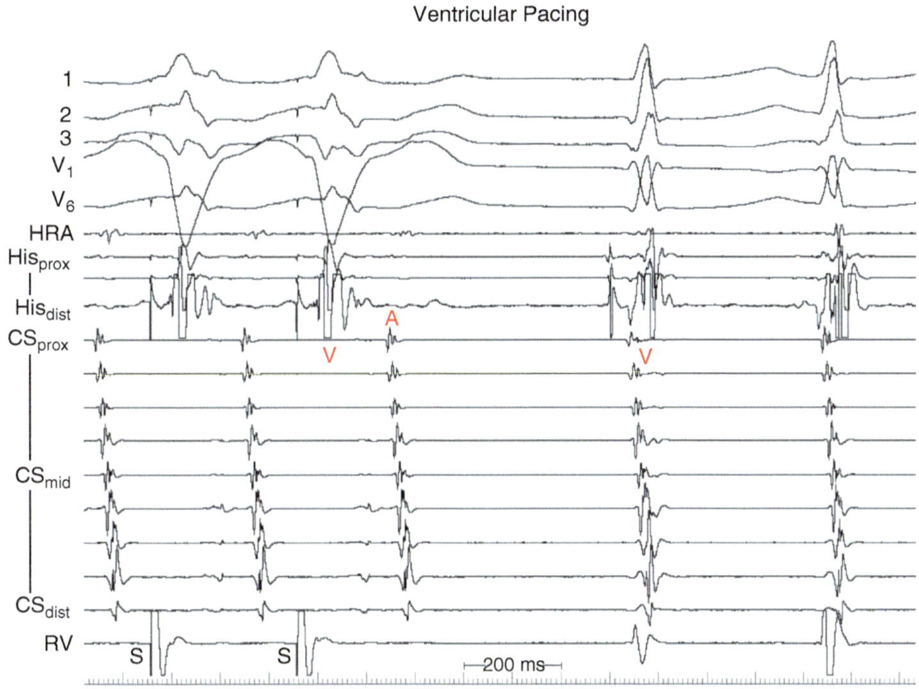

Figure 2-8

Fig. 2-8 is a faster sweep speed of Fig. 2-7, showing the same findings.

Para-Hisian Pacing

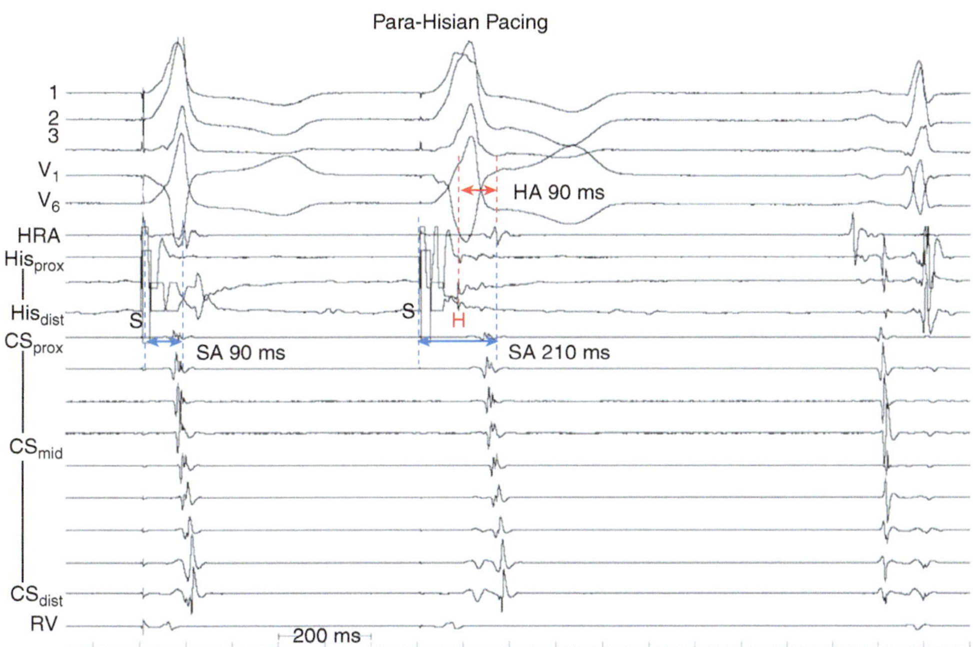

Figure 2-9

The complex at right of Fig. 2-9 shows a normal sinus complex. The complex in middle has a wide QRS suggesting pure ventricular capture. Retrograde conduction is evident. The complex at left is relatively narrow, indicating some element of His capture, though not pure His capture (His + V capture); retrograde conduction is evident with the same pattern as during the wider complex and S-A interval is 90 ms; in the wide complex (V capture only), the S-A interval is 210 ms, indicating conduction only over AV node. The retrograde His is visible (H), with HA still 90 ms.

Ventricular Extrastimuli in Sinus Rhythm

Figure 2-10

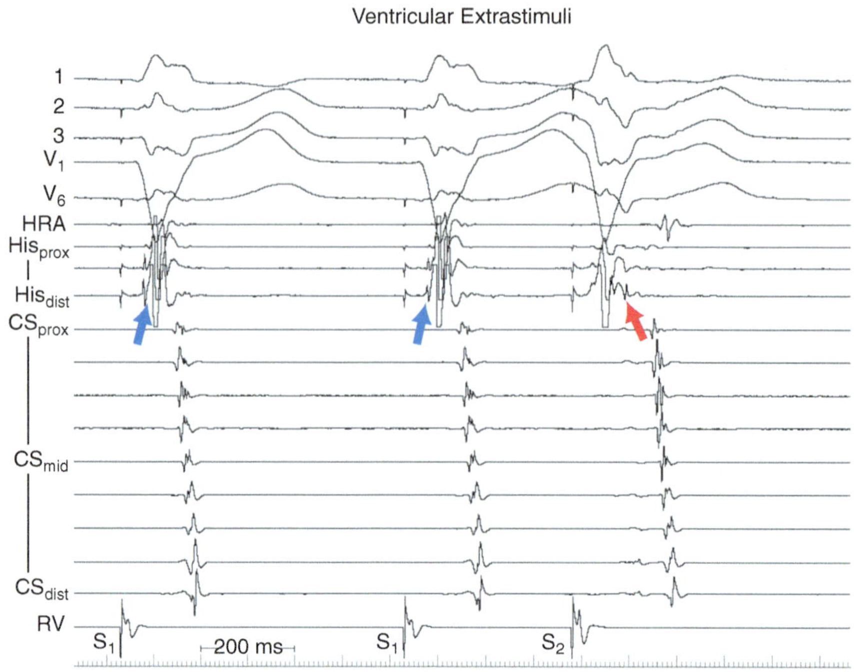

A single ventricular extrastimulus at a drive of 600 ms is shown in Fig. 2-10. A retrograde His *(blue arrow)* is seen before the local ventricular electrogram on drive complexes, whereas the His is "out the back" *(red arrow)* after the extrastimulus complex, as a result of block in the right bundle branch with transseptal conduction to and then up the left bundle to the His. If this relationship (atrial activation dependent on prior His activation) remains constant over a range of coupling intervals, a bypass tract is excluded.

Ventricular Extrastimuli in SVT

Figure 2-11

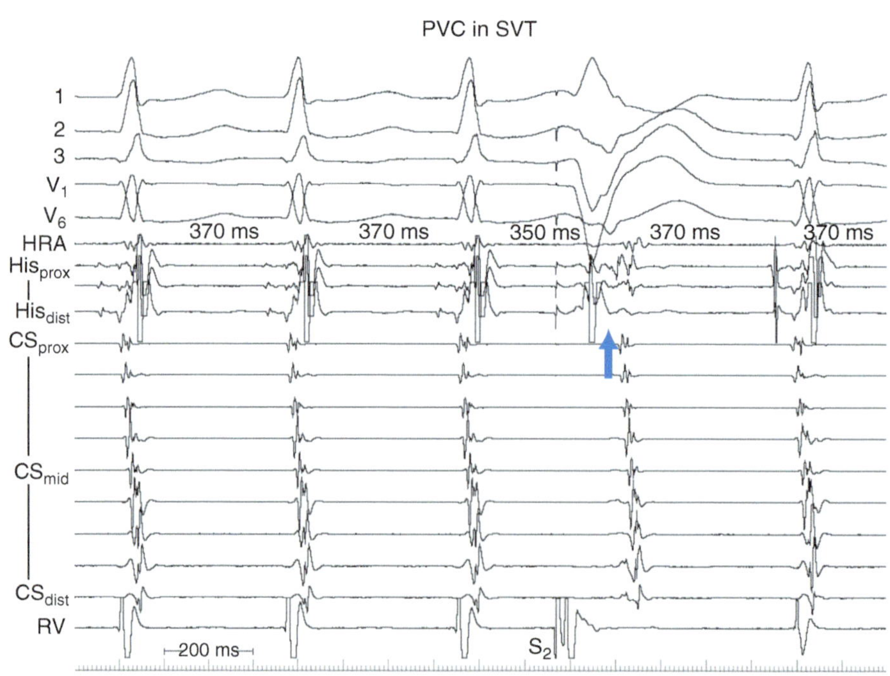

In Fig. 2-11, a ventricular extrastimulus is given during SVT. The A-A interval surrounding the extrastimulus is shorter than the rest of the A-A intervals, but the His was not refractory (*blue arrow*

shows where it would be expected if not for the extrastimulus). Advancement of the timing of atrial activation surrounding a *His-refractory* ventricular extrastimulus demonstrates the existence of a path of conduction extrinsic to the normal conduction system (bypass tract). If the extrastimulus occurs at a time when the His is not refractory (as here), it is feasible that conduction could occur through the His to the AV node and atrium, and would not implicate a bypass tract.

Atrial and Ventricular Pacing and Extrastimuli During SVT

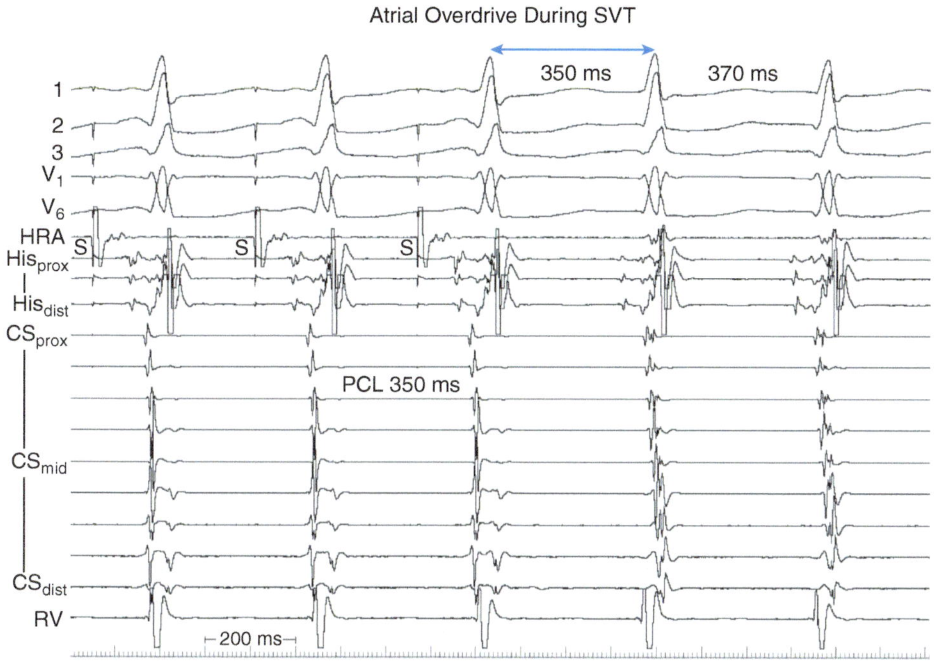

Figure 2-12

Overdrive atrial pacing during SVT is shown in Fig. 2-12. At first glance, the third QRS complex appears to result from the third stimulus. On closer inspection, it is clear that the third stimulus causes the fourth QRS complex because the V-V interval there is the same as the paced cycle length (350 ms). This indicates the presence of slow AV nodal conduction (no surprise, because this type of AV nodal reentry uses an anterograde slowly conducting pathway).

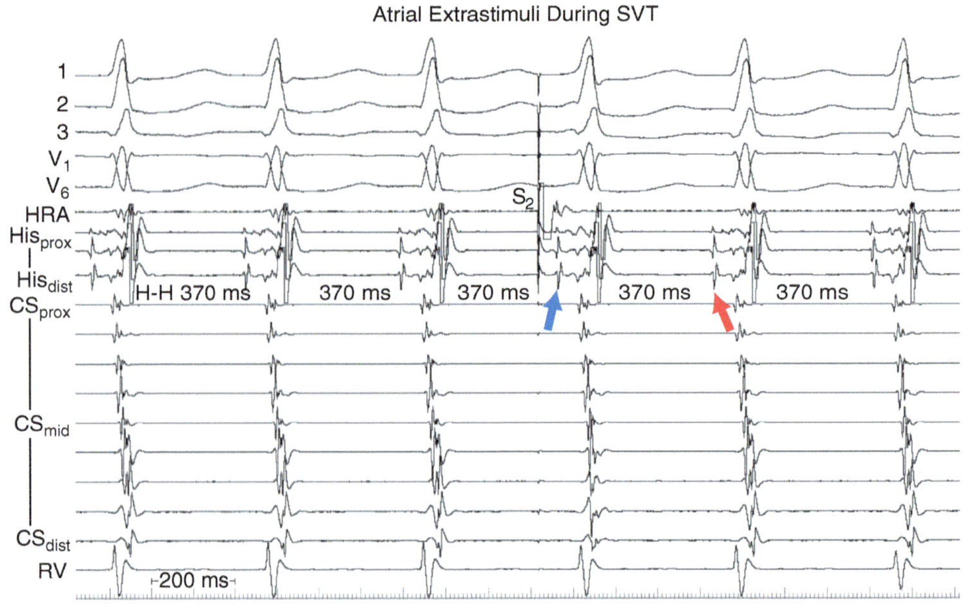

Figure 2-13

In Fig. 2-13, a single atrial extrastimulus is given during SVT. His-His intervals are as indicated; the His immediately after the extrastimulus *(blue arrow)* is on time and unaffected by the stimulus. Thus, if this were a focal junctional tachycardia, it would have already "fired" for that complex and its next occurrence should be right on time. Although this is exactly what happens—the next His *(red arrow)* occurs on time—this finding is also consistent with AV nodal reentry or even AT conducting over a slow AV nodal pathway (the impulse is already on its way down the slow pathway and is unaffected by the atrial extrastimulus). Thus this finding by itself is not diagnostic of focal junctional tachycardia.

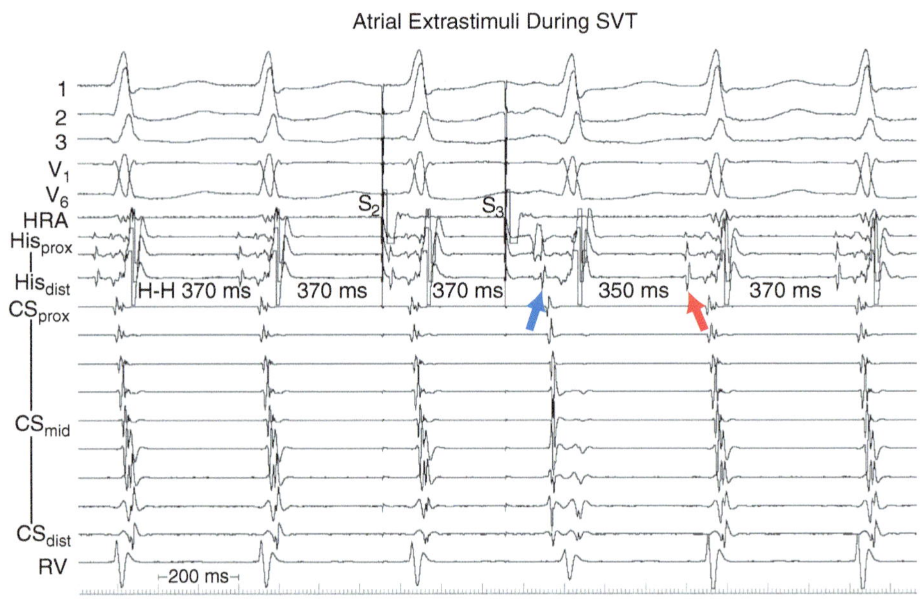

Figure 2-14

Double atrial extrastimuli are now given during SVT (Fig. 2-14). The His potential after second extrastimulus *(blue arrow)* is on time (370 ms), unaffected by the first atrial stimulus (S_2). However, the next His *(red arrow)*, driven by the second atrial stimulus (S_3) is advanced by 20 ms. This shows that focal junctional tachycardia cannot be the diagnosis, because a focal discharge from the His at the red arrow cannot be advanced by an atrial stimulus that did not affect the prior His.

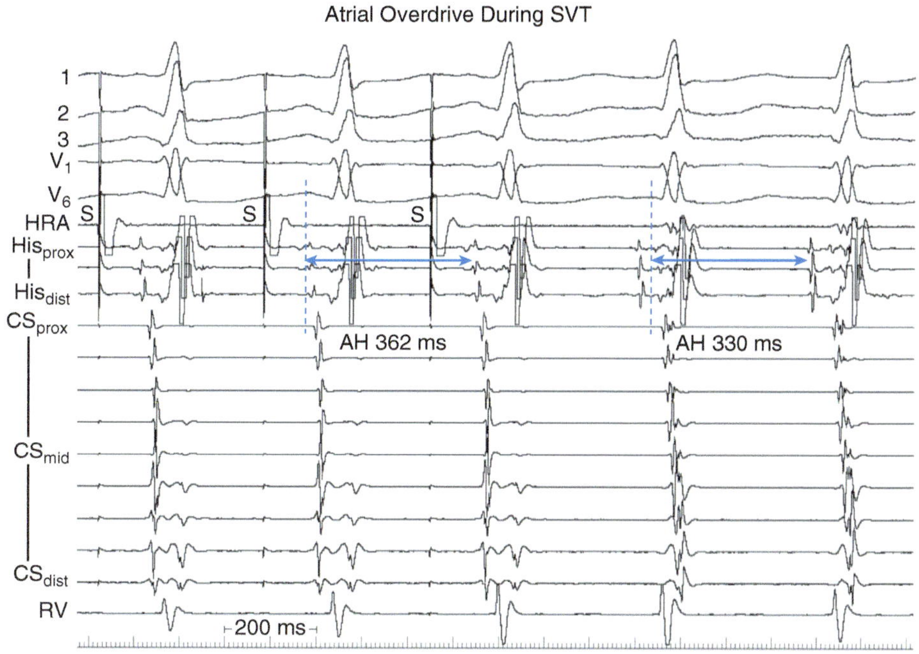

Figure 2-15

Atrial overdrive pacing during SVT is performed again, as shown in Fig. 2-15; the AH interval with pacing (362 ms) exceeds the AH in SVT (330 ms); this is consistent with AV nodal reentry and inconsistent with right AT (in which case the AH intervals should be similar between pacing and SVT).

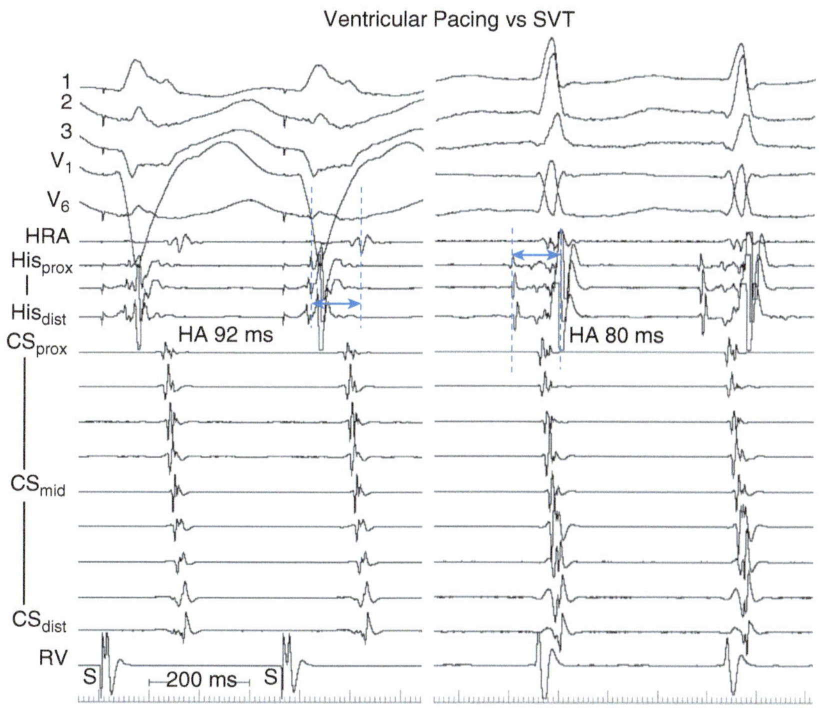

Figure 2-16

The HA interval with ventricular pacing at the SVT cycle length (92 ms) is always the same as or longer than HA in SVT (80 ms), when measured as shown in Fig. 2-16 (end of His to A during pacing, onset of His to A during SVT, with standard 5-mm interelectrode recording catheters). This is not found with very closely spaced, very proximal His recordings, however, where the difference between HA intervals with pacing and SVT narrows as the point of turnaround between anterograde slow and retrograde fast pathways occurs.

Figure 2-17

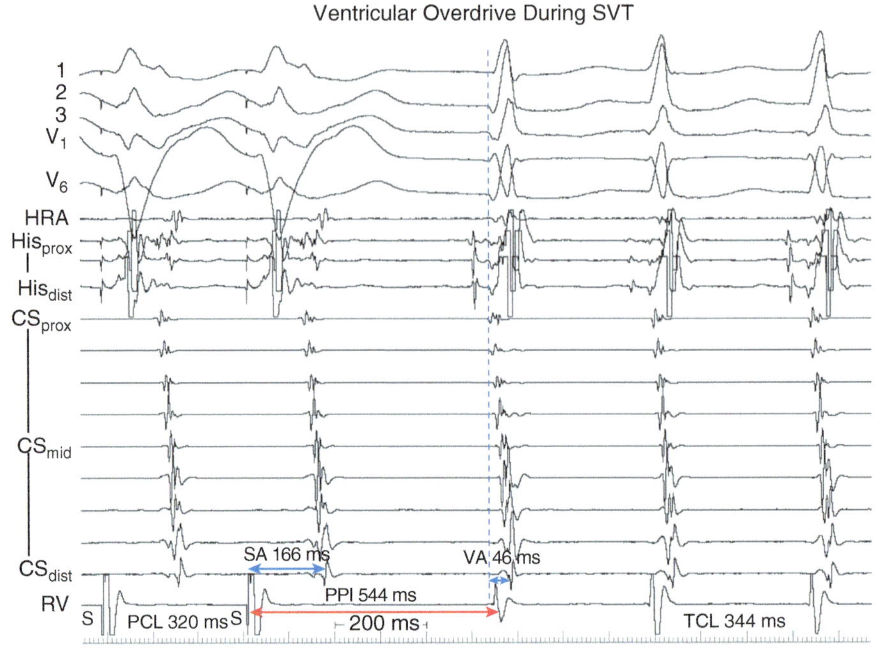

Ventricular overdrive pacing during SVT is shown in Fig. 2-17, with intervals as indicated; the SA-VA difference (120 ms) exceeds 85 ms, and the postpacing interval (PPI)–tachycardia cycle length (TCL) difference (200 ms) exceeds 115 ms; both indices indicate AV nodal reentry rather than orthodromic SVT.

Cartoons and Ladder Diagrams of Pacing

Figure 2-18

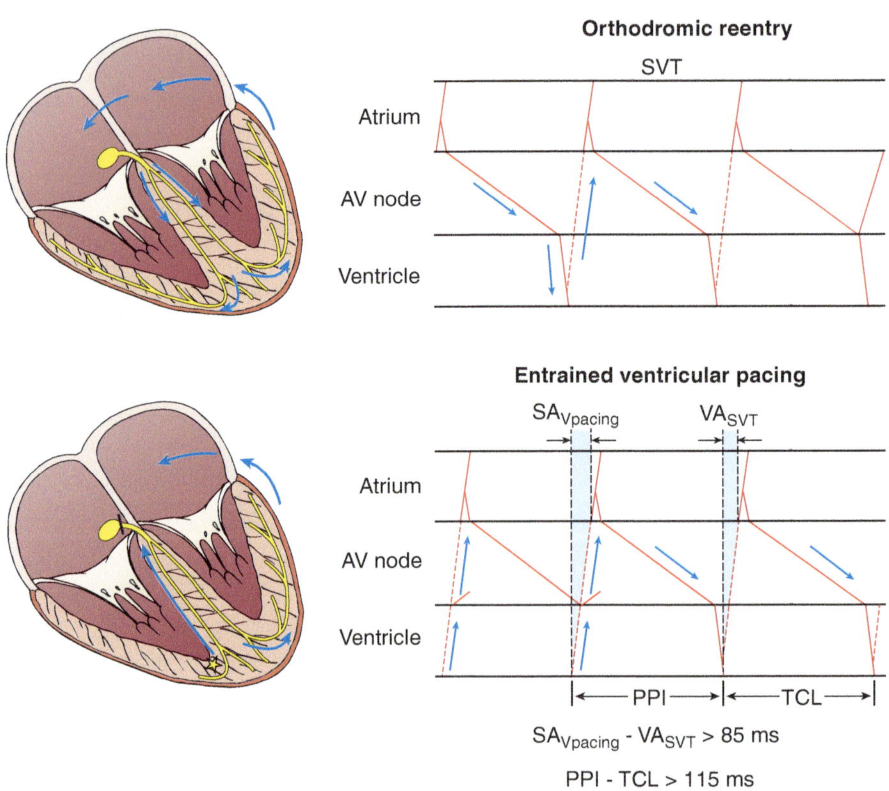

Fig. 2-18 displays entrained ventricular pacing during orthodromic SVT; the bypass tract shown here (connecting left atrium and left ventricle) is indicated in the ladder diagrams as a *dotted line*.

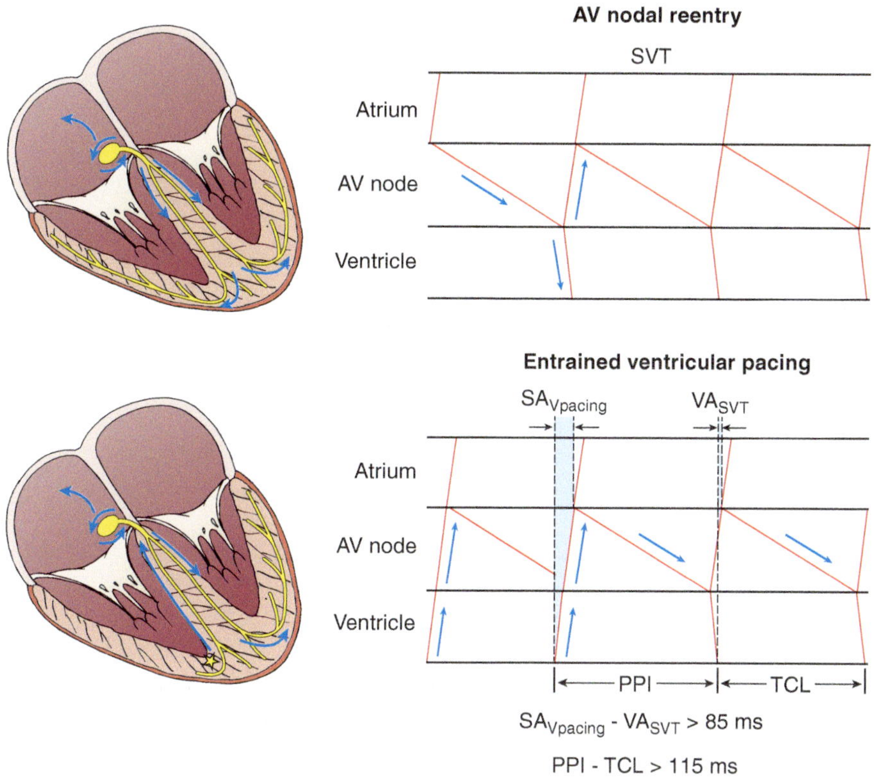

Figure 2-19

Fig. 2-19 shows entrained ventricular pacing during AV nodal reentry.

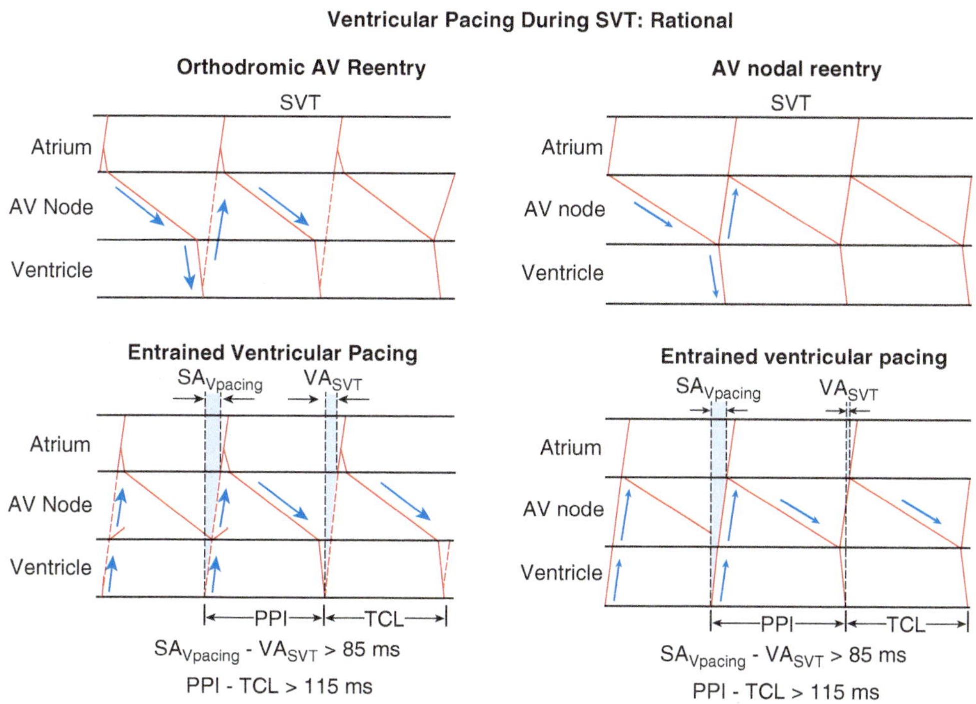

Figure 2-20

(From Michaud et al. Differentiation of atypical atrioventricular node re-entrant tachycardia from orthodromic reciprocating tachycardia using a septal accessory pathway by the response to ventricular pacing. *JACC* 2001;38:1163-7.)

Fig. 2-20 is a comparison of SVT and responses to overdrive ventricular pacing in orthodromic reentry with a bypass tract versus AV nodal reentry. In each case, the paced wavefront must travel from the pacing site to the circuit (stimulus-atrial interval, SA) and back to the pacing site (PPI). Fundamentally, because a right ventricular pacing site is relatively near an orthodromic tachycardia circuit, the SA-VA and PPI-TCL differences are shorter than similar indices in cases of AV nodal reentry, in which the ventricular pacing site is remote from the circuit.

Ventricular and Atrial Pacing in Sinus Rhythm

Figure 2-21

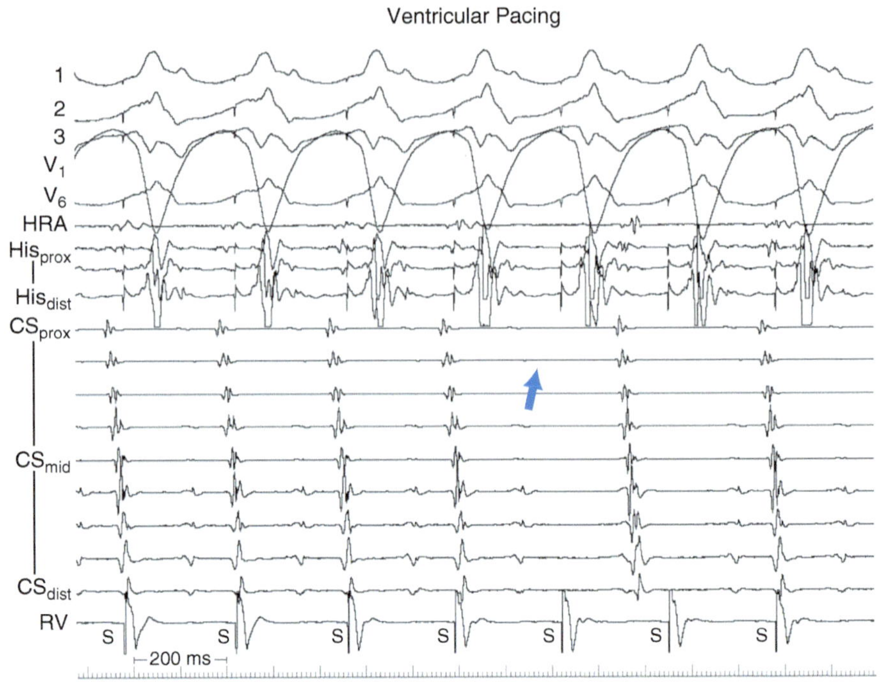

Ventricular pacing to retrograde block in a pattern of Wenckebach is shown in Fig. 2-21 *(blue arrow)*.

Figure 2-22

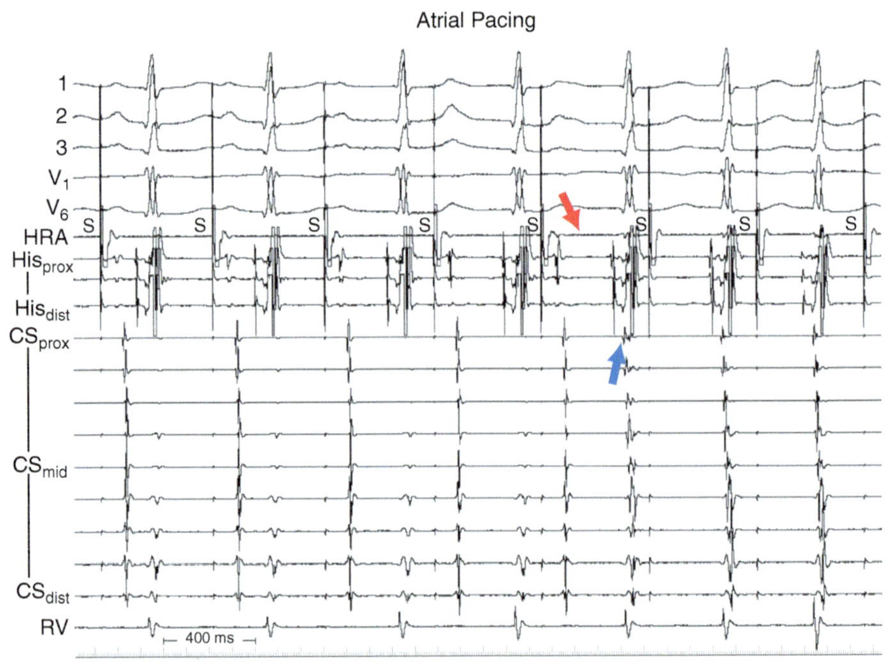

In Fig. 2-22, burst atrial pacing shifts from fast to slow pathway *(red arrow)* and initiates SVT *(blue arrow)*. Subsequent stimuli do not capture because SVT has superseded them.

Atrial Extrastimulus Testing

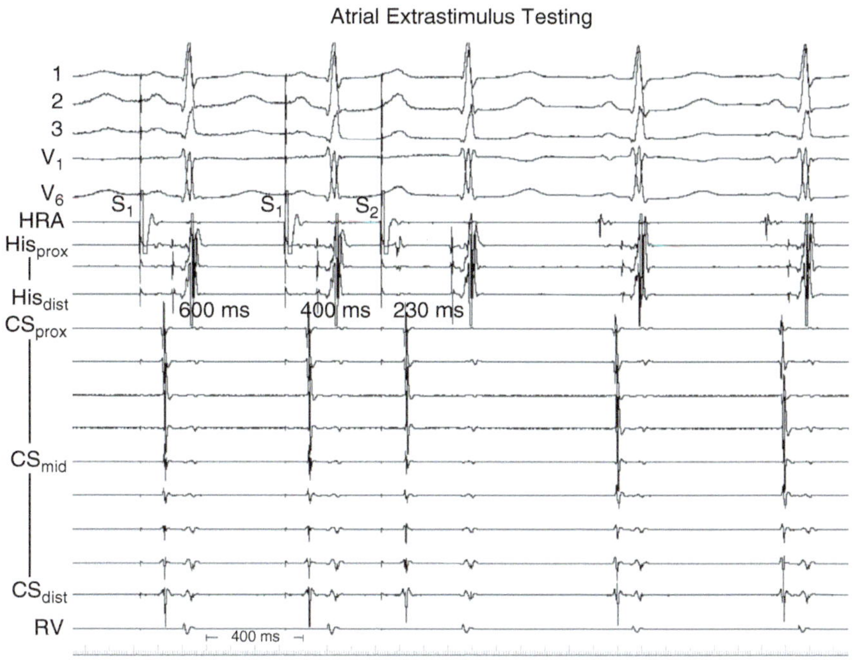

Figure 2-23

Atrial extrastimulus testing 600/400 ms (Fig. 2-23) yields an AH of 230 ms.

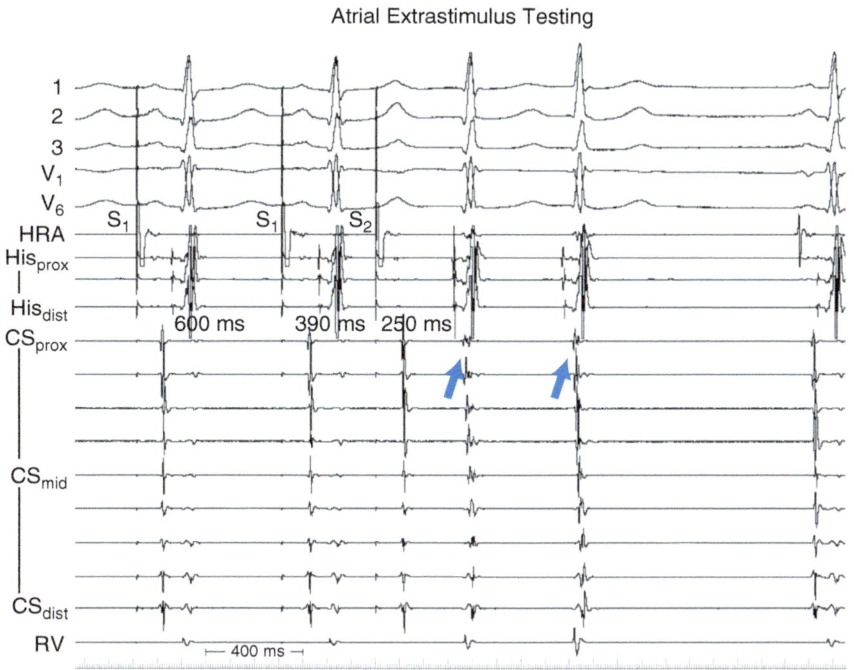

Figure 2-24

Atrial extrastimulus testing 600/390 ms (Fig. 2-24) yields an AH of 250 ms; though not a classic AH "jump" (because the difference in AH intervals resulting from extrastimuli 10 ms apart is <50 ms), the extrastimulus is followed by two echoes *(arrows)*.

Ablation Sites and Assessments

Figure 2-25

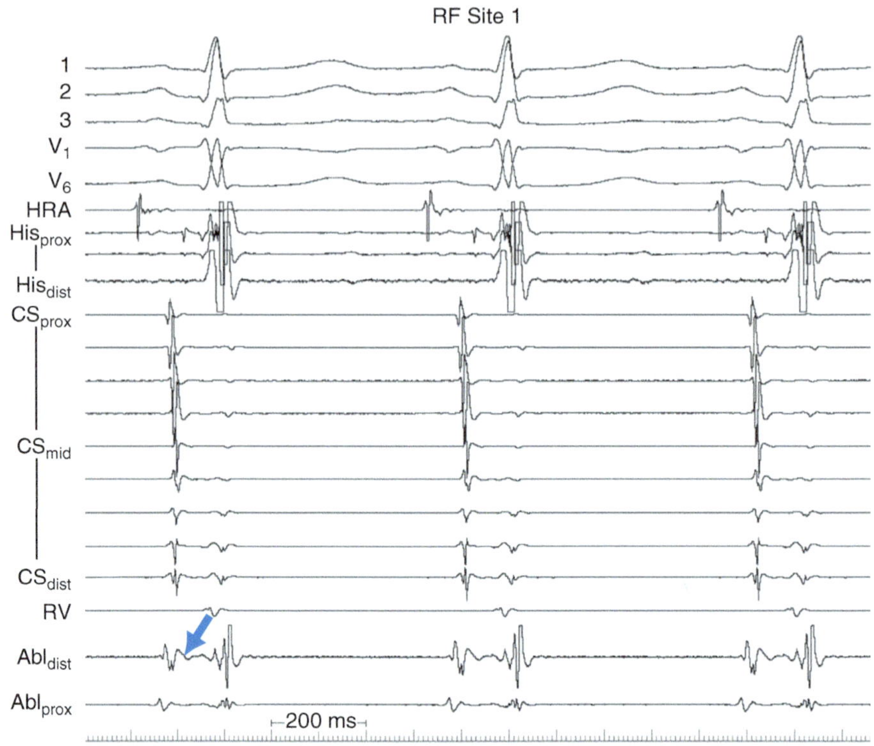

Having established AVNRT as the diagnosis, slow pathway ablation commences, as shown in Fig. 2-25. A typical slow pathway potential *(arrow)* is evident.

Figure 2-26

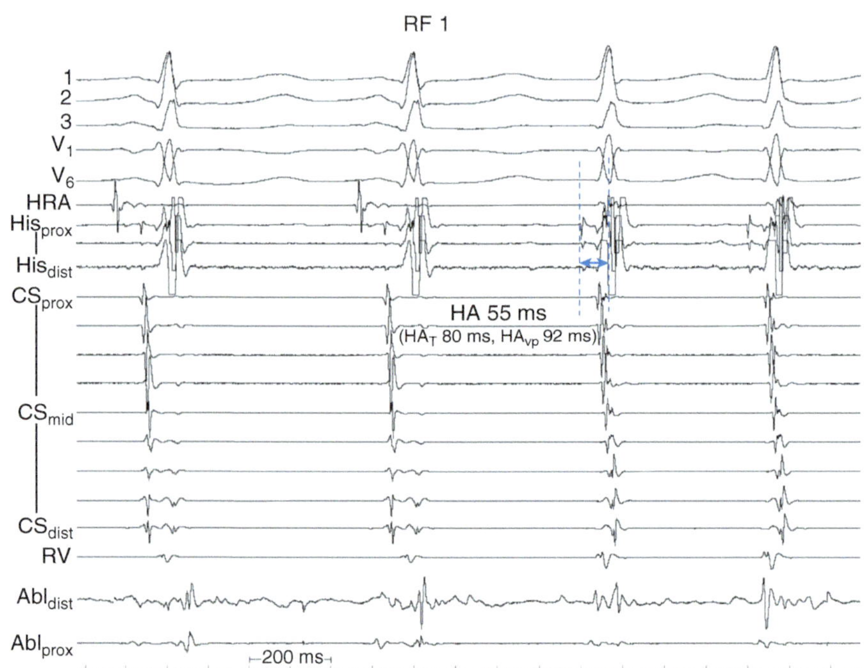

During radiofrequency (RF) energy delivery, accelerated junctional rhythm is seen on the last two complexes at right of Fig. 2-26; the HA interval during junctional rhythm is almost always less than the HA in SVT. This is one way to determine whether a rapid 1:1 VA rhythm during RF energy delivery is caused by accelerated junctional rhythm (successful ablation site) versus initiation and continuation of SVT (unsuccessful ablation site).

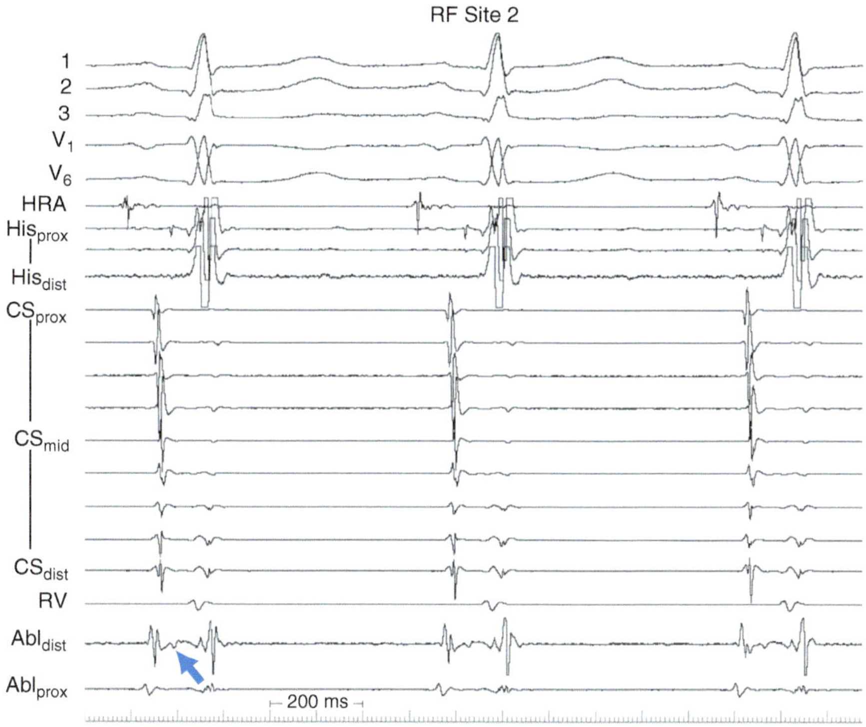

Figure 2-27

After RF 1 (Fig. 2-27), evidence of dual pathways persisted; another site was chosen as shown with another signal compatible with slow pathway activation *(arrow)*.

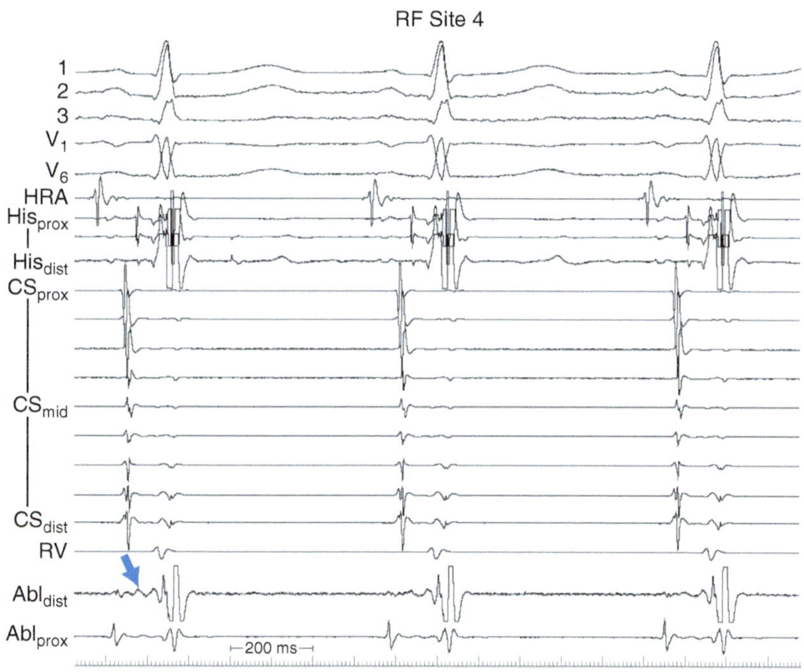

Figure 2-28

As shown in Fig. 2-28, because of persistence of dual pathway physiology, another site of ablation was chosen, with a different type of slow pathway potential *(arrow)*.

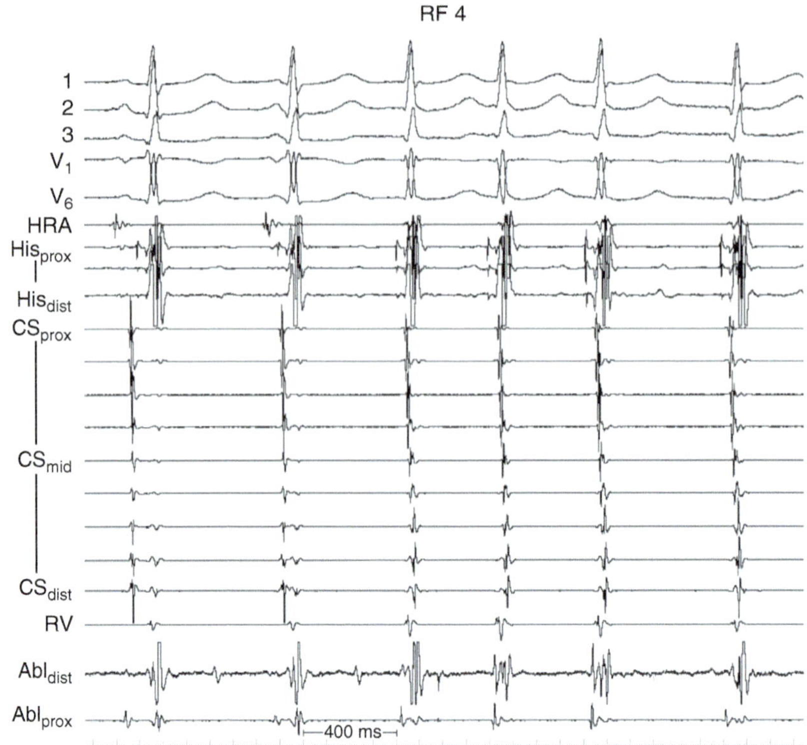

Figure 2-29

At this site in Fig. 2-29, junctional rhythm during RF ablation occurs rather early in the energy application.

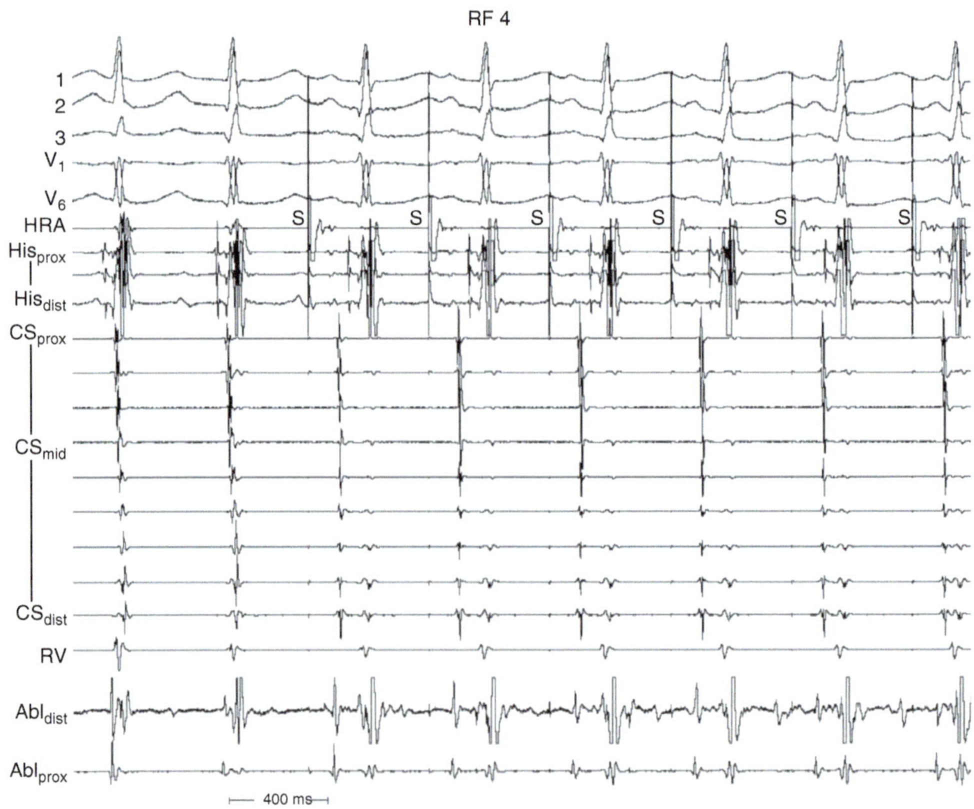

Figure 2-30

Once stable accelerated junctional rhythm is seen, it can be followed by overdrive atrial pacing to ensure the integrity of AV conduction during a more rapid infranodal rhythm (Fig. 2-30). If the PR interval prolongs or AV block occurs, RF delivery can be immediately stopped and almost always conduction returns to what it was before that RF delivery.

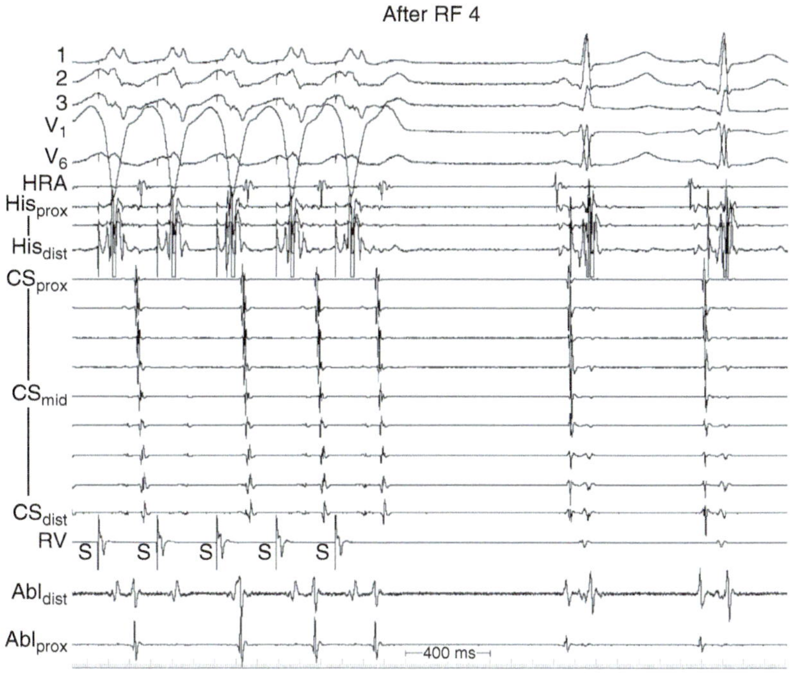

Figure 2-31

Retrograde conduction after RF No. 4 is still good, as is anterograde conduction during sinus rhythm (at right of Fig. 2-31).

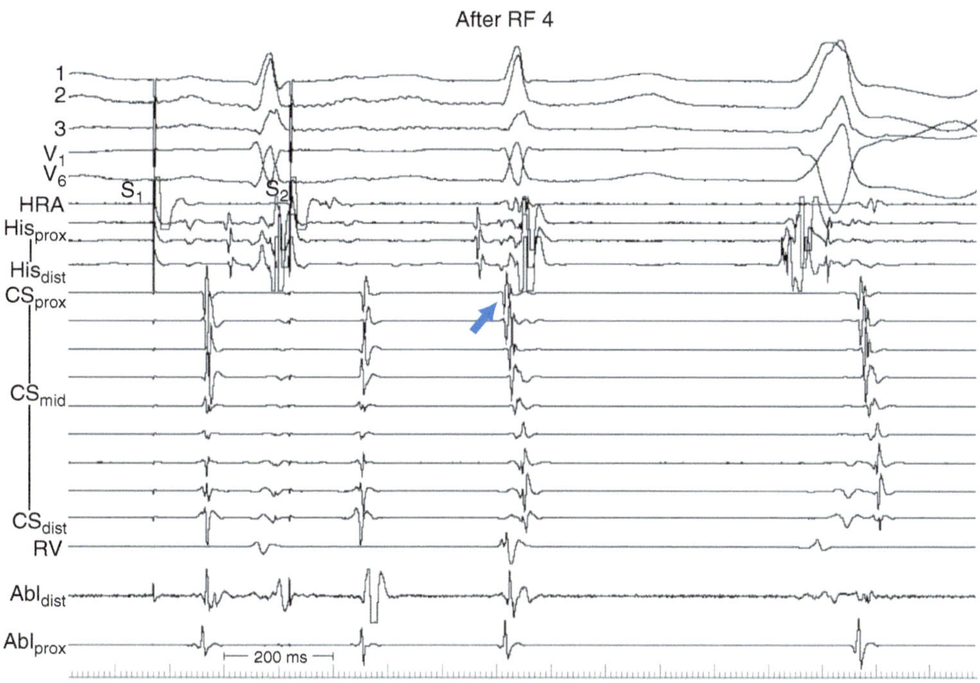

Figure 2-32

Atrial extrastimulus testing after RF 4 still shows an AV nodal echo (only one, *arrow*). A premature ventricular complex (PVC) at the right of Fig. 2-32 shows retrograde His and atrial activation.

SVT Repeatedly Initiated with Atrial Stimulation After Four Attempts at Slow Pathway Ablation,

- No inducible SVT
- Anterograde dual AV nodal pathways and single echoes still
- Preserved AV conduction

What Should You Do Now?

- Try to eliminate dual pathways and echoes?
- End the procedure, risk of AV block is too high?

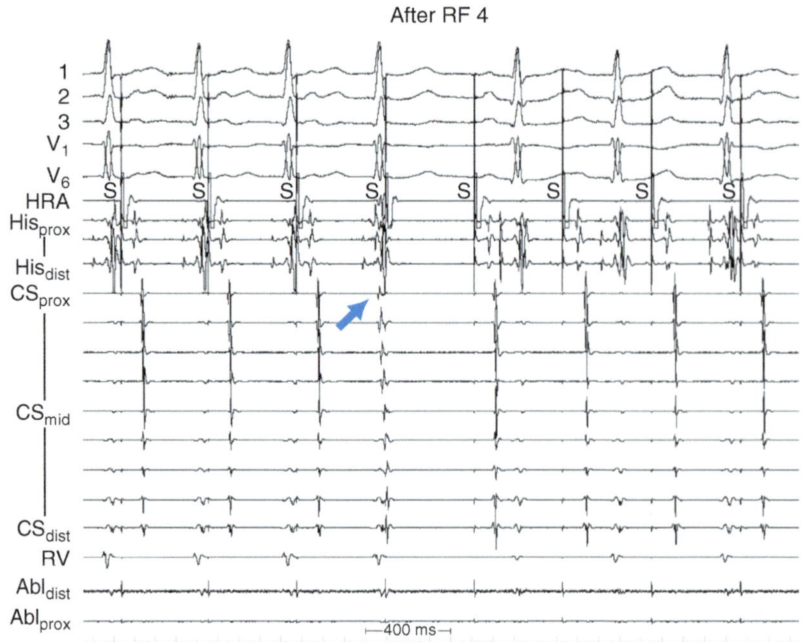

Figure 2-33

In Fig. 2-33, single echoes *(arrow)* remain on atrial drive train; what should be done now? As review, in the baseline state, sustained SVT was easily and repeatedly initiated with atrial pacing, but the slow pathway is still present (although only single echoes are inducible) after four RF applications to the AV nodal slow pathway region. Normal AV conduction is preserved. Is this a good endpoint of the procedure? It would be reasonable to stop here, anticipating a good clinical outcome without risking heart block with additional ablation. We elected to try a little more to eliminate the slow pathway and echoes, however.

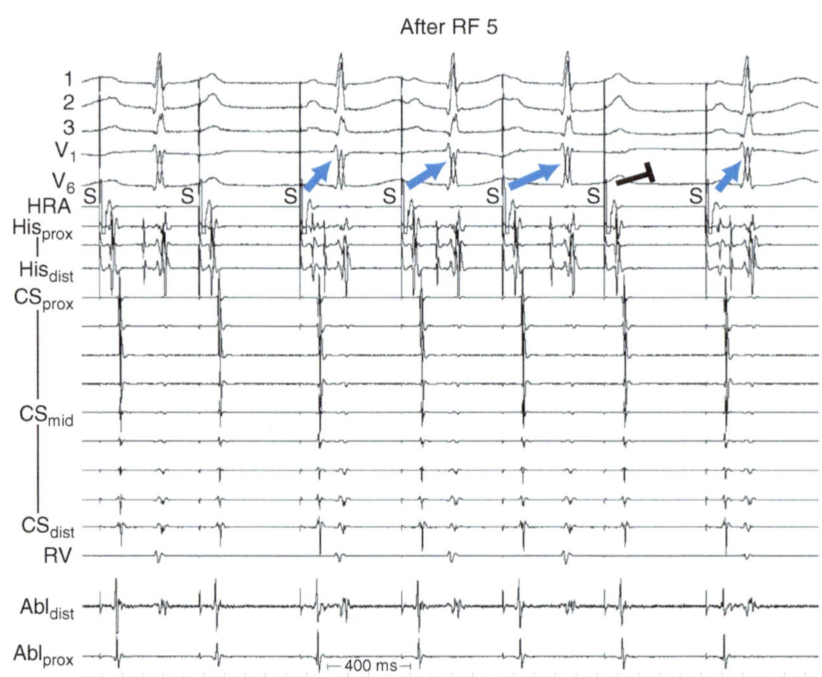

Figure 2-34

In Fig. 2-34, another RF application was given in a similar area, resulting in complete elimination of anterograde slow pathway conduction. (Of note, electroanatomic mapping was not used in this procedure.)

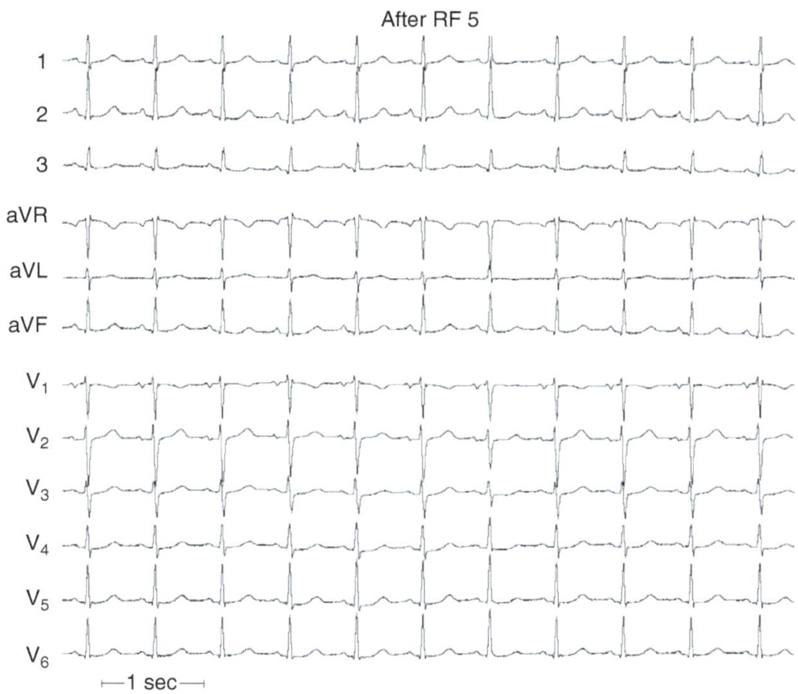

Figure 2-35

Fig. 2-35 demonstrates sinus rhythm after all ablations remains, with normal intervals.

Summary

- AV nodal reentry should be readily distinguished from other SVTs in order to select the appropriate RF targets.
- The vigor of slow pathway ablation should be (Table 2-1)
  - Proportional to the amount of clinical impact SVT has
  - Inversely proportional to the ease of SVT initiation
  - Inversely proportional to the risk of heart block

TABLE 2-1 How Aggressive to be with Slow Pathway Ablation?

Finding	Vigor of Slow Pathway Ablation
Clinical Importance of SVT	
Very bothersome	Relatively safe to be aggressive
Occasional mild nuisance	Be very careful!!!
Ease of SVT Initiation	
Easily reproducible sustained SVT	Eliminate sustained SVT (dual pathways, echoes OK)
Dual pathways + reproducible echoes	Eliminate slow pathway if possible
Dual pathways only	Eliminate slow pathway
Distance from CS os to His Bundle	
Long (≥10 mm)	Relatively safe to be aggressive
Short (<10 mm)	Be very careful!!!

3 Atypical ("Fast-Slow") Atrioventricular Nodal Reentry

Case Presentation

- A 44-year-old man had palpitations for about 2 years. Episodes often occurred during exercise, lasting a few minutes to hours. With one prolonged episode, he went to the emergency room (ER). There, an ECG showed a regular, narrow QRS tachycardia at 180/min, with a long RP interval, which was terminated with intravenous adenosine. Subsequently, metoprolol in tolerated doses was ineffective at preventing recurrent episodes. Findings of physical examination and the resting ECG were normal. Echocardiogram revealed mild global left ventricular hypokinesis. He was referred for EP study and possible ablation.

Baseline ECG and Intracardiac Recordings

Figure 3-1

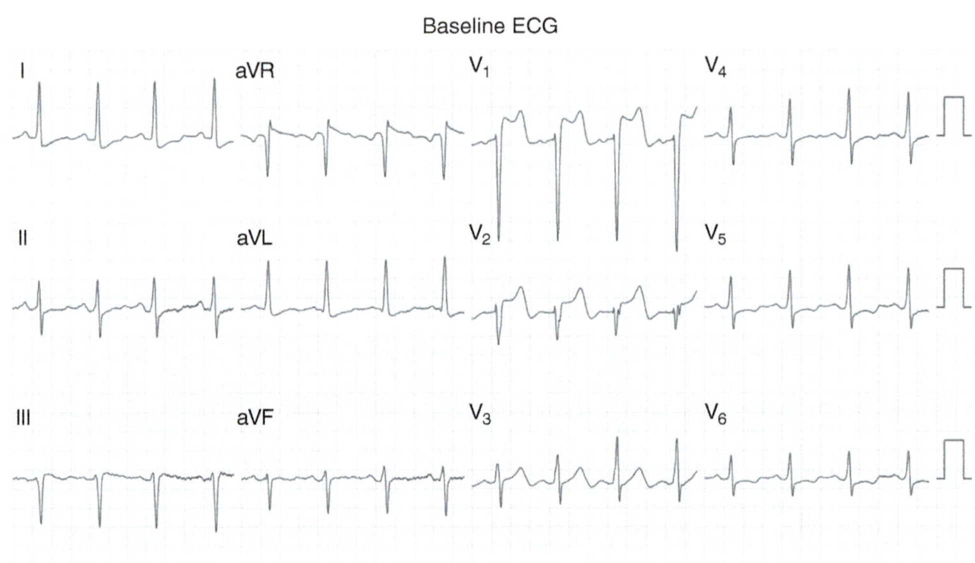

There are no clues from the sinus rhythm ECG (Fig. 3-1) as to what the patient's supraventricular tachycardia (SVT) is. ST elevation in V1-V2 is an artifact of the recording system.

Baseline Intracardiac Recordings

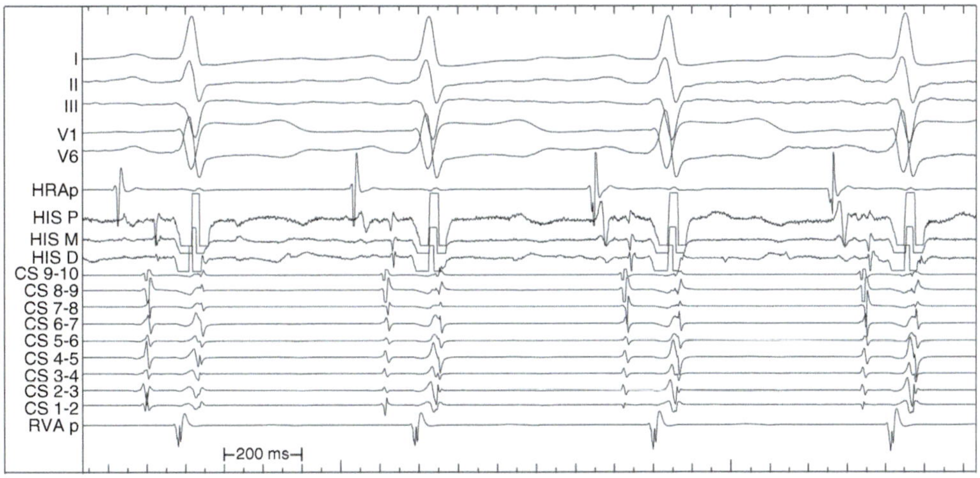

Any Clues as to SVT Diagnosis? [Fig. 3-2]

Figure 3-2

There are likewise no clues from the intracardiac recordings (Fig. 3-2), such as subtle preexcitation, as to the cause of the patient's SVT.

Baseline Ventricular Pacing

Baseline Ventricular Pacing

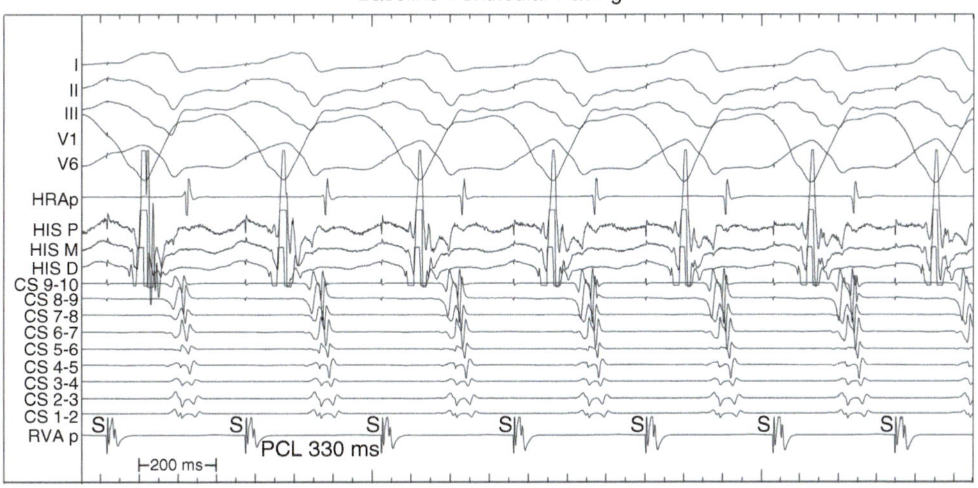

Does This Include/ Exclude Any Diagnoses? [Fig. 3-3]

Figure 3-3

A good way to start investigating for causes of SVT is with ventricular pacing. In Fig. 3-3, it appears that retrograde conduction is rather good and midline (suggesting either a fast atrioventricular [AV] nodal pathway or a septal bypass tract). However, none of the potential causes of SVT is excluded by these findings.

Baseline Coronary Sinus Pacing

Does This Include/ Exclude Any Diagnoses? [Fig. 3-4]

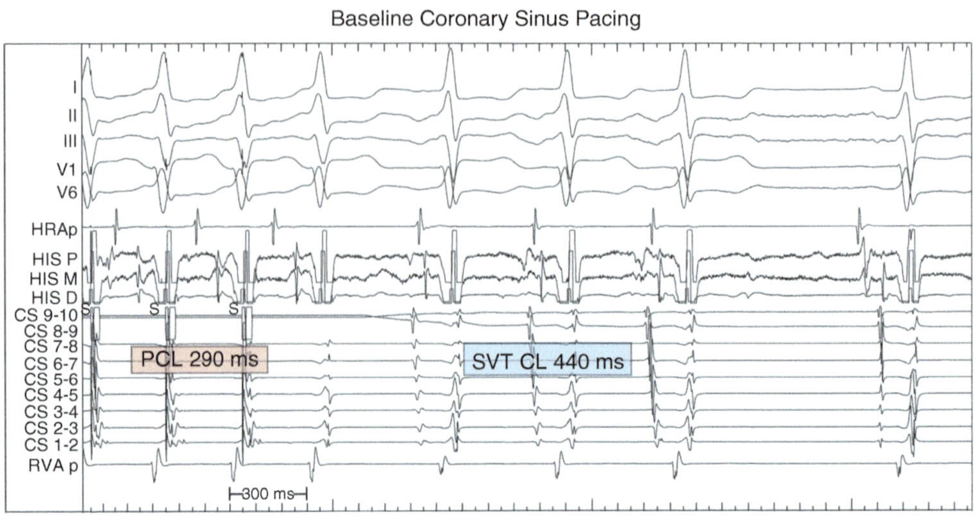

Figure 3-4

Three cycles of a "long-RP" tachycardia are initiated with atrial pacing (Fig. 3-4). The differential diagnosis for this is atrial tachycardia (AT), orthodromic AV reentry using a slowly/decrementally conducting bypass tract as the retrograde limb, or atypical AV nodal reentry (slow pathway retrograde, fast pathway anterograde). Of these diagnoses, a focal AT seems the least good fit because of the prolonged pause between the last stimulated complex and the first tachycardia complex (here, about 550 ms). Nothing in this figure differentiates between the other two possible causes.

SVT Initiation with Ventricular Pacing

What Kinds of SVT Are Initiated With Ventricular Pacing? [Fig. 3-5]

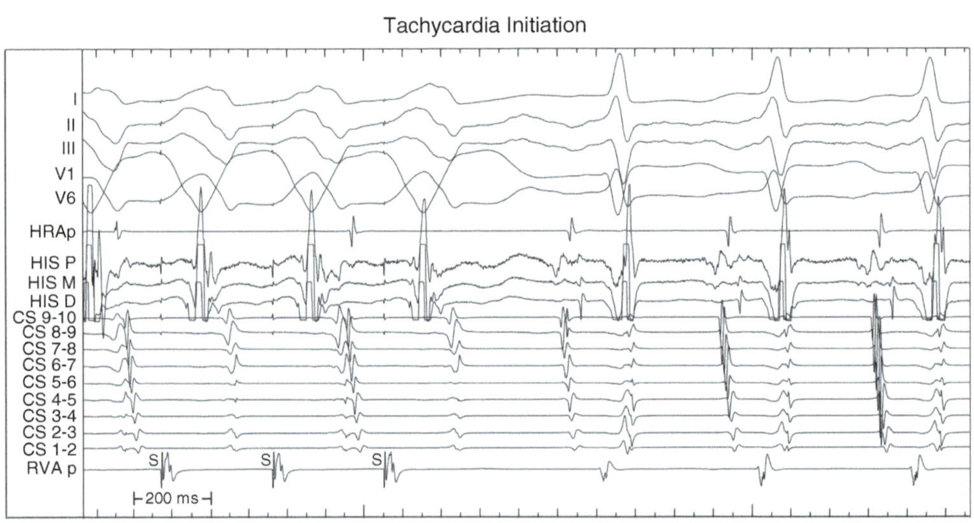

Figure 3-5

In Fig. 3-5, ventricular pacing induces SVT. Several types of SVT can be initiated with ventricular pacing, including orthodromic SVT, atypical AV nodal reentry (AVNRT), and typical AVNRT; even focal ATs (rarely) can be initiated. What information is shown in Fig. 3-5 that could help differentiate among these?

AT initiation with ventricular pacing is rare and likely related to autonomic alterations; it can even occur in the absence of retrograde conduction. The atrial activation sequence is very similar if not the same during ventricular pacing and tachycardia, which would be unusual for AT (not only septal origin—uncommon for AT—but also highly coincidental). Three unlikely events, ventricular pacing induction of AT, tachycardia having the same activation sequence as retrograde conduction, and a septal location, all occurring at once challenge credulity. Thus AT is unlikely. However, there is little here to differentiate between atypical AVNRT and orthodromic SVT using a slowly conducting bypass tract. The longer VA interval after the last ventricular stimulus, compared with the ongoing rhythm, can be seen with either.

SVT ECG and Intracardiac Recordings

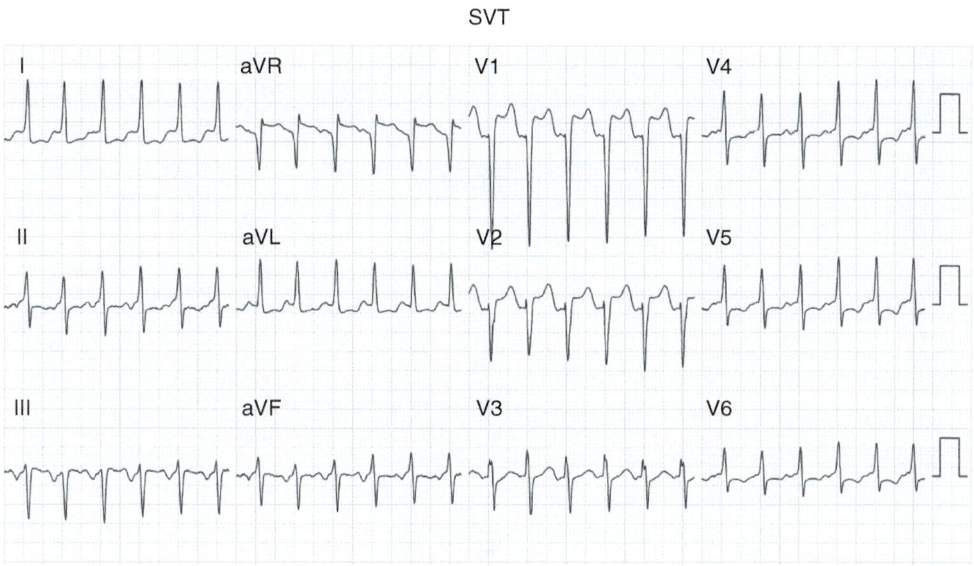

Figure 3-6

Fig. 3-6 shows a 12-lead ECG of SVT, a "long-RP" tachycardia. P-wave morphology suggests a low atrial source of earliest activation.

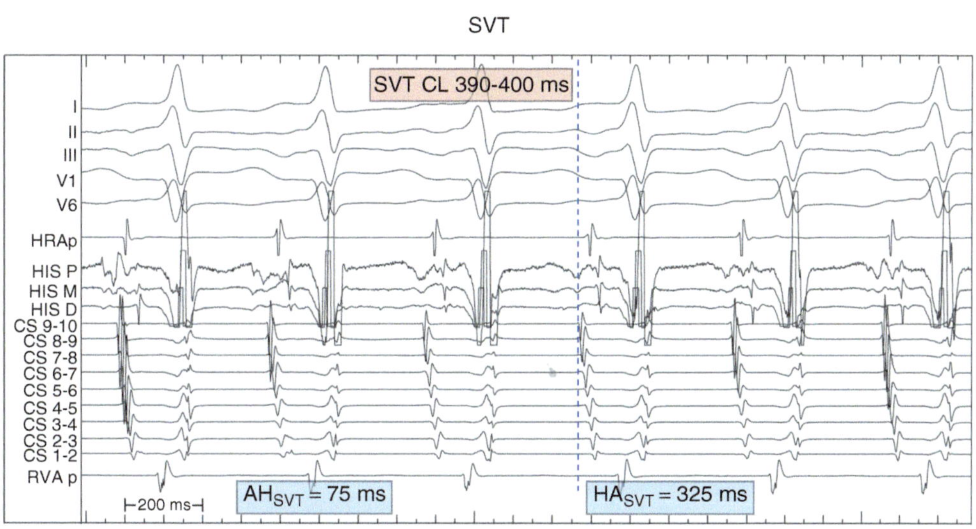

Figure 3-7

Intracardiac recordings during sustained SVT (Fig. 3-7) show an atrial activation pattern with earliest recorded activation near the AV nodal region; measured intervals are as shown for future reference.

Ventricular Extrastimuli and Overdrive Pacing During SVT

Does This Include/ Exclude Any Diagnoses? [Fig. 3-8]

Ventricular Extrastimulus in SVT

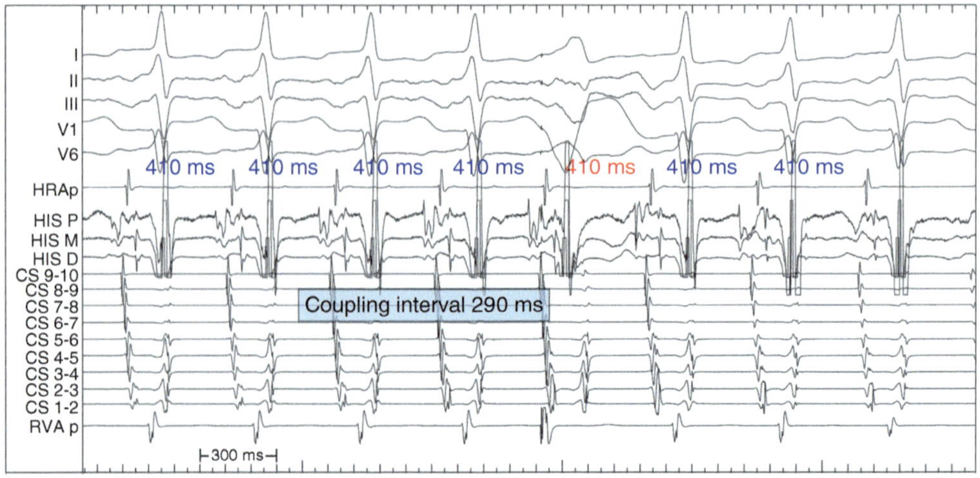

Figure 3-8

A His-refractory has no effect on the timing of subsequent atrial activation; no inference can be made from Fig. 3-8. Closer coupling intervals are needed.

Does This Include/ Exclude Any Diagnoses? [Fig. 3-9]

Ventricular Extrastimulus in SVT

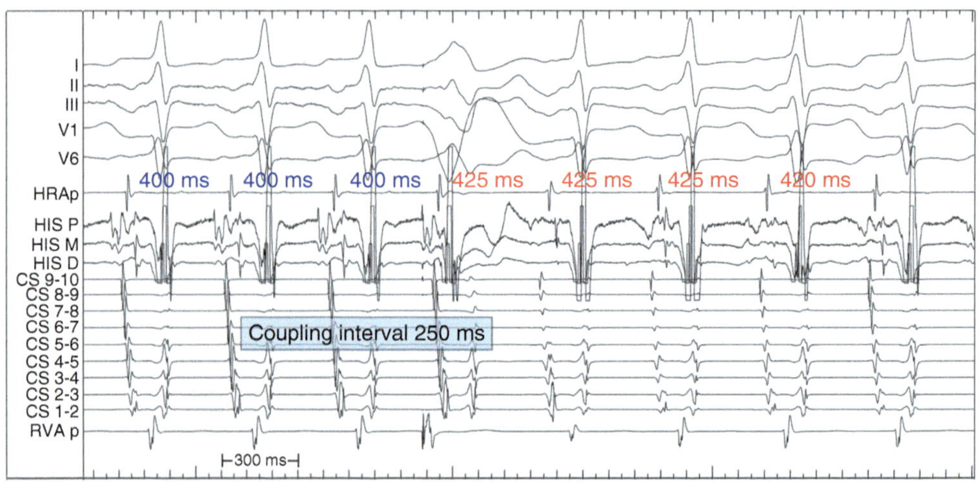

Figure 3-9

In Fig. 3-9, the A-A interval surrounding the more premature (and still His-refractory) ventricular extrastimulus is longer than baseline; however, tachycardia cycle length (TCL) after this stays at the longer A-A interval. Thus the PVC probably did not actually prolong the VA (hence, A-A) interval but happened to occur at a time when TCL was increasing independently. TCL varied during the procedure from 390 to 440 ms. Because the A-A surrounding the PVC did not differ from others during SVT, no inference can be made from it as to the nature of the tachycardia.

Does This Include/ Exclude Any Diagnoses? [Fig. 3-10]

Ventricular Overdrive During SVT

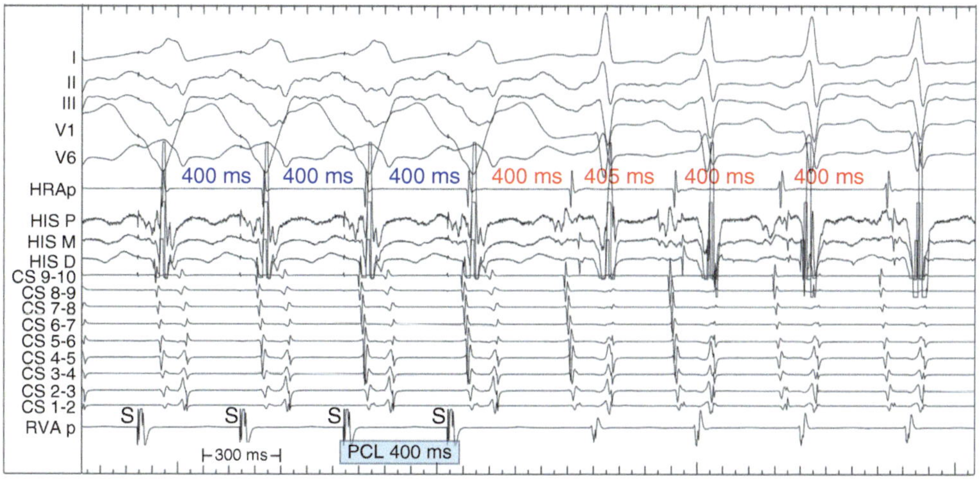

Figure 3-10

Ventricular overdrive pacing during SVT can often yield important information regarding its diagnosis. The chosen ventricular paced cycle length (400 ms) in Fig. 3-10 is about the same as TCL at this time (400–405 ms); thus no inference should be made as to events after cessation of pacing.

Does This Include/ Exclude Any Diagnoses? [Fig. 3-11]

Ventricular Overdrive During SVT

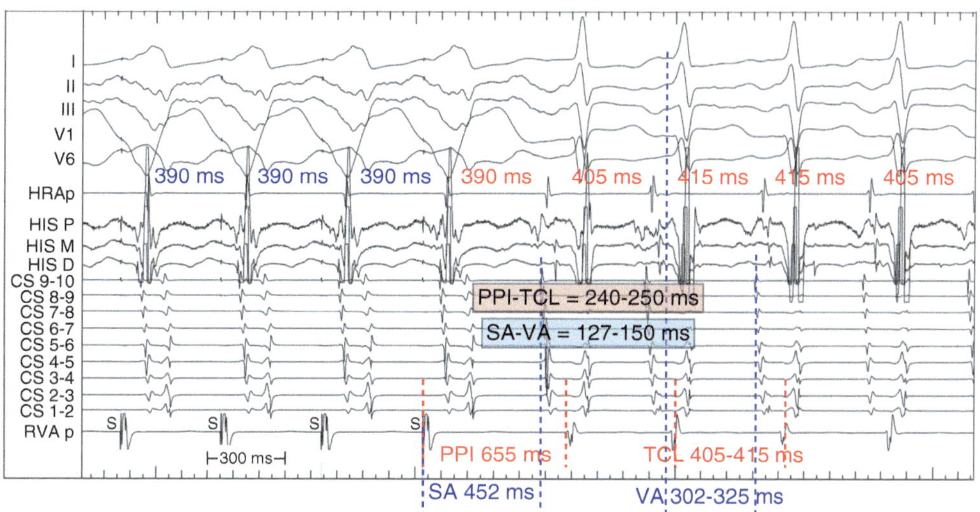

Figure 3-11

The chosen ventricular paced cycle length in Fig. 3-11 is reasonably faster than TCL; now, conclusions can be made as to events after cessation of pacing. The PPI-TCL (>125 ms) and SA-VA (>85 ms) differences are in a range that suggests AV nodal reentry rather than septal bypass tract-based orthodromic reentry.

At Initiation of Ventricular Pacing [Fig. 3-12]

Figure 3-12

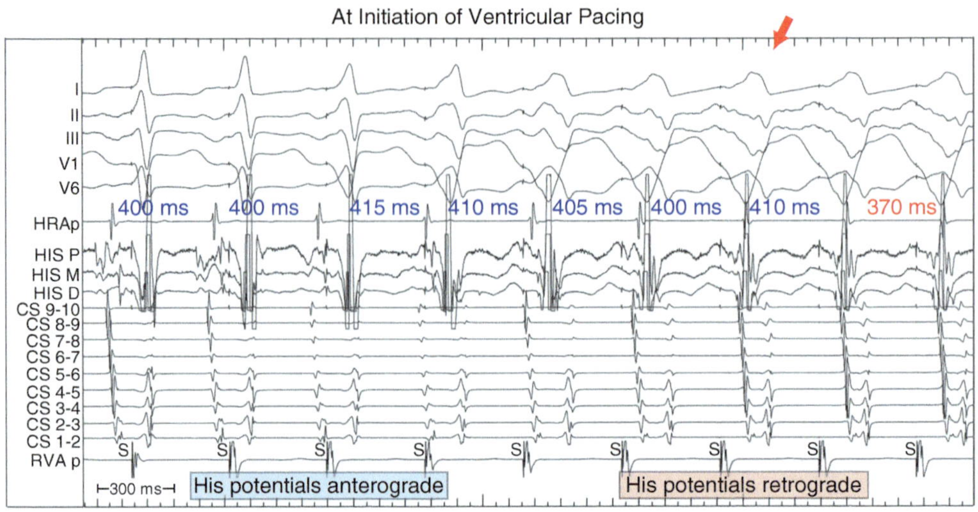

Fully paced complexes are present for the last 3 cycles in Fig. 3-12 (*arrow*); the A-A interval becomes the same as the ventricular paced CL only on the last cycle.

Figure 3-13

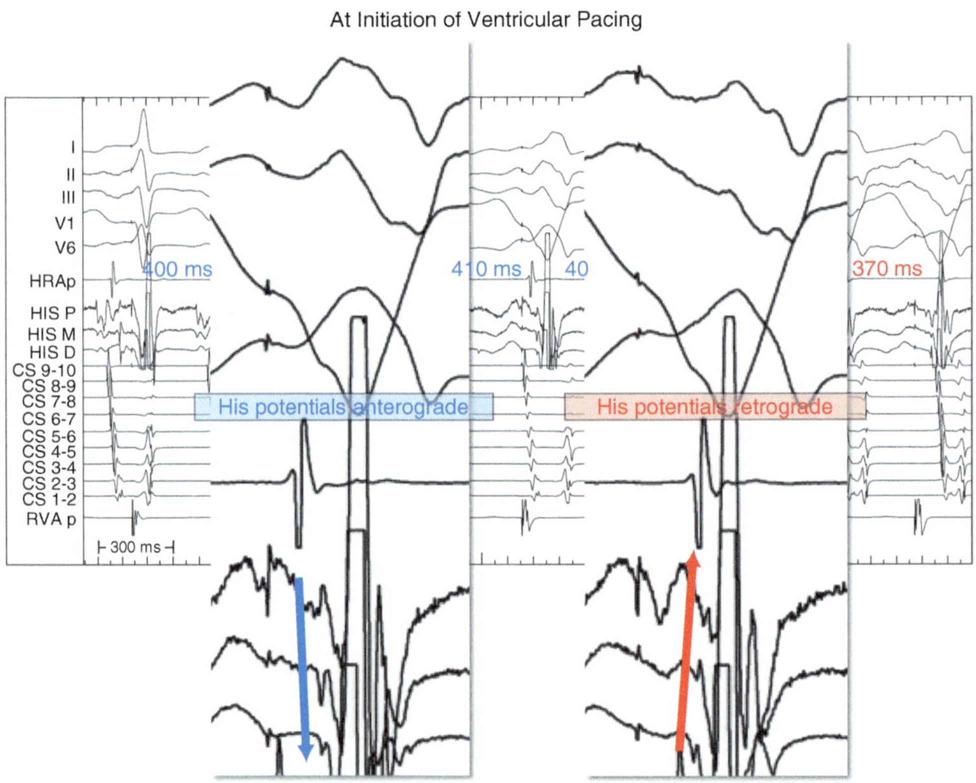

In Fig. 3-13, an enlarged single complex showing anterograde and retrograde His propagation is superimposed on Fig. 3-12.

Initiation of Atrial Fibrillation with Ventricular Pacing

Oops...

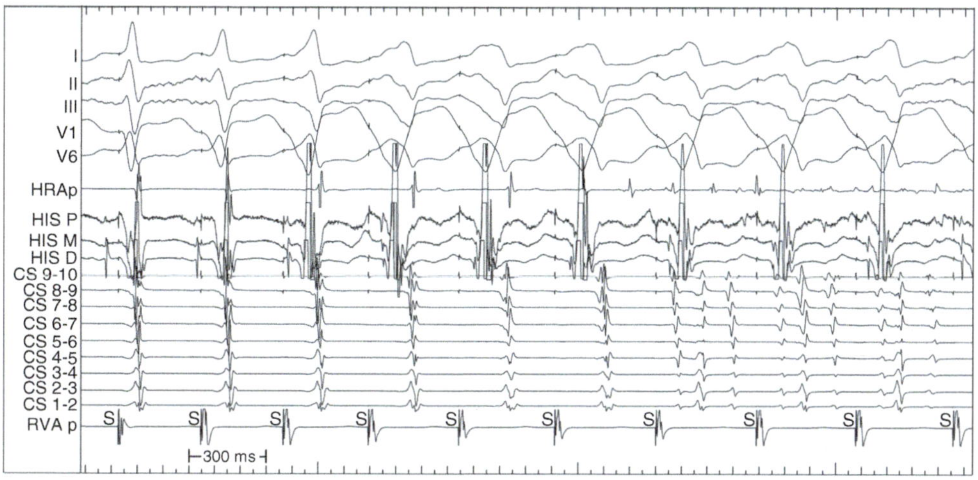

Figure 3-14

As demonstrated in Fig. 3-14, unfortunately, atrial fibrillation (AF) occasionally occurs during ventricular pacing or SVT. This may stop spontaneously or require cardioversion, because it interferes with being able to continue the study. Generally, AF is an artifact of stimulation of the procedure and does not need independent treatment.

Ventricular and Atrial Pacing at TCL During Sinus Rhythm

Does This Help In Any Way? [Fig. 3-15]

Ventricular Pacing at SVT CL

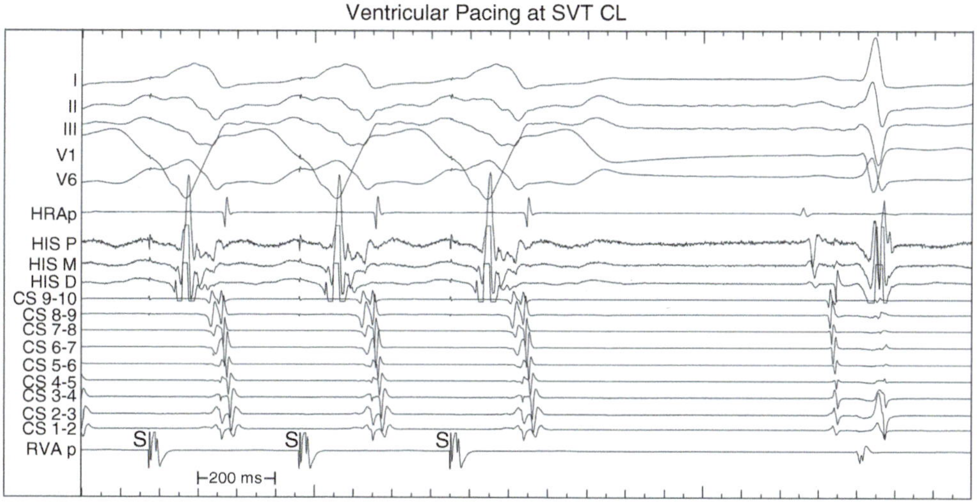

Figure 3-15

Fig. 3-15 shows HA interval during ventricular pacing at TCL 130 ms; however, this is traveling retrogradely up the fast pathway, not the same pathway as is used during SVT. Thus no comparison of HA intervals (pacing vs SVT) can be made.

Does This Include/Exclude Any Diagnoses?

Figure 3-16

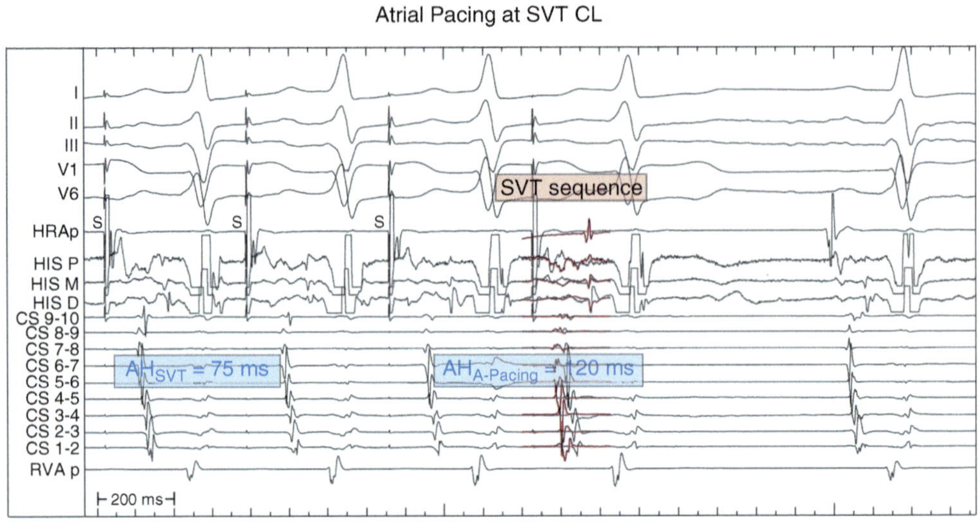

The AH with atrial pacing at TCL is 120 ms, and during SVT (as measured earlier), 75 ms. Fig. 3-16 is the strongest evidence so far that AV nodal reentry is the diagnosis (AH pacing–SVT difference <20 ms for AT, 20–40 ms for slowly conducting bypass tract, >40 ms for atypical AVNRT). A single complex of SVT is superimposed (*red*) to show that this is not pacing during SVT (different activation sequence with pacing than with SVT).

Parahisian Pacing

Figure 3-17

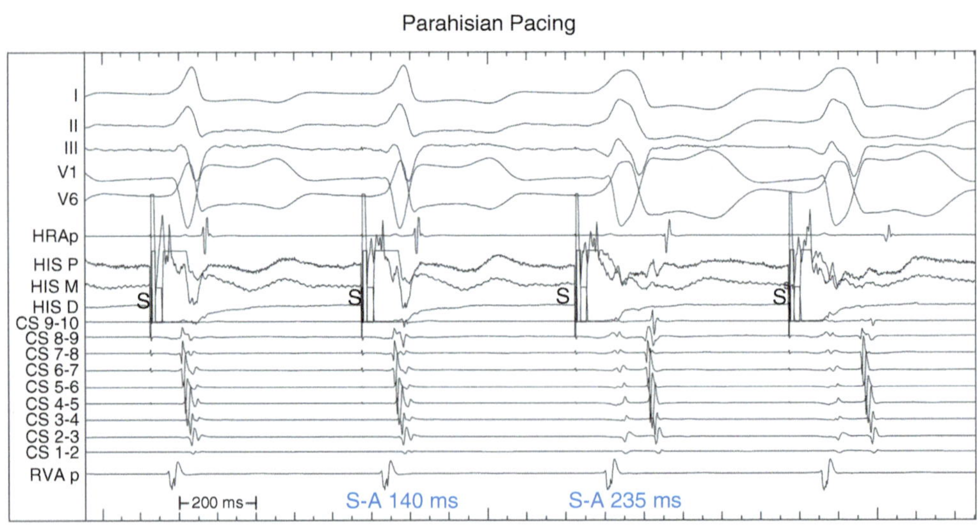

Fig. 3-17 is a nodal pattern (SA in two complexes on the left with a component of His capture shorter than SA with only ventricular capture in two complexes at right) and unfortunately sheds no light for us because any retrograde pathway operative during SVT has a long (rather than short) conduction time and is not evident here, because the retrograde AV nodal fast pathway conducts quite well.

Atrial Extrastimuli in SVT

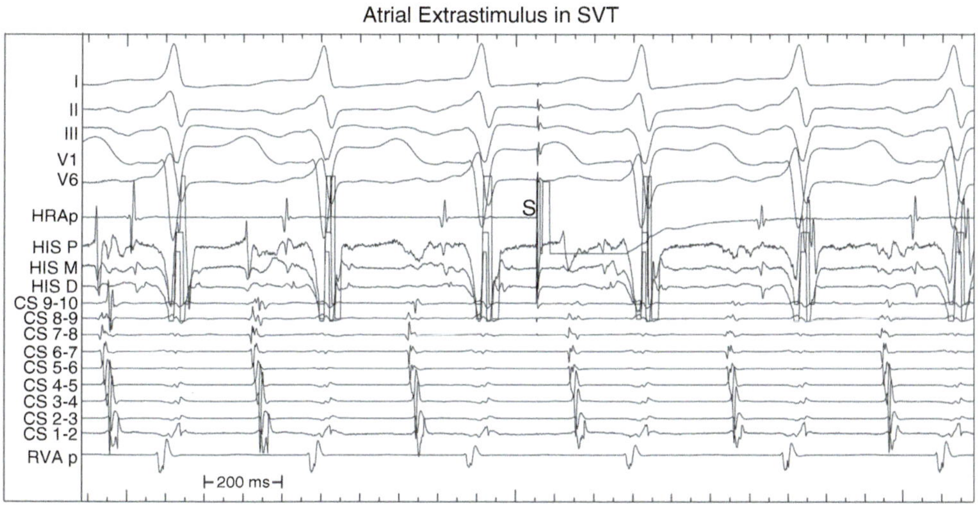

Figure 3-18

Fig. 3-18 is the most premature coupling interval obtainable during SVT (earlier ones met atrial refractoriness). The atrial recording in the His catheter as well as high right atrium are advanced but there is no effect on tachycardia. An AT would not be expected to behave thus.

Ablation Site

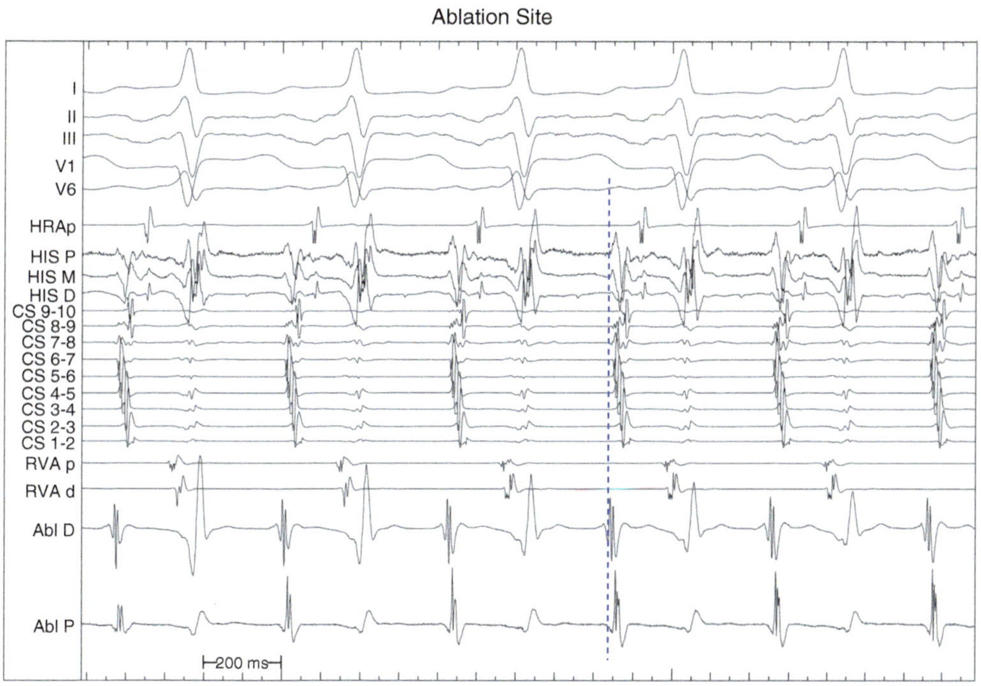

Figure 3-19

Having accumulated a substantial amount of data pointing to atypical AV nodal reentry as the tachycardia diagnosis, mapping for an ablation site is begun around the low atrial septum and coronary sinus os. The electrogram at the site shown in Fig. 3-19 begins slightly before all other atrial activations as well as the surface P wave (difficult to discern because of T wave).

Status

At this time, the patient has been diagnosed with atypical (anterograde fast-retrograde slow) AV nodal reentry. An ablation target site below coronary sinus (CS) ostium has been selected, but SVT is now incessant (despite pacing termination, it immediately resumes) and thus ablation cannot be performed during sinus rhythm. How best to proceed? We need to eliminate SVT and not endanger normal AV conduction. Table 3-1 illustrates the advantages and disadvantages of several possible strategies.

TABLE 3-1 Strategies for Ablation During Tachycardia

Ablation Strategy	Advantages	Disadvantages
During tachycardia	Can tell when ablation is successful	Sudden change in heart rate when SVT stops may displace catheter
During sinus rhythm	Can monitor AV conduction	Can't tell when ablation is successful
During ventricular pacing	None	Can't tell when ablation is successful Can't monitor AV conduction
During SVT/ventricular pacing	Can tell when ablation is successful	Can't monitor AV conduction
During SVT/atrial pacing	Can tell when ablation is successful Can monitor AV conduction	Hard to do

Atrial Entrainment During SVT

Atrial Entrainment During SVT

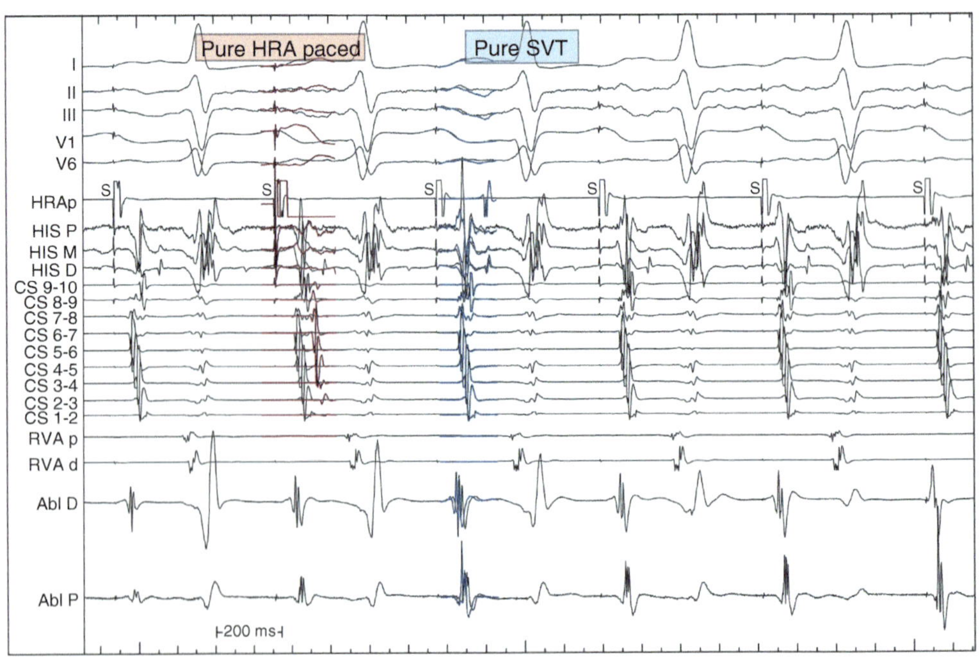

Figure 3-20

The patient had incessant SVT by this time (Fig. 3-20) in the procedure, and so ablation during sinus rhythm was not an option and ablation during SVT was required. If ablation is successful, SVT will terminate and with a sudden heart rate change, the ablation catheter may be displaced from the ablation site, leading to inadequate power delivery at the target. To prevent this, pacing the atrium at the SVT cycle length can help by maintaining the heart rate during successful ablation; the activation sequence will suddenly change when SVT is terminated but there is no sudden change in heart rate that could result in catheter movement. Pacing has to be performed very carefully to prevent SVT termination by pacing itself. As shown in the figure, the complexes during SVT entrained by right atrial pacing are neither the same as pure atrial pacing (superimposed in *red*) nor SVT (superimposed in *blue*).

Ablation Begins

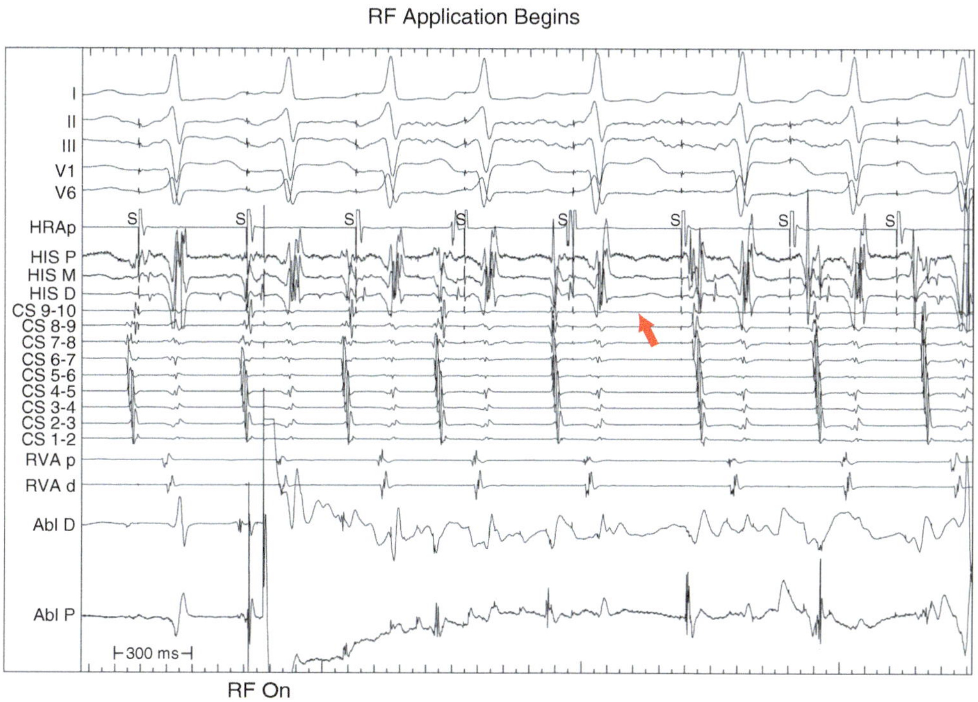

Figure 3-21

SVT terminates (Fig. 3-21, *arrow*) just over 1 second after onset of RF delivery, but the heart rate changes minimally; the ablation catheter position remains stable throughout the time of RF delivery.

Final Recordings

Figure 3-22

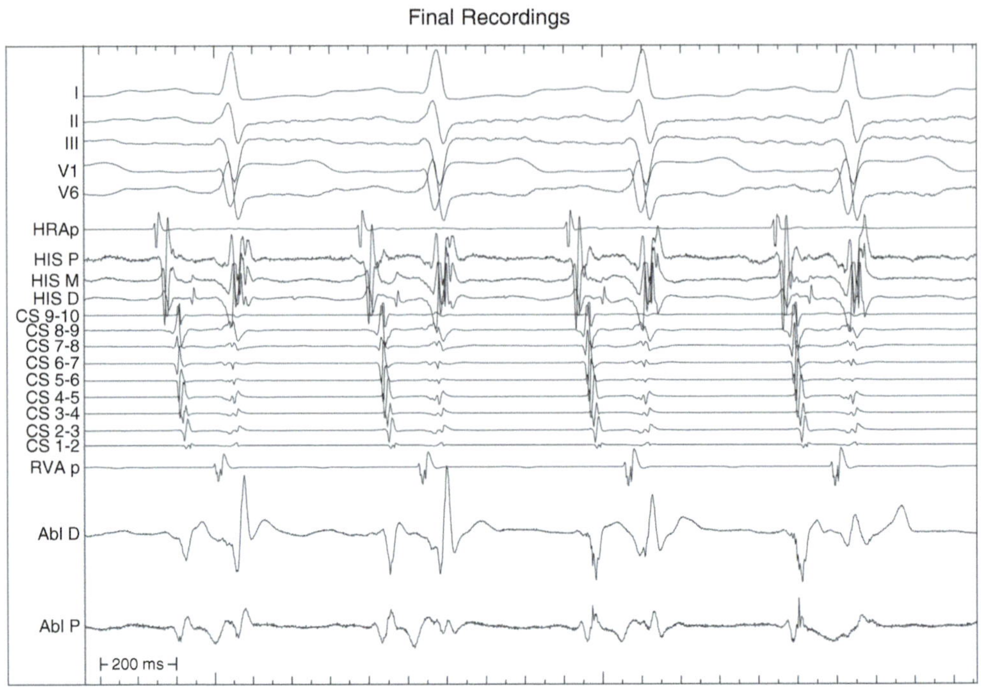

As shown in Fig. 3-22, SVT is no longer inducible, and AV conduction is unchanged (normal).

Summary

- Long R-P tachycardias can be challenging to diagnose, but using standard methods the right answer is usually clear:
    - Atrial tachycardia
    - Atypical (fast-slow) AV nodal reentry
    - Orthodromic AV reentry (slowly conducting bypass tract)
    - Rarely, junctional tachycardia with retrograde conduction
- Atypical (fast-slow) AV nodal reentry can occur at any age
- Ablation during incessant tachycardia has several options:
    - *Ablate during tachycardia:* can tell when successful but sudden change in HR with termination may displace ablation catheter
    - *Ablate during SR:* can't tell success but can monitor conduction
    - *Ablate during ventricular pacing:* can't see success during ablation or monitor AV conduction
    - *Ablate during SVT/ventricular pacing:* can tell when successful but AV conduction may suffer
    - *Ablate during SVT/atrial pacing:* can tell when successful as well as monitor AV conduction

Accelerated Junctional Rhythm

4

Case Presentation

A 29-year-old woman has a history of palpitations and dizziness since age 13. ECGs during episodes showed narrow QRS tachycardia at 190/min. She eventually underwent electrophysiology (EP) study 4 months ago, at which time typical atrioventricular (AV) nodal reentry was initiated and successful slow pathway ablation performed. She had recurrent symptoms within days that became nearly constant. Exam showed heart rate 75/min; large A waves in the jugular veins; soft S1; and was otherwise normal. ECG showed junctional rhythm at 75/min with retrograde P waves. An ambulatory monitor showed junctional rhythm 75 to 90/min most of the time; occasionally, with exertion, sinus tachycardia at 130/min overrode the otherwise constant junctional rhythm. Echocardiogram was otherwise normal. Her symptoms were refractory to beta blockade, propafenone, and flecainide and she was referred for repeat EP study and possible ablation.

Baseline ECG and Intracardiac Recordings

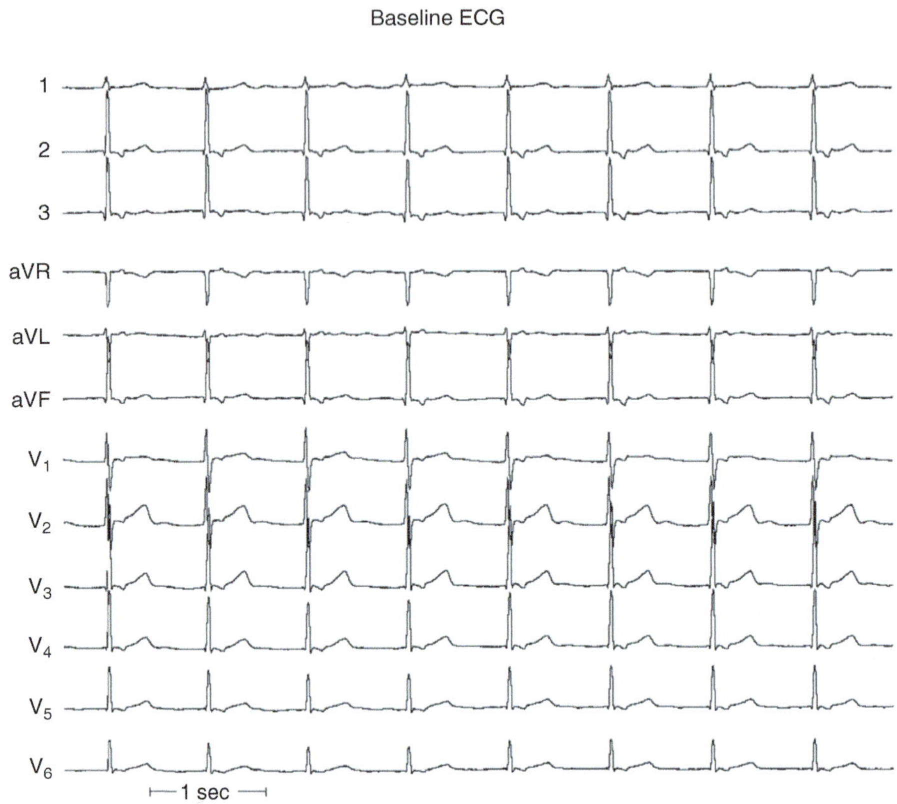

Figure 4-1

Baseline ECG (Fig. 4-1) appears to show narrow complex junctional rhythm at 75/min with retrograde P waves. This was present nearly constantly and caused a functional pacemaker syndrome (nearly simultaneous atrial and ventricular contraction).

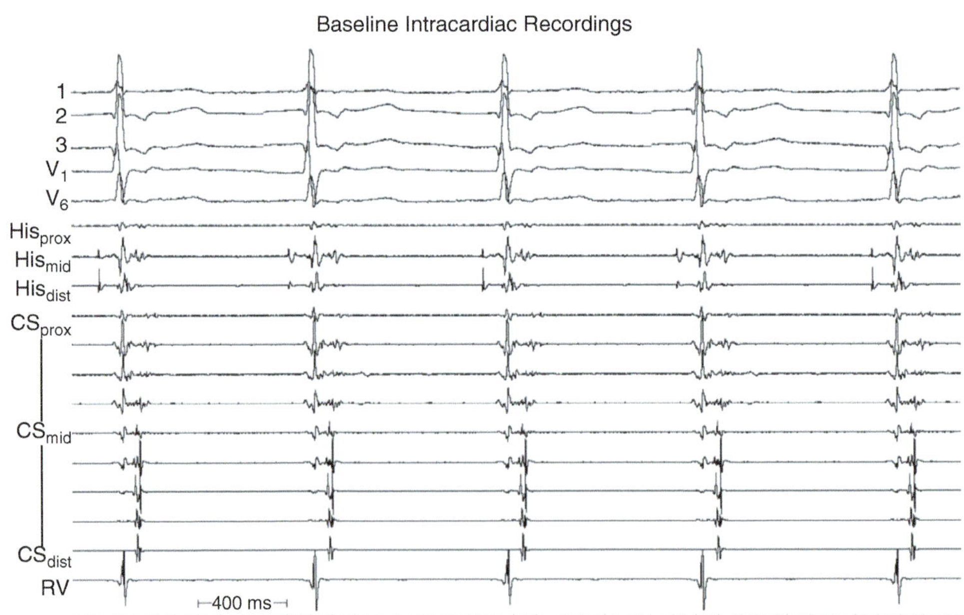

Figure 4-2

Intracardiac recordings during the baseline rhythm (Fig. 4-2) show a His potential before each QRS complex with a normal HV interval (43 ms). Atrial activation is midline and compatible with use of an AV nodal fast pathway. The differential diagnosis for this is automatic accelerated junctional rhythm, AV nodal reentry with a very slow anterograde pathway, or (least likely) atrial rhythm with very slow anterograde AV nodal conduction.

Atrial Extrastimuli in Rhythm

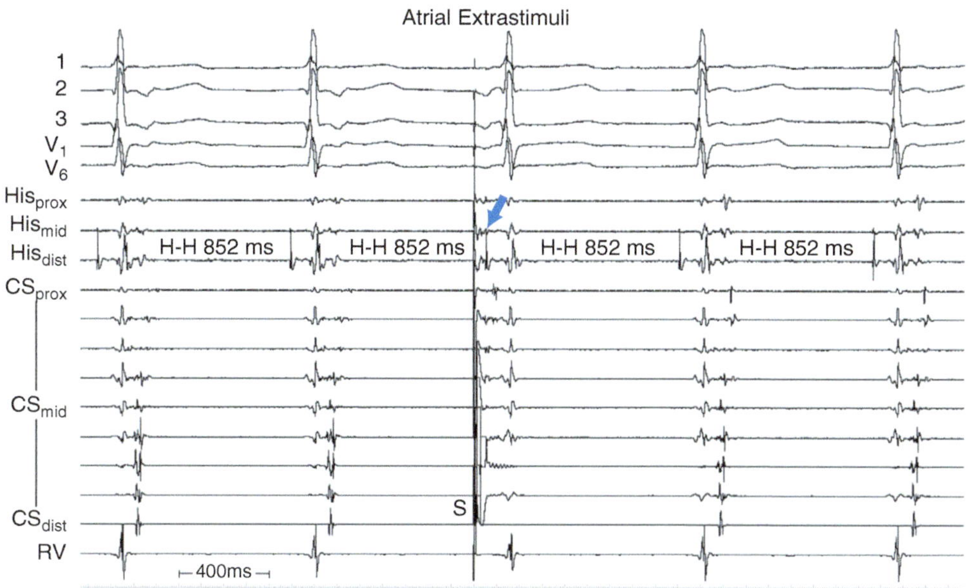

Figure 4-3

To investigate the nature of the rhythm, single atrial extrastimuli are delivered from the coronary sinus. Fig. 4-3 shows that a late-coupled extrastimulus (S), delivered when the His potential has already occurred on time *(arrow)*, captures and advances the timing of atrial activation but does not alter the timing of the next His potential (occurs on schedule at 852 ms). If the rhythm were AV nodal reentry or an atrial rhythm, the timing of the next His potential would have either been advanced or delayed (because in either case its inscription would be dependent on AV nodal conduction). Thus the rhythm is neither AV nodal reentry or atrial in origin.

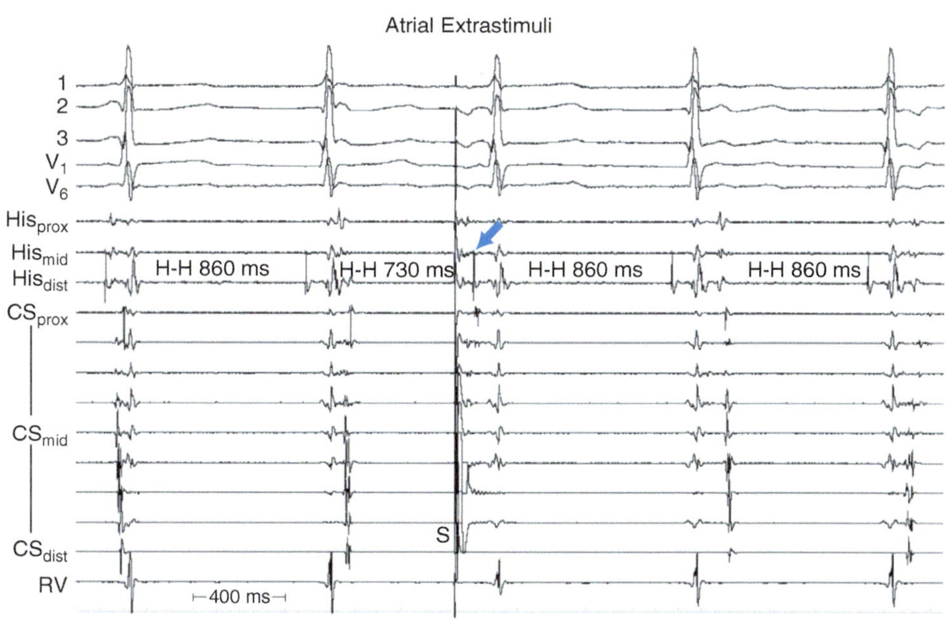

Figure 4-4

In Fig. 4-4, a more premature extrastimulus (S) not only captures and advances the timing of atrial activation, but also conducts over the fast AV nodal pathway to activate the His bundle *(arrow)*. This resets the timing of the rhythm and the next His potential occurs at the same discharge interval (860 ms now) and the rhythm continues on thereafter.

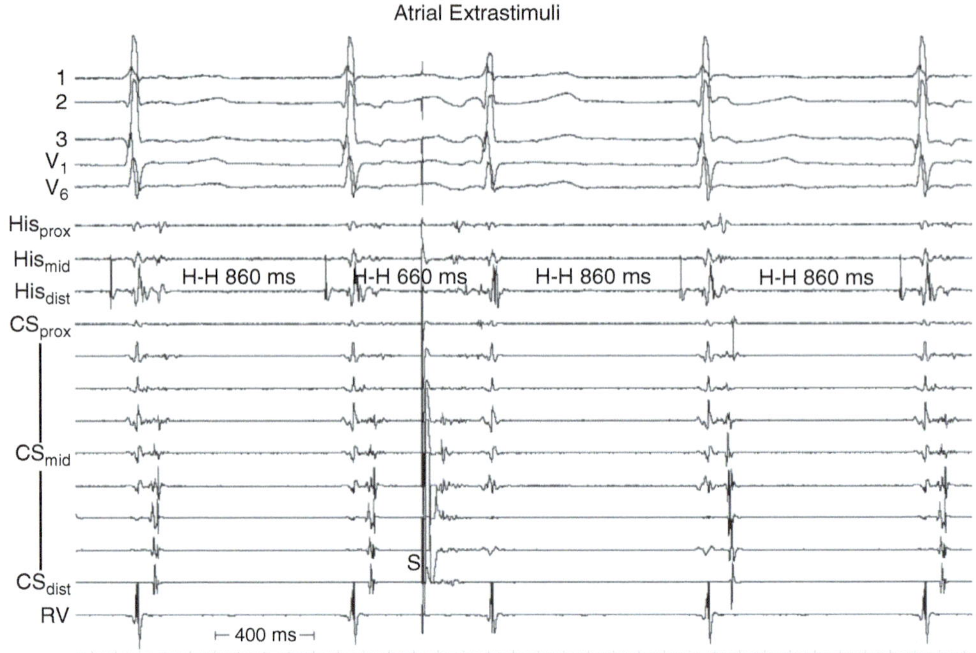

Figure 4-5

A still more premature extrastimulus (S, Fig. 4-5), the earliest one that captured, advances atrial and His activation even more than previously. The next His potential on resumption of the rhythm is at the same discharge interval (860 ms). This is all consistent with accelerated junctional rhythm.

Ventricular Extrastimuli in Rhythm

Where Is the Exact Source of the Abnormal Rhythm? [Fig. 4-6]

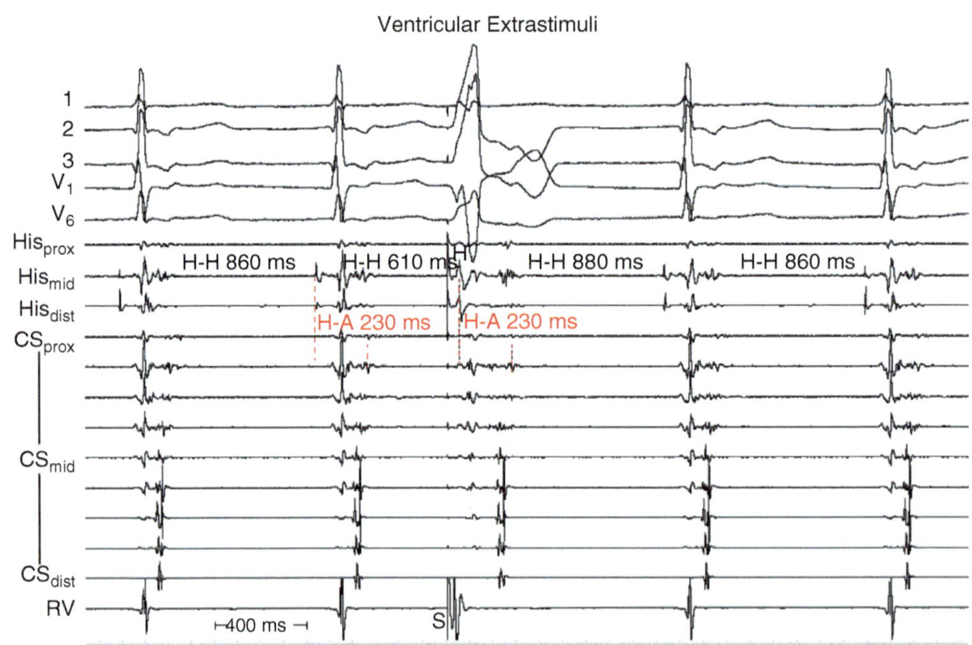

Figure 4-6

From where is the junctional rhythm arising? His propagation is anterograde, indicating somewhere proximal to the His recording site, but where? To investigate this, HA intervals can be analyzed (Fig. 4-6). Here, a ventricular extrastimulus during the baseline rhythm conducts retrogradely to the His (H); the resulting HA interval as shown is the same as during the baseline rhythm, indicating that the site of impulse formation is not far from the

His recording site: if the rhythm originated from a site significantly more proximal in the AV conduction axis, some time would be required to travel from the focus to the His recording site during the rhythm, and thus the "HA" measured would be shorter than the actual time from focus to atrium. Likewise, after ventricular stimulation, the "HA" would be longer than the actual time from the focus to the atrium. A site not far from the proximal His recording can now be sought with the mapping catheter. In this example also, the focus has been prematurely excited to the extent that it shows some overdrive suppression (HH interval after the extrastimulus 880 ms, slightly longer than the baseline interval).

Ablation Site

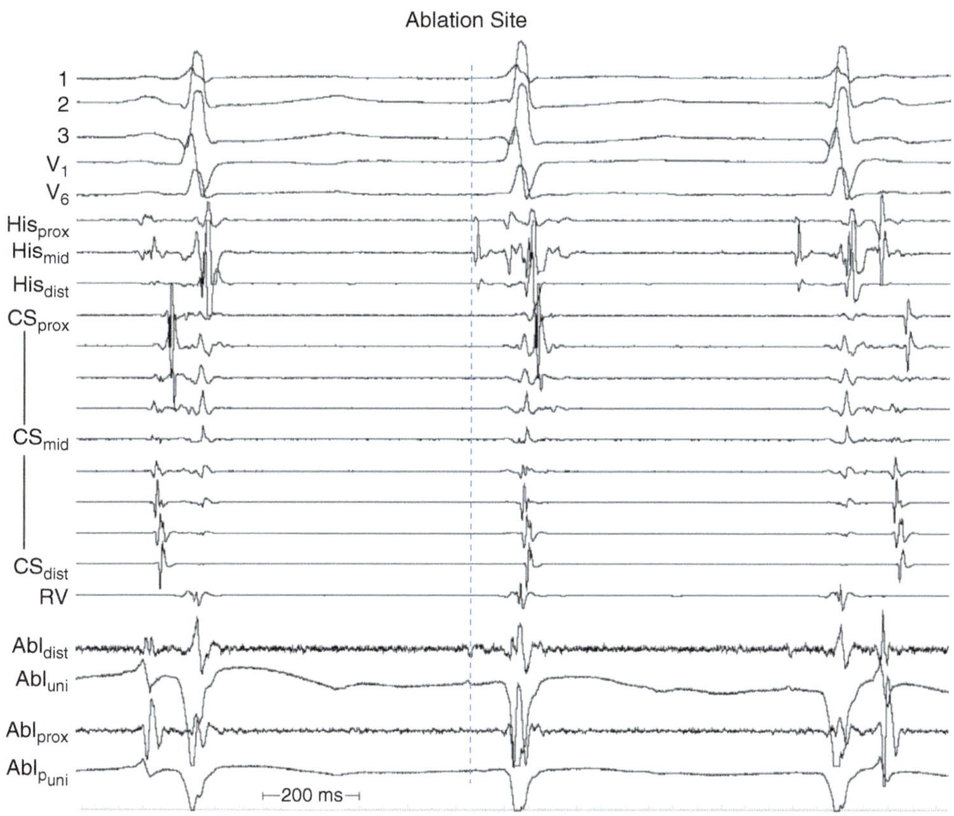

Figure 4-7

The desired ablation target should be the earliest possible His recording, often in the region of the compact AV node. In Fig. 4-7, a potential on the ablation catheter occurs about 10 ms before the earliest activation on the His catheter. At this time in the procedure, the sinus rate had accelerated somewhat accounting for the positive P waves in inferior leads.

RF Ablation Begins

Figure 4-8

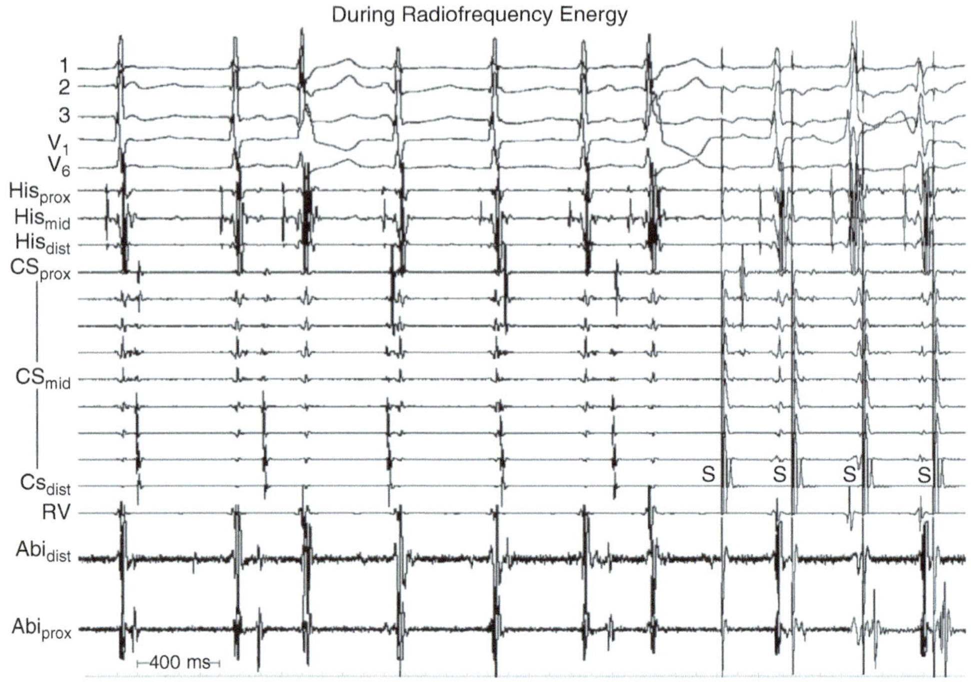

RF ablation at this site resulted in acceleration of the junctional discharge rate as well as retrograde conduction block (Fig. 4-8). As is often done during accelerated junctional rhythm with AV nodal reentry slow pathway ablation, atrial pacing (S, on *right* side of figure) is begun to ensure that anterograde AV conduction remains intact during the accelerated junctional rhythm. If the PR lengthens or conduction fails for even one cycle, RF energy delivery can immediately be stopped. Conduction remained intact with a mildly prolonged but stable PR interval throughout a 1 min RF application.

Final Recordings

Figure 4-9

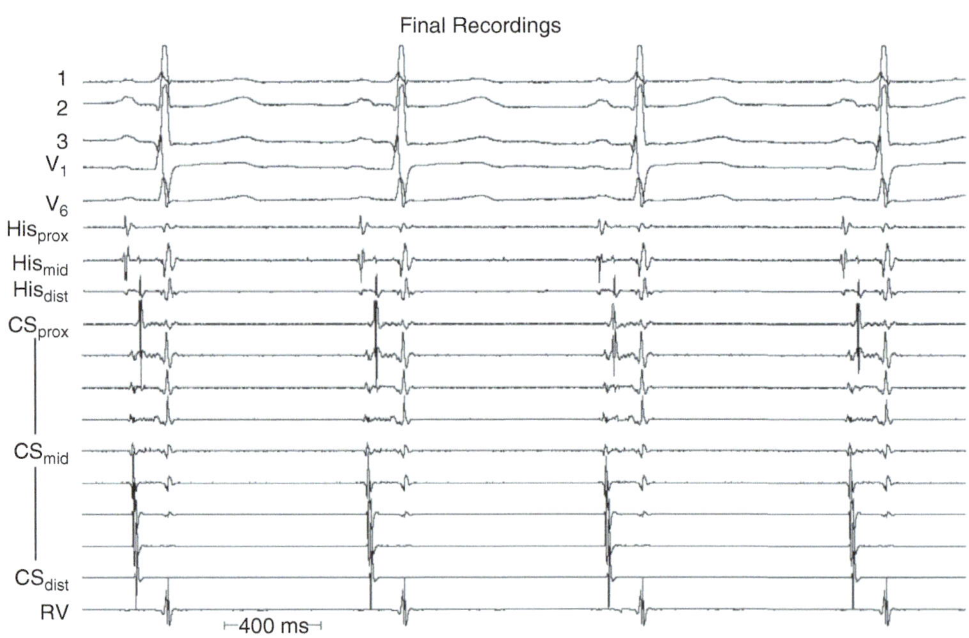

As seen in Fig. 4-9, after ablation, sinus rhythm with intact conduction and normal intervals is present, CL 950 to 1000 ms. With isoproterenol, the sinus rate accelerated and AV conduction remained consistent. No accelerated junctional rhythm was observed.

Fluoroscopy of Catheter Positions

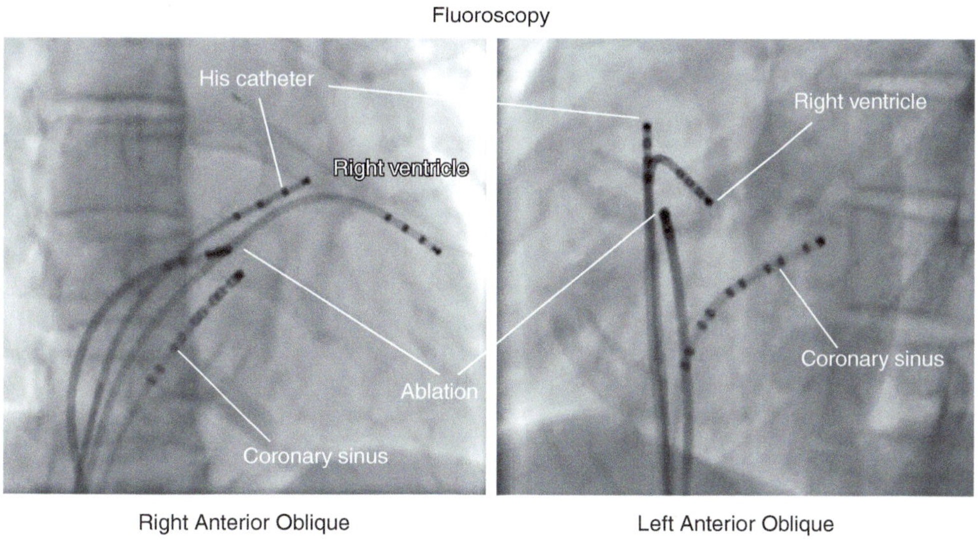

Figure 4-10

Fig. 4-10 displays fluoroscopic images of the ablation catheter at the site of successful ablation, where the compact AV node would be expected to reside.

Summary

- Accelerated junctional rhythm is rare but can be very symptomatic, resulting in functional "pacemaker syndrome"
- It must be distinguished from AV nodal reentry and atrial rhythm with long PR interval
- The site of impulse formation is in the conduction system and must be targeted very carefully to avoid heart block:
  - Site of earliest His potential
  - Often occurs in slow pathway region
  - Further acceleration of junctional rhythm occurs with RF application—a sensitive, but not specific, indicator
  - Atrial pacing to monitor anterograde conduction can help avoid heart block

5 Left Lateral Concealed Pathway Supraventricular Tachycardia

Case Presentation

A 21-year-old man with a lifelong history of palpitations and supraventricular tachycardia (SVT) was referred for catheter ablation. He began having episodes as a child, only occasionally at first but more frequently as a teenager. He was diagnosed with SVT at age 10; episodes were characterized as sudden onset with palpitations, lightheadedness, and dyspnea. Medical therapy with beta blockers failed to control episodes and he underwent an attempt at catheter ablation. A concealed left lateral bypass tract was diagnosed but ablation (retrograde aortic approach) failed despite multiple radiofrequency (RF) applications, and the procedure was stopped because of prolonged fluoroscopy time. Three years later another ablation attempt likewise failed (retrograde aortic approach).

He also had a history of cyanosis and a heart murmur at birth and was diagnosed with tetralogy of Fallot. A Blalock-Taussig shunt was constructed at age 2 weeks and he underwent complete intracardiac repair at age 15 months (shunt taken down at that time). He has had progressive pulmonic regurgitation in the ensuing years but a normal physical capacity.

Baseline ECG in Sinus Rhythm: SVT ECG

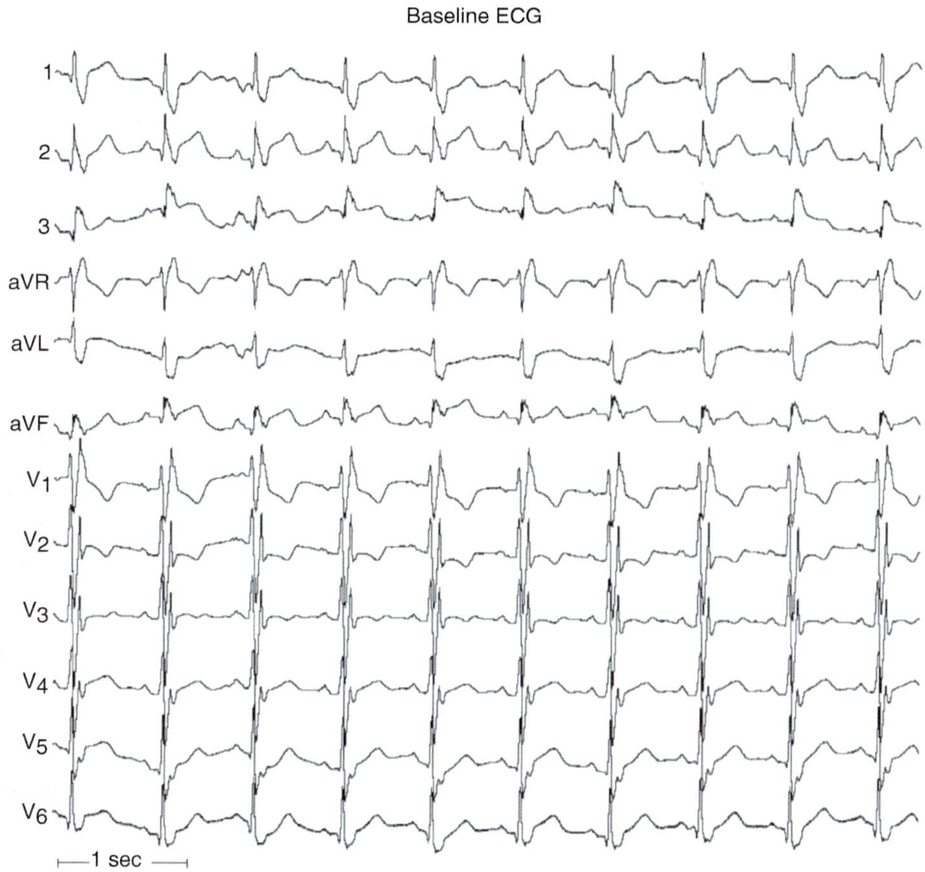

What Questions Should You Ask About History and Prior Procedures?

Figure 5-1

In Fig. 5-1, right bundle branch block (RBBB) is evident during sinus rhythm, consistent with right ventriculotomy for tetralogy repair.

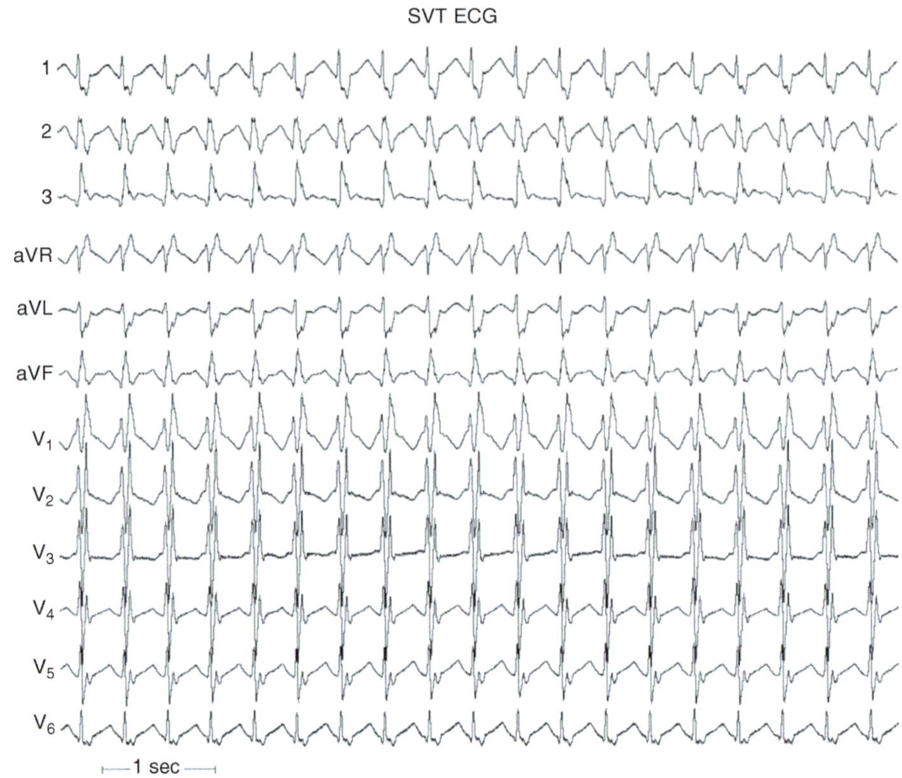

Figure 5-2

In Fig. 5-2, SVT has the same QRS configuration and no discernible P waves. This could thus be atrioventricular (AV) nodal reentry or atrial tachycardia with P waves hidden in the QRS complex. Orthodromic SVT using a left-sided bypass tract could also appear the same way (P wave inside the widened, RBBB QRS complex). However, the P wave should be visible after the RBBB QRS in orthodromic SVT using a right lateral pathway.

Baseline Intracardiac Recordings in Sinus Rhythm

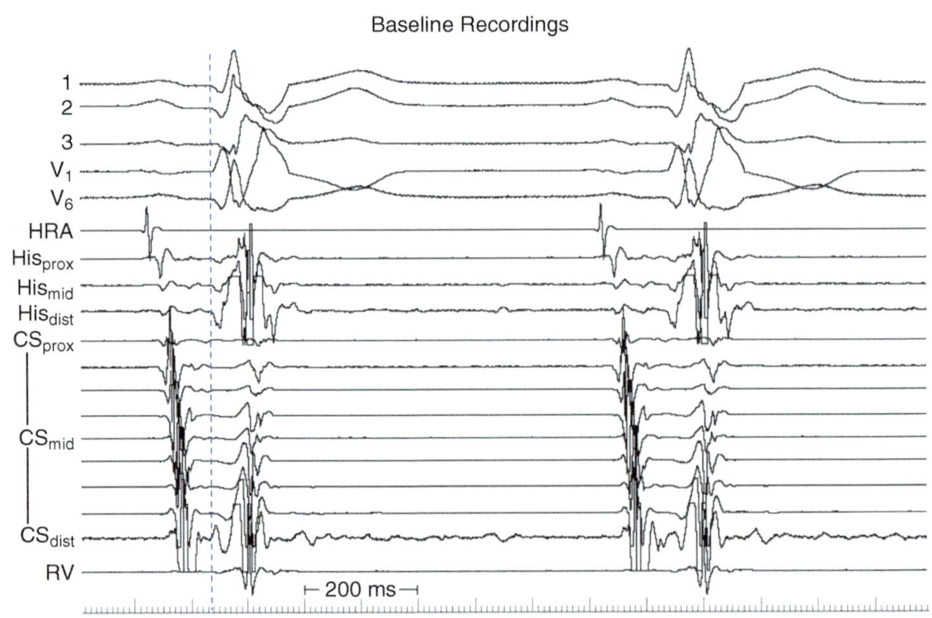

Figure 5-3

Fig. 5-3 shows no evidence of left lateral (or other location) preexcitation on intracardiac recordings in sinus rhythm; *dashed line* denotes QRS onset.

Ventricular Pacing at Progressively Rapid Rates During Sinus Rhythm

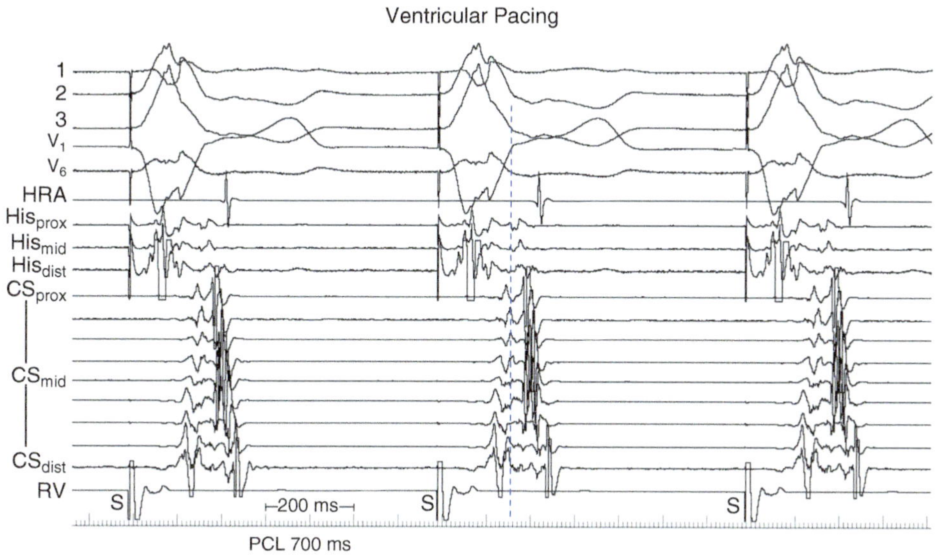

Figure 5-4

With ventricular pacing at 700 ms (Fig. 5-4), it is evident that retrograde conduction is present; the His bundle atrial activation appears earliest *(dashed blue line)*, but the distal coronary sinus (CS) recordings are difficult to interpret (likely because of prior ablation in this area).

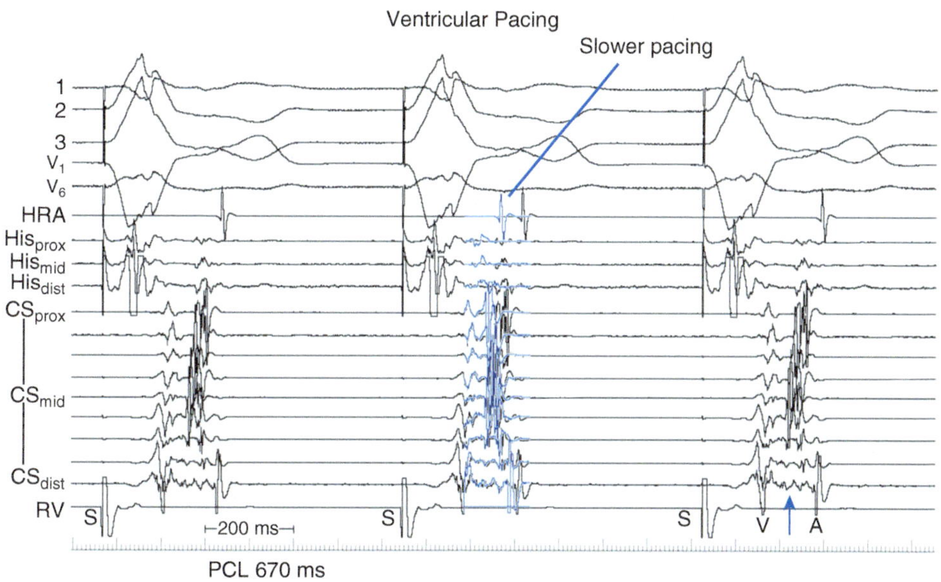

Figure 5-5

With slightly more rapid pacing (670 ms; Fig. 5-5), there is a change in the atrial activation sequence (slower pacing sequence shown superimposed in *blue*). The most obvious change is in the high right atrium (HRA) and His atrial recordings, which are delayed with more rapid pacing, signifying loss of AV nodal conduction, whereas most of the CS recordings are largely unchanged (consistent with conduction over a left lateral bypass tract). A series of complex signals *(blue arrow)* is present in between what is clearly ventricular (V) and what is clearly atrial activation (A); because of prior ablation, these could represent slow conduction in either ventricular or atrial tissue, or recordings from the bypass tract itself.

Figure 5-6

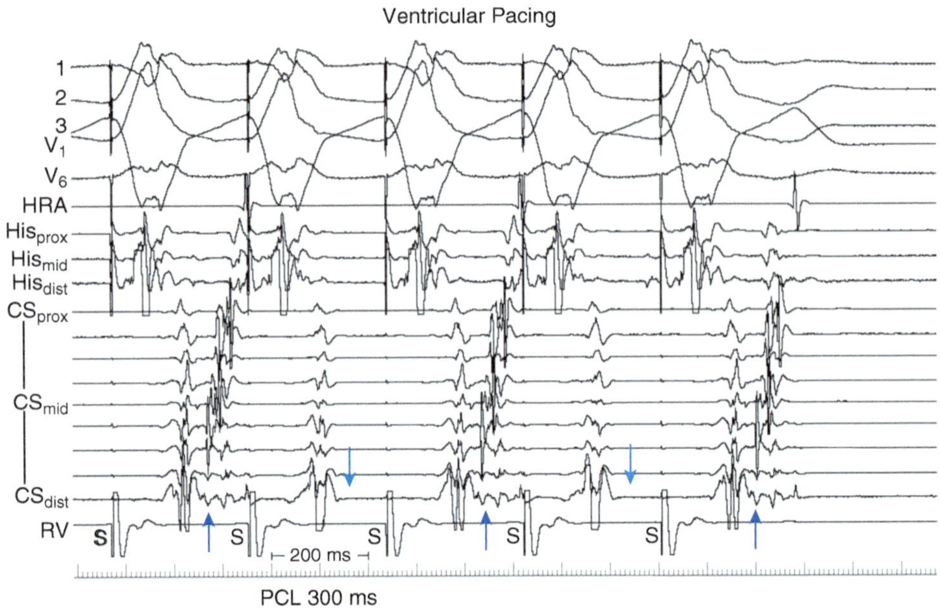

To investigate the nature of these signals, some way must be devised to clearly separate atrial from ventricular activation. In Fig. 5-6, rapid ventricular pacing at 300 ms results in 2:1 retrograde conduction. On cycles without atrial recordings *(light blue downward arrows)*, the signals in question are absent *(upward blue arrows)*—signifying that they are not ventricular in origin, because there is a ventricular electrogram on each of the paced complexes.

Ventricular Pacing Initiates SVT

Figure 5-7

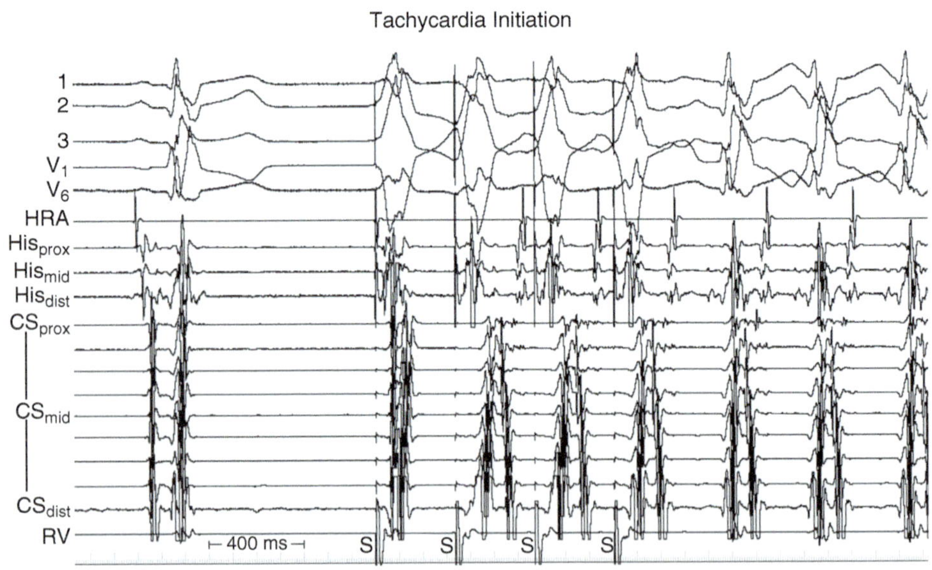

Fig. 5-7 shows a burst of rapid ventricular pacing initiating an episode of SVT.

Ventricular Extrastimuli in SVT

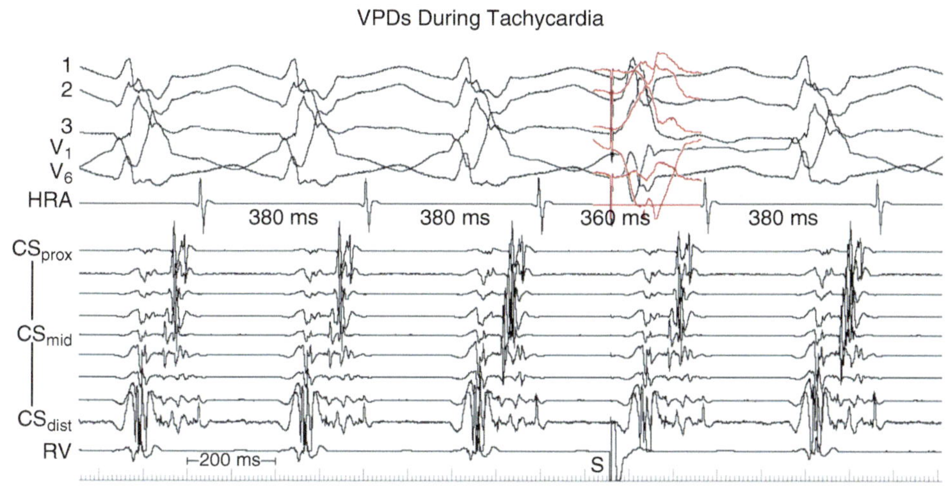

Figure 5-8

In Fig. 5-8, a single extrastimulus (S) is delivered from the right ventricle during SVT. A-A intervals in the HRA recordings are as indicated. The A-A interval surrounding the premature complex is shorter than any other during tachycardia, suggesting bypass tract conduction; however, this is only valid if the His bundle is refractory at the time the extrastimulus is delivered. A complex of pure right ventricular pacing is superimposed in red atop the complex associated with the extrastimulus. It is clear that simulation during tachycardia yields a QRS complex different from both pure pacing and SVT, and is thus a fusion complex between these two. Because the fusion derives from some element of a conducted QRS complex, the His bundle must have already been activated on that complex, and thus by definition the extrastimulus is His-refractory. Thus the fact that the A-A interval surrounding this complex is shorter than all others can be interpreted to indicate that a bypass tract is present, but not necessarily participating in tachycardia.

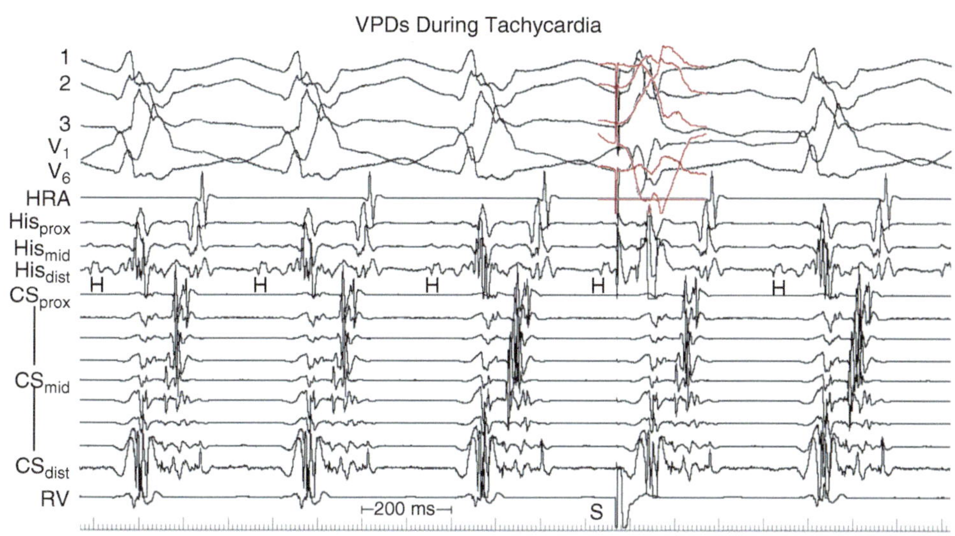

Figure 5-9

The same event is shown in Fig. 5-9, this time including the His recordings where it can be seen that the His bundle (H) had indeed already been activated on the complex in question and was thus refractory.

Ventricular Overdrive Pacing in SVT

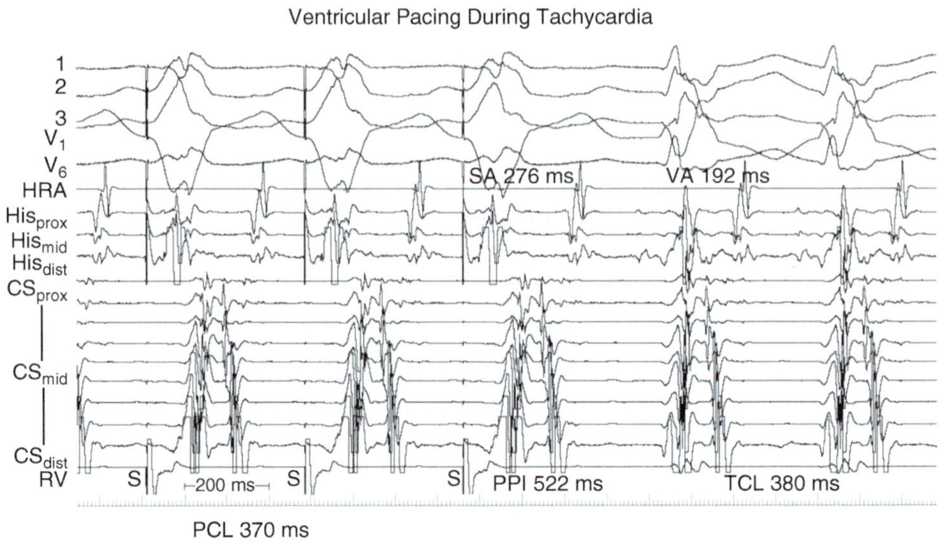

Figure 5-10

The results of ventricular overdrive pacing during SVT are shown in Fig. 5-10; the stimulus-atrial minus ventricular-atrial (SA-VA) difference (84 ms) is just less than 85 ms and suggests orthodromic SVT, whereas the post-pacing interval–tachycardia cycle length (PPI-TCL) difference (158 ms) is more suggestive of AV nodal reentry. Some of the disparity can be accounted for by the longer AH interval after the last paced complex, but the conflicting numbers is one reason that these intervals should be interpreted with caution in situations in which a far left-sided bypass tract is involved. Note also that the CS activations have changed—the catheter has been advanced somewhat (more distally in the CS). Finally, the SA interval during right ventricular pacing—simulating left bundle branch block (LBBB)—is much longer than the VA during SVT, strongly suggesting participation of a left free wall bypass tract during tachycardia.

Ventricular Pacing with Different Coronary Sinus Catheter Positions

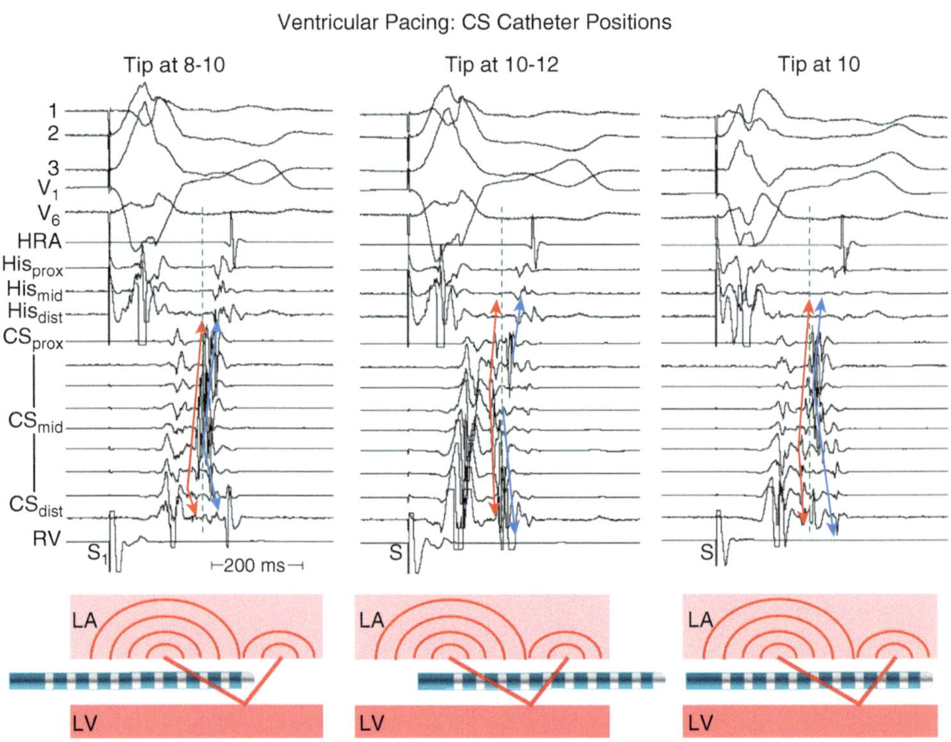

Figure 5-11

It is sometimes useful to "bracket" the site of earliest atrial activation in CS recordings. In Fig. 5-11A, recordings are shown with the catheter tip at site "8-10" (directly lateral on the mitral annulus), site "10-12" (anterolateral mitral annulus), and site "10" (intermediate between these two). A *dashed green line*, placed at the same interval before the HRA recordings in each panel, serves as a reference for comparison of activation sequences (Fig. 5-11B). Two activation sequences are evident within the coronary sinus recordings, indicated by *red arrows* and *blue arrows* (Fig. 5-11C). Whether these represent propagation over a bypass tract or partially insulated strands of atrial muscle within scar from prior ablation is not clear. One possible resolution to the different propagation patterns is shown in the diagram at bottom, where a multipolar electrode catheter is moved along the mitral annulus between the left atrium (LA) and left ventricle (LV). It is possible that there are two atrial insertions of the bypass tract, as indicated.

Nature of "Funny Spikes" Explored

Atrial Extrastimuli During Fixed-Rate Ventricular Pacing

Are the Funny Spikes A, V, or BT? [Fig. 5-12]

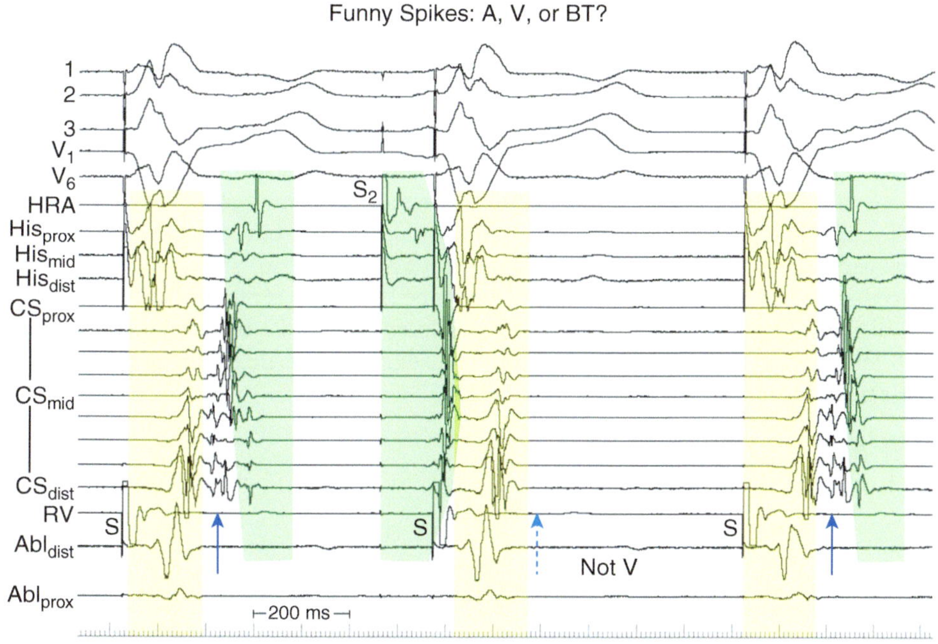

Figure 5-12

In Fig. 5-12, to further investigate the nature of the peculiar signals (*blue*) between what is thought to clearly ventricular *(shaded yellow)* and clearly atrial *(shaded green)*, an atrial extrastimulus (S2) is introduced during fixed-rate ventricular pacing (S). This draws the atrial electrograms earlier, whereas the ventricular electrogram is unaffected. Because the complex potentials are no longer seen, they cannot be part of the ventricular recording.

Onset of Ventricular Pacing at Time of Sinus Complex

Figure 5-13

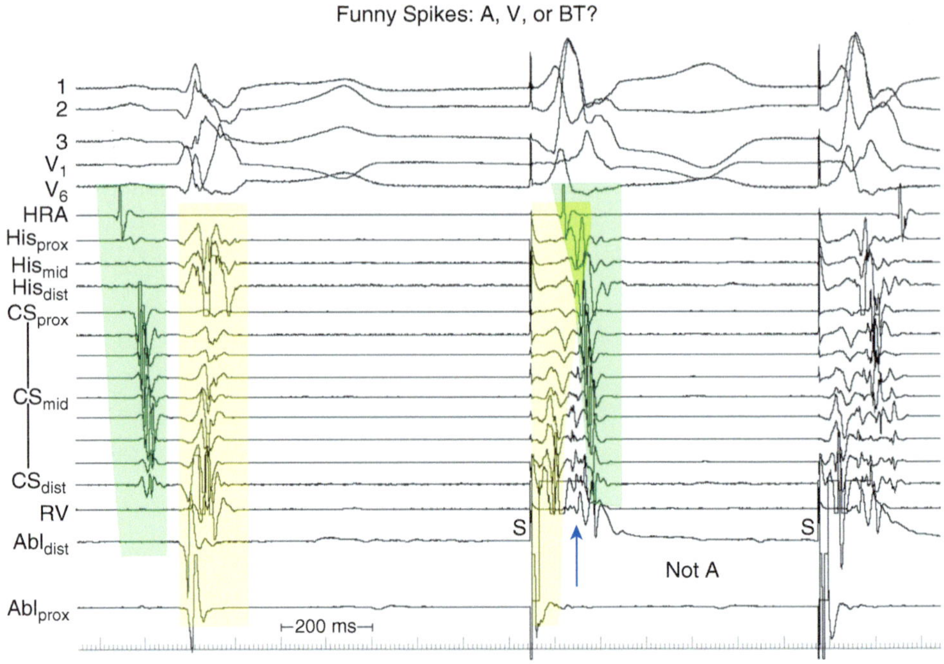

Similarly, a ventricular stimulus introduced during atrial pacing (or, as in Fig. 5-13, sinus rhythm) that causes the potentials in question to appear while the atrial recording is unchanged indicates that the questionable potentials are also not atrial in origin. Because they are neither atrial nor ventricular, they must be bypass tract recordings.

Mapping and Ablation Sites and Results

First Ablation Site

Is This Mapping Site a Good Site to Deliver RF Energy? [Fig. 5-14]

Figure 5-14

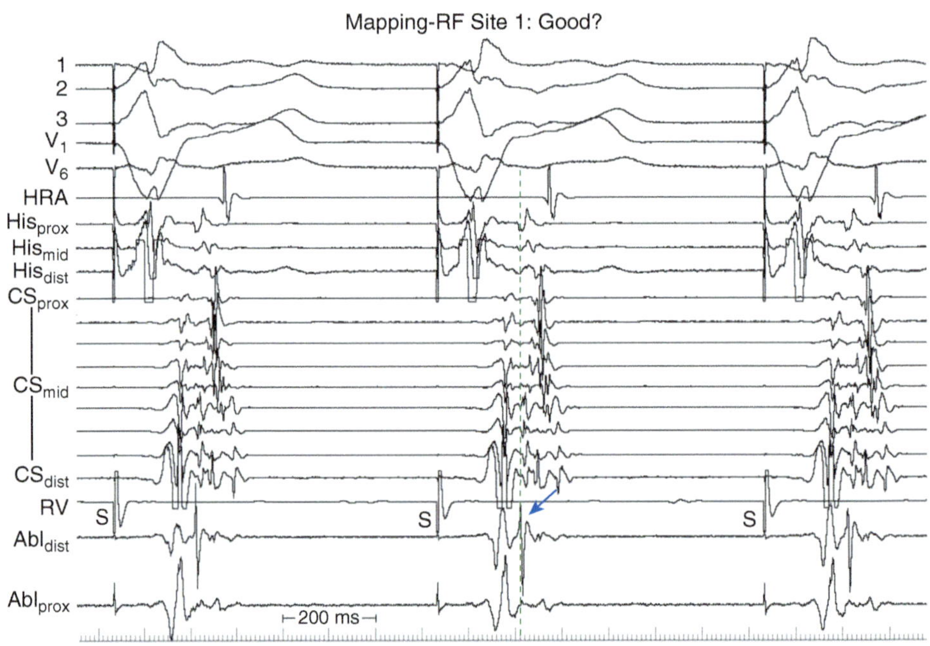

Now that the nature of the potentials in the CS recordings is clear, mapping can begin, targeting the bypass tract potentials as the most vulnerable site. Notice in Fig. 5-14, after transseptal catheterization, the ablation catheter records a sharp potential *(arrow)* that precedes all others in the CS *(dotted green line)*. With a large, stable electrogram, this looks like a good site to deliver RF energy.

Effect of First Ablation, Second Mapping Site

Is This Mapping Site a Good Site to Deliver RF Energy? [Fig. 5-15]

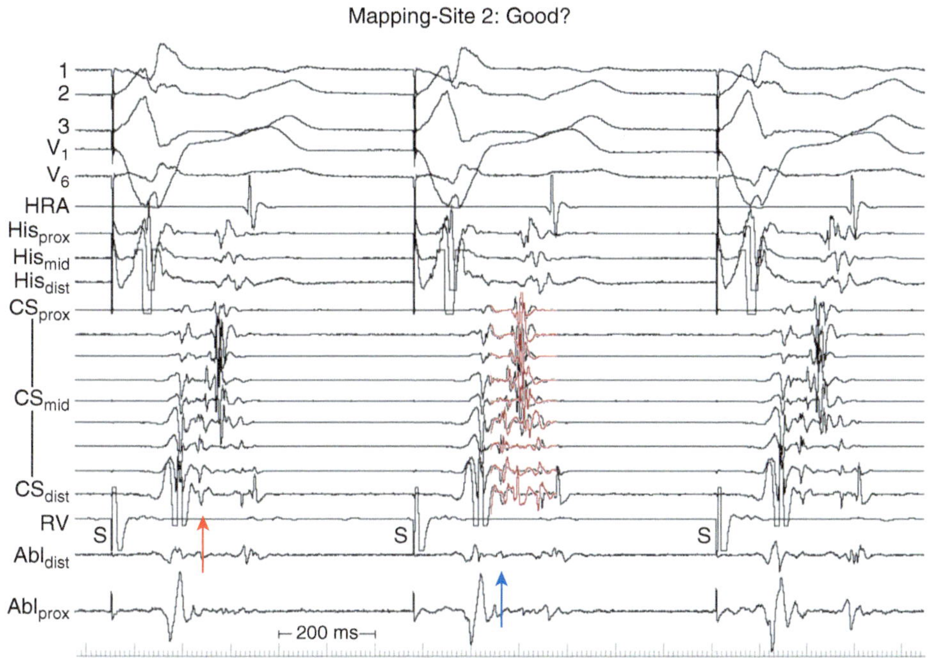

Figure 5-15

After ablation at the first site, retrograde conduction remains; however, the atrial activation sequence has changed (prior sequence superimposed in red on Fig. 5-15). The early bypass tract potentials *(red arrow)* persist, but atrial electrograms in the more distal CS recordings have been delayed. This could be because of ablation of one of two atrial insertions of the pathway, or of a branch of the pathway itself. The mapping site is not particularly attractive because of the small, far-field appearance of the bypass tract potential recording *(blue arrow)*.

Mapping Site No. 4 and Ablation

Is This Mapping Site a Good Site to Deliver RF Energy? [Fig. 5-16]

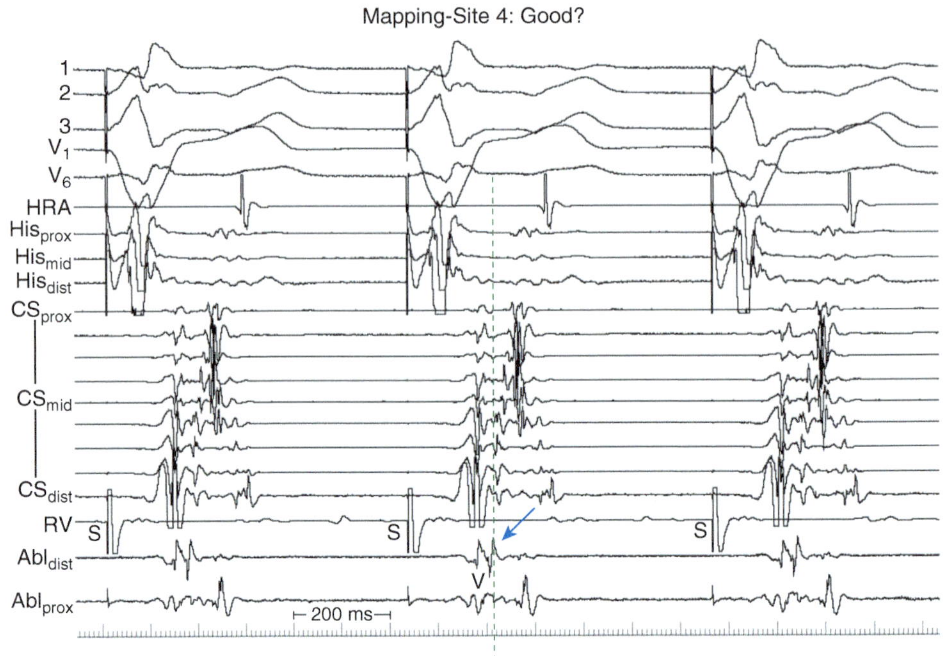

Figure 5-16

Other nearby sites were sampled, this one showing sharp ventricular (V) and bypass tract (*blue arrow*, Fig. 5-16) recordings during ventricular pacing. The *dashed green line* indicates timing of bypass tract potentials recorded in CS electrodes.

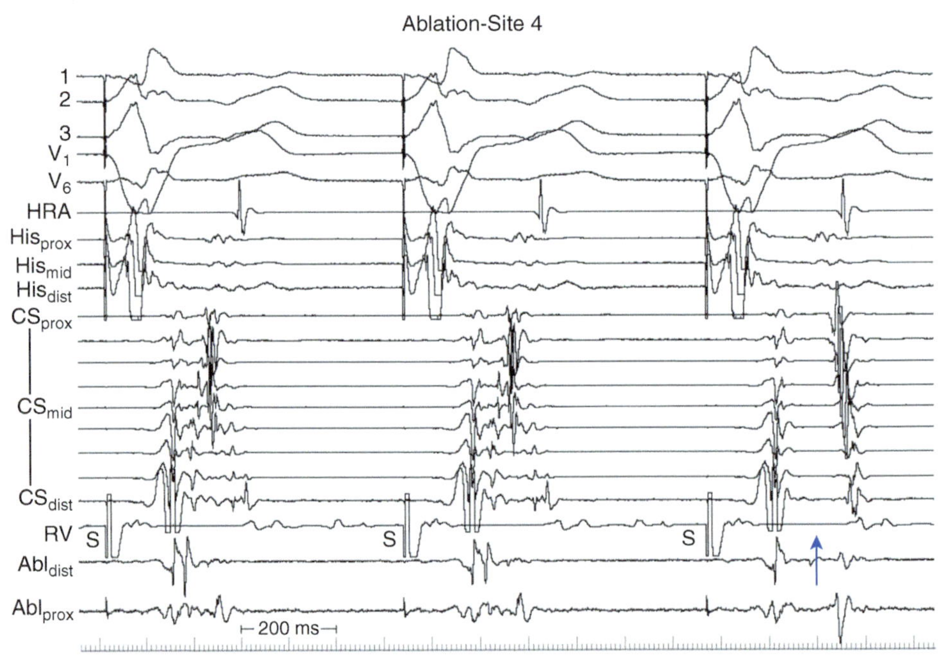

Figure 5-17

During RF energy delivery at this site (Fig. 5-17), retrograde conduction over the bypass tract suddenly fails *(arrow)*, instead now proceeding over the AV node.

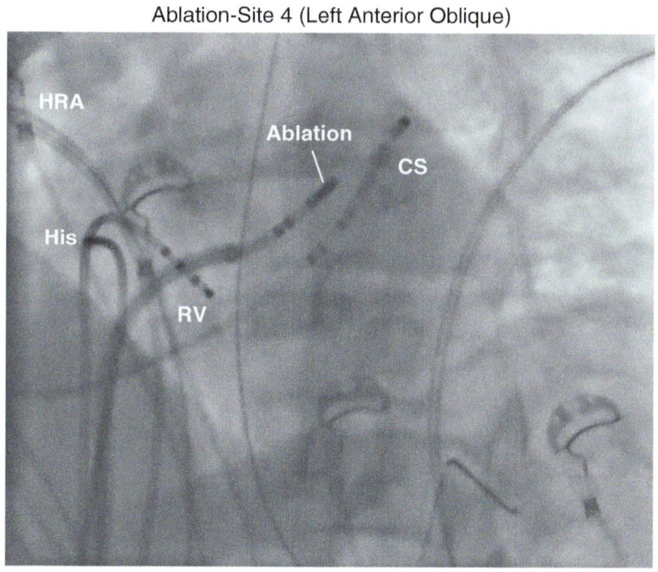

Figure 5-18

A left anterior oblique fluoroscopic image of the ablation site is displayed in Fig. 5-18.

Ventricular Pacing Postablation (AV Nodal Conduction Only)

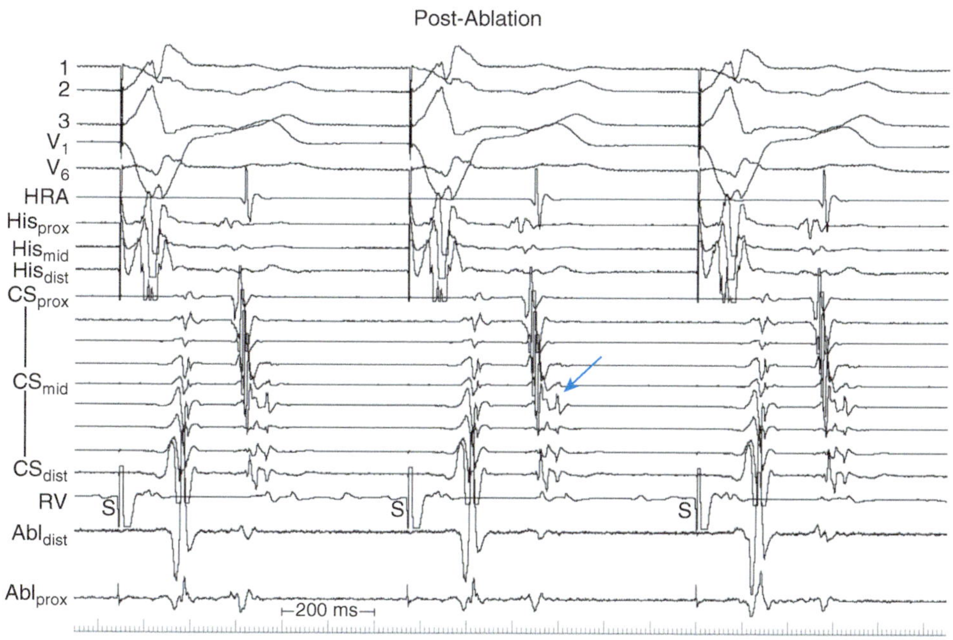

Figure 5-19

After ablation, ventricular pacing in Fig. 5-19 shows retrograde conduction with a midline activation sequence. In addition, small potentials *(arrow)* are now seen after the atrial electrogram in the middle and distal CS, possibly representing activation of the bypass tract after (rather than before) atrial activation. Retrograde conduction over the pathway did not recur during a 45-min waiting period or after isoproterenol provocation. The patient has not had recurrent tachycardia.

Summary

- AV bypass tracts typically cross the AV groove at an angle, with the ventricular insertion more proximal along the coronary sinus than the atrial insertion
- Prior ablation disrupts atrial electrograms, sometimes making interpretation of electrograms difficult
- Searching for and proving the identity of a bypass tract potential may be preferable to looking for earliest atrial activation, especially after prior ablation
- In general, the retrograde and transseptal approaches yield equivalent outcomes, but in any given case, one might be better suited to success than the other

6 Antidromic Supraventricular Tachycardia

Case Presentation

A 52-year-old man developed wide-complex tachycardia (WCT) after coronary artery surgery. He had a history of refractory hypertension and complained of palpitations and chest discomfort. Evaluation ultimately showed an anomalous left coronary artery from the right sinus of Valsalva, coursing between great vessels. He underwent open surgical reconstruction of the left main coronary artery. He reportedly had both severe bradycardia and tachycardia (possibly ventricular fibrillation) coming off the heart-lung machine. He was given amiodarone, and a dual-chamber pacemaker. He had an episode of wide QRS complex tachycardia 5 days postoperatively and was asymptomatic with this; pacemaker interrogation showed a 1:1 A:V relationship in tachycardia. He was treated with metoprolol but continued to have palpitations and tachycardia episodes on pacemaker interrogation. He was referred for electrophsyiology study.

ECG in Sinus Rhythm

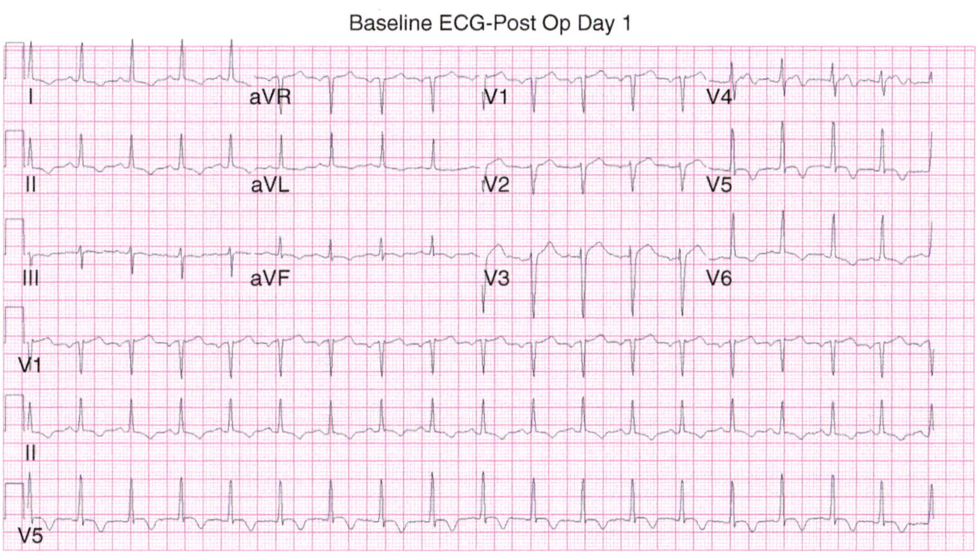

Figure 6-1

The early postoperative sinus rhythm ECG (Fig. 6-1) is relatively normal; there are no normal septal q waves, probably because of longstanding hypertension. Nonspecific ST and T-wave abnormalities may be related to the postoperative state. There is certainly no infarct pattern.

Wide-QRS Tachycardia ECG

Figure 6-2

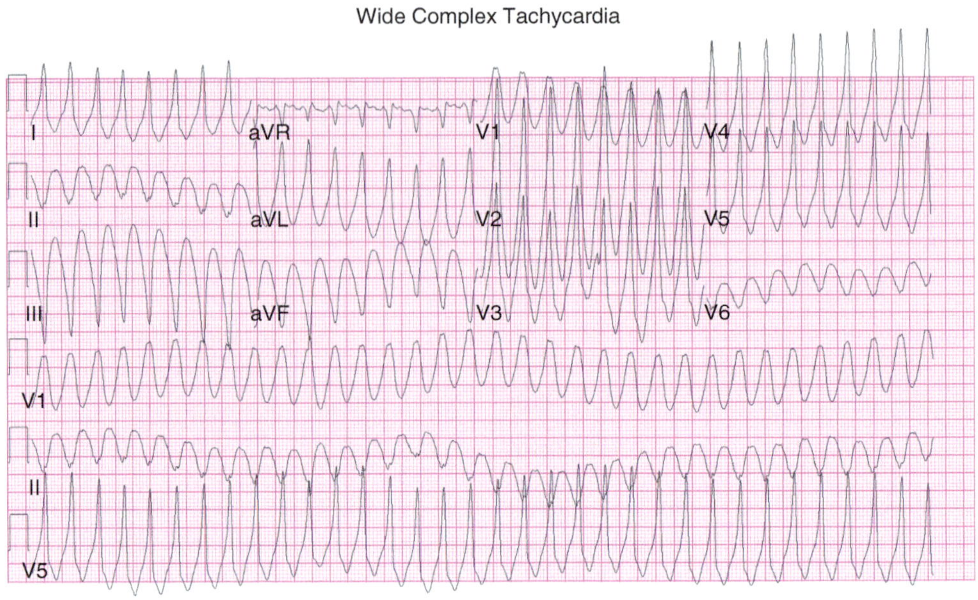

Fig. 6-2 displays the WCT recorded on day 5 postoperatively. It has a right bundle branch block (RBBB), left superior axis morphology, and no clearly discernible P waves. Q waves are evident in the inferior leads as well as V6 (slightly suspect as to its location because of the great disparity between V5 [all positive] and V6 [all negative]; this may be because of postoperative bandaging). The differential diagnosis of this WCT consists of broad categories, including supraventricular tachycardia (SVT) with aberration, a preexcited tachycardia, or ventricular tachycardia. The pattern is not particularly consistent with aberration of any form, and he does not have a reason to have either ventricular tachycardia (no prior scar) or preexcited tachycardia (no delta waves during sinus rhythm). He does have a pacemaker, which can pace the ventricle rapidly in response to atrial flutter or fibrillation, and could account for a wide-QRS tachycardia; however, the pacing lead is in the right ventricle and should yield a left bundle branch block pattern (also, no pacemaker stimulus artifacts are evident).

At this time, additional history from the patient revealed that he had Wolff-Parkinson-White syndrome and had undergone ablation about 12 years earlier that was thought to have been successful. He had nearly forgotten this in all the events surrounding his bypass surgery.

Intracardiac Recordings and Atrial Pacing

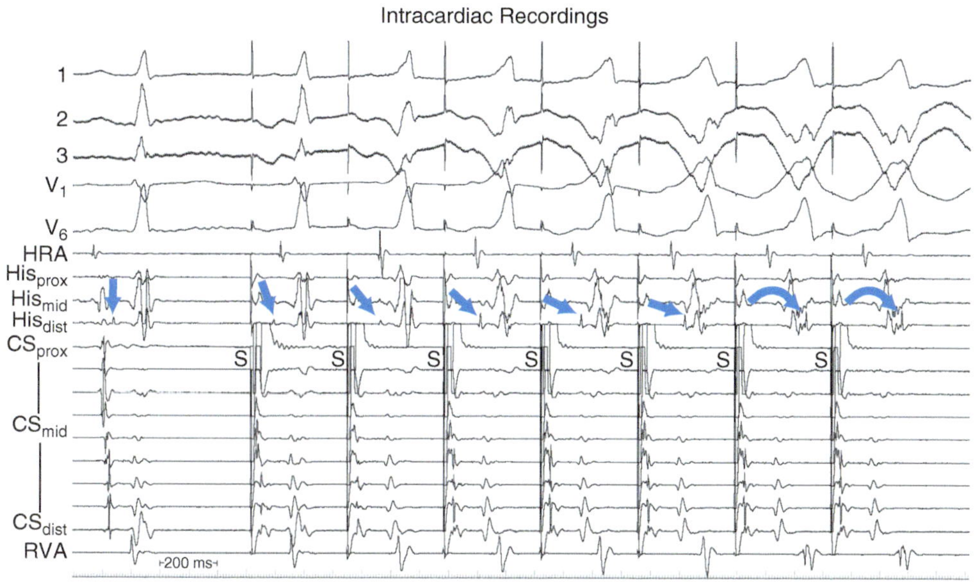

Figure 6-3

At the time of electrophysiologic study 2 months after surgery, catheters were placed in standard intracardiac locations as shown in Fig. 6-3. There is no strong evidence of preexcitation on the surface or intracardiac recordings during the sinus rhythm complex shown at left (*blue arrows* indicate His potential with normal AH and HV intervals on this complex). However, with rapid atrial pacing, the QRS complex shows progressive widening until it assumes a configuration similar to that of the WCT. In addition, the interval from stimulus to the His potential *(blue arrow)* shows progressive delay, with the His potential occurring at or after the QRS onset following the third to last stimulus. Furthermore, the His potential actually becomes retrograde, occurring toward the end of the QRS complex after the last two stimuli *(curved arrows)*. This behavior (progressive widening of the QRS complex with His potential occurring after QRS onset) is seen with ventricular tachycardia or preexcitation. Here, it seems most consistent with preexcitation.

WCT Initiation (Atrial and Ventricular Pacing)

Figure 6-4

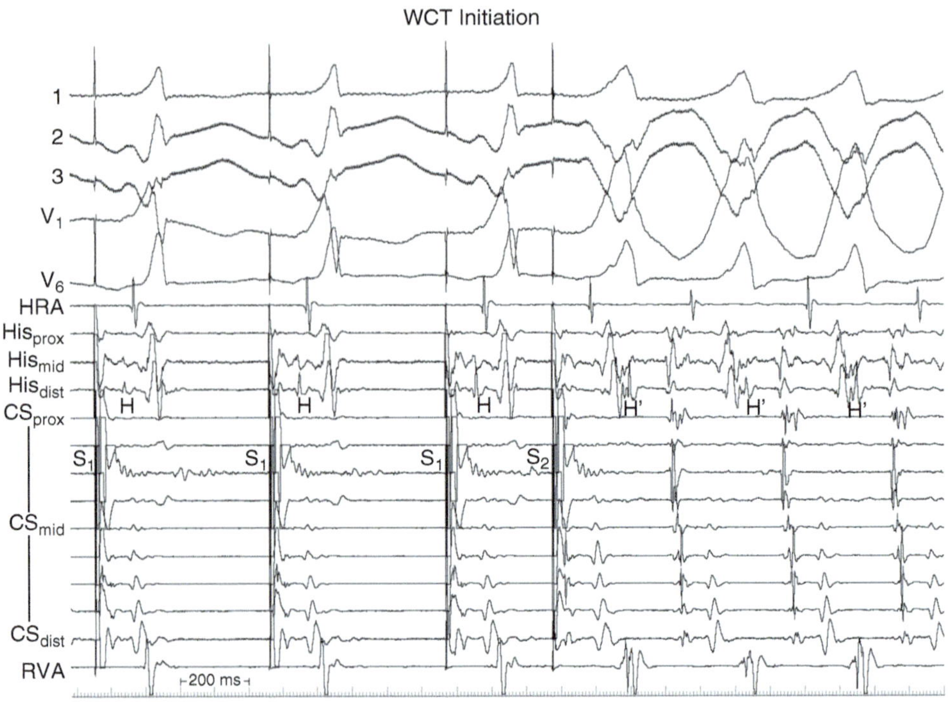

With an atrial drivetrain from the proximal coronary sinus, a preexcited QRS complex is evident in Fig. 6-4. An anterograde His potential (H) is still seen. After the extrastimulus (S2), WCT is initiated. A His potential (H′) is seen after the local ventricular electrogram in each complex. This preexcited tachycardia could be true antidromic reentry or the pathway may be a bystander with preexcited AV nodal reentry or atrial tachycardia.

Figure 6-5

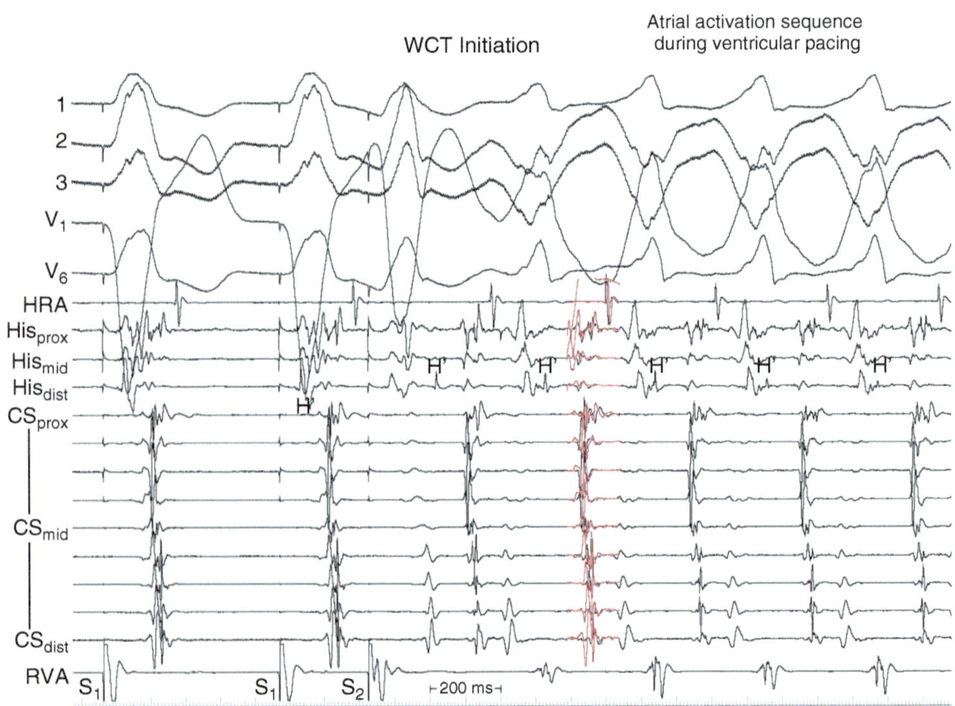

The tachycardia was also inducible with ventricular pacing and extrastimuli. In Fig. 6-5, an atrial activation sequence during ventricular pacing is superimposed in red over the atrial activation during tachycardia, showing an identical pattern. Thus it is reasonable to assume that conduction in each instance is over the same pathway, which is compatible with the

AV node (evidenced by His potential [H′] occurs at the same interval before each atrial recording; midline activation sequence; relatively long VA interval).

WCT vs Right Ventricular Pacing at Tachycardia Cycle Length

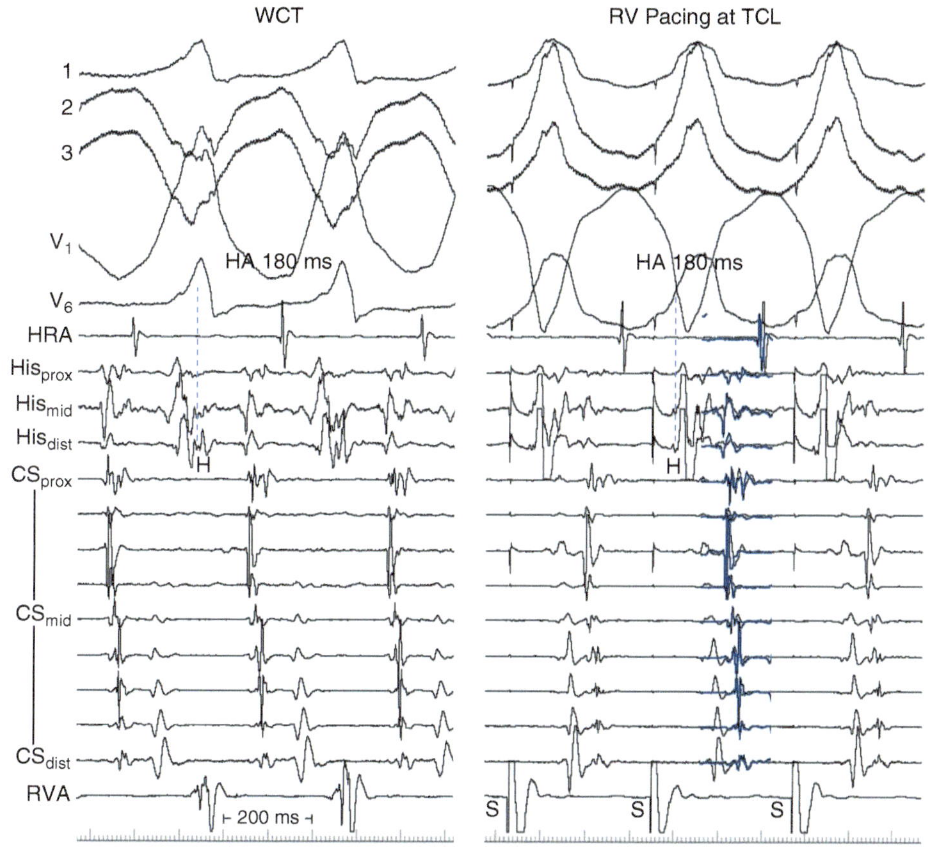

Figure 6-6

In Fig. 6-6, comparison of HA intervals (H denotes His potential) during tachycardia and ventricular pacing at the tachycardia cycle length shows the same atrial activation sequence (WCT activation sequence *superimposed in blue* over that during ventricular pacing at right) and identical HA intervals. If another bypass tract were used in the retrograde direction in either situation, the His and atrium would be activated in parallel during ventricular pacing (in series during tachycardia), leading to an artificially shorter apparent HA interval. Because the HA intervals are identical, conduction is probably proceeding over the same pathway in each situation.

Para-Hisian Pacing

These Findings:

A. Exclude a retrogradely conducting bypass tract (BT)

B. Demonstrate exclusive BT conduction

C. Show AV nodal and BT conduction

D. Show AV nodal conduction

E. Show atrial capture

[Fig. 6-7]

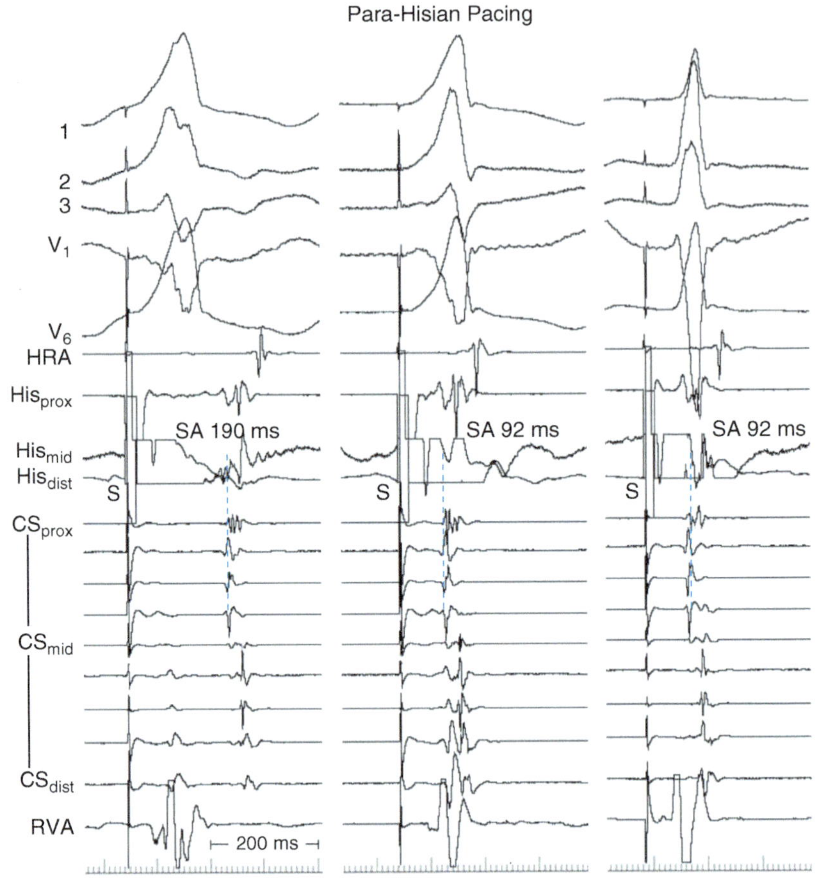

Figure 6-7

Para-Hisian pacing is performed from the His catheter (Fig. 6-7). At left, the widest resulting QRS complex is associated with a stimulus-A (SA) interval 280 ms. The complex at center shows a slightly narrower QRS complex, indicating His + ventricular capture; the SA interval is much shorter (180 ms). At right is an almost totally normal QRS complex, with a long stimulus-QRS interval likely indicating no or minimal ventricular capture ("pure" His capture). Here, the SA interval is also 180 ms. These findings are compatible with retrograde conduction over the AV node, but do not exclude the presence of a bypass tract, especially one with a long conduction time (longer than the retrograde AV nodal conduction time).

Atrial Extrastimuli (Premature Atrial Complex [PAC]) in WCT

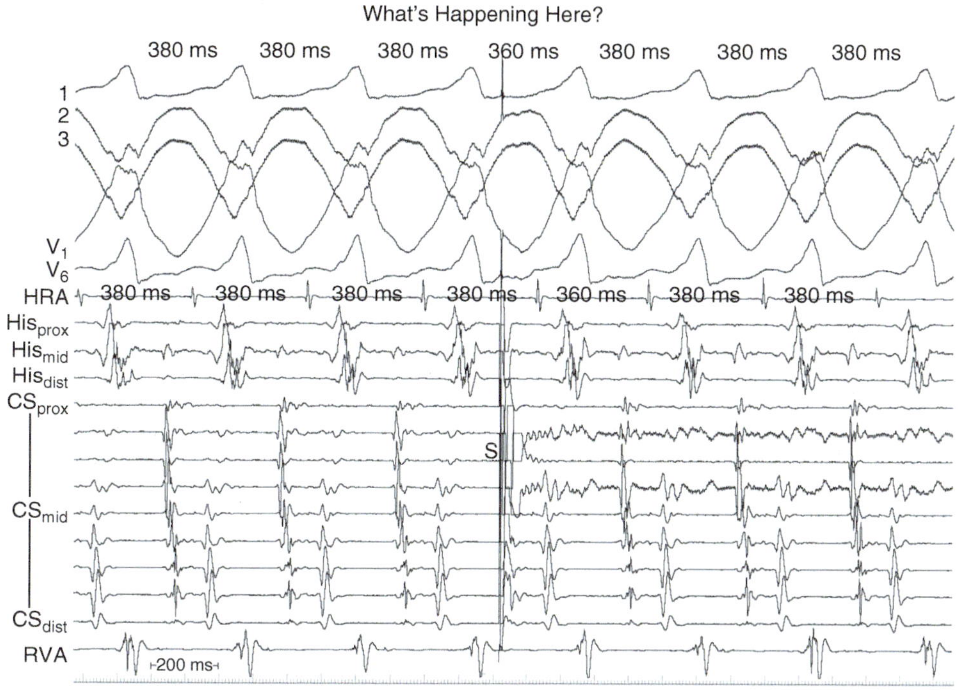

Figure 6-8

During sustained, stable WCT (Fig. 6-8), a single atrial extrastimulus (S) is introduced from the coronary sinus at a time when the atrial electrogram in the His bundle region is being inscribed (and that tissue is thus refractory). Intervals shown at the top are QRS-QRS intervals, showing that the QRS complex immediately after the extrastimulus is advanced by it. This cannot happen with ventricular tachycardia, but can with a preexcited tachycardia. In addition, the intervals shown in the middle are A-A intervals measured in the high right atrium (HRA) recording. These show advancement of the timing of the subsequent atrial electrogram, after the QRS complex that had been advanced. This indicates dependence of atrial activation on the prior QRS complex, and thus an atrial tachycardia is excluded. In addition, the fact that the stimulus occurred while the AV nodal region was refractory shows that this cannot be preexcited AV nodal reentry. Thus true antidromic tachycardia (anterograde bypass tract, retrograde AV node) is favored.

Figure 6-9

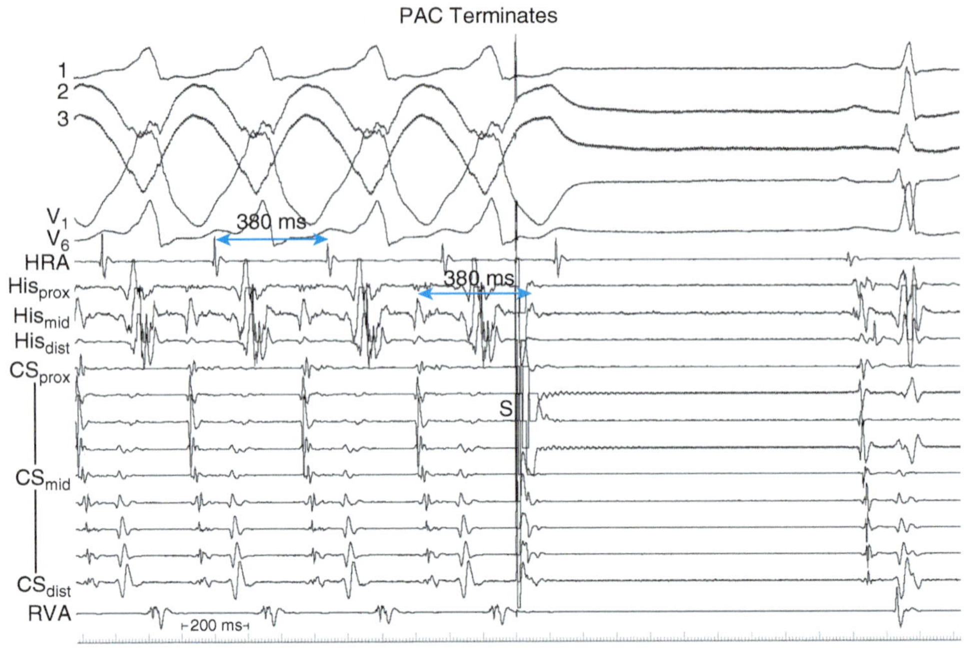

As shown in Fig. 6-9, another atrial extrastimulus delivered during stable tachycardia again occurs at a time when the AV nodal region is refractory (*arrows* on atrial recordings). In this case, atrial capture occurs (as indicated by HRA recording), but tachycardia terminates without ventricular activation. This again excludes ventricular tachycardia, as well as forms of SVT in which the bypass tract was a bystander (such as atrial tachycardia or AV nodal reentry), because simply blocking in the bypass tract with the atrial extrastimulus should eliminate preexcitation but the tachycardia should continue with narrow QRS complexes. Thus antidromic tachycardia is the diagnosis.

Investigating Possible Accessory Pathway Potential

Figure 6-10

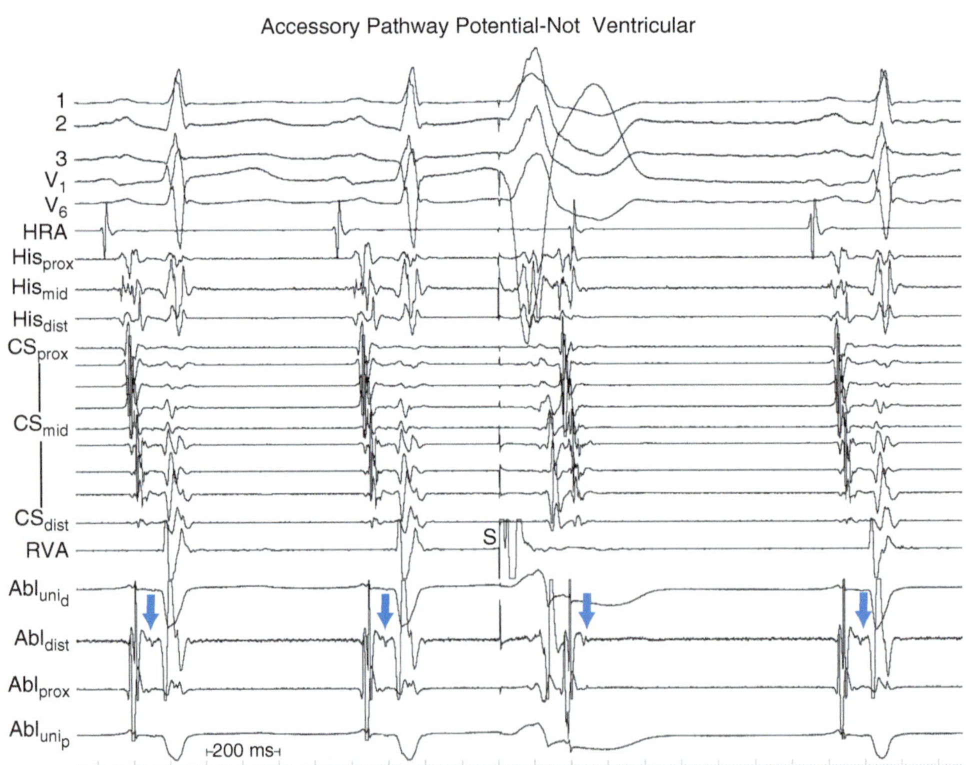

Now that a diagnosis has been established, mapping can proceed. At a site around the coronary sinus os, a recording is made that has a large atrial potential, a large ventricular potential, and a small potential between these (*blue arrows*, Fig. 6-10) that may represent the bypass tract. This is tested by introducing a ventricular extrastimulus (S) during sinus rhythm. The small potential remains with a fixed relationship to the atrial recording and is thus not part of the ventricular electrogram.

Preexcited SVT Initiation

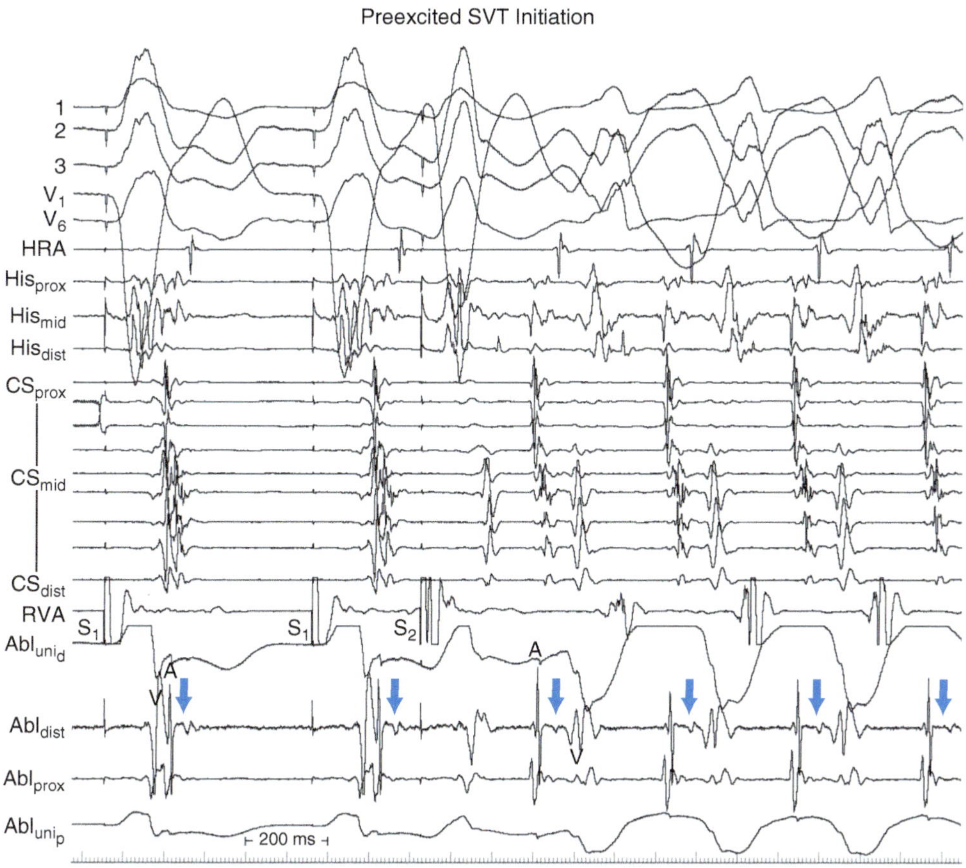

Figure 6-11

During another induction of preexcited tachycardia (Fig. 6-11), the interesting potential *(blue arrow)* remains between atrial (A) and ventricular (V) electrograms during preexcited tachycardia. However, during ventricular pacing, the potential follows the atrial electrogram. This indicates that the pathway has no retrograde conduction (retrograde conduction occurs through the AV node and activates the atrium and the pathway thereafter).

Ablation Site and Ablation Delivery

Figure 6-12

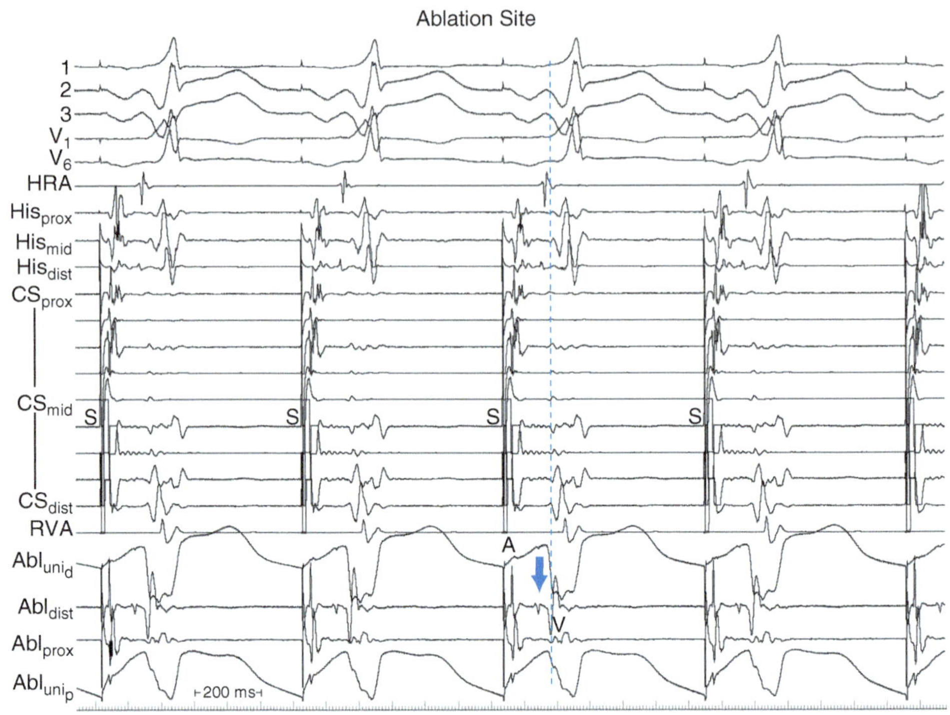

A site for possible ablation is chosen as indicated in Fig. 6-12. The surface QRS/delta wave onset is shown by a *dashed blue line*; the recording at this site shows a large atrial potential (A), bypass tract potential *(blue arrow)*, and ventricular electrogram (V). In addition, the unipolar recording shows a "QS" configuration; this and the bipolar ventricular recording precede the onset of the delta wave by about 20 ms.

Figure 6-13

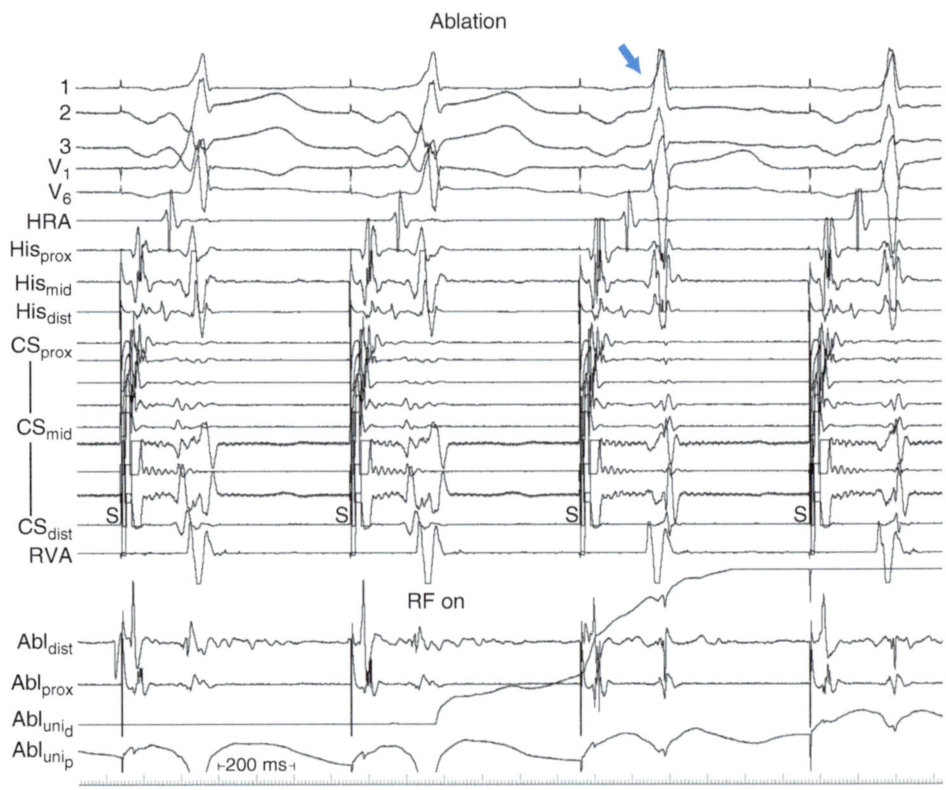

Radiofrequency energy application at this site (as indicated in middle of Fig. 6-13) during atrial pacing to maximize the delta wave shows a nearly immediate loss of preexcitation (see surface ECG leads, *arrow*).

Pre- and Postablation ECGs Compared

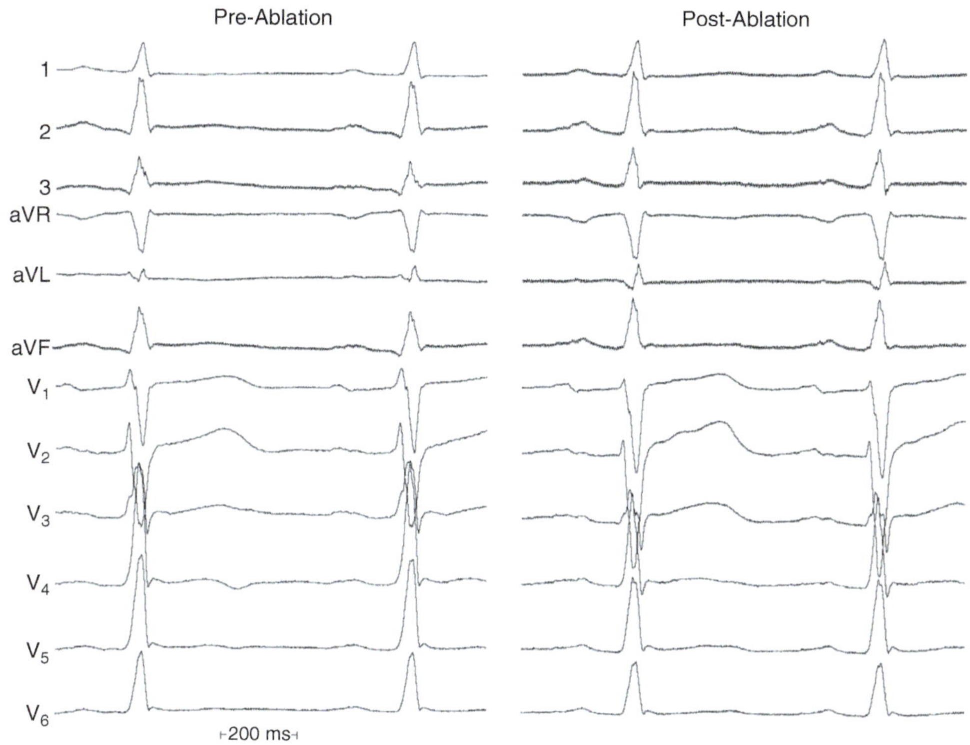

Figure 6-14

In Fig. 6-14, 12-lead ECG recordings before ablation and immediately postablation show subtle differences, suggesting that preexcitation really was present to a very minor degree before ablation (small Q wave in leads 2, 3, and aVF, and larger R wave before ablation in leads V1 and V2).

Bypass tract conduction did not recur during a waiting period, with or without isoproterenol provocation. Electroanatomic mapping was not used during this procedure (only electrogram-based mapping). The patient has done well on long-term follow-up without recurrence of preexcitation or tachycardia for several years.

Summary

- Not all WCTs after coronary artery surgery are ventricular tachycardia
- History is important (remote ablation recalled)
- Usually, partially successful ablation eliminates anterograde pathway conduction; here, it was retrograde conduction that had been ablated successfully at the first procedure. The patient still had the capability of having preexcited tachycardias such as atrial flutter/fibrillation, atrial tachycardia or AV nodal reentry (in which the bypass tract is a bystander), or, as here, antidromic tachycardia
- It is both possible and important to distinguish true antidromic SVT (which will be eliminated by successful pathway ablation) from other preexcited tachycardias (which need additional ablation of the cause of the tachycardia, not just of the pathway, which is a bystander)

7 Atriofascicular Pathway Supraventricular Tachycardia

Case Presentation

A 30-year-old woman had been bothered by sustained palpitations for the last 8 years; there had been a recent (2 years) increase in frequency of episodes. She had several emergency room (ER) visits for palpitations; ECGs consistently showed left bundle branch block (LBBB) tachycardia at ~200/min that terminated reliably with adenosine. Following tachycardia termination, the QRS was normal. She was diagnosed with supraventricular tachycardia (SVT) with LBBB aberration. Physical examination and non-invasive evaluation were completely normal. Because of increased frequency of episodes refractory to beta blockers, an electrophysiology (EP) study and ablation were performed:

EP study 1/11: Atrioventricular (AV) nodal reentrant SVT was diagnosed, leading to extensive slow pathway ablation; the operator noted that the catheter kept falling into a large coronary sinus ostium. A long vascular sheath was used but tachycardia was still inducible at the end of the procedure.

EP study 5/11: AV nodal reentrant SVT was again diagnosed, further ablation in the slow pathway region was performed with "transient success".

In the months following her second ablation, she experienced a "crescendo" in frequency of episodes, resulting in 16 ER visits (each with tachycardia having LBBB pattern, almost all readily terminated with adenosine). She was referred for repeat EP study and possible ablation.

ECG During Tachycardia

ECG From ER Visit

Figure 7-1

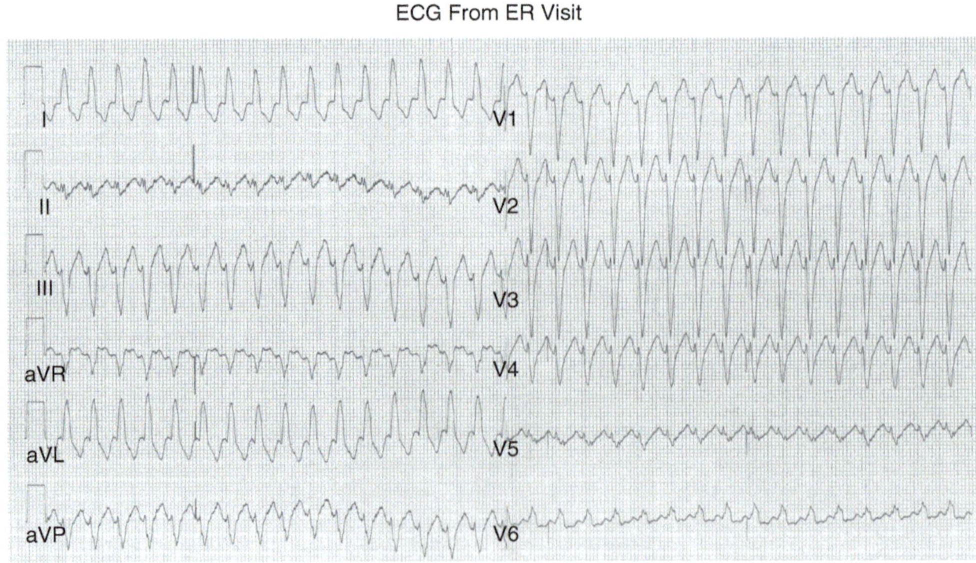

The ECG in Fig. 7-1 is representative of those obtained at each of several emergency room visits over the prior months, showing a regular tachycardia with a left bundle branch block pattern. This was reliably terminated with adenosine injection, resulting in a sinus rhythm ECG that showed no abnormalities (narrow QRS complex).

Differential Diagnosis of LBBB-Appearing Tachycardia

What About Left Bundle Branch Block (LBBB) Tachycardias?

Although right bundle branch block (RBBB) aberration is more common in younger individuals, LBBB-type tachycardias can certainly occur, with a certain relatively short list of possibilities as noted below:

- Differential diagnosis of typical LBBB tachycardia in patients with a normal resting ECG and no structural heart disease includes the following:
  - Orthodromic supraventricular tachycardia (SVT) with left lateral concealed bypass tract
  - Any type of SVT with LBBB aberration
  - Antidromic SVT using atriofascicular pathway
  - Right ventricular papillary muscle focal VT
- Typical LBBB tachycardia in patients *with* structural heart disease includes the following:
  - SVT of any type and preexisting LBBB
  - Bundle branch reentry
- *Atypical* LBBB may be seen in the following:
  - Preexcited SVT using an atrioventricular pathway anterogradely
  - VT

Baseline ECG and Intracardiac Recordings

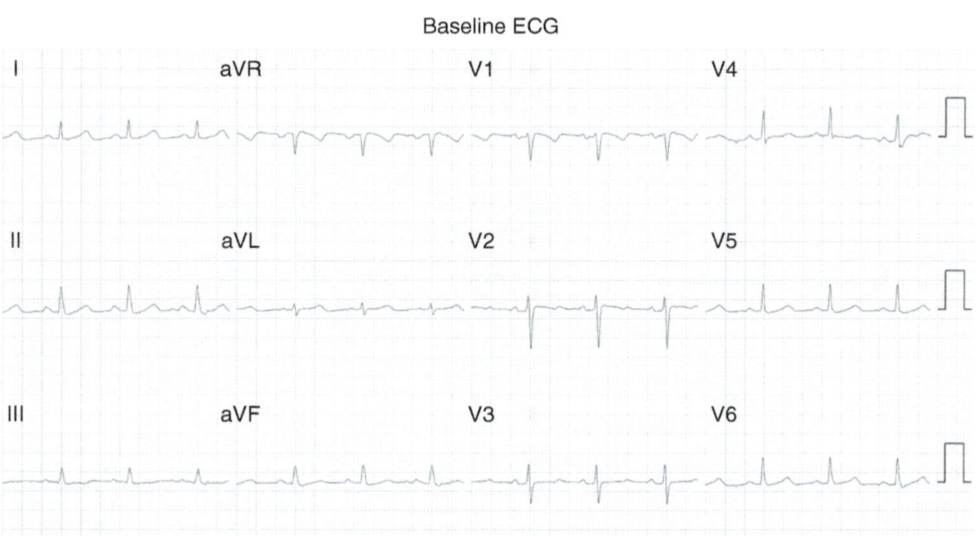

Figure 7-2

The baseline ECG (Fig. 7-2), as indicated previously, was entirely normal without bundle branch block.

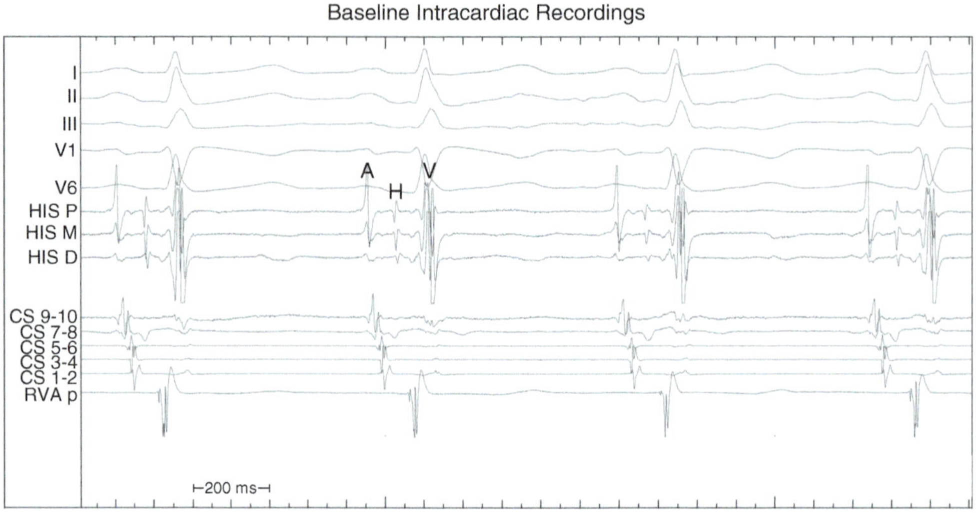

Figure 7-3

Baseline intracardiac recordings (Fig. 7-3) were likewise entirely normal, with AH and HV intervals within the normal range.

Atrial Pacing with Change in QRS and Tachycardia Induction

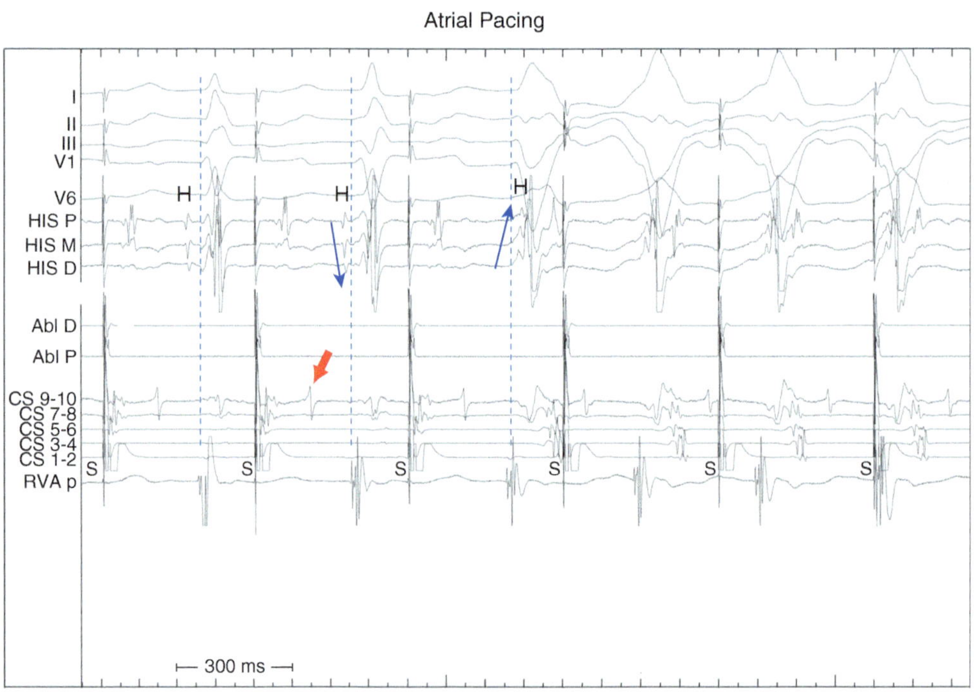

Figure 7-4

With atrial pacing from the distal coronary sinus, some unusual features are observed in Fig. 7-4. The *red arrow* indicates an odd potential in the region of the coronary sinus ostium; this may have been a "split potential" caused by repeated ablation in this region. Additionally, the surface ECG shows changes with a progressive increase in QRS duration until tachycardia with a left bundle branch block pattern ensues. Before this, while the AH interval changes little, the His potential (H) moves further toward and even into the QRS complex (*dashed line* denotes onset) until its direction of propagation becomes retrograde *(upward blue arrow)*. Note also that the right ventricular recording, which has a right bundle branch potential, precedes the onset of the surface QRS complex as well as the His potential. All of these taken together make a strong case for the presence of an atriofascicular bypass tract (BT); gradual development of left bundle branch block is related to progressive delay in the atrioventricular (AV) node, allowing slow conduction down the atriofascicular pathway to its insertion in the distal right bundle branch; conduction is then retrograde to the His bundle, recording of which occurs after the onset of the QRS complex. Conduction back to the atrium is typically over the normal AV node, and tachycardia then proceeds with conduction through the atrium to the atriofascicular pathway's atrial portion (which behaves physiologically like an AV node).

Wide QRS Tachycardia

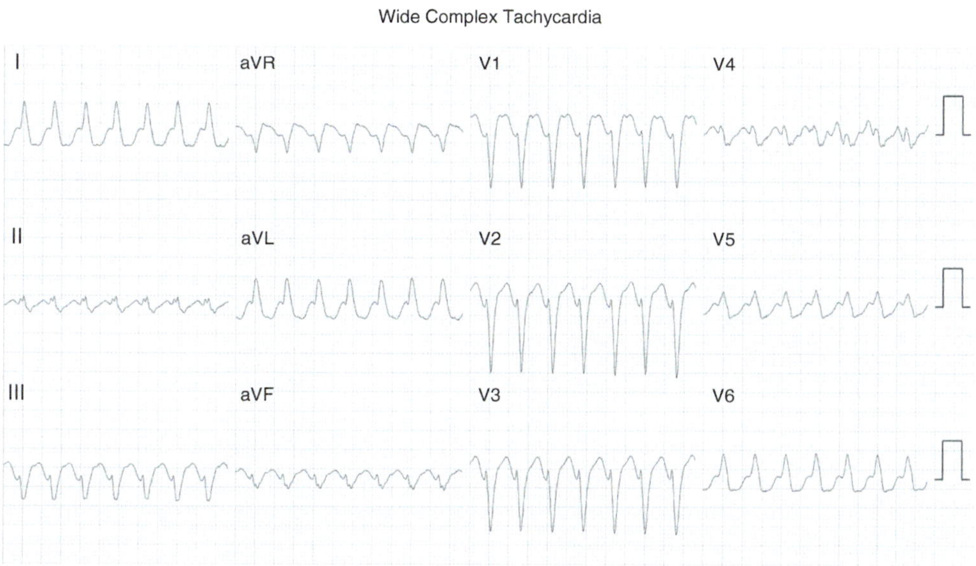

Figure 7-5

A full ECG of the induced tachycardia is shown in Fig. 7-5, matching that of spontaneously occurring episodes with left bundle branch block.

Atrial Extrastimuli During Tachycardia

Is Any Diagnosis Excluded? [Fig. 7-6]

Figure 7-6

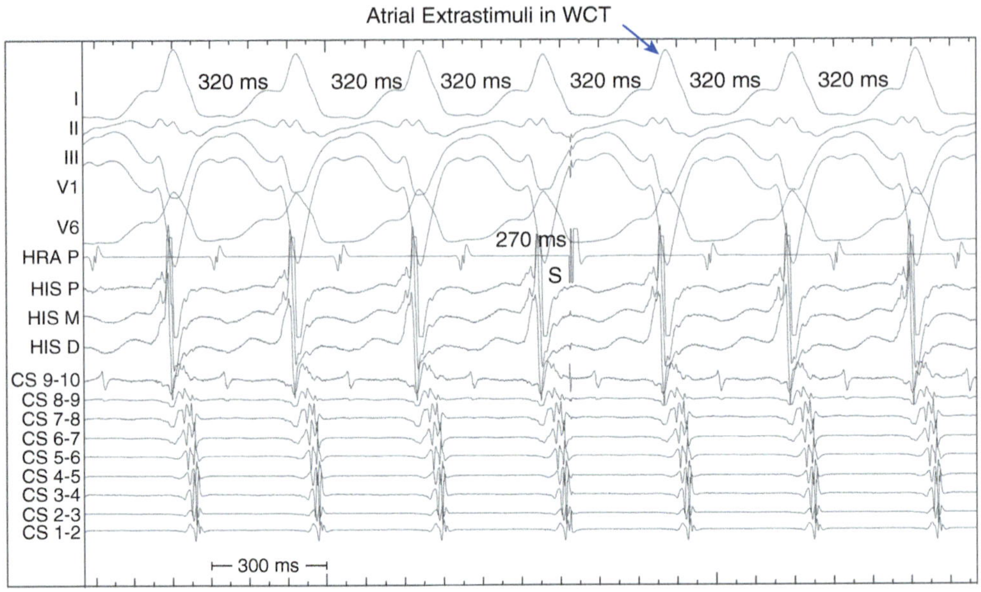

To prove that an atriofascicular pathway is present and participating in tachycardia, as well as to exclude other potential causes, atrial extrastimuli are introduced (Fig. 7-6) along the lateral tricuspid annulus at a time when the atrial electrogram in the region of the normal AV node is refractory (such that the AV node cannot be affected by the extrastimulus). The location at which the extrastimuli are delivered is important, because it is desirable to have a relatively small amount of atrium to traverse before arriving at the pathway. In the example shown, numbers of the top indicate intervals between QRS complexes. When the extrastimulus (S) is delivered at 270 ms from the prior atrial recording, the next QRS complex *(arrow)* occurs exactly on time (320 ms). Because there was no effect on the tachycardia, no conclusions can be drawn as to its nature and none of the potential causes is excluded.

Next QRS Advanced While AVJ-A is Refractory: [Fig. 7-7A]

- Excludes ventricular tachycardia
- An accessory pathway present
- Not nodofascicular or nodoventricular

Figure 7-7A

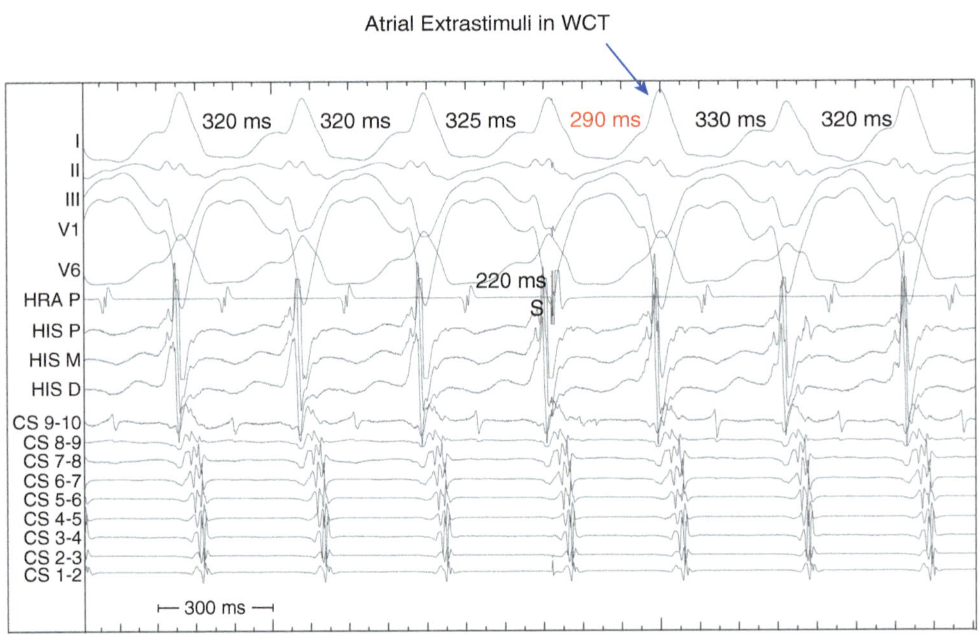

When the atrial extrastimulus (S) is delivered at an interval of 220 ms, the subsequent QRS complex *(blue arrow)* is advanced (290 ms) (see Fig. 7-7A). This excludes ventricular tachycardia, because there is no way an atrial premature event should affect the timing of ventricular activation when the AV node is refractory.

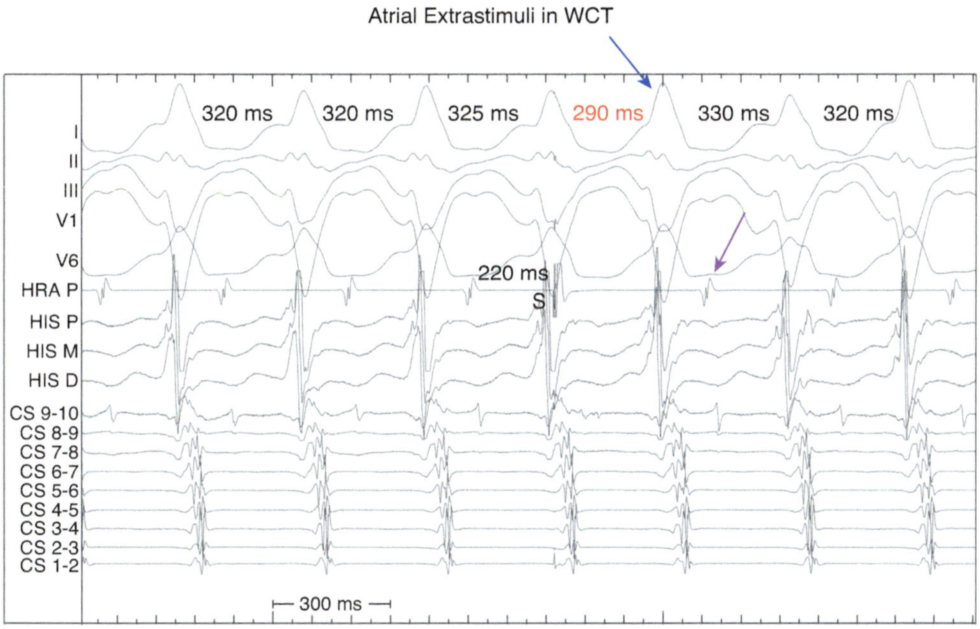

Next A Advanced Only to Same Extent as QRS:

- Not preexcited AVNRT [Fig. 7-7B]
- Not preexcited atrial tachycardia
- Second BT not excluded

Figure 7-7B

In addition, the first atrial event (*purple arrow*, Fig. 7-7B) after the QRS complex that was advanced *(blue arrow)* is likewise earlier than expected. If this tachycardia were AV nodal reentry or an atrial tachycardia, the atrial complex indicated by the *purple arrow* should have occurred exactly on time. However, because its occurrence appears to depend on the timing of the prior QRS complex, this appears to be true antidromic atrioventricular reentry proceeding down the atriofascicular pathway and up the AV node. In addition, a nodofascicular or nodoventricular pathway cannot be involved, because the AV node was refractory when the extrastimulus was delivered.

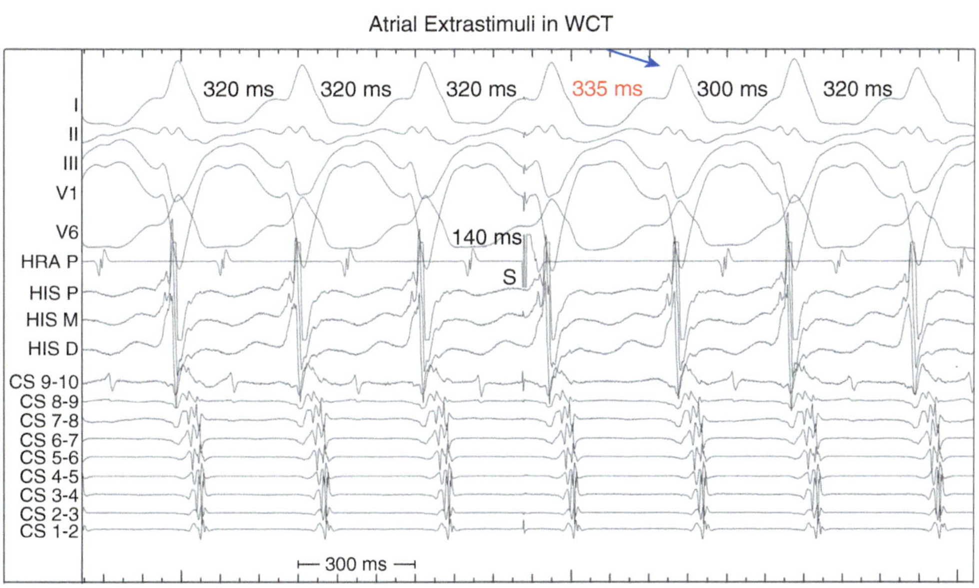

Next QRS Delayed (Not While AVJ-A is Refractory): [Fig. 7-8A]

- Excludes ventricular tachycardia

Figure 7-8A

As the atrial extrastimulus (S, Fig. 7-8A) is made to be more premature (140 ms now), the subsequent QRS complex *(blue arrow)* is actually delayed from when it would be expected to occur. This atrial stimulus is so premature that the AV node cannot be considered to be refractory; however, the fact that the next QRS complex is delayed again excludes ventricular tachycardia.

Next A Linked to Next QRS: [Fig. 7-8B]

- Not preexcited AVNRT
- Not preexcited atrial tachycardia
- Second BT not excluded

Figure 7-8B

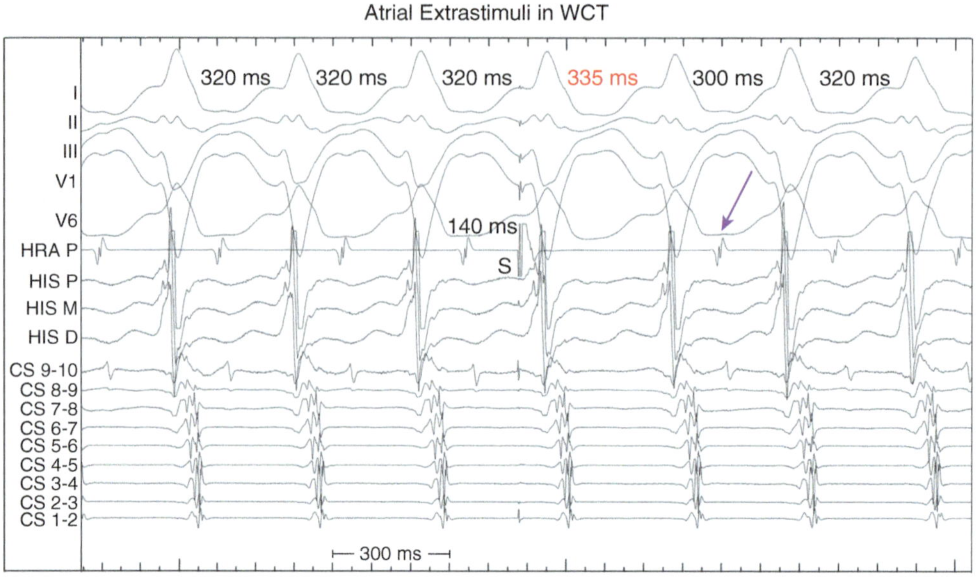

As seen previously, the first atrial complex (*purple arrow*, Fig. 7-8B) that follows the delayed QRS complex *(blue arrow)* occurs at a time later than expected and is linked to the prior QRS complex. This once again excludes atrial tachycardia or a bystander atriofascicular pathway with AV nodal reentry as the main arrhythmia diagnosis. However, retrograde conduction over a second, septal bypass tract is not necessarily excluded thereby.

Next QRS Absent (Not While AVJ-A is Refractory): [Fig. 7-9]

- Excludes ventricular tachycardia

Figure 7-9

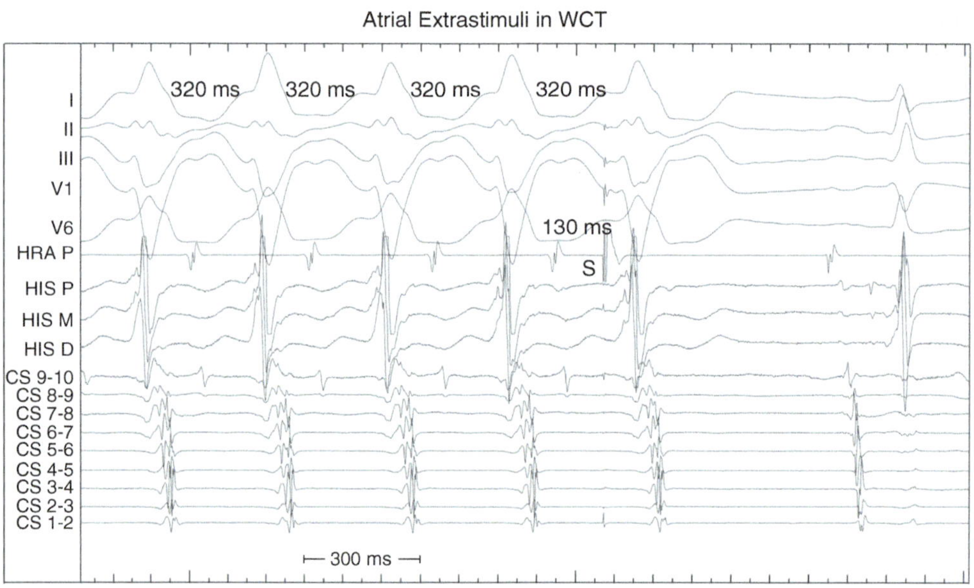

Finally, as shown in Fig. 7-9, with an even more premature atrial extrastimulus (S), at 130 ms from the prior atrial complex, the atrium is captured but there is no subsequent QRS complex. Again, this excludes ventricular tachycardia as a potential diagnosis. Because the AV node is not refractory at the time this extrastimulus is delivered, AV nodal-dependent tachycardias could conceivably have been terminated with this and cannot be excluded on the basis of this finding alone.

Atriofascicular Pathways

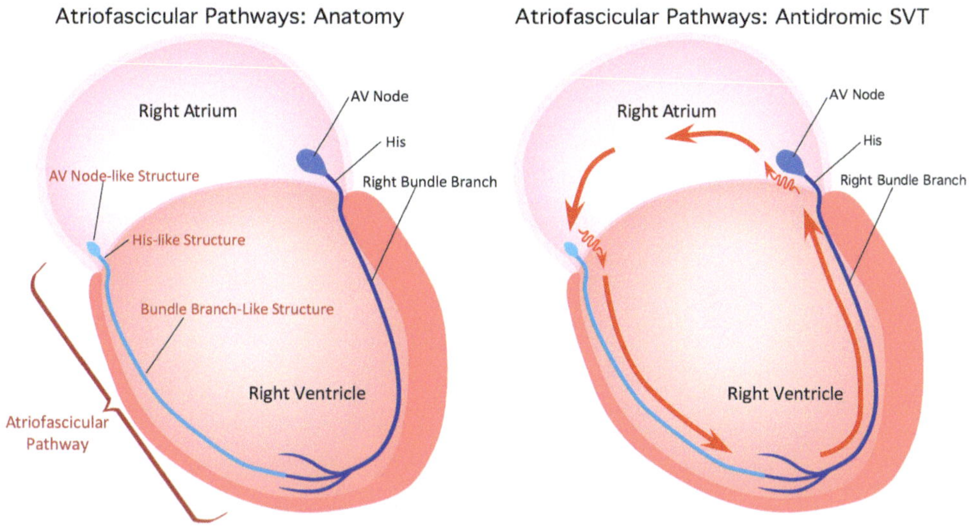

Figure 7-10

The diagram on the left in Fig. 7-10 shows the anatomy of atriofascicular pathways that have several components: an AV node–like structure in the lateral right atrium near the tricuspid annulus, a His bundle–like structure that crosses the annulus, and a long fiber-like right bundle that connects the His-like portion to the true distal right bundle. In this sense, the entire pathway is like a duplication of the normal conduction system. During antidromic tachycardia, as shown at right, the impulse travels down the atriofascicular pathway and up the normal conduction system. Zigzag lines denote slow conduction encountered in the normal AV node and the node-like part of the atriofascicular pathway.

More Baseline Recordings (with Halo Catheter)

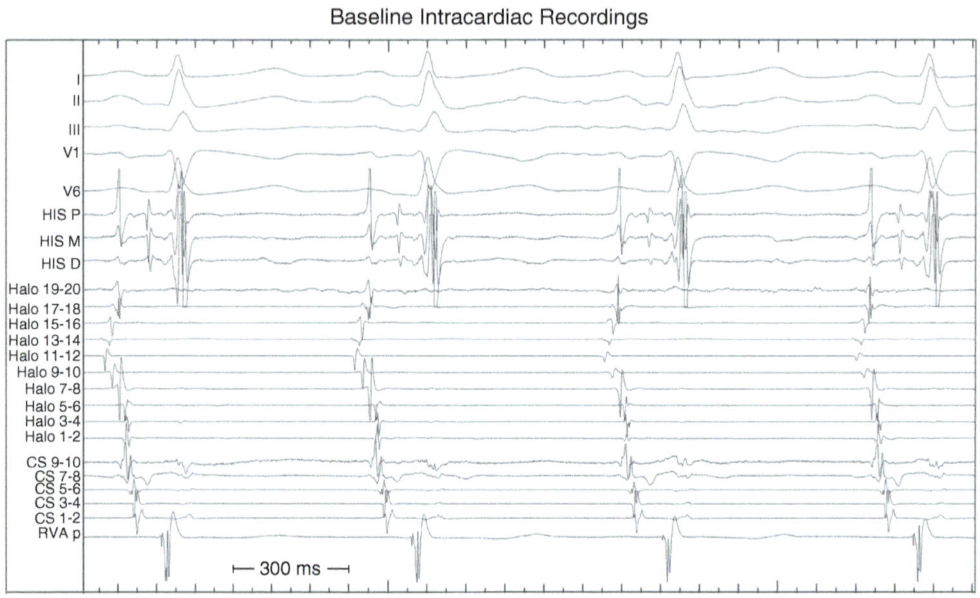

Figure 7-11

Now that a diagnosis of an atriofascicular pathway–mediated atrioventricular reentrant tachycardia has been made, selection of target sites for ablation can begin. At the beginning of the procedure, a multipolar electrode catheter ("Halo") was placed around the tricuspid annulus to facilitate mapping. The recording that had been labeled "HRA" in prior figures was in fact one of the electrodes of this catheter. During sinus rhythm as shown in Fig. 7-11, it is not possible to determine the atriofascicular pathway's location.

Ventricular Pacing

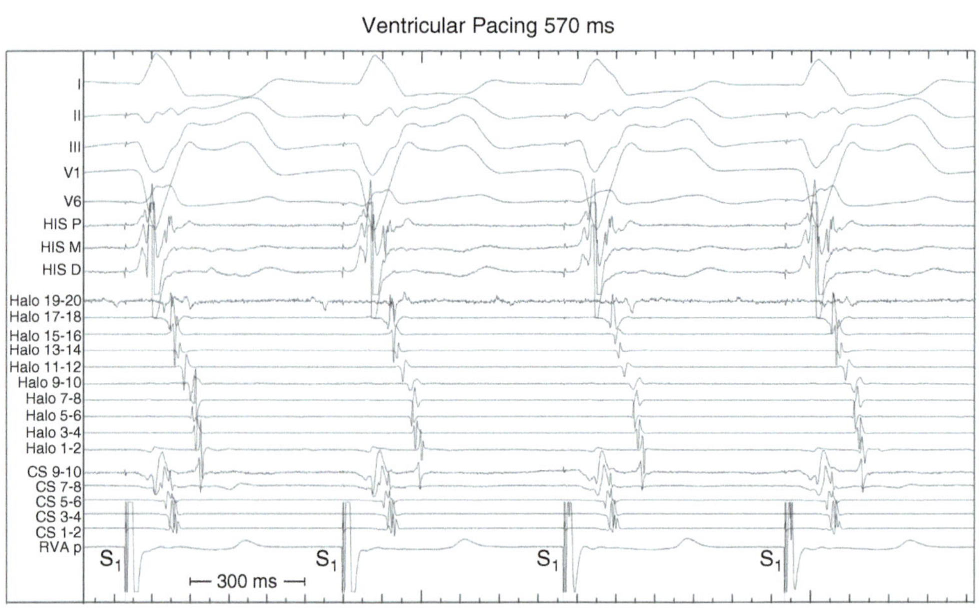

Figure 7-12

Ventricular pacing at a slow rate shows an atrial activation pattern consistent with retrograde conduction over the AV node (Fig. 7-12).

Ventricular Pacing 360 ms

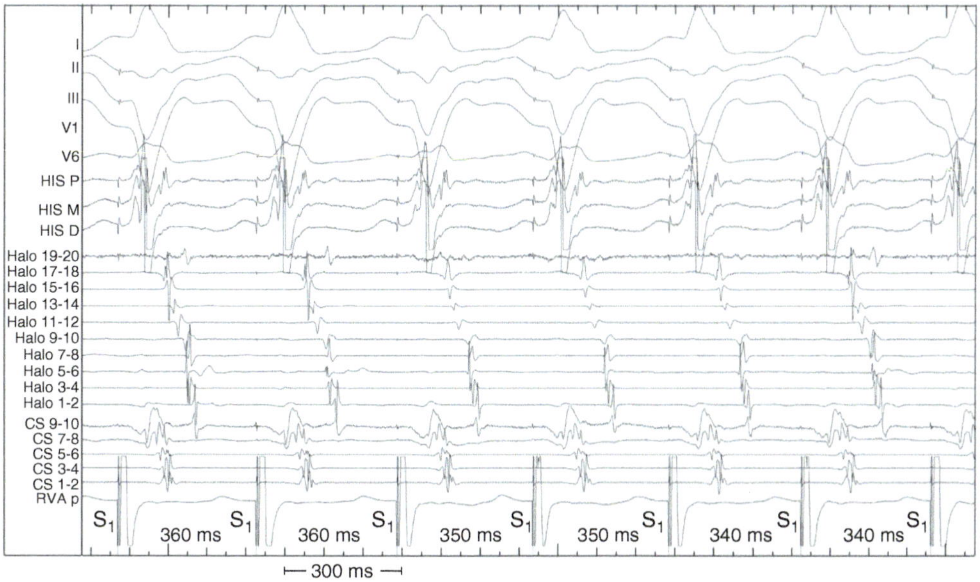

Figure 7-13

The same atrial activation pattern is maintained with ventricular pacing at a more rapid rate in Fig. 7-13.

Ventricular Pacing 240 ms

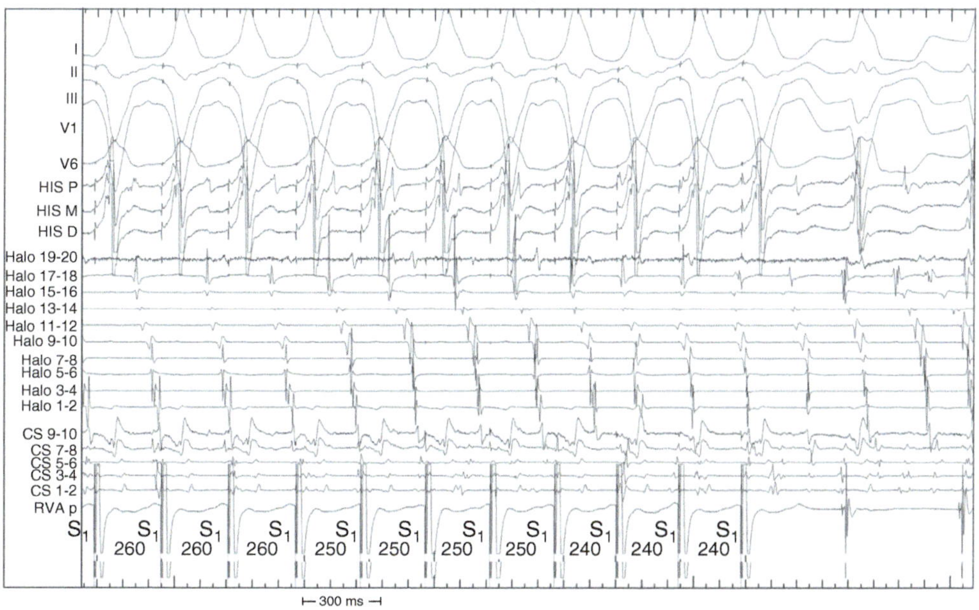

Figure 7-14

With still more rapid ventricular pacing (Fig. 7-14), conduction over the AV node persists. However, atrial fibrillation ensues.

Atrial Fibrillation ECG and Intracardiac Recordings

Figure 7-15A

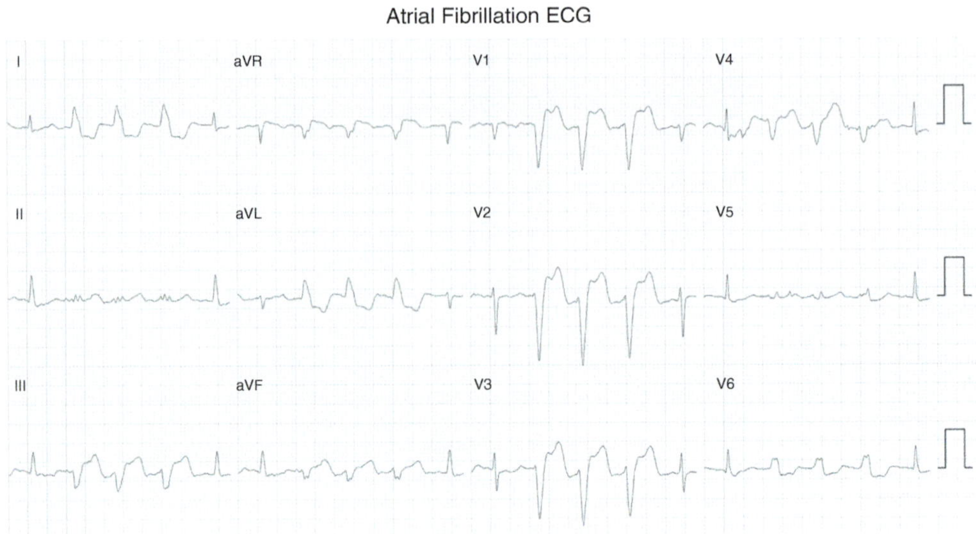

An ECG of atrial fibrillation, partially conducted over the atriofascicular pathway, is shown in Fig. 7-15A.

Figure 7-15B

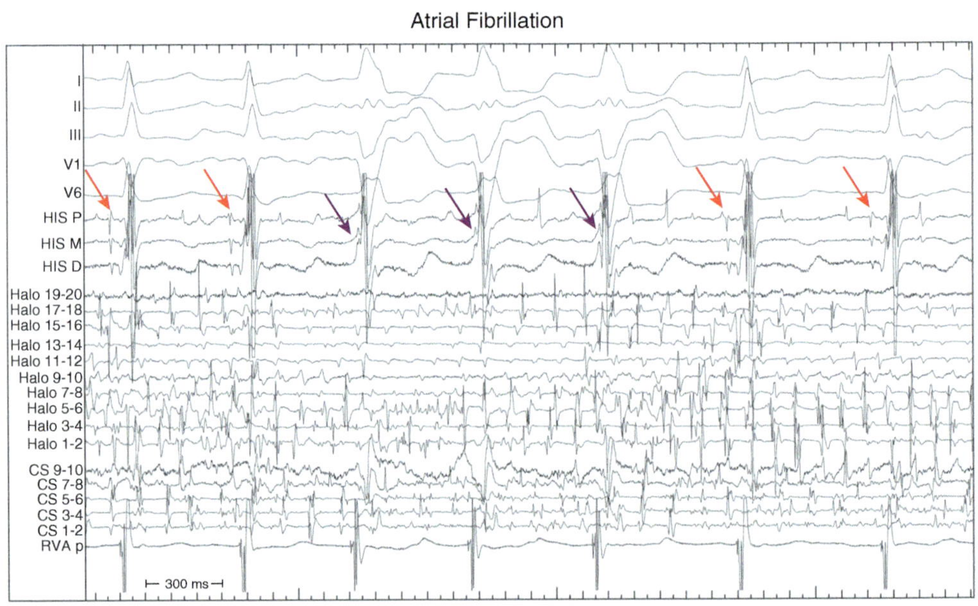

In Fig. 7.15B, intracardiac recordings during atrial fibrillation show narrow QRS complexes with an anterogradely activated His potential *(red arrows)*, as well as wide QRS complexes with retrogradely activated His recordings *(purple arrows)*, because of anterograde conduction over the atriofascicular pathway on these complexes rather than the AV node.

Atrial Pacing and Premature Stimulation

Atrial Pacing 460 ms

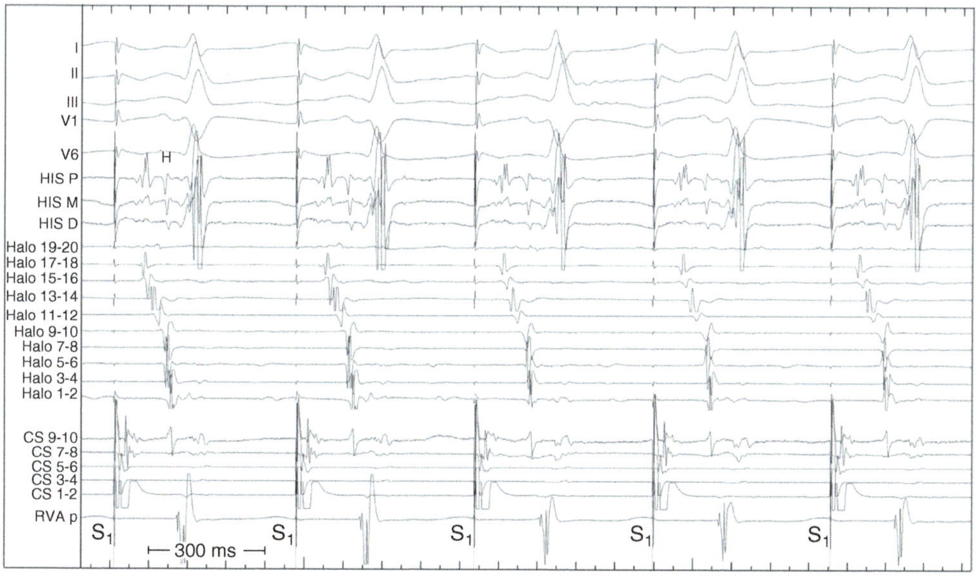

Figure 7-16

Cardioversion was necessary to terminate atrial fibrillation and continue with the procedure. Thereafter, with atrial pacing at 460 ms, ventricular activation is still largely mediated over the normal AV node-His Purkinje system (H), with a relatively narrow QRS complex (Fig. 7-16).

Atrial Pacing 400 ms

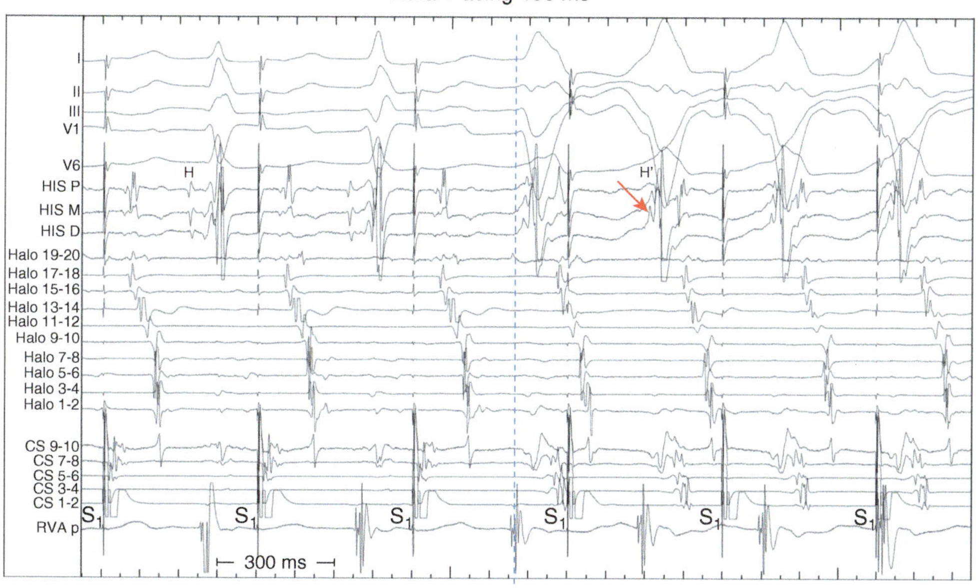

Figure 7-17

As the atrial pacing cycle length is decreased to 400 ms (Fig. 7-17), the AV node fatigues and the atriofascicular pathway becomes the mode of ventricular activation. The His potential (H′, *red arrow*) is activated retrogradely. The onset of the first preexcited QRS is indicated by a *dashed line*; note the RV electrogram and sharp spike (right bundle branch potential) precede the QRS onset.

Figure 7-18

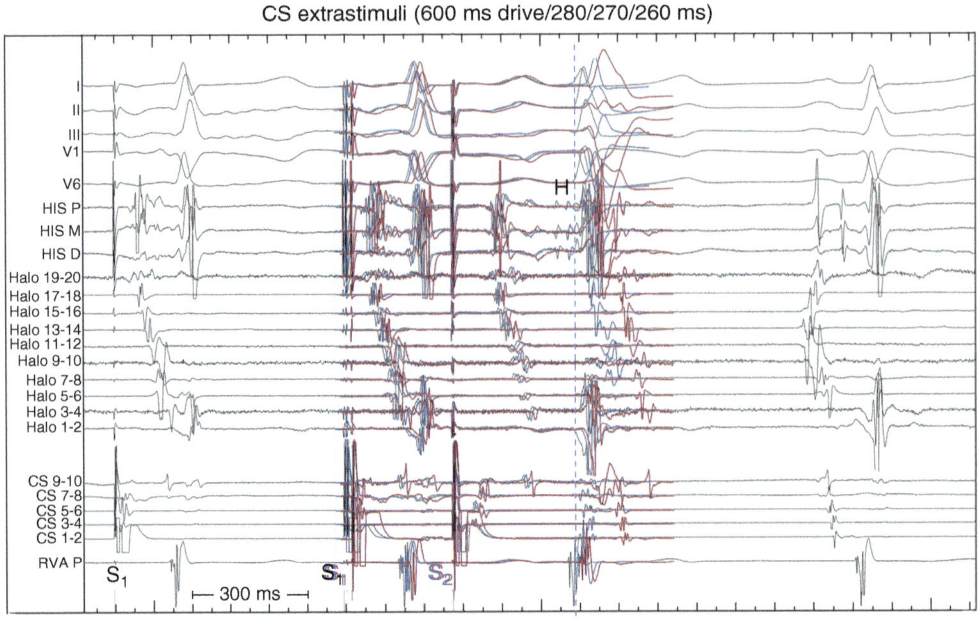

The effect of increasing prematurity of atrial stimulation on atrioventricular conduction is illustrated in Fig. 7-18 by superimposing successive coupling intervals (black, 280 ms; blue, 270 ms; red, 260 ms). It can be seen that the His bundle recording (H) is progressively delayed while the timing of the onset of the QRS complex *(dashed line)* does not change significantly, and the QRS duration progressively increases as more of the ventricular muscle is activated over the atriofascicular pathway and less over the AV node.

Mapping Atriofascicular Potential

Figure 7-19

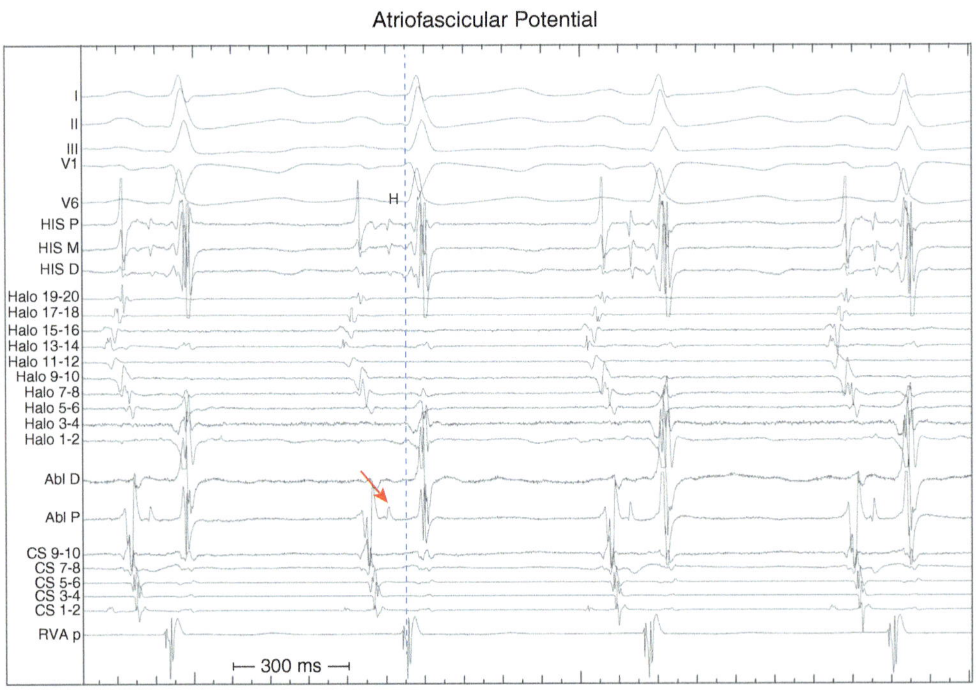

A site along the lateral tricuspid annulus is sampled, at which a recording is obtained (Fig. 7-19) that looks very much like the recording from the His catheter at the septum (atrial electrogram, His-like potential *[red arrow]*, ventricular electrogram). This is compatible with the atriofascicular pathway potential.

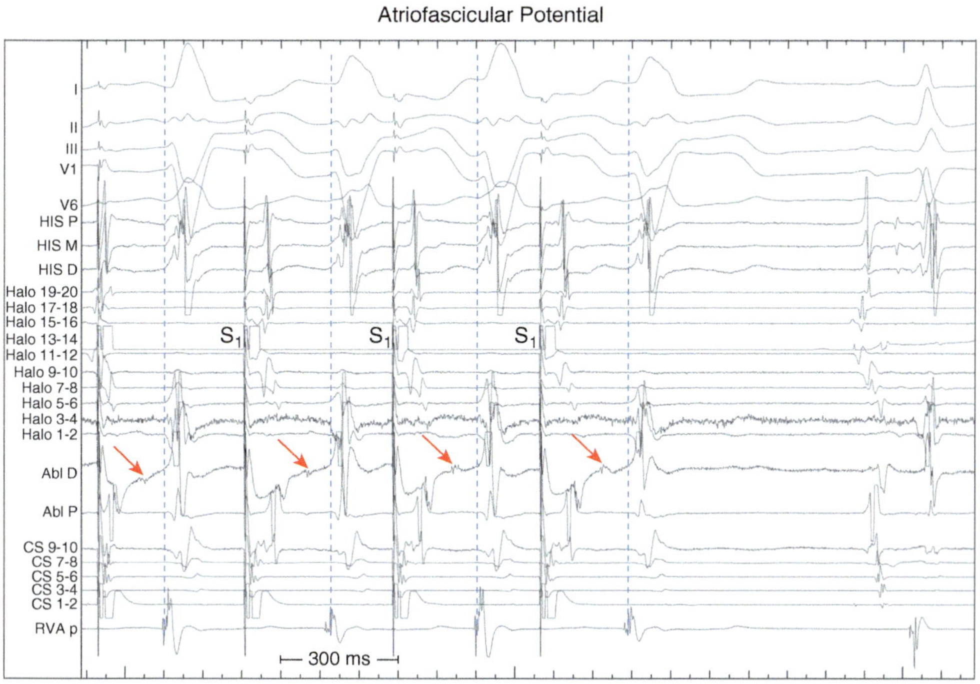

Figure 7-20

To validate the signal at the *red arrows* as a true atriofascicular pathway potential, pacing is performed (Fig. 7-20). If an actual atriofascicular potential, it should always be present during preexcited complexes and at a consistent interval before the QRS onset *(dashed line)*, which it does appear to be.

Figure 7-21

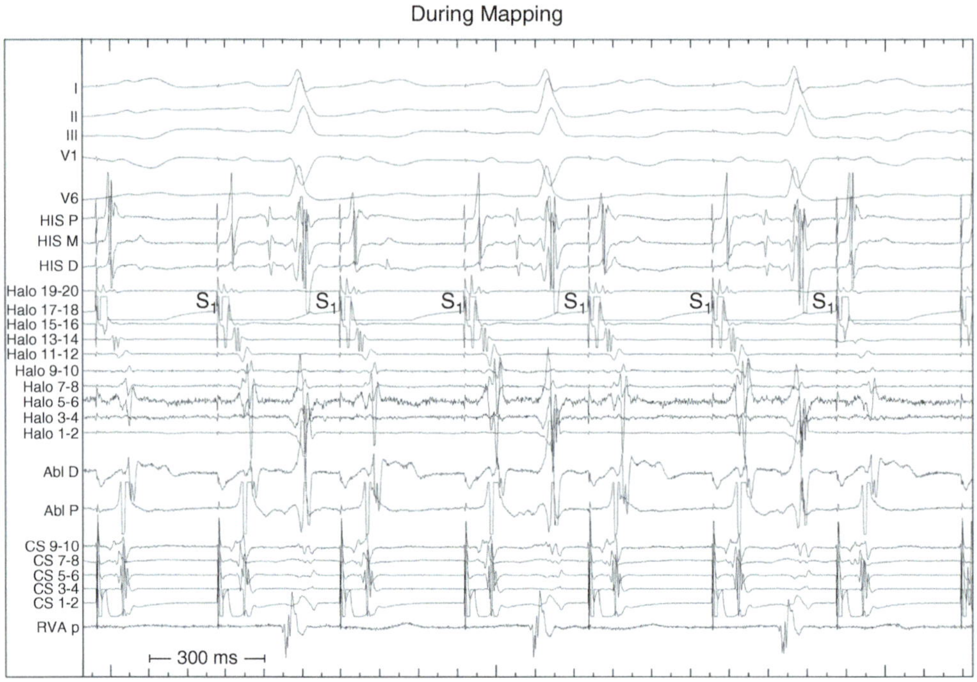

As often occurs in cases of atriofascicular pathways, small movements of the catheter tip in the vicinity of the pathway can "bump" into it and render it unexcitable for extended periods. In Fig. 7-21, under the same conditions as in Fig. 7-20, preexcitation is suddenly lost as is recording of the pathway potential. Although this is further corroboration of being at the correct site, it is not very helpful if pathway conduction does not resume. It is thus important to be very careful and deliberate with movement of the ablation catheter as it nears the anticipated location of the pathway, either to not cause trauma that temporarily eliminates conduction or, if it occurs nonetheless, to be able to ablate at the site where it occurred if the catheter has not moved from that site. Too often, however, the ablation catheter bumps the pathway while brushing past its location, and when the operator observes this and then looks at where the catheter tip is, it is no longer at the location at which mechanical interruption of pathway conduction occurred. Obviously, ablation at this other site will do no good.

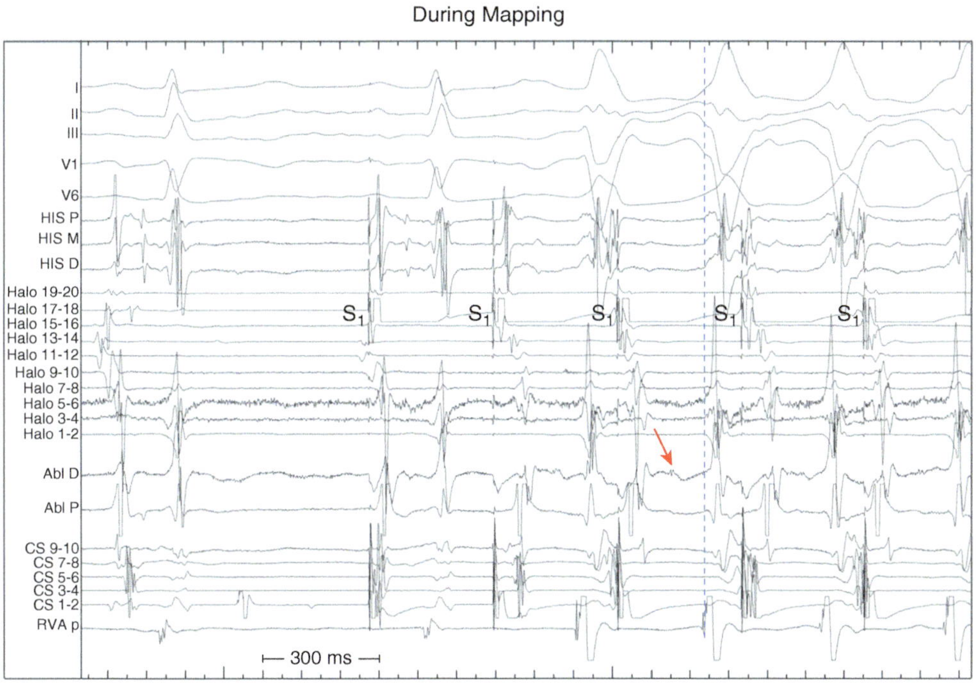

Figure 7-22

Fortunately, pathway conduction did come back a few minutes later, and the catheter was at the same location as shown (Fig. 7-22; *red arrow* shows pathway potential before preexcited QRS with *dashed line* at onset). If it had not resumed, moving the catheter away from there or administering isoproterenol or even adenosine may facilitate resumption of pathway conduction.

Pacing Ablation Site

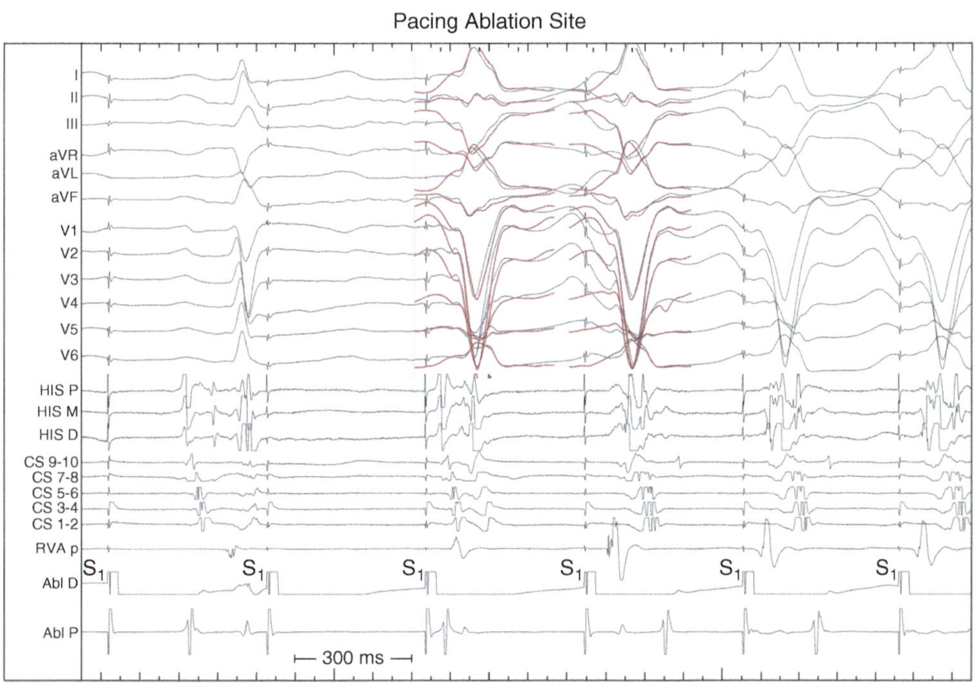

Figure 7-23

As one final corroboration, pacing from the ablation catheter nearly entirely mimicked QRS complexes during SVT (superimposed in red, Fig. 7-23), indicating that the catheter was at the site of the pathway. Importantly, if a significant amount of local ventricular capture had occurred, the QRS complex (pacing from the tricuspid annulus) would be significantly different from SVT complexes (with activation beginning closer to the apex).

Ablation Site and Radiofrequency Delivery

Figure 7-24

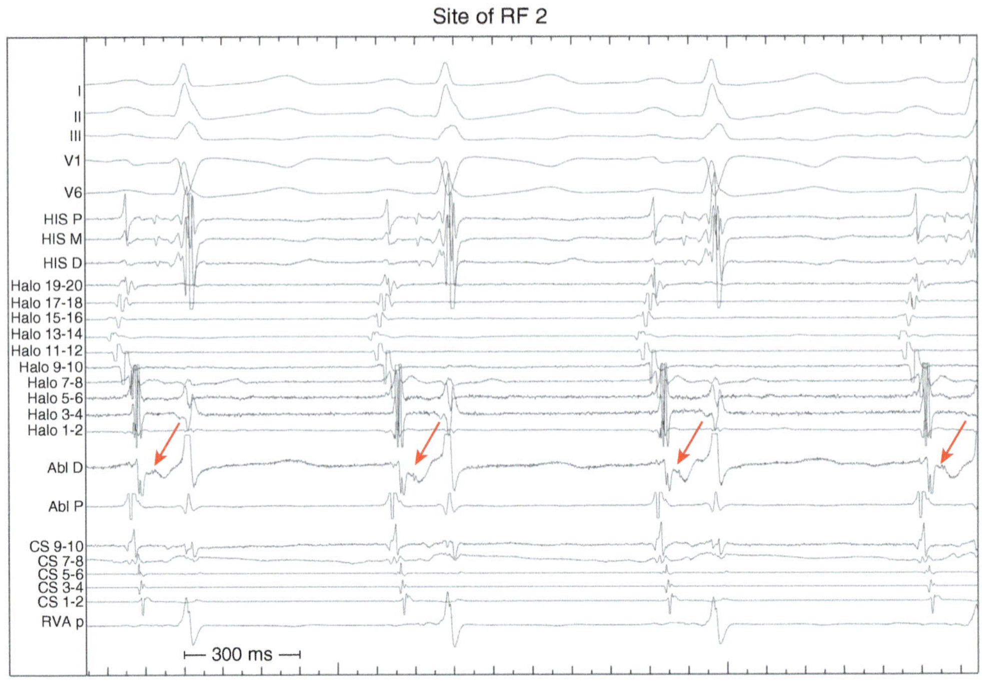

The first radiofrequency (RF) application was stopped after a few seconds because of catheter movement. The catheter was repositioned as shown in Fig. 7-24, for a second attempt at RF application. The *arrow* shows a tiny potential, indicating the atriofascicular pathway recording, just after the atrial signal at an annular site (both atrial and ventricular recordings clearly seen).

Figure 7-25

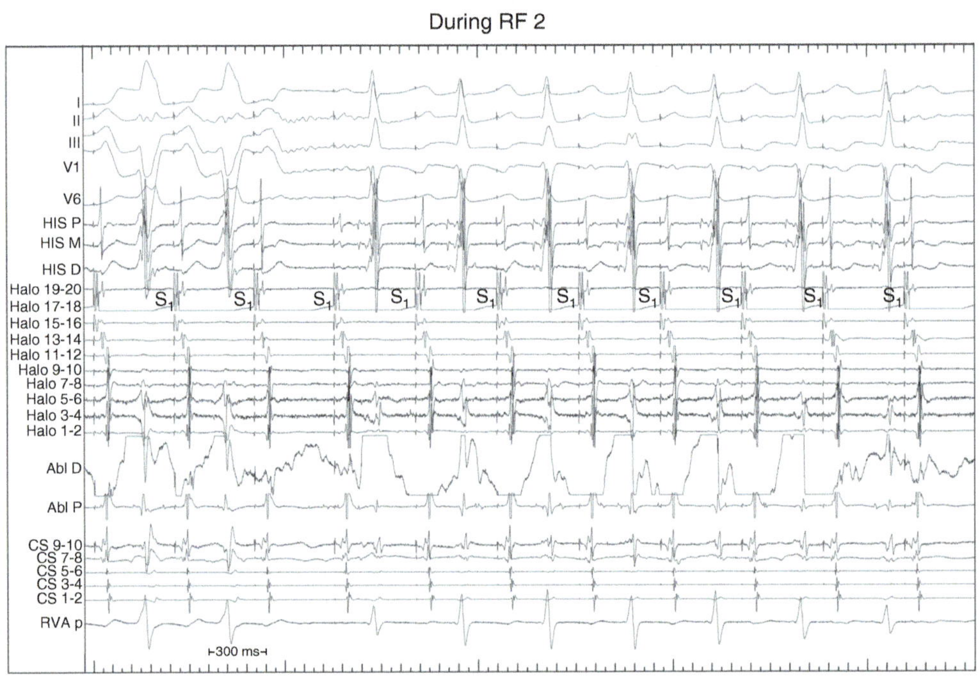

Shortly after beginning RF application during atrial pacing, preexcitation suddenly disappears as the pathway has been eliminated (Fig. 7-25).

Atrial Pacing Postablation

Atrial Extrastimuli (600 ms/350 ms)

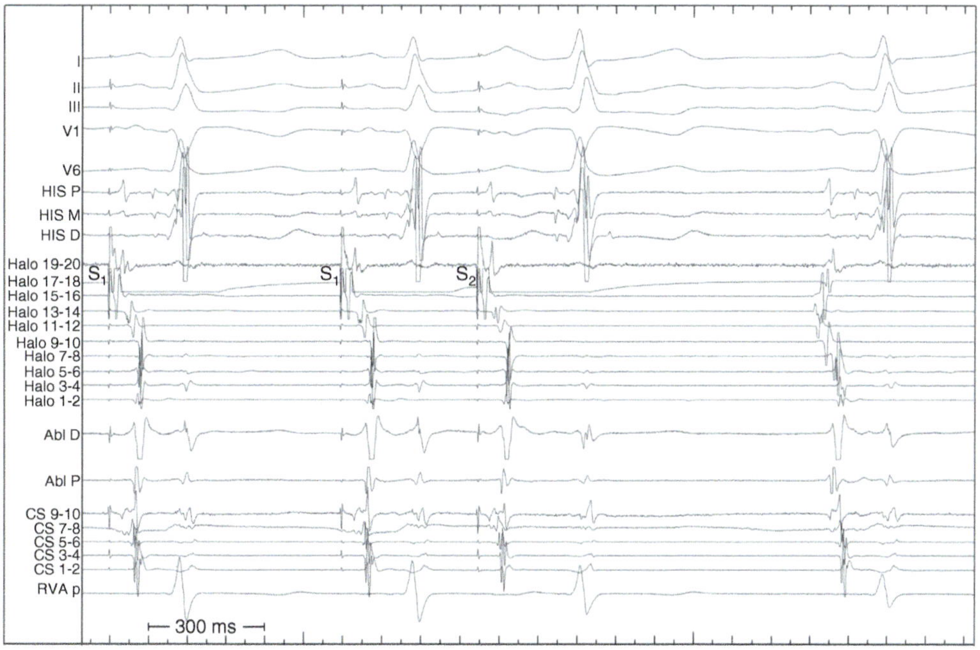

Figure 7-26

In Fig. 7-26, atrial extrastimuli delivered after successful ablation show only conduction over the AV node–His-Purkinje system and no preexcitation.

Atrial Extrastimuli (600 ms/320 ms)

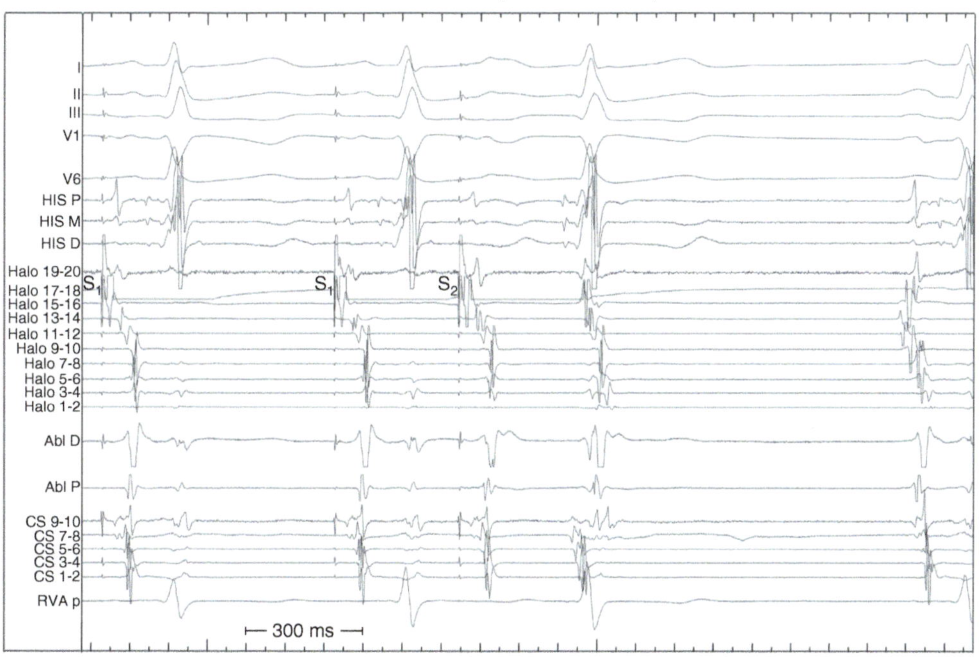

Figure 7-27

The same coupling intervals as had shown preexcitation before ablation no longer do so, as shown in Fig. 7-27.

Figure 7-28

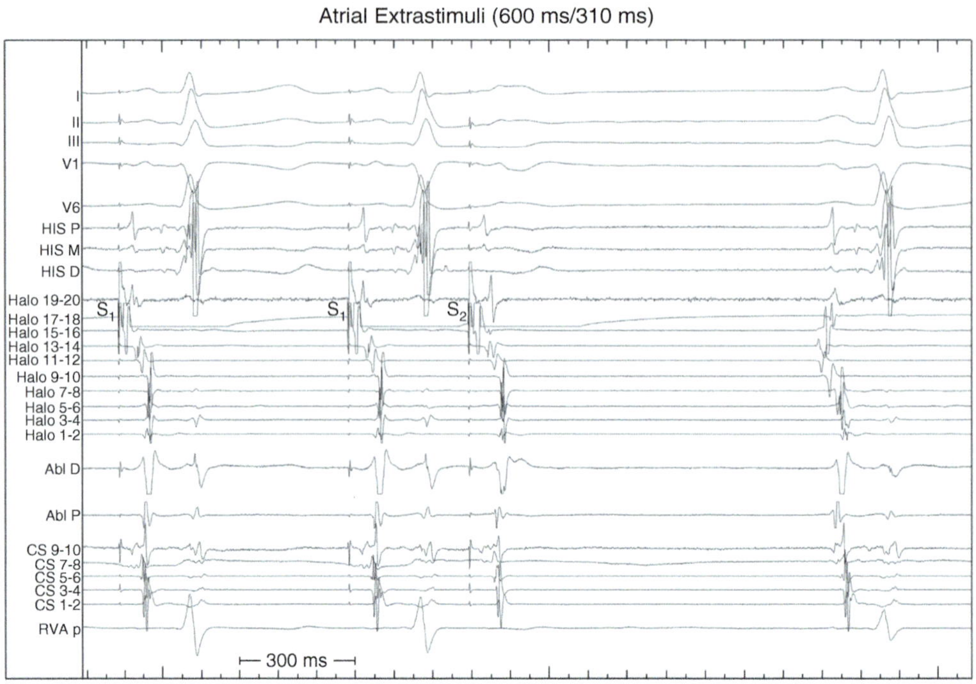

An atrial extrastimulus results in AV nodal refractoriness; before successful ablation, this would have conducted over the atriofascicular pathway to the ventricle (Fig. 7-28).

Figure 7-29

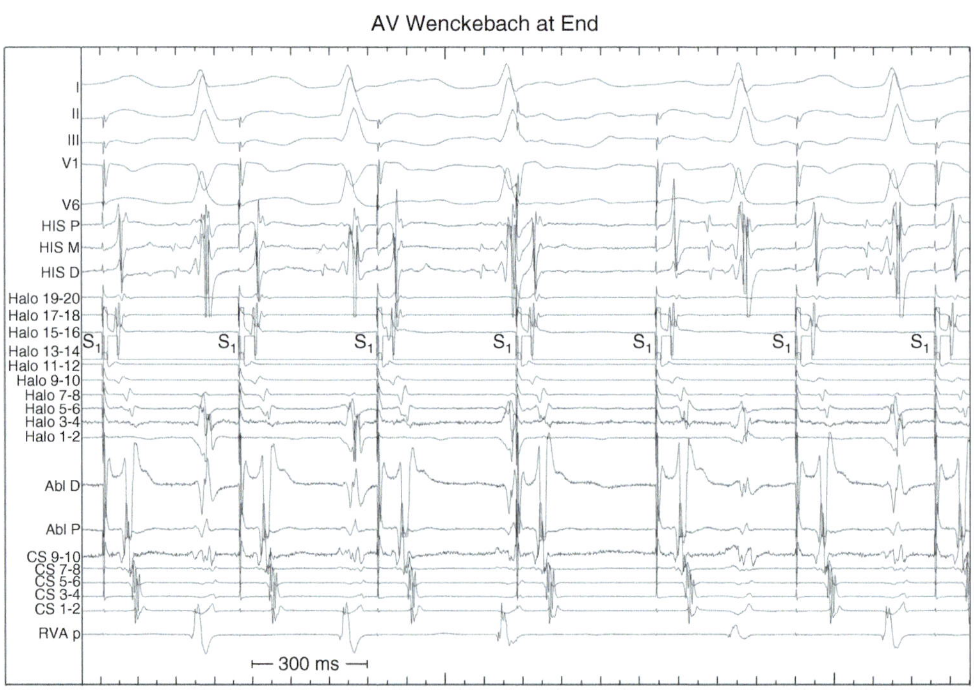

At the end of the procedure, AV conduction was exclusively over the AV node–His-Purkinje system. Atrioventricular Wenckebach is shown in Fig. 7-29.

Final Fluoroscopy

Fluoroscopy

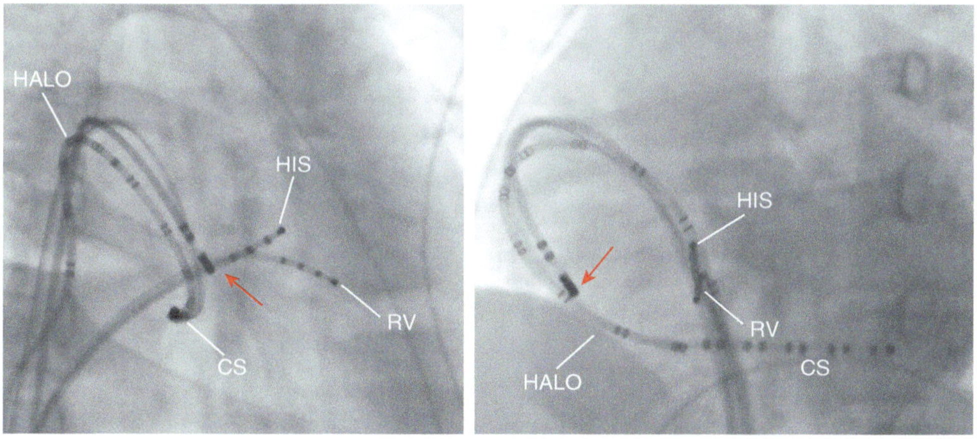

Right Anterior Oblique   Left Anterior Oblique

Figure 7-30

Fluoroscopic views of catheter positions at the time of successful ablation are shown in Fig. 7-30. The mapping/ablation catheter (tip indicated by a *red arrow*) is looped around the tricuspid annulus, a technique that is sometimes helpful for maintaining catheter stability. The coronary sinus catheter was also looped around the tricuspid annulus, as was the Halo catheter.

Principles of Mapping Atriofascicular Pathways

Methods for mapping/ablation of atriofascicular pathways include targeting the following:

- Pathway potential
  - At tricuspid annulus
  - In ventricle, be careful (if RBBB occurs this results in longer path length, incessant SVT)
- Site at which longest atrial extrastimulus coupling interval during SVT advances next QRS
- Site at which shortest S-QRS with atrial pacing is seen
- Site at which pace mapping at tricuspid annulus exactly replicates preexcitation pattern
- Site at which catheter manipulation damages pathway
  - Be VERY careful—trauma may somnify pathway for prolonged periods

Summary

- Atriofascicular pathways are rare but full of physiology
- Clues to diagnosis:
  - Multiple episodes of LBBB SVT
  - Delayed R-wave progression in LBBB SVT
- Antidromic reciprocating tachycardia (ART) can mimic AVNRT with LBBB
  - ECG looks like LBBB; His position may be unstable (thus not consistently seen)
  - Earliest retrograde activation is at AVN fast pathway
  - Differentiation:
    - His occurs before (AVNRT) or after (ART) QRS onset
    - ΔHA interval (AVNRT $> +10$ ms, ART ≈ 0 ms)
      - His activation in ART is retrograde (anterograde in AVNRT)
      - Second bypass tract is excluded by ΔHA interval (ART ≈ 0 ms, preexcited ORT < -10 ms)

8 Slowly Conducting Bypass Tract Supraventricular Tachycardia

Case Presentation

A 20-year-old woman had been experiencing palpitations and near syncope with increasing frequency over the last 2 years. Beta blockers were used in the past but to no avail. She had several emergency room (ER) visits in the interim where supraventricular tachycardia (SVT) episodes were terminated with intravenous adenosine termination. The electrophysiologist was called at 2 AM one day when the patient was in incessant SVT at an outside hospital ER (despite multiple adenosine doses) and hypotensive. She was also 30 weeks pregnant with her third child. She was transferred to our hospital for further therapy. Options considered: medical therapy (but what medications are effective and safe during pregnancy?) or catheter ablation (but what about fluoroscopic exposure to the unborn child?).

Prior SVT ECG

What Is the Differential Diagnosis? [Fig. 8-1]

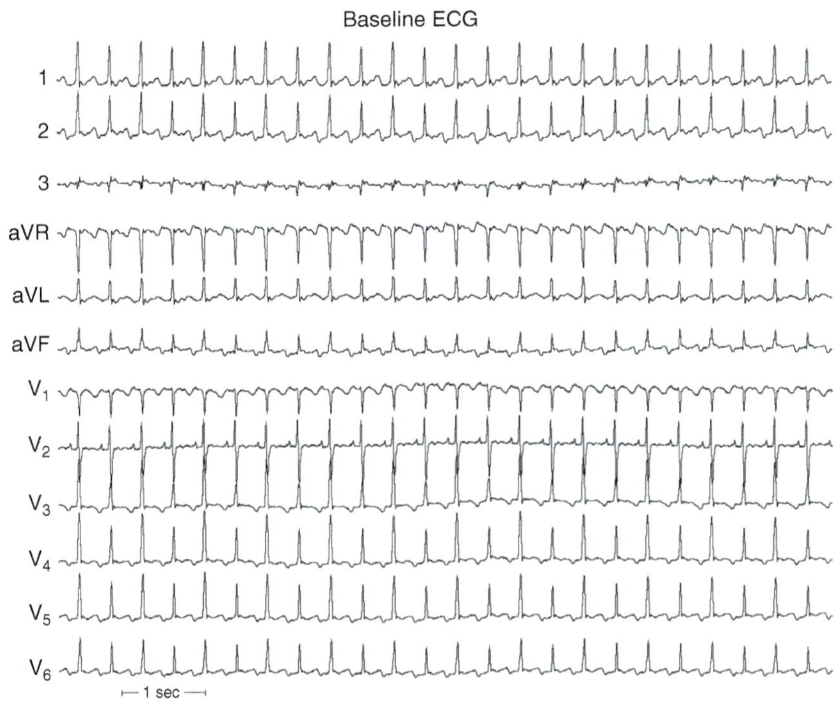

Figure 8-1

Figure 8-1 displays a so-called "long-RP" supraventricular tachycardia with inverted P waves in inferior leads. The differential diagnosis for this rhythm includes atrial tachycardia from the low septum/region of the coronary sinus ostium; atypical "fast-slow" AV nodal reentry; automatic junctional tachycardia; and orthodromic SVT using a slowly conducting bypass tract. She clearly needs some treatment not only for her but also for her baby's health.

Her SVT stopped by the time of arrival to our hospital, without recurrence for several hours. She and her family were uncertain about ablation. Medical therapy with sotalol (relatively safe in pregnancy) was recommended. After one dose of sotalol (80 mg), nearly incessant SVT occurred, lasting 20 to 30 min at a time, stopping for a few seconds and resuming; episodes started with either P or QRS. Because of the poor response to medical therapy, catheter ablation was then recommended.

Electroanatomic "Shell" [Fig. 8-2]

Electroanatomic Mapping

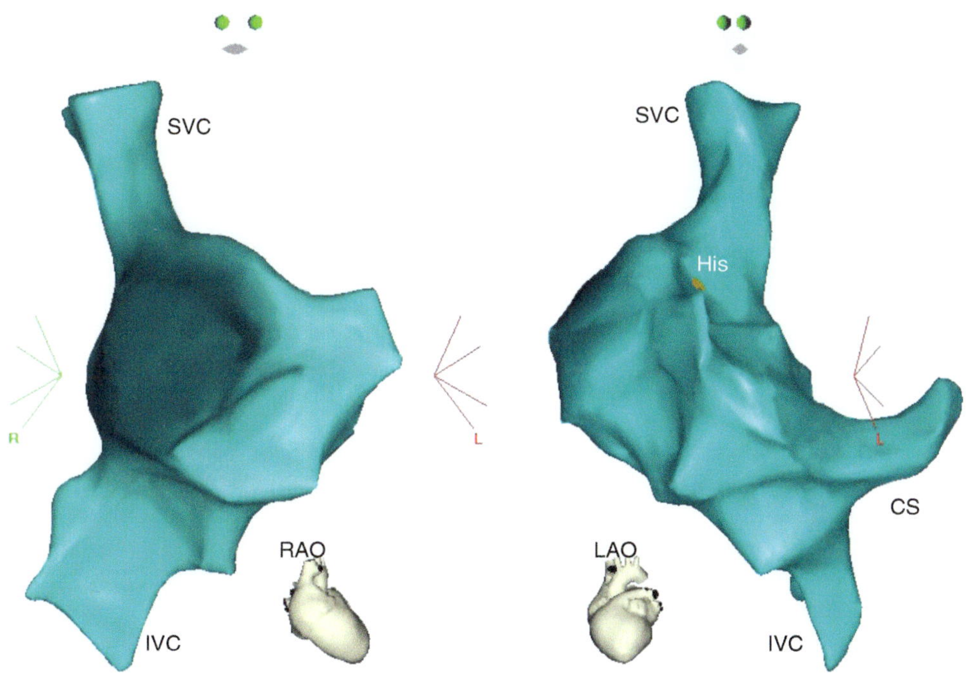

Figure 8-2

At the electrophysiology (EP) study, electroanatomic mapping and stereotactic remote magnetic catheter navigation were used. First, the mapping/ablation catheter was used for delineation and recording of anatomy on an electroanatomic mapping system (navigating to His, coronary sinus (CS), and characterizing the extent of the RA chamber; Fig. 8-2). SVC, superior vena cava; IVC, inferior vena cava; CS, coronary sinus; RAO, right anterior oblique; LAO, left anterior oblique.

Figure 8-3

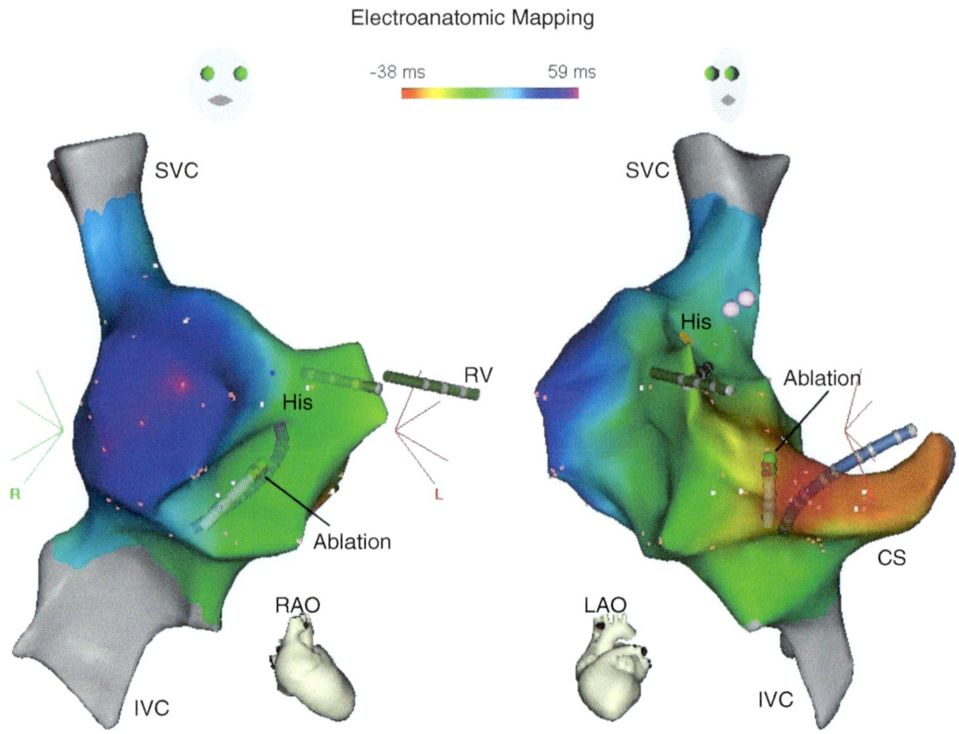

Once the anatomy was clear, other electrode catheters were guided into place at previously determined locations (CS, high RA, RV, His) using the electroanatomic map (Fig. 8-3). Representations of the electrode catheters in these locations are as shown. Activation mapping was performed, using a stable CS electrogram as timing reference; all of this was accomplished without use of fluoroscopy. Mapping showed earliest atrial activation at the proximal CS (*red area*). Of note, this is consistent with any of the diagnostic possibilities and does not differentiate among them. Thus EP testing was performed to determine the precise diagnosis. RA, right atrium; RV, right ventricle.

Baseline Intracardiac Recordings During Sinus Rhythm and SVT

Figure 8-4

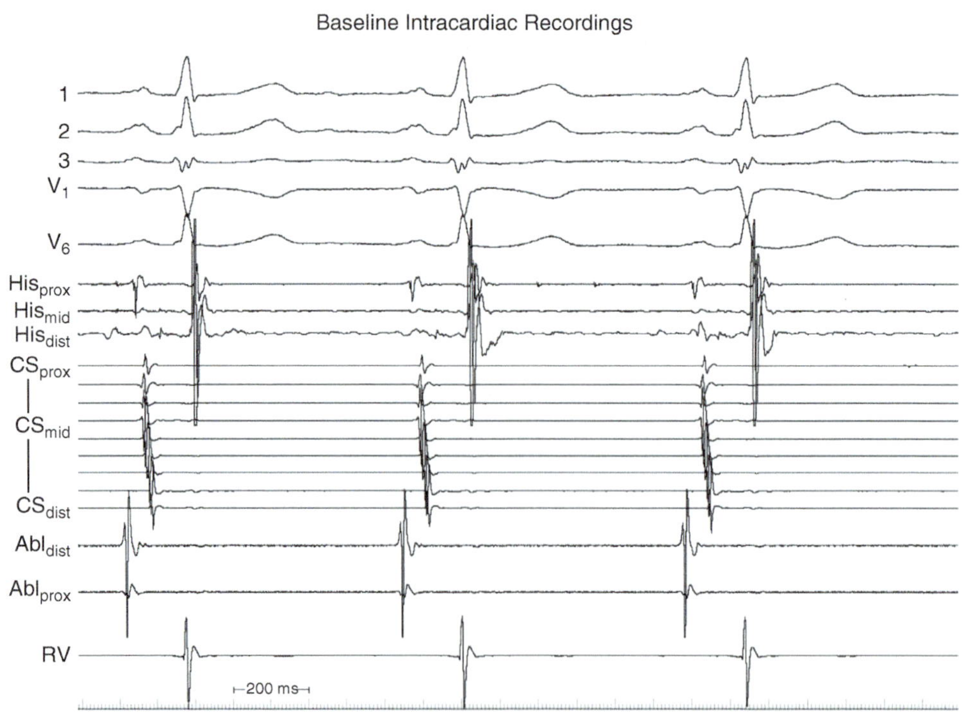

Baseline intracardiac recordings are as shown in Fig. 8-4 during sinus rhythm; as anticipated, SVT was readily initialed by a variety of means including spontaneously or following ventricular (VPC) or atrial (APC) premature complexes.

What Can You Diagnose From This, If Anything? [Fig. 8-5]

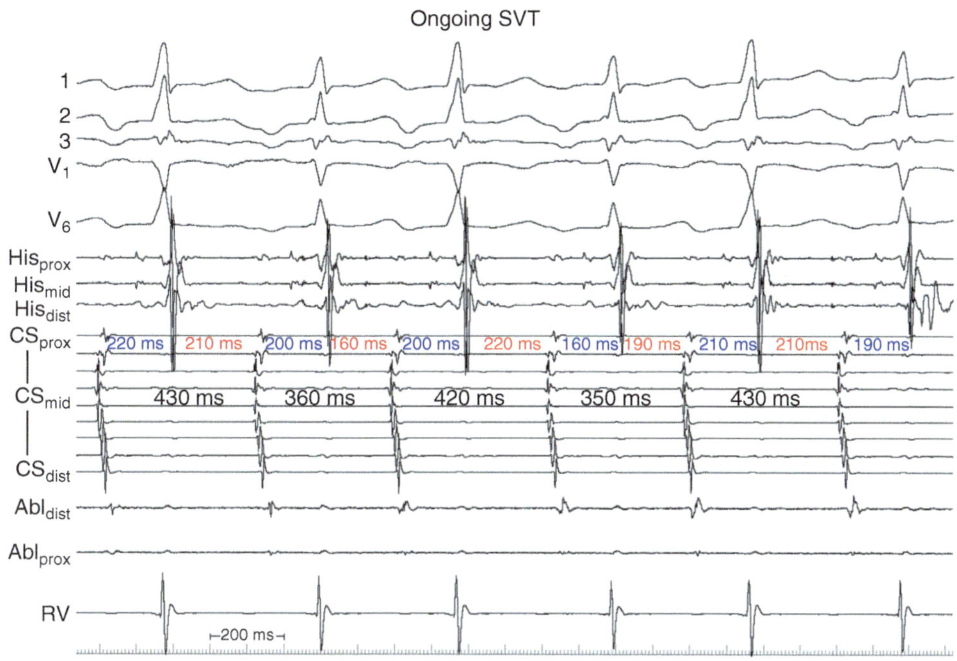

Figure 8-5

SVT was rather irregular. Whenever this is the case, it is an opportunity to determine which electrograms depend on others and which are "leaders" that other recordings follow. In Fig. 8-5, cycle length (A-A) intervals are shown in *black*, A-V intervals in *blue*, and VA intervals in *red*. There does not seem to be a consistent relationship of one recording definitely leading to another. Irregularity of tachycardia cycle length significantly hampers use of pacing maneuvers, most of which implicitly rely on a regular cycle length to provide a predictable occurrence of the next SVT complex after a pacing-induced perturbation (such as single extrastimuli or trains of pacing). For instance, if the SVT CL is very irregular, it is very difficult to compare the postpacing interval (PPI) to tachycardia CL (TCL) as an indicator of proximity of the pacing site to a tachycardia circuit.

Ventricular Extrastimuli and Overdrive Pacing in SVT

Does This Help? [Fig. 8-6]

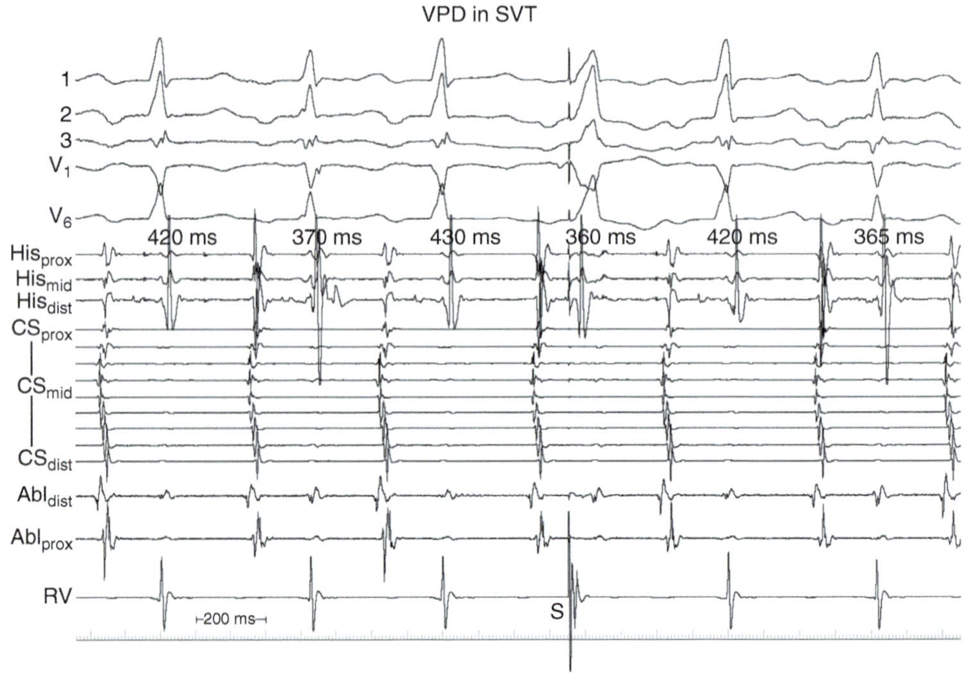

Figure 8-6

In Fig. 8-6, a single ventricular extrastimulus is delivered during SVT. This was difficult to do because the CL was very irregular and timing a ventricular extrastimulus to occur at a time when the His bundle was refractory was a matter of chance. Though one such event is shown here (His-refractory extrastimulus, Fig. 8-6), can anything be inferred from its effect? The atrial recording after the extrastimulus occurs earlier than others and in fact has a slightly shorter A-A interval than any others. The interval surrounding the extrastimulus has to be meaningfully shorter than any other A-A interval in order to use it as evidence for the presence of an atrioventricular bypass tract. The difference between this A-A interval (360 ms) and the shortest spontaneously occurring interval during SVT (365 ms) is very small, and so this should not be the only evidence used to make a diagnosis of a bypass tract.

Does This Help? [Fig. 8-7]

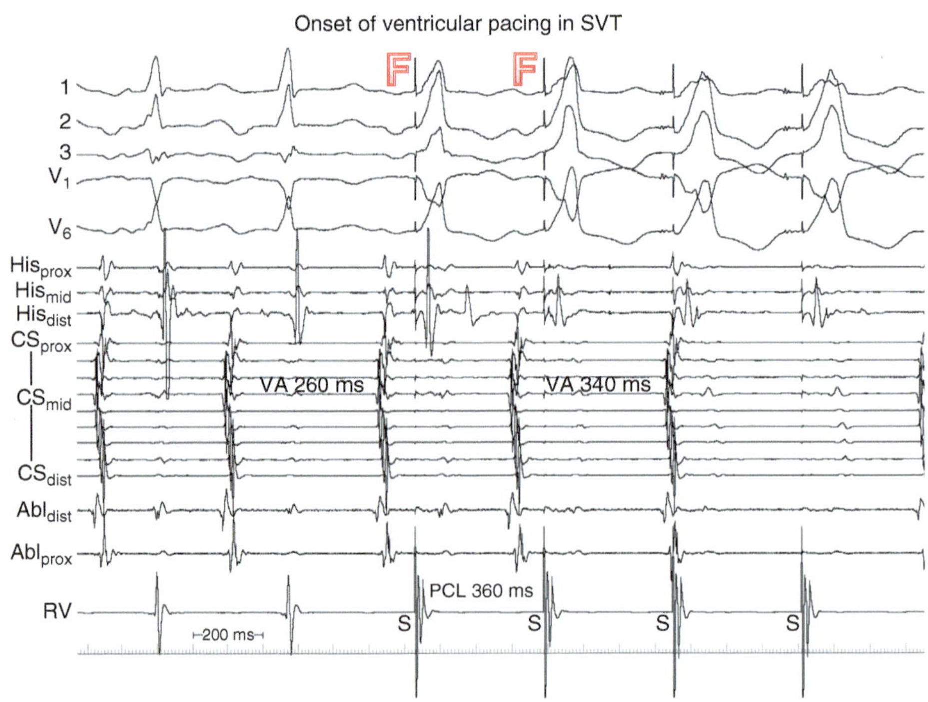

Figure 8-7

Similarly, interpreting the results of overdrive pacing during SVT can be difficult in the presence of significant CL variability. In Fig. 8-7, at the initiation of overdrive ventricular pacing, the second stimulus is followed by an atrial electrogram that occurs much later than anticipated (VA interval 340 ms). This occurred in response to a paced complex that is a fusion (F) between tachycardia and fully paced complexes (the last two). Because the timing of atrial activation was altered at time when the His had been anterogradely activated, this indicates that there is an extranodal pathway over which atrial activation can occur in response to ventricular stimulation. Further, the fact that the atrial activation is delayed from when it would be expected to occur shows that the pathway is not only present but also participates integrally in SVT. Thus a diagnosis of orthodromic SVT is established (stronger if this is a reproducible finding). Note that SVT terminated during continued pacing (no atrial electrogram after the second to last QRS complex).

Does This Help? [Fig. 8-8]

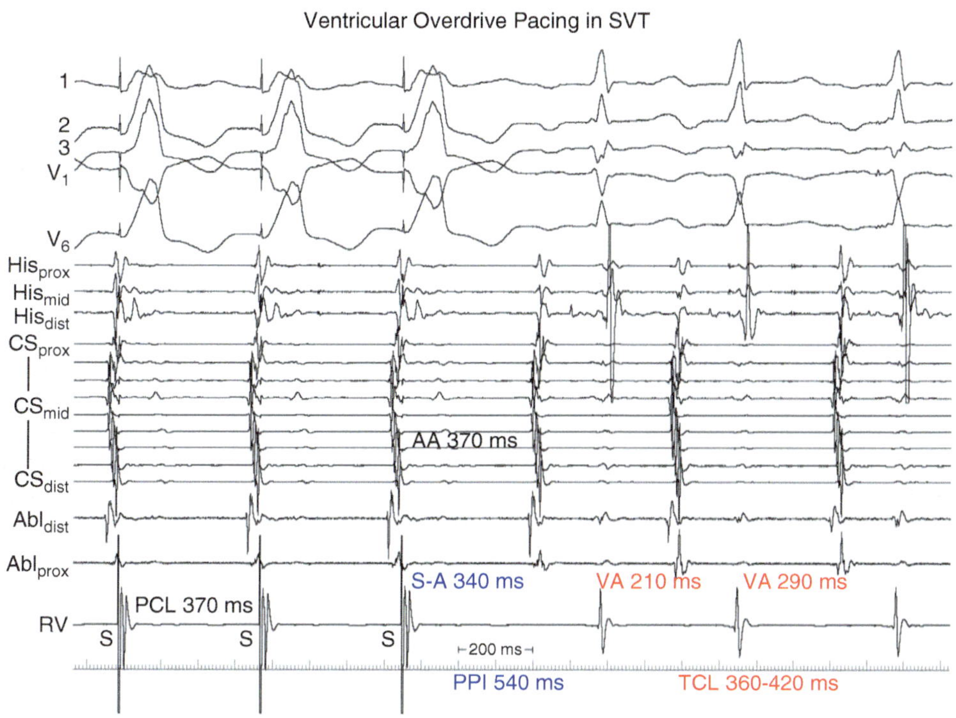

Figure 8-8

At the end of another attempt at ventricular overdrive pacing, SVT resumes. The usual interval measurements are made, with uninterpretable results: the PPI-TCL difference ranges from 120 ms (consistent with bypass tract SVT) to 180 ms (inconsistent with bypass tract SVT) (Fig. 8-8). Similarly, the stimulus-atrial (SA) minus ventriculoatrial (VA) interval difference ranges from 50 ms (consistent with bypass tract SVT) to 130 ms (not consistent with bypass tract SVT). The problem is that the retrograde limb has cycle length–dependent slowing of conduction ("decremental conduction") that invalidates the measurements.

Atrial Pacing at SVT Cycle Length Compared with SVT

Does This Help? [Fig. 8-9]

Figure 8-9

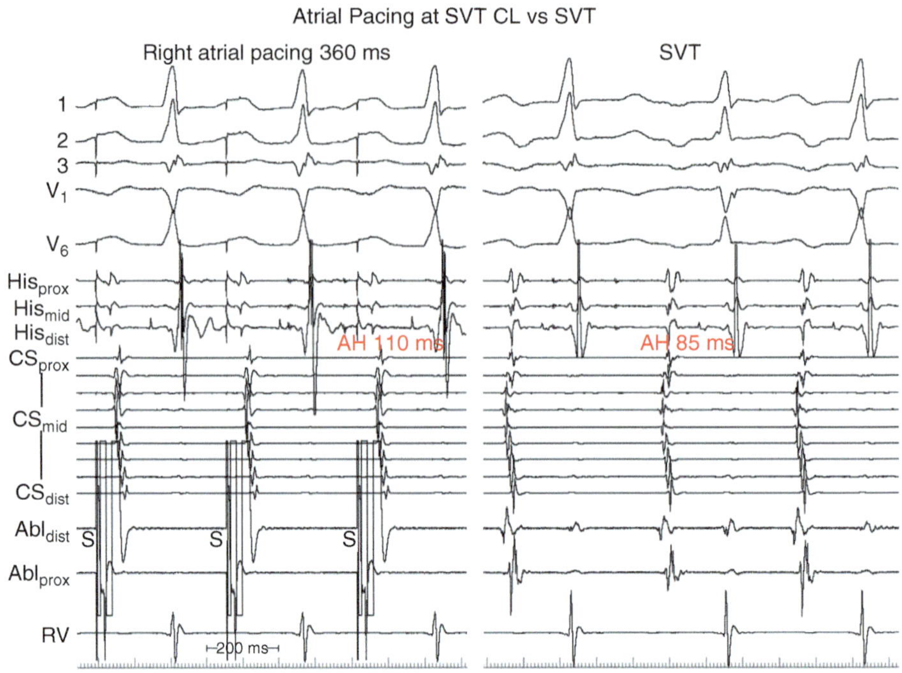

To exclude an (unlikely) atrial tachycardia, the atrio-His (AH) interval is compared between that during SVT and during atrial pacing at the SVT CL. If a right atrial tachycardia, the AH intervals should be similar; with orthodromic SVT, the difference between paced and SVT AH intervals is typically 20 to 40 ms, whereas with atypical AV nodal reentry the difference is usually ≥40 ms. Here, the difference of 35 ms is consistent with orthodromic SVT (Fig. 8-9).

Spontaneous SVT Termination

Does This Help? [Fig. 8-10]

Figure 8-10

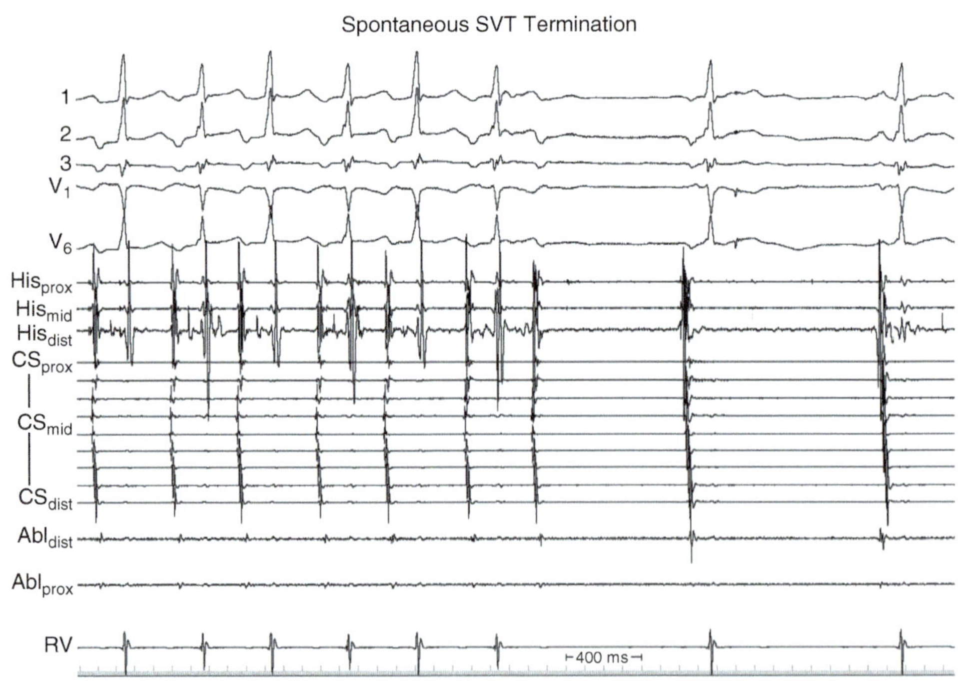

Another means of excluding atrial tachycardia as a diagnosis occurred spontaneously here—tachycardia terminates spontaneously with the last event being atrial. An atrial tachycardia with 1:1 AV conduction would not be likely to terminate suddenly at the same instant as AV block occurred (Fig. 8-10).

Comparison of Features and Behavior of Different SVTs

TABLE 8-1 Truth Table

	Atrial Tachycardia	Orthodromic SVT	Atypical (F-S) AVNRT	Junctional Tachycardia
Onset	A first	A or V first	A or V first	V first
Irregularity	A predicts V	V predicts A	V predicts A	V predicts A
His-refract. VPC	No effect	Adv. or delay A	No effect	No effect
Post-V overdrive	No VAC/VAAV	VAV	VAV	VAV
V entrainment	(NA)	$SA - VA < 85$ ms $PPI - TCL < 115$ ms	$SA - VA > 85$ ms $PPI - TCL > 115$ ms	$SA - VA > 85$ ms $PPI - TCL > 115$ ms
Post-A overdrive	AVAV	AVAV	AVAV	AVVA
Delta HA	(NA)	$HA_{SVT} > HA_{Pace}$	$HA_{SVT} < HA_{Pace}$	$HA_{SVT} = HA_{Pace}$
Delta AH	$AH_{SVT} \leq AH_{Pace}$ (10–20 ms)	$AH_{SVT} < AH_{Pace}$ (20–40 ms)	$AH_{SVT} < AH_{Pace}$ (>40 ms)	$AH_{SVT} > AH_{Pace}$
Termination	After V	After A or V	After A or V	After A

A, atrial; AH, atrio-His interval; AHpace, AH during atrial pacing at tachycardia cycle length; AHSVT, AH during SVT; AVAV, sequence of atrial and ventricular events after overdrive pacing; AVNRT, atrioventricular nodal reentrant tachycardia; AVVA, sequence of atrial and ventricular events after overdrive pacing; HA, His-atrial interval; HASVT, HA during SVT; HApace, HA during ventricular pacing at tachycardia cycle length; PPI, post-pacing interval; SA, stimulus-atrial interval; SVT, supraventricular tachycardia; TCL, tachycardia cycle length; V, ventricular; VA, ventriculo-atrial interval; VAV, sequence of atrial and ventricular events after overdrive pacing; VAAV, sequence of atrial and ventricular events after overdrive pacing; VPC, ventricular premature complex.

Table 8-1 is a comparison of features of different types of SVT that are in the differential diagnosis of this SVT. Based on the preponderance of data, orthodromic reentry was diagnosed.

Site of Ablation

Figure 8-11

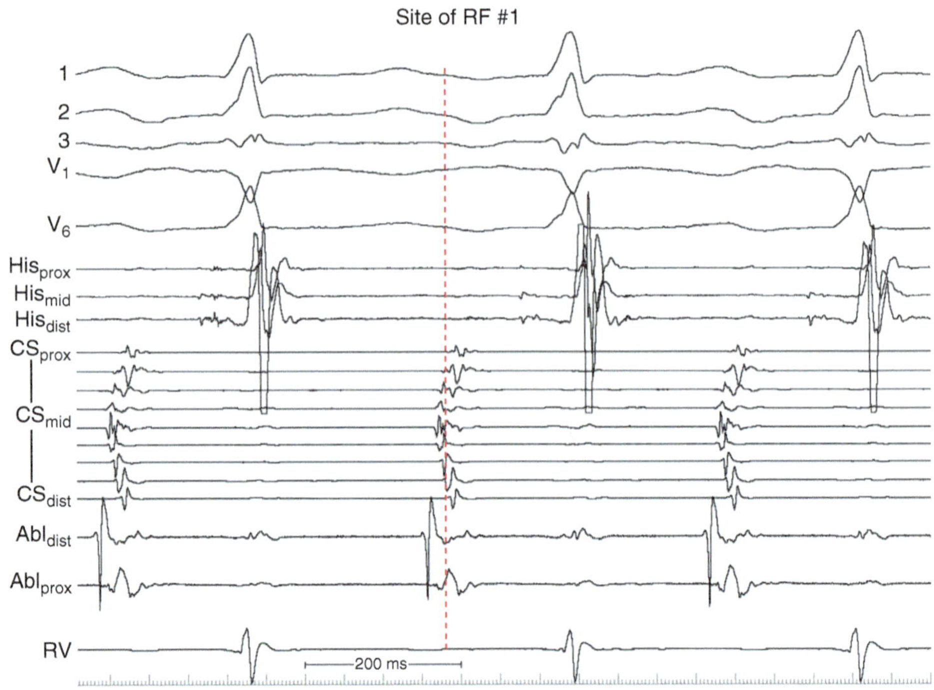

With a secure diagnosis, an ablation site may be sought; slowly conducting/decrementally conducting bypass tracts are usually located around the coronary sinus ostium, where more precise mapping began. In Fig. 8-11, a large, sharp potential on the ablation distal recording is seen followed by a more far-field potential. The atrial recording in the proximal electrode suggests that this far-field recording is atrial. The ventricular recording is small and similarly relatively far-field appearing. Because the large potential appears separate from the atrial potential, it is a good candidate for a bypass tract potential. Because of the constraints of cycle length variability, it was not feasible to perform pacing maneuvers to validate this as a true bypass tract potential.

During Ablation SVT Ceases

Figure 8-12

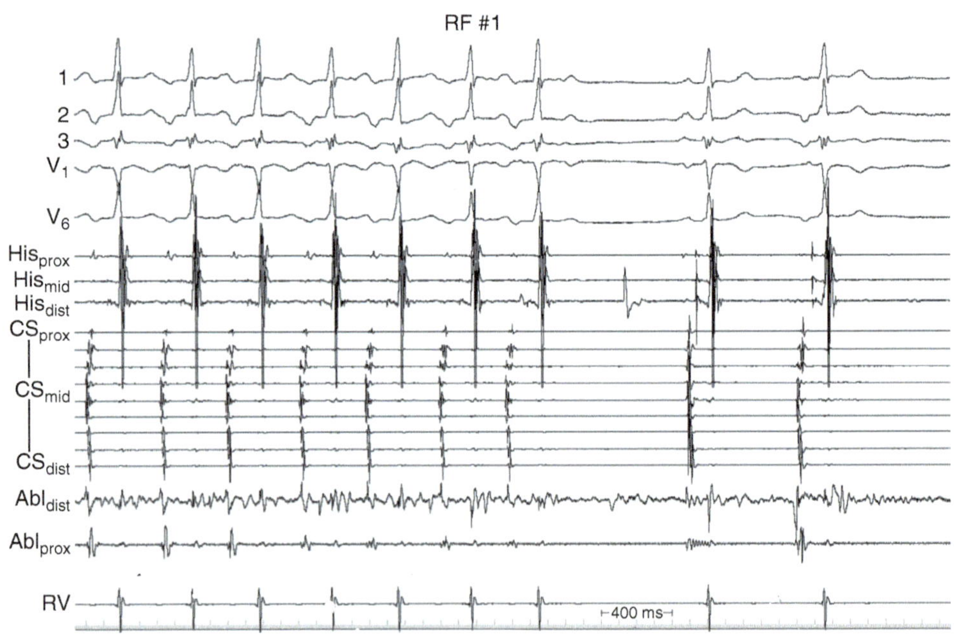

RF application at this site terminated SVT within 8 seconds of onset of power delivery (Fig. 8-12). Additional applications were made during sinus rhythm to consolidate the damage.

Ventricular Pacing Postablation

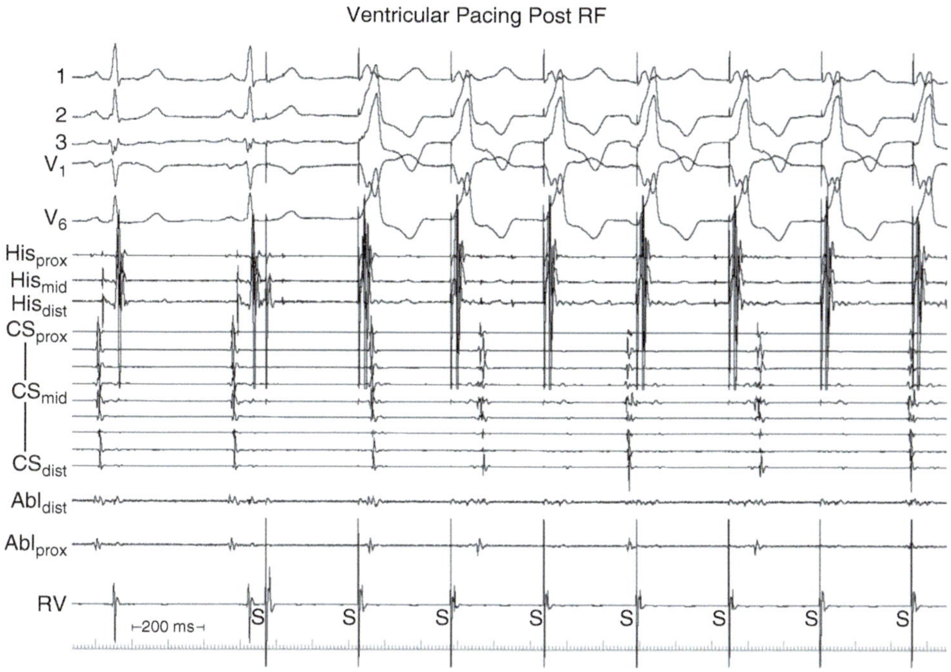

Figure 8-13

After ablation (Fig. 8-13), retrograde conduction was poor and concentric; in contrast to the preablation situation, SVT could not be initiated baseline or after isoproterenol infusion.

Final ECG

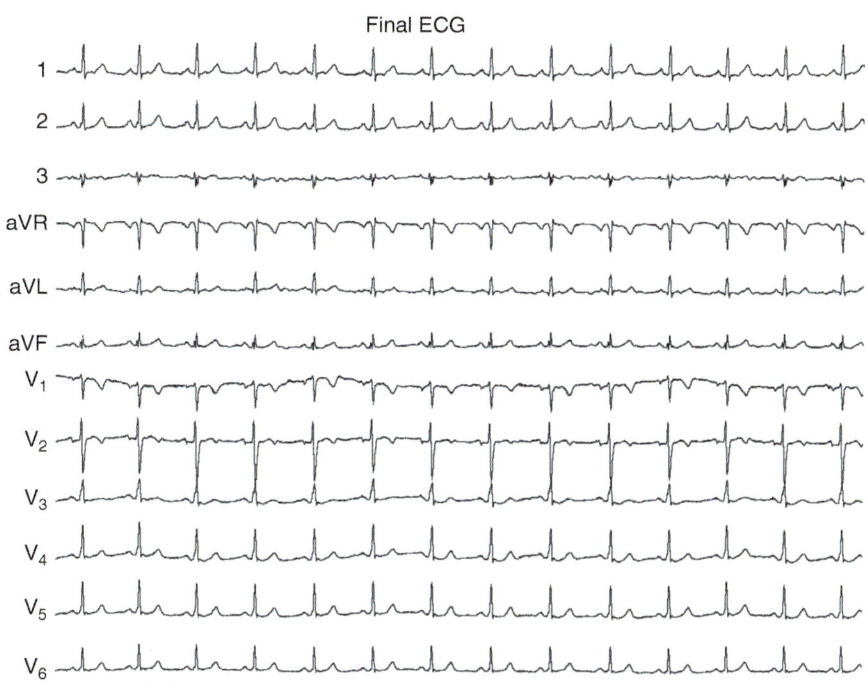

Figure 8-14

Sinus rhythm was present at the end of the procedure and SVT has not recurred (Fig. 8-14). Fetal monitoring throughout the procedure showed no adverse effects on the unborn child (a healthy baby girl, born 8 weeks later).

Electroanatomic Map

Figure 8-15

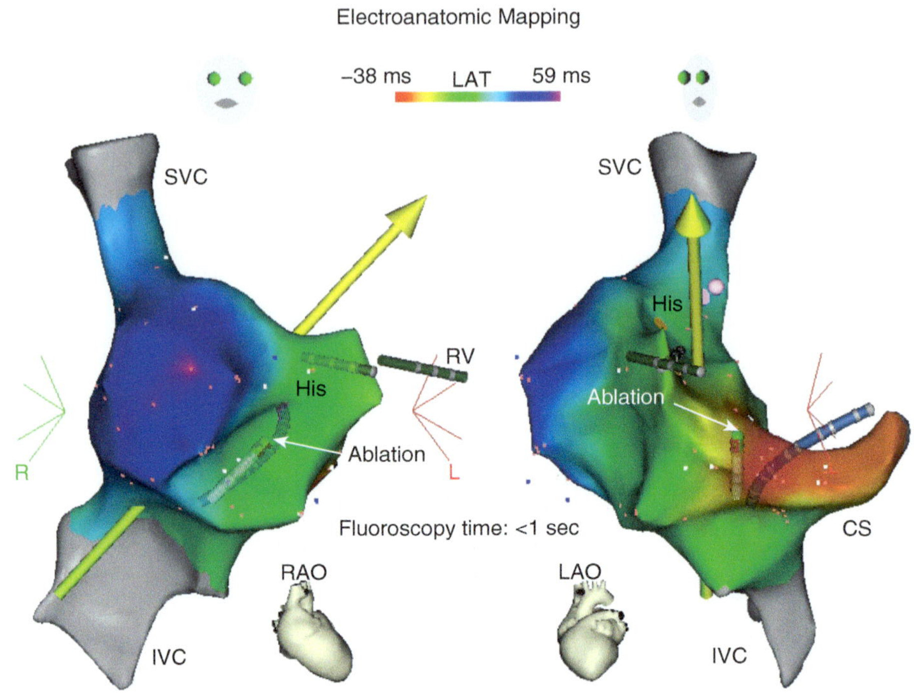

The *red area* on the image at the right of the previously shown activation map during SVT (Fig. 8-15) indicates the ablation site. Fluoroscopic exposure was <0.5 seconds (for registration of the patient and electroanatomic system at the beginning of the procedure; no fluoroscopy was used thereafter).

Summary

- A correct diagnosis can almost always be made if the correct tools are used and correct interpretations made
- Significant cycle length variability hampers diagnosis, but can make mapping easier (it is usually clear whether the electrogram of interest leads or follows other recordings)
- Current tools allow drastic limitation in fluoroscopic exposure, including <1 minute in some cases

9 Fasciculoventricular Pathway

Case Presentation

A 13-year-old girl presented with palpitations and lightheadedness for 2 years. She is an orphan, adopted shortly after birth. A muscular ventricular septal defect was detected in early childhood and repaired surgically. She did well until the current syndrome of palpitations developed; these increased in frequency and severity over the 2 years leading up to this evaluation. Physical exam was normal without residual murmur. Her resting ECG showed sinus rhythm with preexcitation. An event monitor was obtained, showing supraventricular tachycardia (SVT) at 250/min. At a prior electrophysiology (EP) study, atrial tachycardia at 250/min was induced, but not mapped or ablated; dual atrioventricular (AV) nodal pathways were observed; preexcitation was noted but not ablated due to proximity to the normal conduction system. Due to continued episodes of palpitations, she was referred for repeat EP study and possible ablation.

Baseline ECG and Intracardiac Recordings

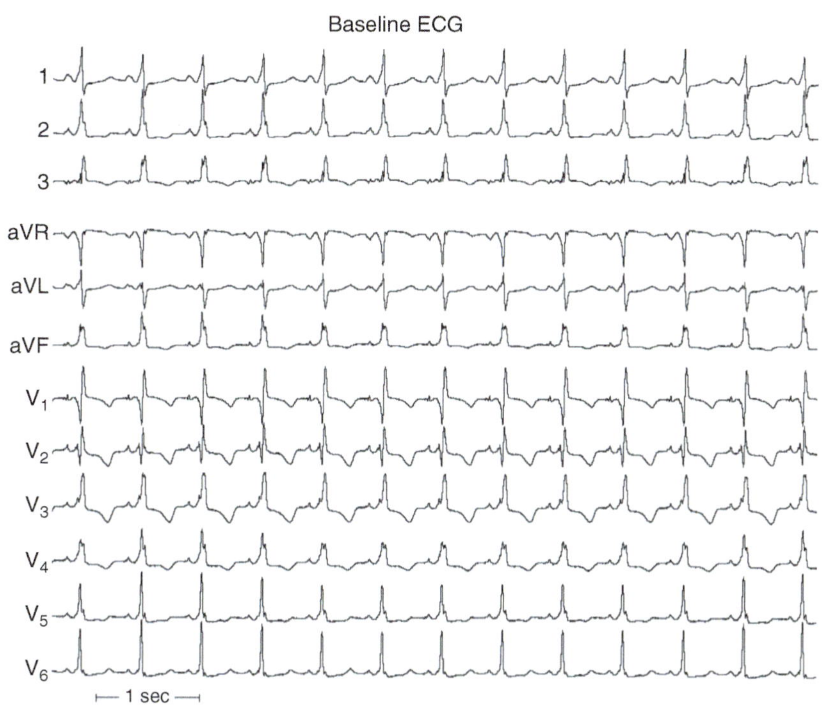

Figure 9-1

The baseline ECG in Fig. 9-1 shows a short PR interval and preexcitation with a pattern suggesting a midseptal pathway insertion. The terminal R′ in V1 and V2 hints that there may be right bundle branch block when preexcitation is absent.

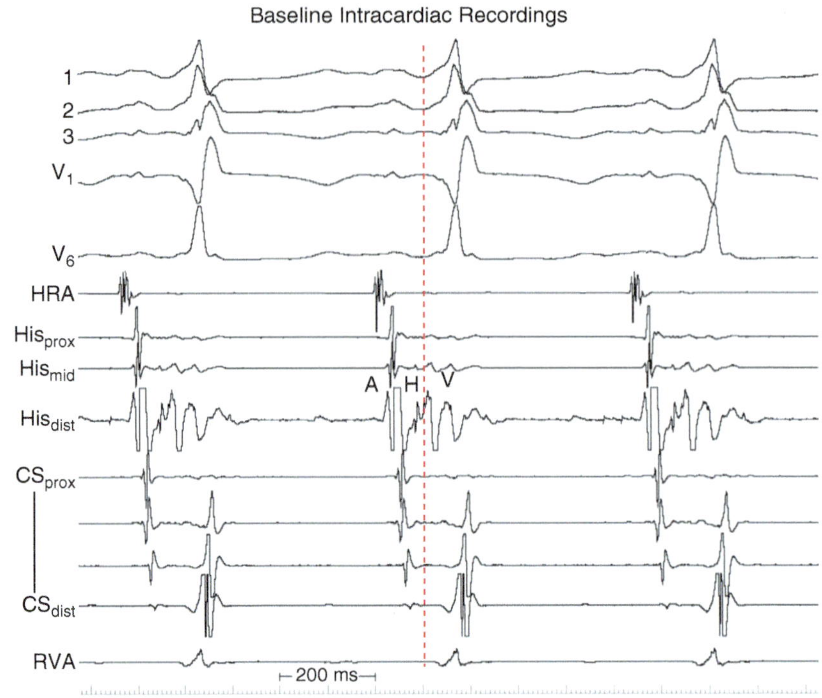

Figure 9-2

Baseline intracardiac recordings confirm preexcitation and show a His potential (H) just before the QRS onset *(dotted line)* with an HV interval 22 ms (Fig. 9-2).

Ventricular Pacing

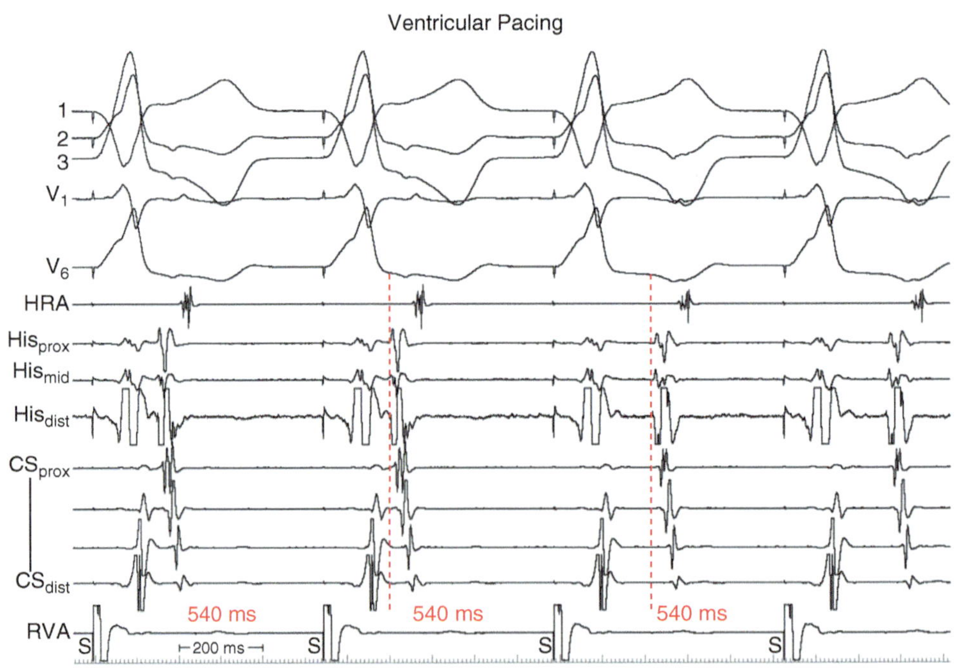

Figure 9-3

Decremental ventricular pacing (Fig. 9-3) shows a concentric activation sequence with a sudden increase in the ventriculo-atrial (VA) interval *(arrows)* without change in pacing rate. Wenckebach VA block occurred at paced cycle length 470 ms. After isoproterenol, VA

Wenckebach block occurred at cycle length 440 ms. Thus because VA conduction characteristics are those of the AV node, the bypass tract either has AV nodal-like properties (very rare) or does not appear to have retrograde conduction.

Atrial Pacing

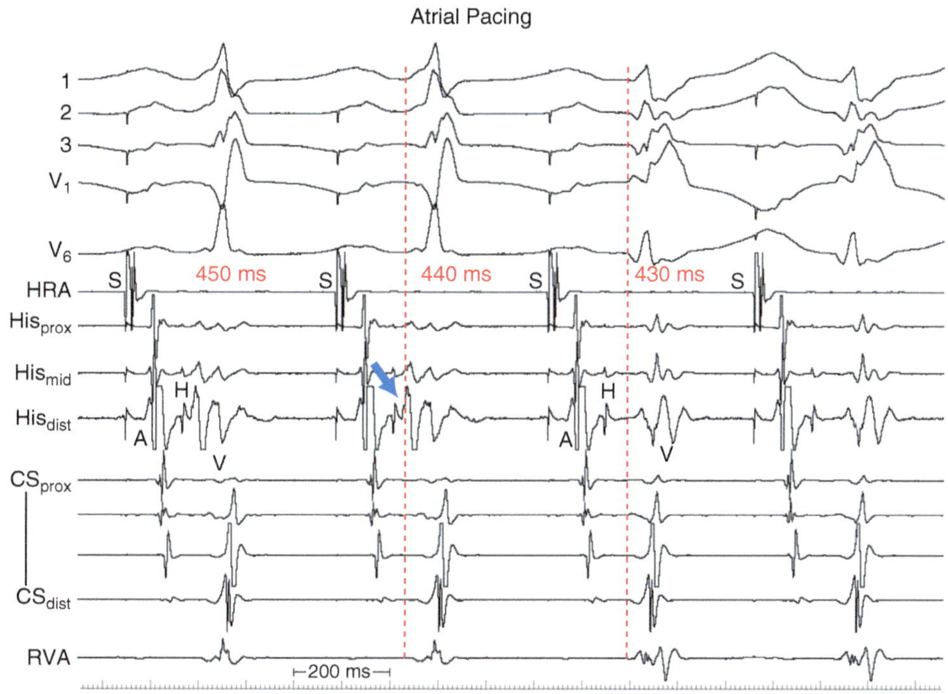

Figure 9-4

With progressively rapid atrial pacing (Fig. 9-4), sudden block in the bypass tract is observed (third and fourth complexes). Coincident with this, the HV interval prolongs from 22 to 50 ms. Of note, right bundle branch block is present in the nonpreexcited beads, as anticipated from the original surface ECG. With the loss of preexcitation, it is evident that early ventricular activation over the pathway had occurred near the His bundle *(arrow)*.

Atrial Extrastimuli

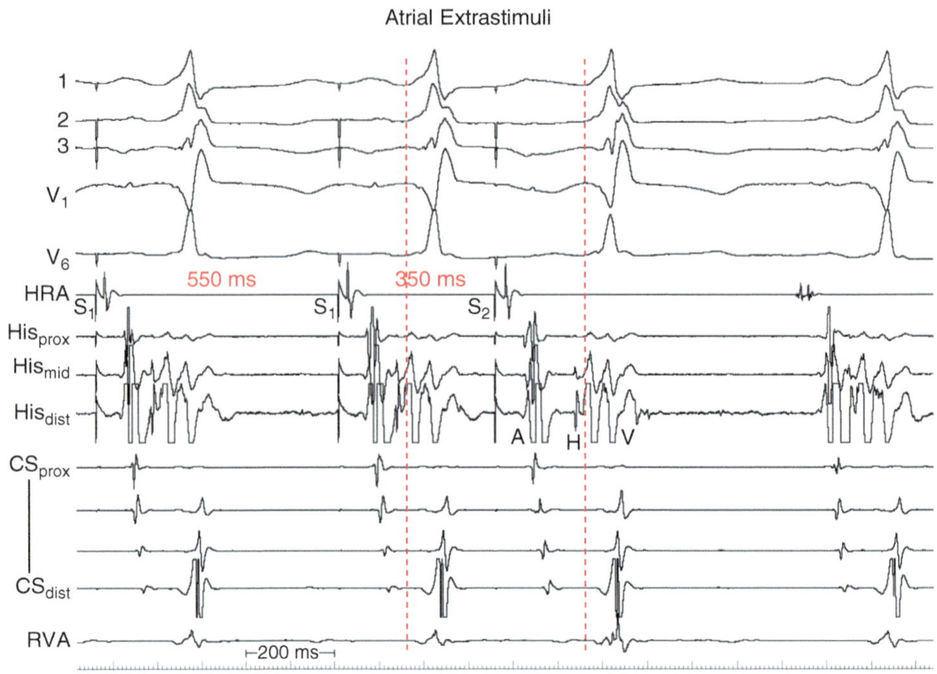

Figure 9-5

In response to atrial premature stimulation, preexcitation persists; the AH interval increases by an anticipated amount consistent with AV nodal behavior (Fig. 9-5). However, the HV interval and preexcitation pattern are unchanged from the drive complexes. *Dashed lines* indicate onset of QRS complexes.

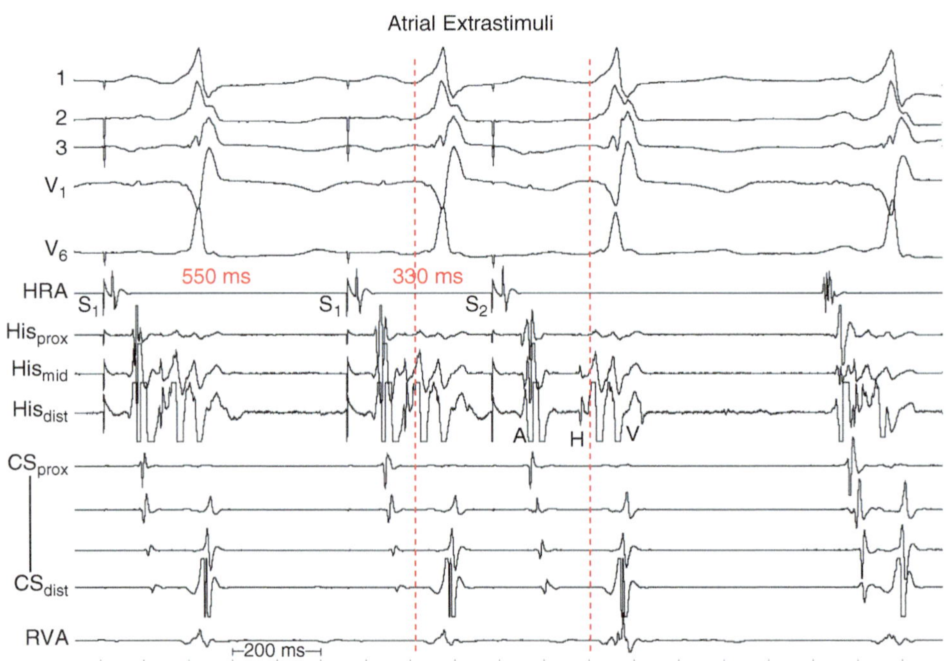

Figure 9-6

With more premature stimulation, preexcitation again persists; the AH interval also increases but the HV interval and preexcitation pattern are unchanged from the drive complexes (Fig. 9-6). This is not typical for the usual atrioventricular pathway, with which the stimulus-delta interval is largely fixed, such that prolongation of the AH interval results in a greater degree of preexcitation and shorter (or even negative) HV interval. Instead, in this case, the HV remains fixed and short, and preexcitation is constant regardless of the AH interval. These are characteristics of a fasciculoventricular pathway. *Dashed lines* indicate onset of QRS complexes.

Atrial Pacing at Various Rates

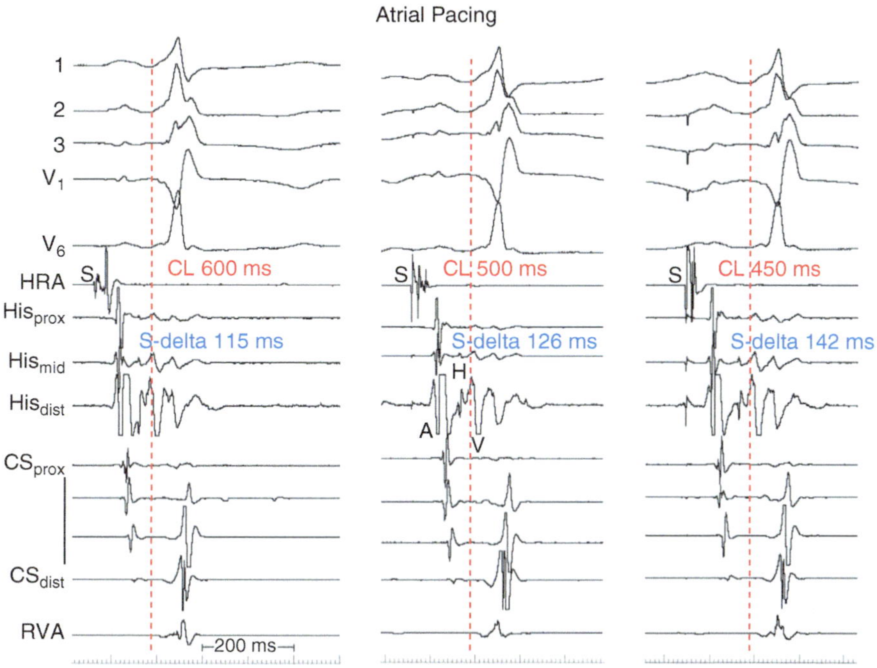

Figure 9-7

In Fig. 9-7 a single complex of atrial pacing at different cycle lengths is shown. It is evident that with progressive shortening of the atrial-paced cycle length, an increase in the S-delta interval occurs. This is because of increase in the AH interval, whereas the HV interval remains fixed at 22 ms and the degree of preexcitation remains unchanged. With standard atrioventricular bypass tracts, there is little if any change in the stimulus-delta interval with faster atrial pacing; because the AH interval lengthens under these conditions, but bypass tract conduction remains rather fixed, a greater proportion of ventricular activation is controlled by bypass tract conduction leading to greater degrees of preexcitation and shortening of the HV interval. The findings in this figure are again most consistent with a fasciculoventricular pathway—one that connects the His bundle with ventricular muscle. With these pathways, the amount of preexcitation does not vary regardless of rate of stimulation or prematurity, and unless there is block in the pathway, whenever the His is activated anterogradely, a preexcited complex ensues.

Junctional Escape Complex

Figure 9-8

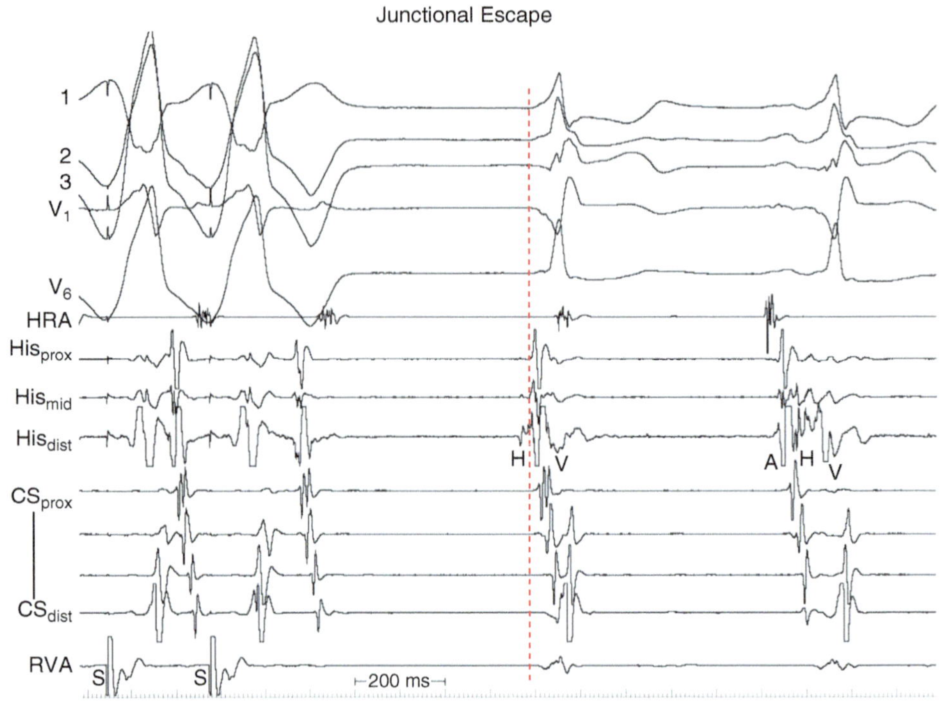

One of the strongest lines of evidence for the existence of a fasciculoventricular pathway is shown in Fig. 9-8, with a junctional (His bundle) escape complex after a burst of rapid ventricular pacing. (This technique, when retrograde conduction is present, can suppress the sinus node such that a junctional escape complex may occur.) The junctional escape complex has a pattern of preexcitation identical to that of complexes conducted from the atrium, indicating that the pathway connection is between His bundle and ventricle. With standard atrioventricular bypass tracts, a junctional escape complex will not be preexcited, because preexcited complexes in such cases result from conduction from the atrium to the ventricle over a pathway outside the normal conduction system.

Final ECG

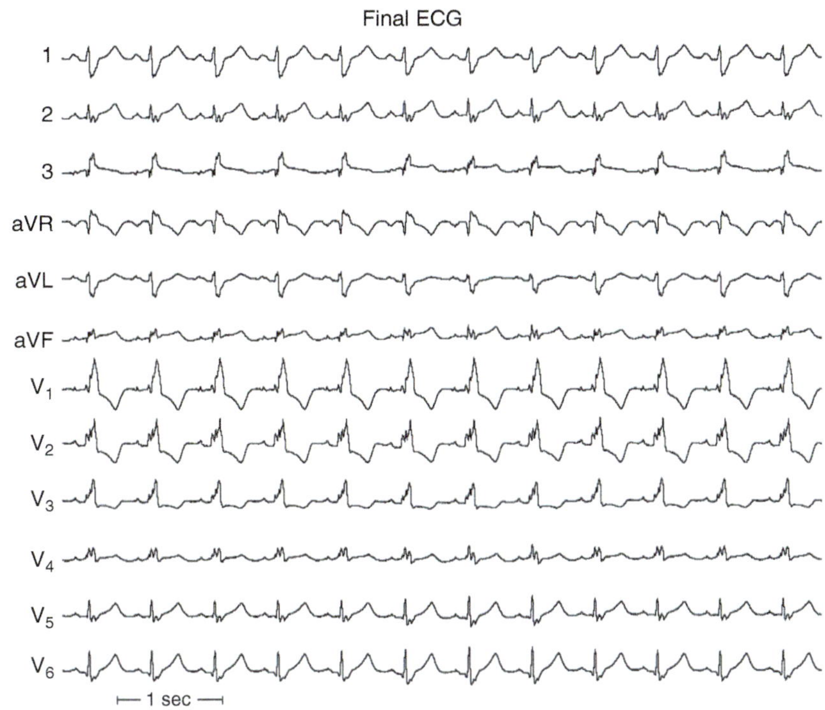

Figure 9-9

Catheter manipulation around the upper septum resulted in "bumping" of the pathway (Fig. 9-9), leading to loss of preexcitation. After the fasciculoventricular pathway was thus traumatized, the QRS complex showed RBBB as anticipated.

The cause of preexcitation in this case was thus a fasciculoventricular pathway; because these do not integrally participate in arrhythmias, this was not targeted for ablation. The patient had inducible typical right atrial cavotricuspid isthmus-dependent atrial flutter at 250 ms cycle length, consistent with the prior findings. Successful ablation was performed for this arrhythmia. At the end of the procedure, after catheter trauma, fasciculoventricular pathway conduction was absent. However, it returned the following day. The patient has done well in follow-up without recurrent arrhythmias.

Summary

- Fasciculoventricular pathways have unique properties:
  - A moderate degree of preexcitation is present
  - Preexcitation does not vary over a range of paced rates
  - The HV interval likewise remains constant
  - Junctional complexes are preexcited
  - These pathways are not integral participants in arrhythmias
- Catheter ablation of bypass tracts is not always necessary, for example:
  - Pathways that do not conduct rapidly enough under any conditions to result in patient risk
  - Pathways with intermittent conduction
  - Pathways that do not participate in arrhythmias (ie, fasciculoventricular pathways)
- This patient had another cause of palpitations unrelated to the bypass tract and consistent with prior data; simple ablation of the bypass tract in this case not only would not have yielded a successful outcome, but could also have risked damage to the normal conduction system

10 Focal Right Atrial Tachycardia

Case Presentation

An 18-year-old woman who was 36 weeks pregnant with her first child presented with dyspnea; she was found to have heart failure (HF), with heart rate 130–170/min, which was believed to be compensatory sinus tachycardia. Echocardiogram showed left ventricular dilation (5.2 cm in diastole), fractional shortening of 0.13, ejection fraction 30%, mild mitral regurgitation, and 4-chamber dilation (or upper-normal size for stage of pregnancy). She was started on standard HF medications (no ACE inhibitor because of pregnancy).

ECG of Tachycardia

What Is the Differential Diagnosis? [Fig. 10-1]

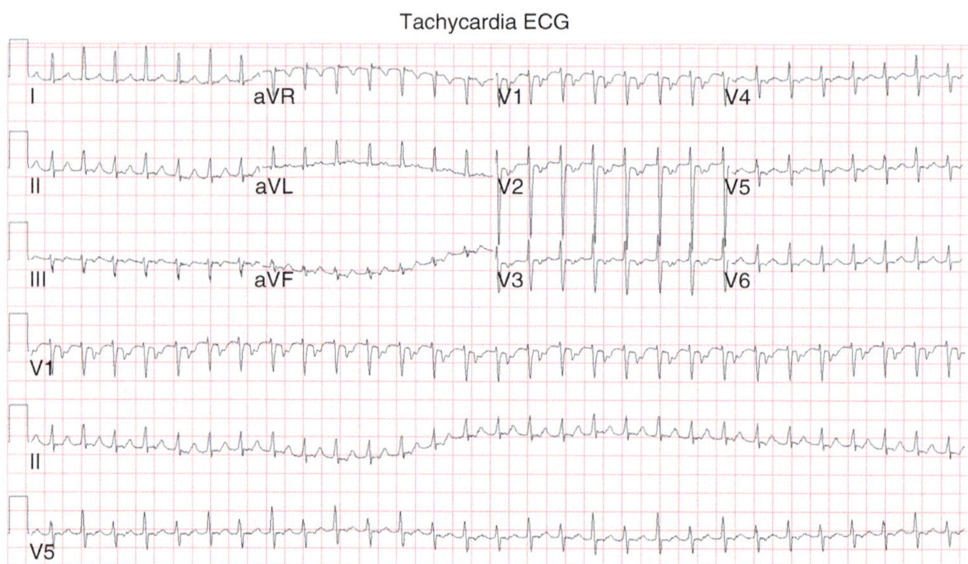

Figure 10-1

The baseline ECG in Fig. 10-1 shows regular supraventricular tachycardia (SVT) about 145/min. The P waves (best seen in lead V1) are very unusual and the PR interval is slightly long for this heart rate, if it were sinus tachycardia. The differential diagnosis includes atrial tachycardia or accessory pathway tachycardia using a right-sided bypass tract for retrograde conduction (from the P-wave vector in the inferior leads and V1). She was given an injection of adenosine that yielded transient 2:1 atrioventricular (AV) block, with continuation of the rapid atrial rhythm. Her child was delivered (cesarean section); tachycardia continued thereafter. She underwent direct-current cardioversion, but reverted to SVT nearly immediately. She was then scheduled for electrophysiology (EP) study and ablation. The response to adenosine excludes orthodromic SVT, in which a 1:1 AV relationship must be maintained, and because the P-wave vector is not consistent with exit from the AV nodal region, AV nodal reentry is excluded; thus, an atrial tachycardia is present.

Subsequent ECG

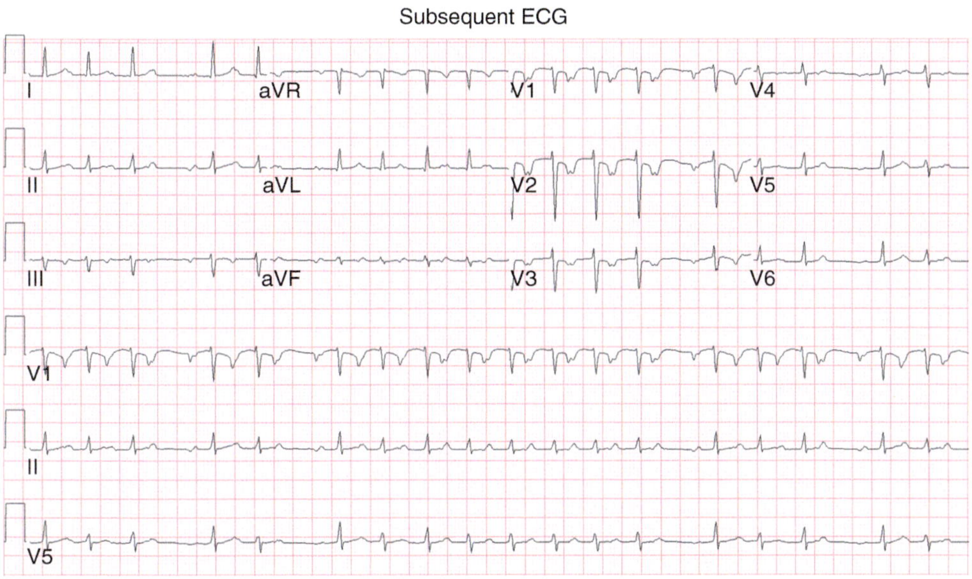

Figure 10-2

An ECG taken after administration of a beta blocker (Fig. 10-2) shows a slightly slower atrial rate along with periods of AV Wenckebach block. This again is indicative of atrial tachycardia and affords a better look at the P-wave morphology (positive in leads 1 and aVL, initially negative in inferior leads and V1–3).

Baseline ECGs and Intracardiac Recordings in SVT

Tachycardia ECGs [Fig. 10-3]

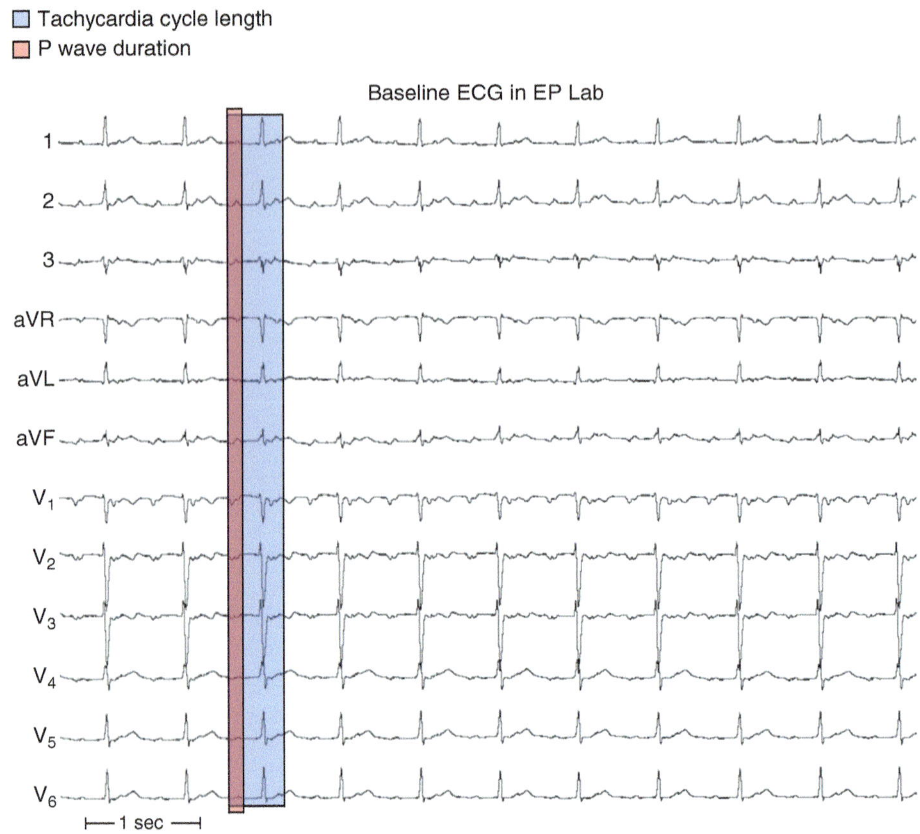

Figure 10-3

The patient was brought to the electrophysiology laboratory for catheter ablation of an atrial tachycardia. The question now is what type of atrial tachycardia: focal or macroreentrant? In most young people with a structurally normal heart, a focal process is present. Macroreentry generally requires some degree of scarring, which is not present in a structurally normal heart. However, because she has HF with early chamber dilatation, perhaps she has scarring in the atrium leading to macroreentry (it is also possible that the arrhythmia has caused a tachycardia-related cardiomyopathy). Because the ablation target is determined by the tachycardia mechanism, it is important to separate focal from macroreentrant causes. In Fig. 10-3, the P-wave duration is shown in *red* and the tachycardia cycle length in *blue* (2:1 AV conduction is present). Generally, the smaller the proportion of the tachycardia cycle length that is occupied by the P wave, the more likely that a focal process is present. In the example here, a focal process seems more likely.

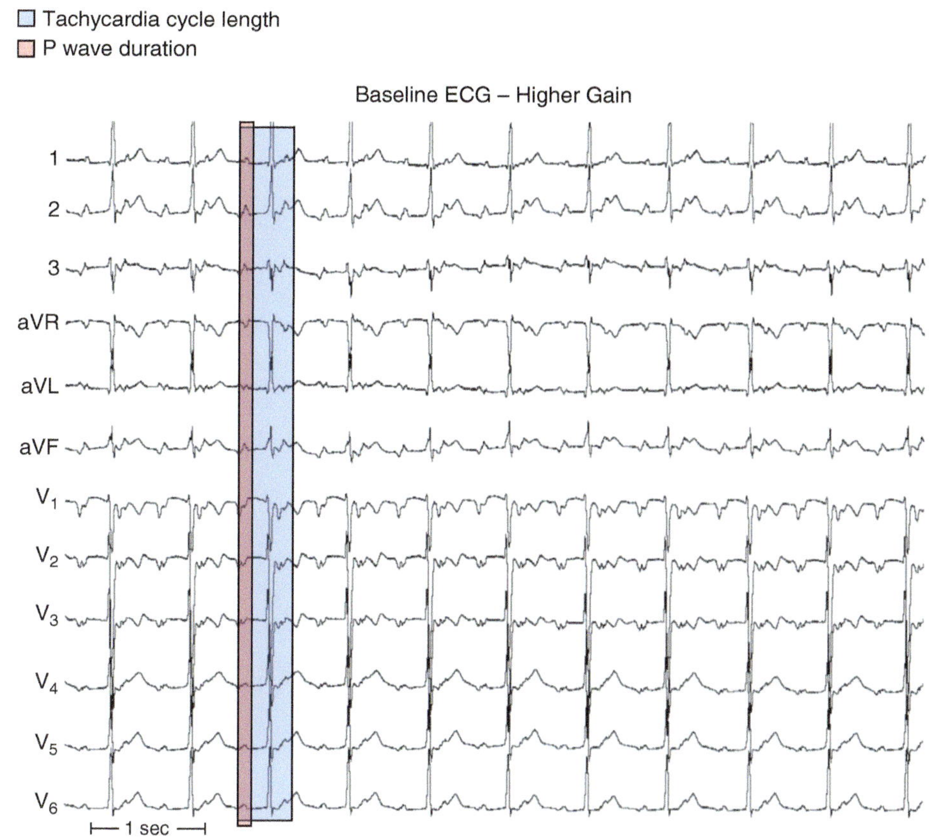

Figure 10-4

Sometimes it is helpful to increase the gain on recordings to be able to see more of the duration of the P wave (Fig. 10-4). In this case the conclusion is the same as before.

Intracardiac Recordings [Fig. 10-5]

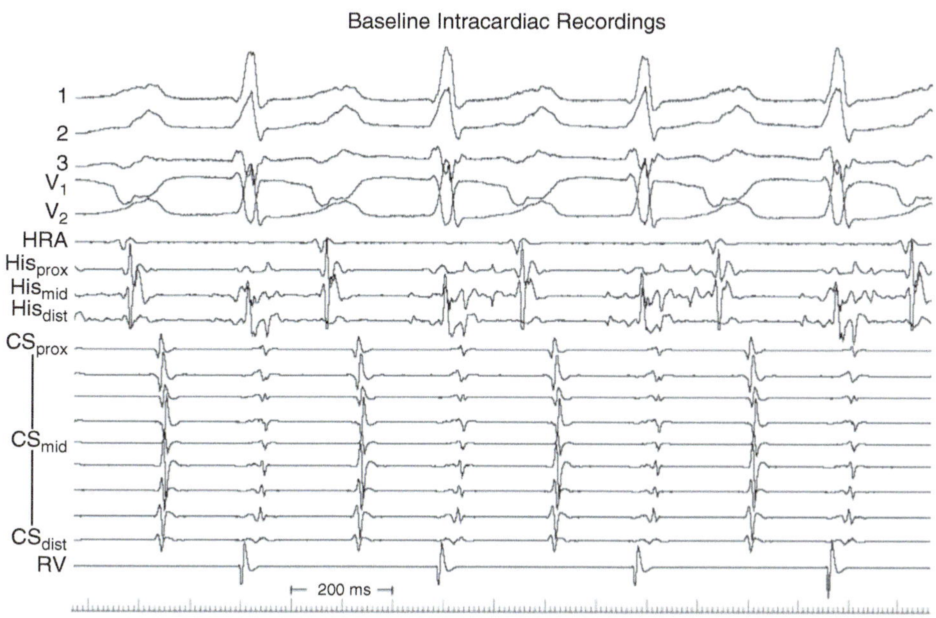

Figure 10-5

Intracardiac recordings during tachycardia are shown in Fig. 10-5. Of the recordings shown, earliest activation appears to occur in the high right atrium (HRA).

TABLE 10-1 Atrial Tachycardias

	Focal			
	Automaticity	Triggered Activity	Microreentry	Macroreentry
Onset	Spontaneous	Induced (burst > PES)	Induced (PES >> burst)	Induced (PES >> burst)
Occurrence	Incessant; bursts	Variable	Sporadic, sustained	Sporadic, sustained
P wave vs TCL	Small fraction	Small fraction	Small fraction	Large portion
Atrial activation	Small fraction	Small fraction	Small fraction	Large portion
Isoproterenol	Facilitates onset; acceleration	Facilitates onset; acceleration	Minimal effect	Minimal effect
Adenosine	Variable effect	Termination	Minimal effect	No affect/ acceleration
Response to single premature extrastimuli	Reset or fusion; flat/ increasing	Reset or fusion; decreasing	Reset or fusion; flat/ increasing	Reset + fusion; flat/ increasing
Overdrive pacing response	Suppression; ↑RC with ↓PCL	Acceleration; ↓RC with ↓PCL	Entrainment; No Δ RC w/↓PCL	Entrainment; No Δ RC w/↓PCL
Ablation target	Late diastolic; unipolar QS	Late diastolic; unipolar QS	Prolonged diastolic	Middiastolic
Response to RF	Accelerate/stop	Accelerate/stop	Slow/stop	Slow/stop

PES, programmed electrical stimulation; TCL, tachycardia cycle length; RC, return cycle of tachycardia; PCL, paced cycle length; QS, completely negative wave in unipolar recording.

Table 10-1 shows differences between three categories of tachycardias with apparent focal propagation from what seems to be a point source (automatic, triggered because of delayed after depolarizations, and microreentry) vs macroreentry.

Overdrive Coronary Sinus Pacing in SVT

Midcoronary Sinus Pacing [Fig. 10-6]

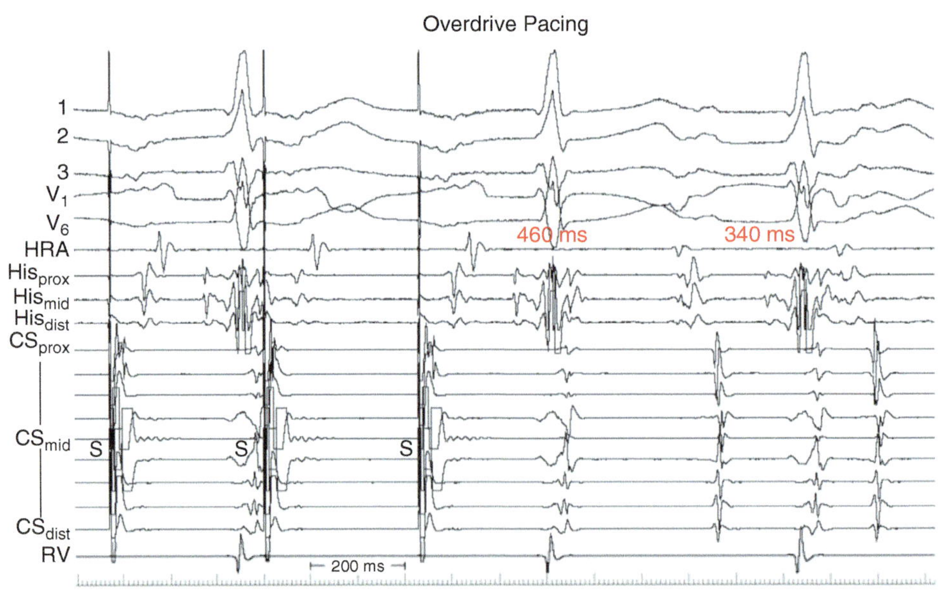

Figure 10-6

The result of overdrive spacing from the midcoronary sinus is shown here, after which the tachycardia resumes. This information, by itself, is not very helpful because both focal tachycardias and macroreentry will have this response. However, the fact that the interval from the last paced complex to the first beat of tachycardia (460 ms) is substantially longer than tachycardia cycle length (340 ms) would be very unusual for macroreentry, in which the interval consists of propagation time from the pacing site to the circuit, around the circuit once, and back to the pacing site (Fig. 10-6). In most cases of macroreentry, this should ordinarily not be >100 ms or so longer than tachycardia cycle length.

Proximal Coronary Sinus Pacing [Fig. 10-7]

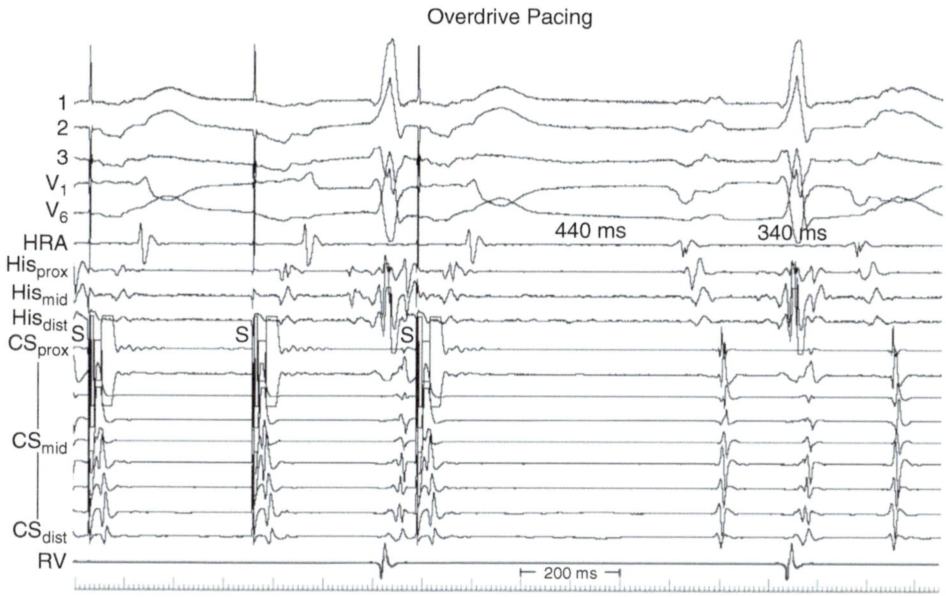

Figure 10-7

Pacing from the proximal coronary sinus yields a slightly shorter interval until the tachycardia resumes, suggesting that this spacing site is slightly closer to the exit from what now appears to be a focus (Fig. 10-7). Ideally, overdrive pacing from several sites could be used looking for fusion (indicating macroreentry), or its absence (suggesting a focal process); however, because the tachycardia is incessant, knowing what pure pacing looks like for comparison to pacing during tachycardia is not possible, making this technique less helpful at this time. Pacing from right atrium and distal coronary sinus yielded similar results. All the evidence taken together suggests a focal process.

Activation Mapping

Various Sites

Activation Mapping [Fig. 10-8]

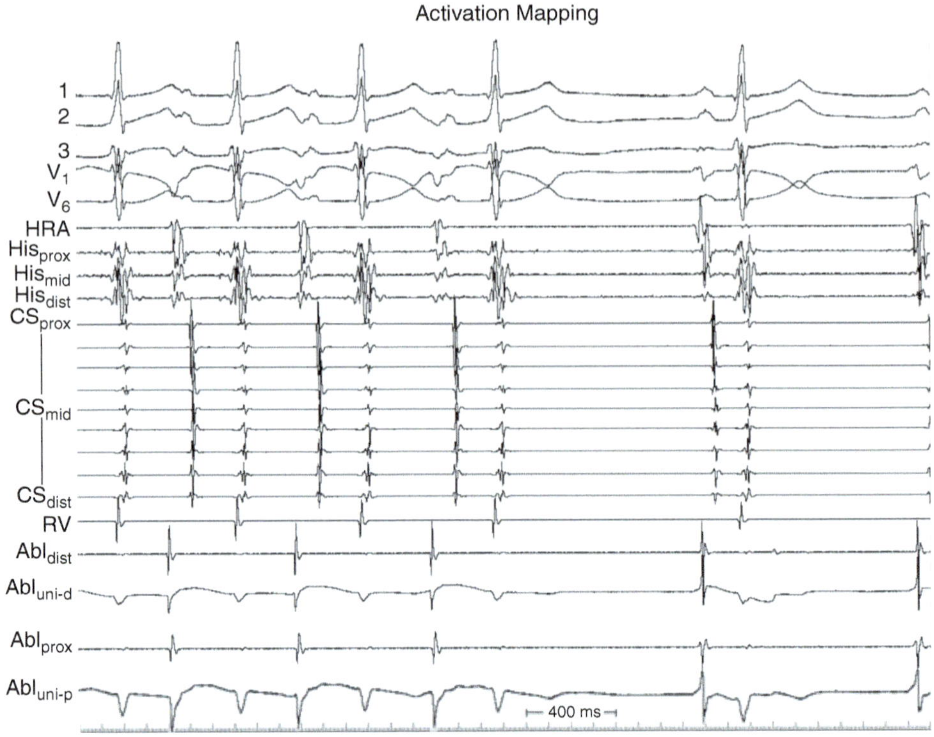

Figure 10-8

Now that a focal process has been identified as the likely cause of the tachycardia, activation mapping can begin. During the process of mapping, the tachycardia suddenly terminated when moving the catheter along the lateral tricuspid annulus (Fig. 10-8). This so-called "bump-mapping" has important implications: it signifies that (1) a critical site for continuation of the tachycardia has been "bumped" by the catheter (thus, where the catheter was at the time of this encounter is important); (2) the amount of tissue necessary for continuation of the tachycardia is quite small, because the effect of trauma with the catheter tip is spatially quite limited; and, finally, (3) the source is on the endocardial surface, because mechanical effects of the catheter on the endocardium would not be expected to affect deep myocardial or epicardial sources. Of note, this phenomenon does not distinguish between a focal process and macroreentry because tachycardias of either type may be terminated by catheter contact.

Activation Mapping [Fig. 10-9]

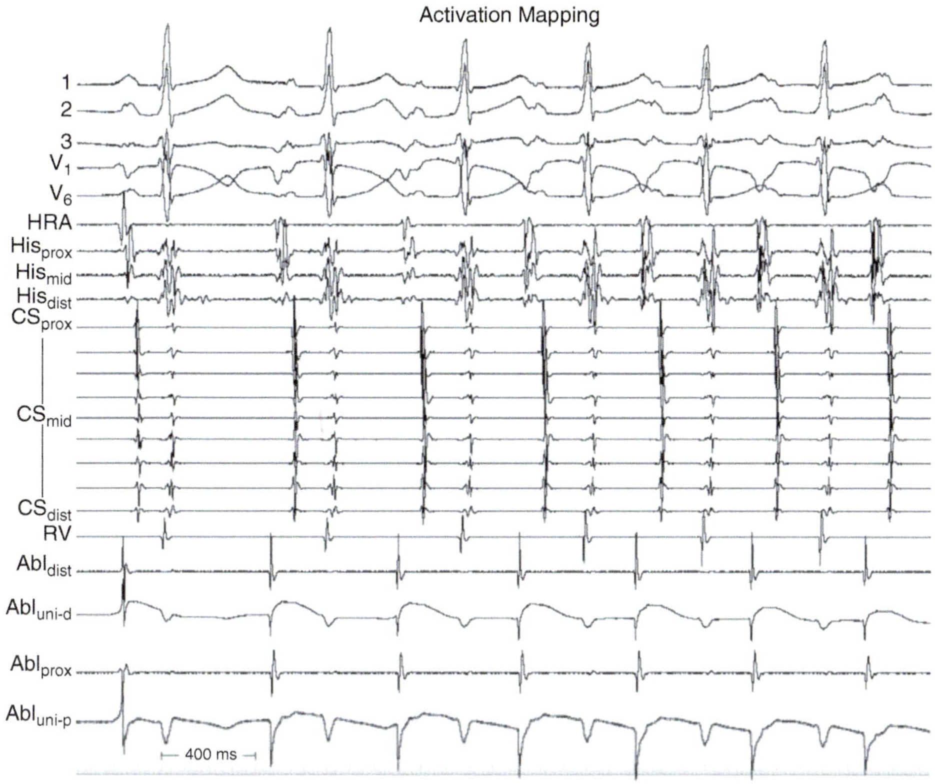

Figure 10-9

Fortunately, tachycardia resumes in Fig. 10-9, and gradually "warms up" (gradual rate increase after the onset). This is most consistent with a focal, automatic process.

Activation Mapping [Fig. 10-10]

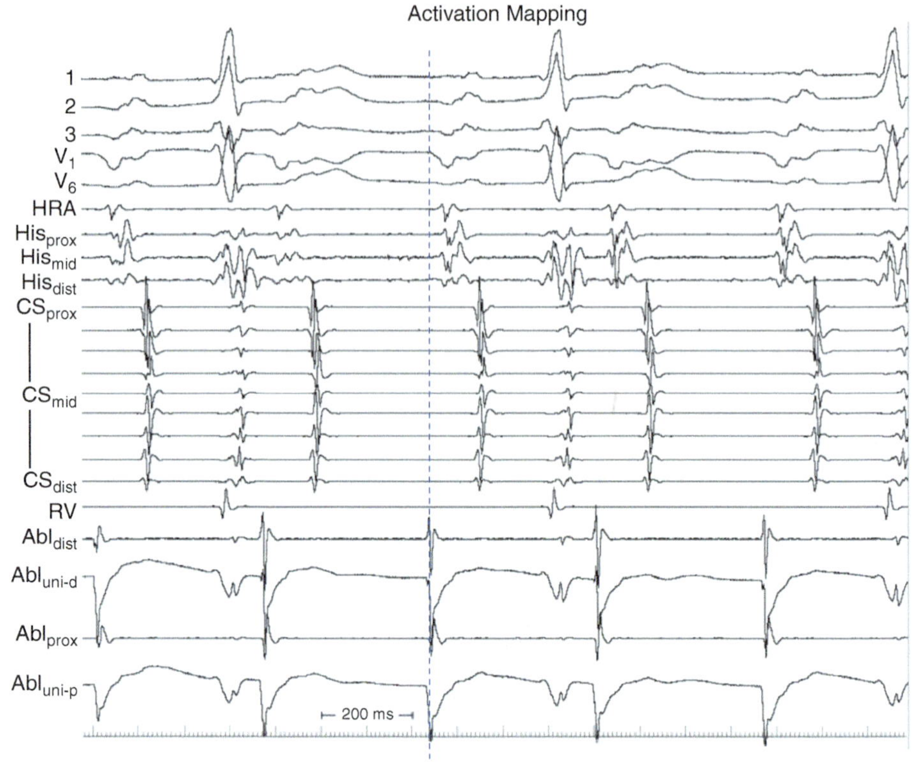

Figure 10-10

A site on the lateral tricuspid annulus is sampled during mapping (Fig. 10-10). The P-wave onset is designated by a *dashed line*; the ablation/mapping electrograms occur slightly (about 5 ms) before the P-wave onset; the distal bipolar electrode and unipolar signal have similar timing, and the unipolar has a "QS" configuration. Although the electrogram parameters are encouraging, the timing is not; ordinarily, propagation from a focus takes 20–40 ms before the onset of the P wave occurs, and so additional mapping is necessary.

Activation Mapping [Fig. 10-11]

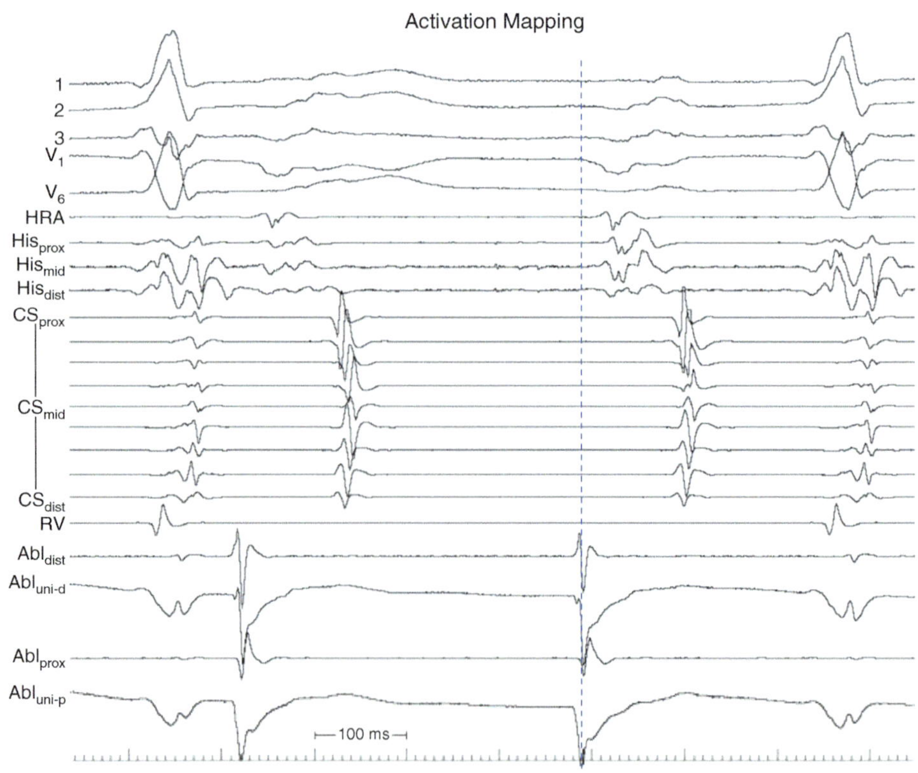

Figure 10-11

At a faster sweep speed (Fig. 10-11), it is clear that this site is not very early before the P-wave onset.

Electroanatomic Map

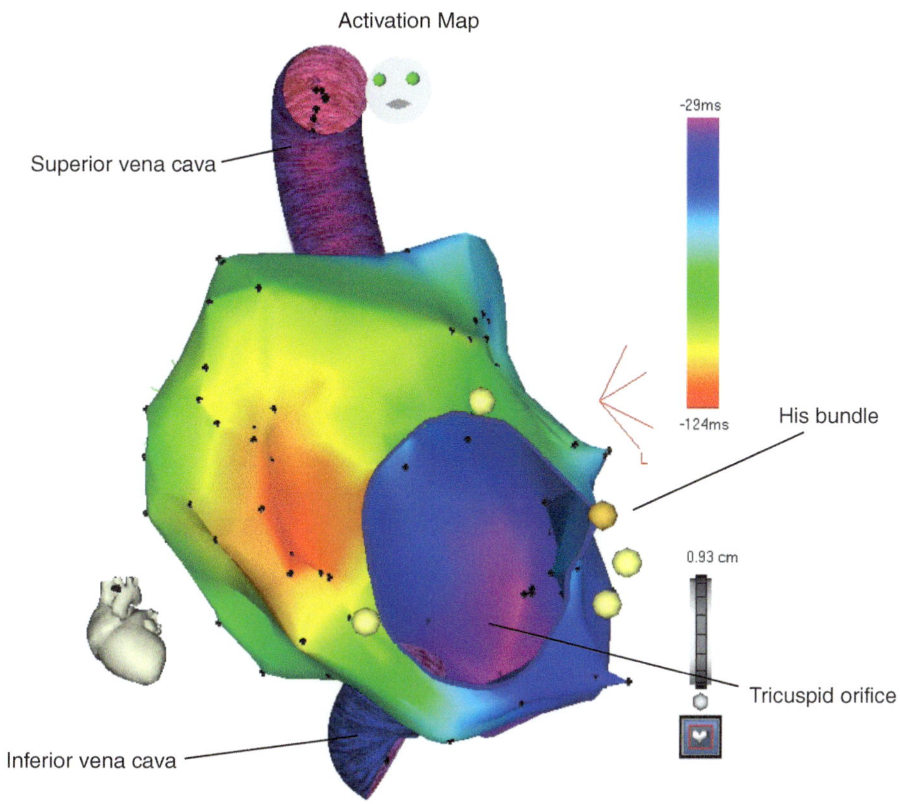

Figure 10-12

An electroanatomic map of right atrial activation during the tachycardia is shown in Fig. 10-12, indicating focal propagation from a site on the lateral tricuspid annulus (red area, surrounded by orange, yellow, etc.).

Additional Sites Sampled and Pace Mapping

Activation Mapping [Fig. 10-13]

Figure 10-13

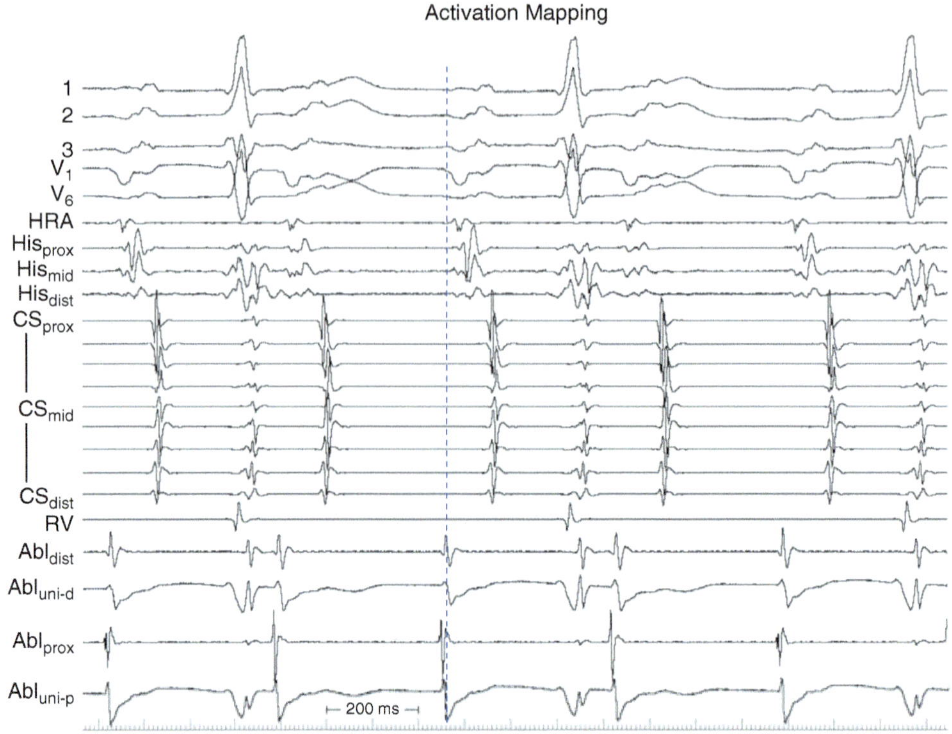

Additional mapping is performed; at this site (Fig. 10-13), the proximal bipolar electrogram has a timing before the distal, and is thus not a good site for ablation.

Pace Mapping [Fig. 10-14]

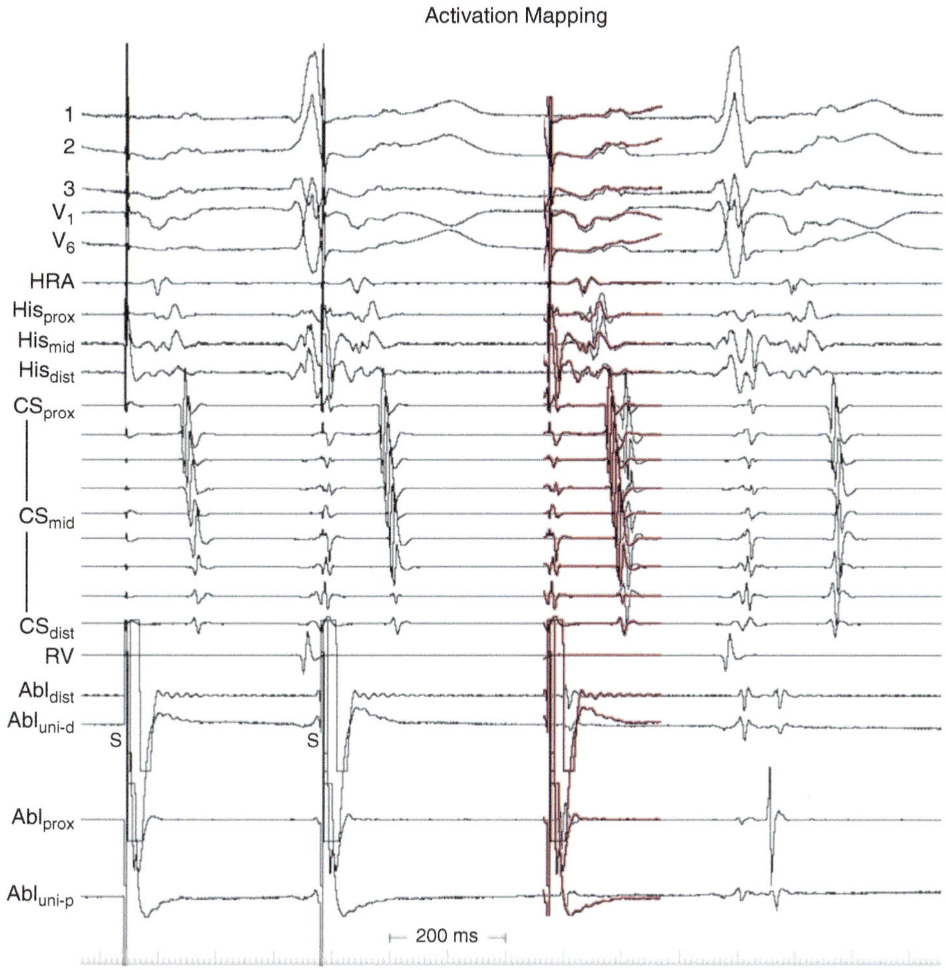

Figure 10-14

Pacing at this site (Fig. 10-14) yields a poor match with tachycardia (paced activation sequence in *red* superimposed on first tachycardia cycle after pacing). When the pacing electrode is at the actual site of impulse formation in a focal tachycardia, pacing should exactly match the activation sequence of the tachycardia.

Activation Mapping [Fig. 10-15]

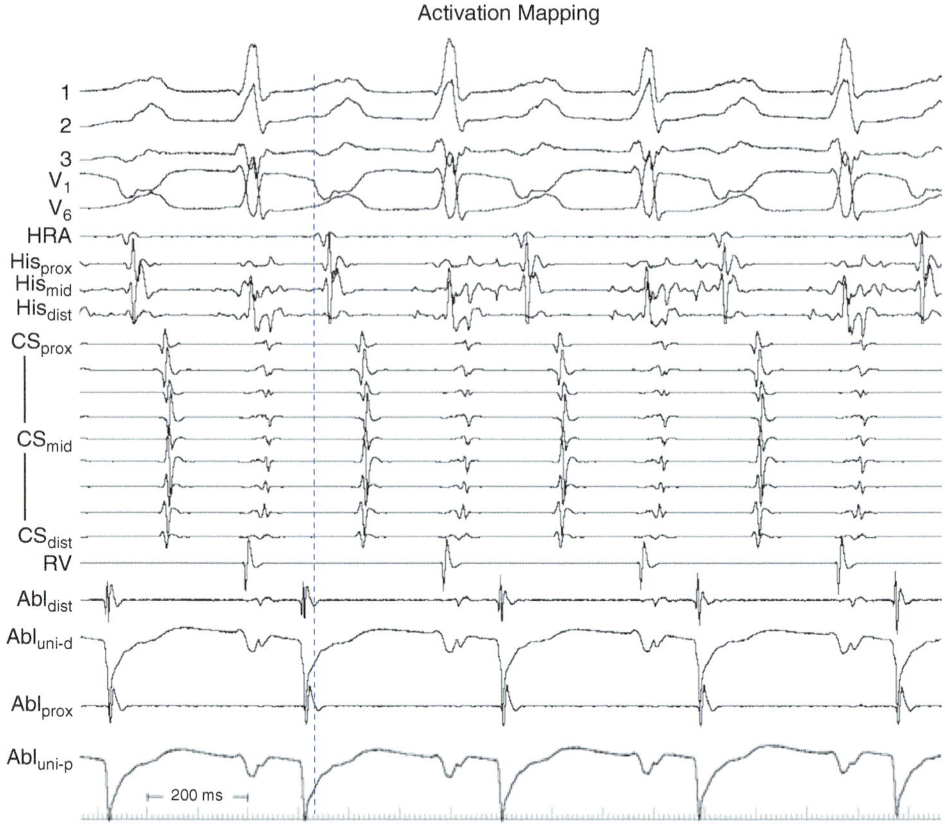

Figure 10-15

Another site is sampled; in Fig. 10-15, local activation in both the bipolar and the unipolar recordings substantially precedes P-wave onset (*dashed line*, inferred from its timing relationship to the HRA recording, because tachycardia now has a 1:1 AV relationship and the onset of the P wave is not as clear). The site is now 40 ms before P-wave onset, with unipolar–bipolar "agreement" and a "QS" unipolar configuration.

Activation Mapping [Fig. 10-16]

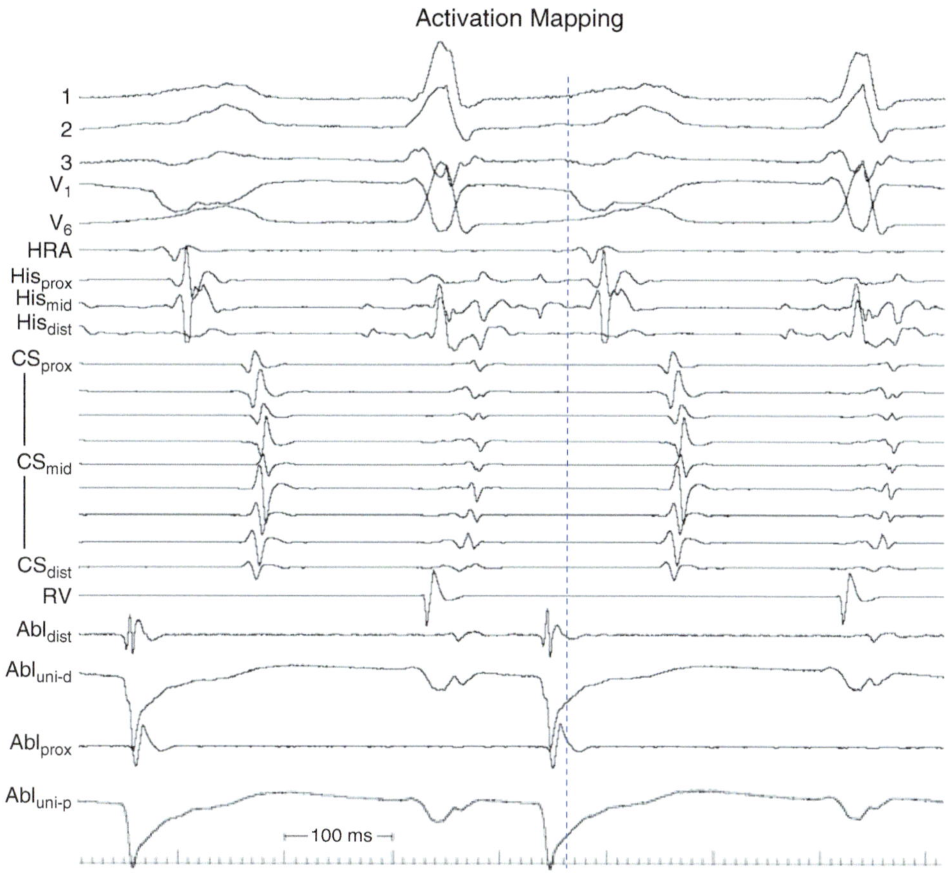

Figure 10-16

In Fig. 10-16, the same site is shown at a faster sweep speed, showing the site is 40 ms before P-wave onset.

Pace Mapping [Fig. 10-17]

Figure 10-17

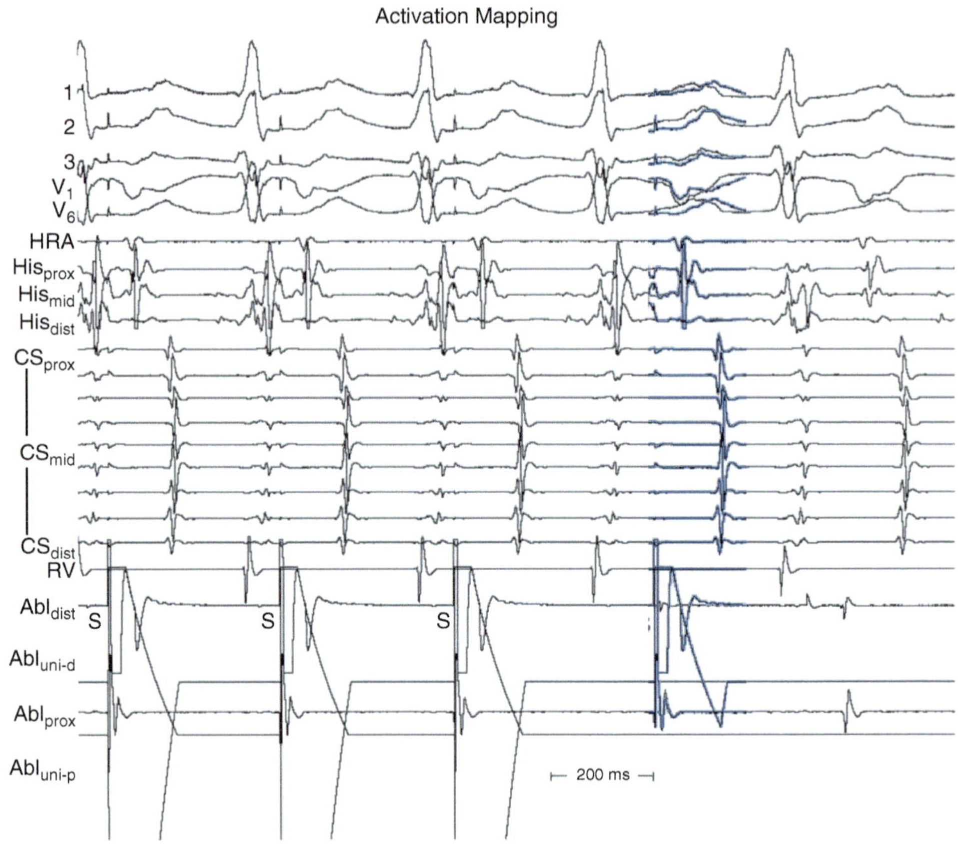

Pacing at this site (Fig. 10-17) yields a perfect match with tachycardia (paced complex in blue superimposed on first tachycardia complex after pacing). This corroborates the early local activation time recorded at this site.

Ablation

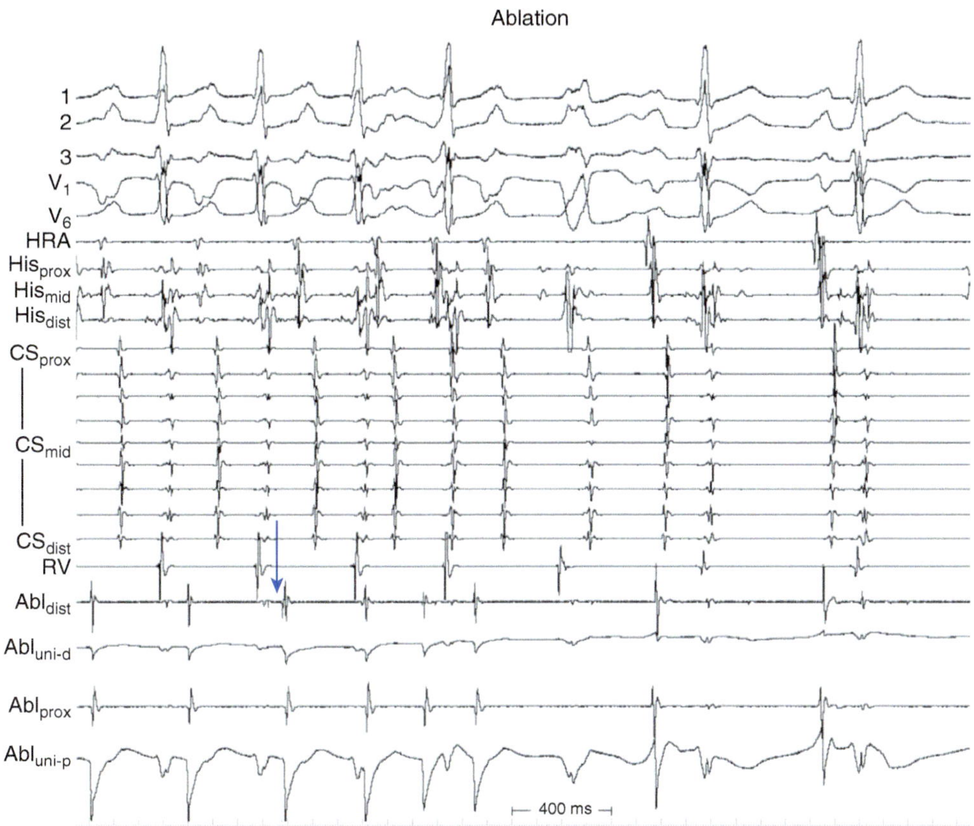

Figure 10-18

Radiofrequency energy application at this site (Fig. 10-18, starting at the *blue arrow*) results in a rapid acceleration of tachycardia followed by abrupt termination to sinus rhythm.

ECG Postablation

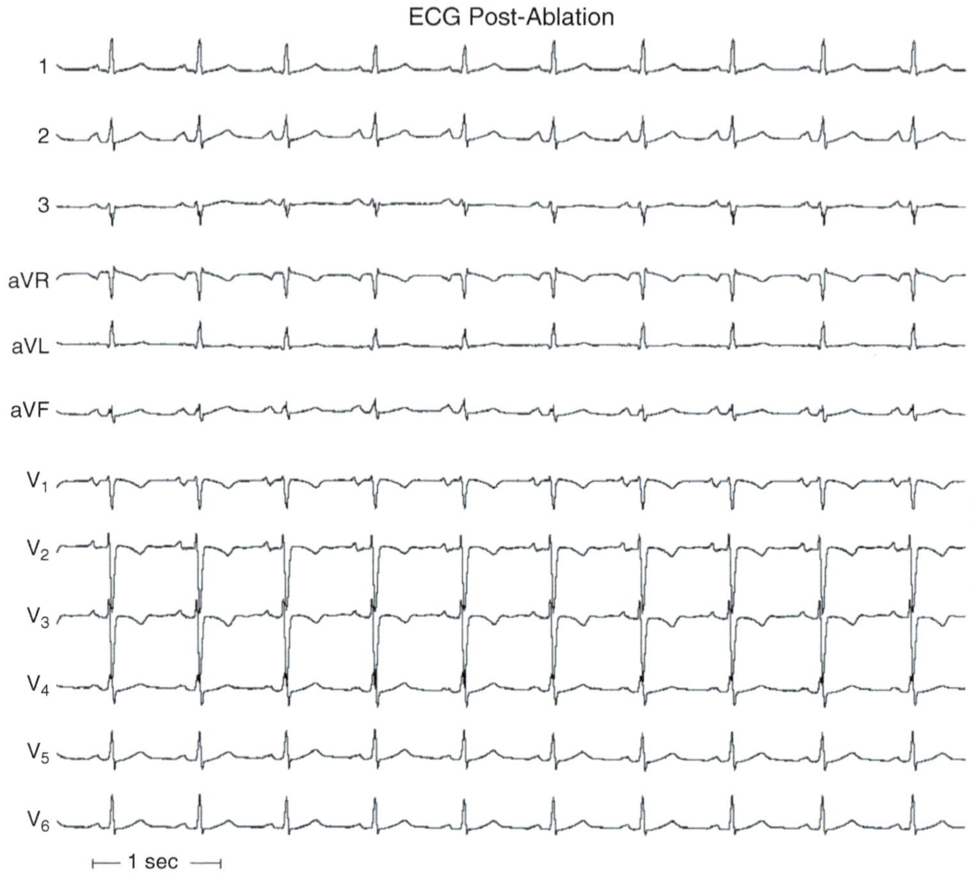

Figure 10-19

Sinus rhythm persisted through the waiting period. The P wave shown in Fig. 10-19 is not particularly abnormal despite the prolonged high rate and mild HF.

Atrial Activation Sequence with Various Sites of Coronary Sinus Pacing vs SVT

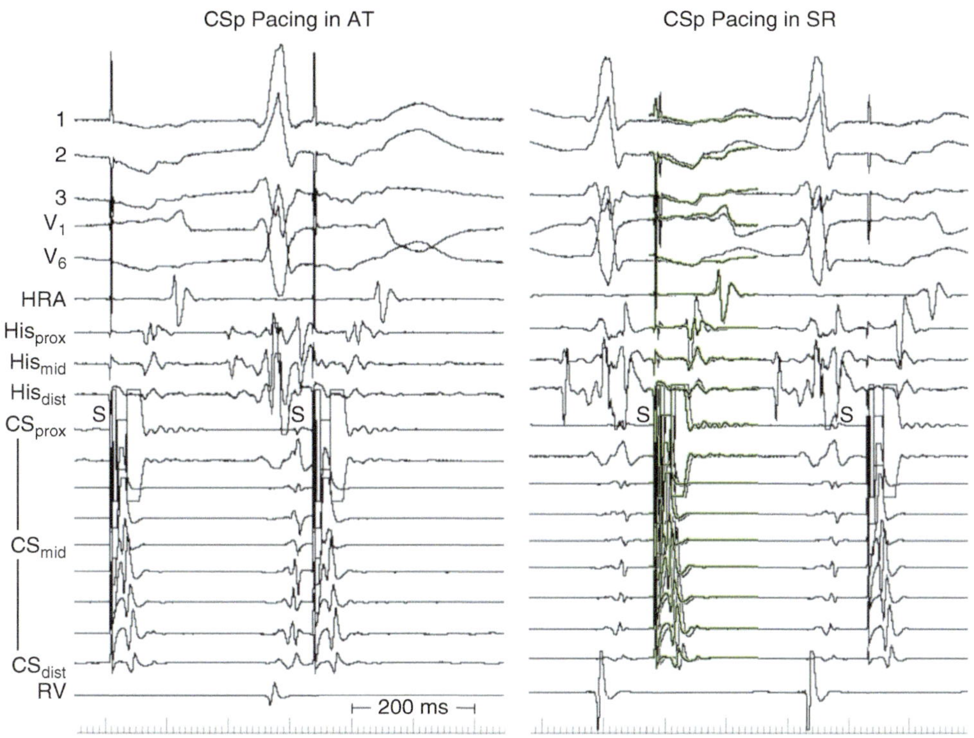

Figure 10-20

After restoration of sinus rhythm, pacing from different sites can be performed to determine what "pure" pacing from these sites looks like, compared with pacing during tachycardia. If there is a difference between these, fusion is present and macroreentry can be diagnosed. If pacing during tachycardia and pure pacing have identical activation sequences, a focal process is more likely. In Fig. 10-20, pacing from the proximal CS (CSp) during SVT at left is compared with pure pacing during sinus rhythm at right. A complex of pacing during SVT *(green)* is superimposed on a pure paced complex; these are identical.

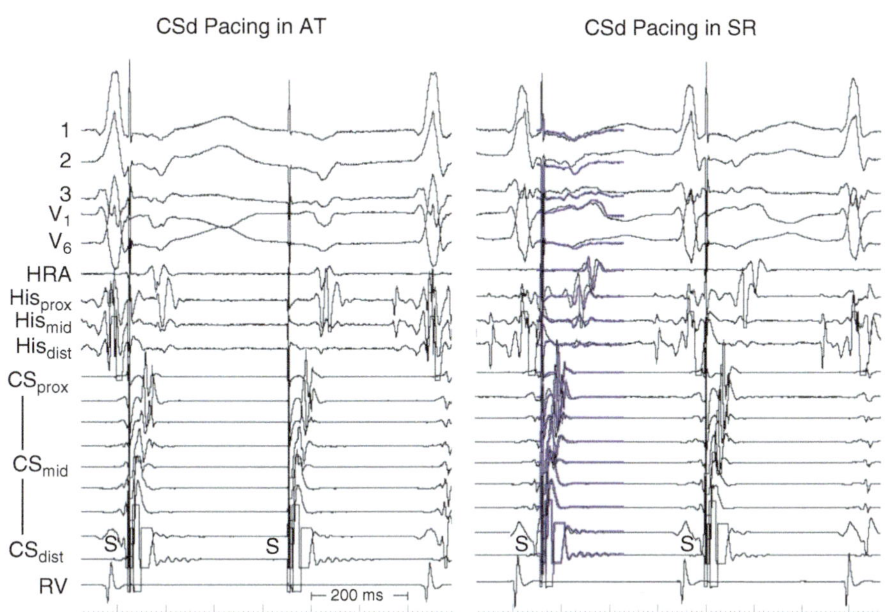

Figure 10-21

Similarly, pacing from the distal CS electrodes is compared when performed during tachycardia vs sinus rhythm. Again, in Fig. 10-21, pacing during tachycardia *(purple)* is superimposed on pure pacing, showing no difference.

Figure 10-22

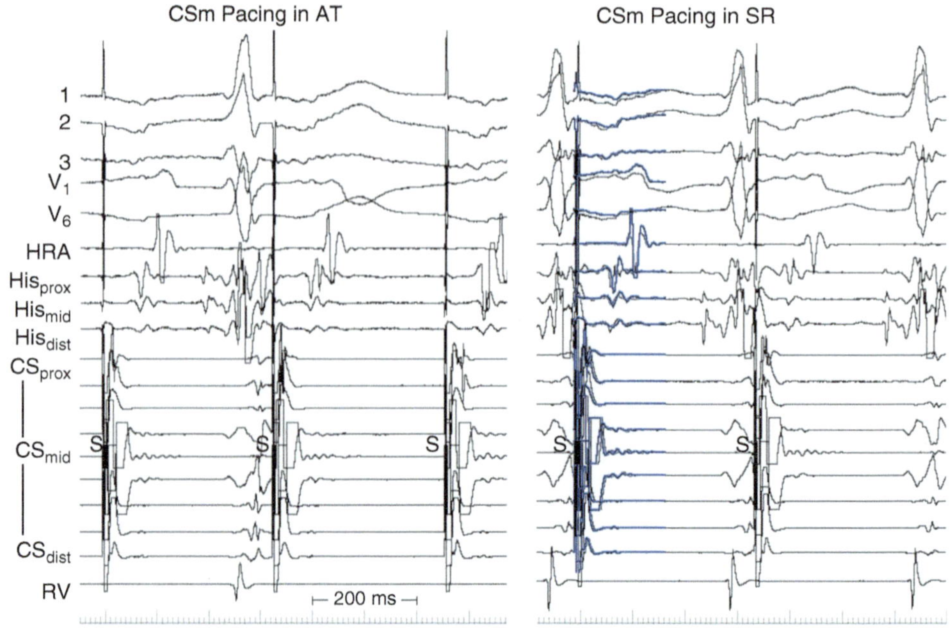

Pacing from the middle CS electrodes (Fig. 10-22) again shows no difference in atrial activation whether during tachycardia or sinus rhythm. Again, pacing during tachycardia *(blue)* is superimposed on pure pacing, showing no difference. Had this lack of evidence of fusion despite pacing at several sites been available earlier in the study, it would have helped exclude macroreentry.

Ventricular Pacing During Sinus Rhythm

Figure 10-23

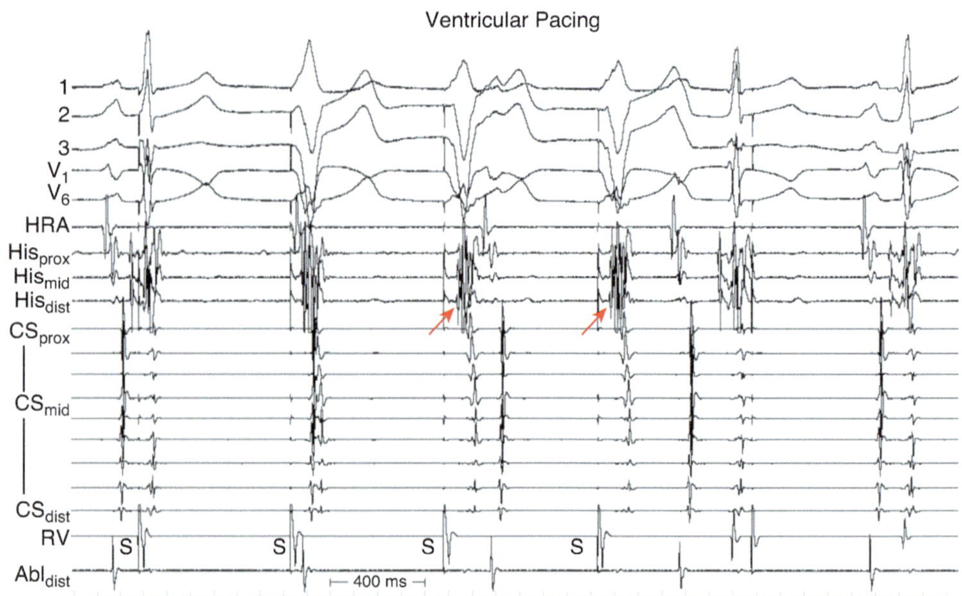

In Fig. 10-23, ventricular pacing immediately after ablation shows no retrograde conduction, with block in the AV node (retrograde His seen on third and fourth complexes [*arrow*]).

Tachycardia 1 h After Ablation

Tachycardia [Fig. 10-24]

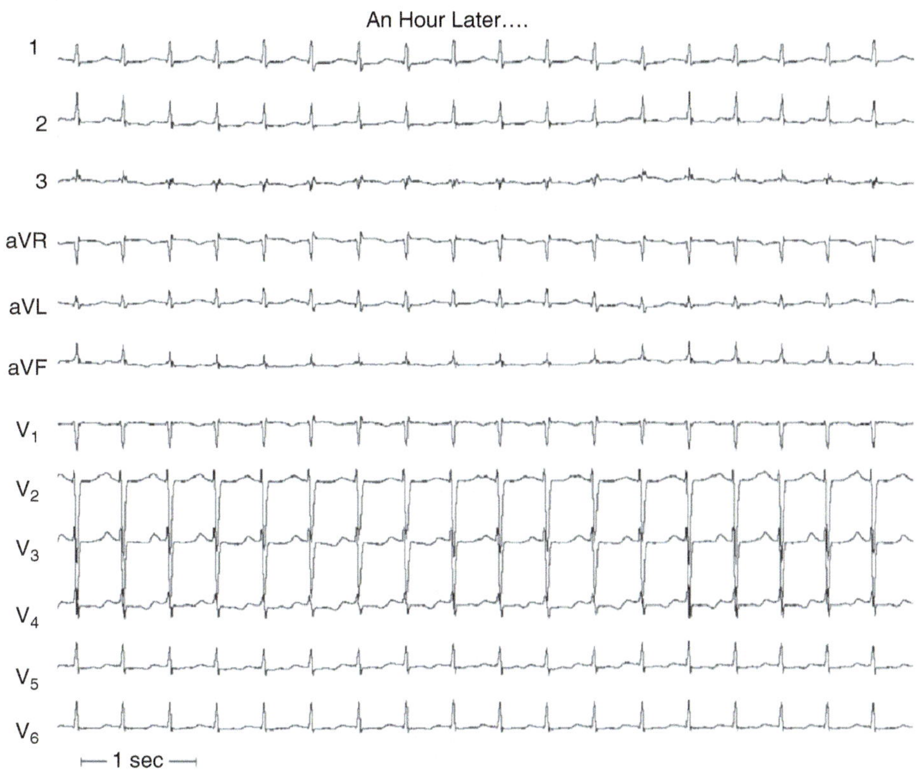

Figure 10-24

Isoproterenol was administered during the waiting period to try to reinitiate atrial tachycardia, which did not occur; however, this arrhythmia was noted in Fig. 10-24.

Atrial Pacing Induces SVT

Figure 10-25

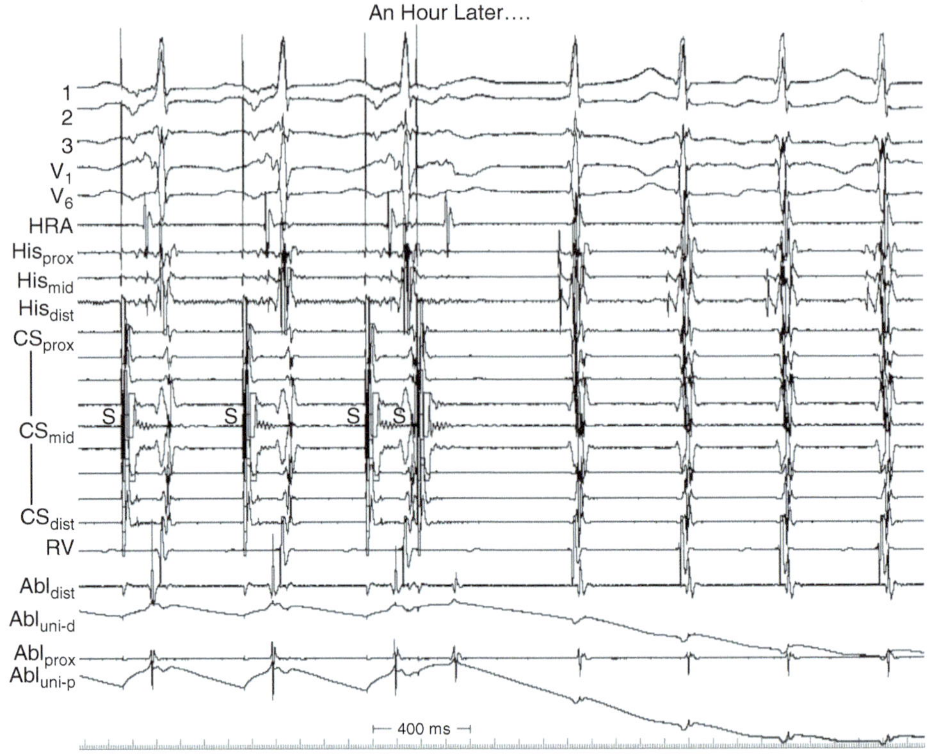

Atrial extrastimulus testing, to try to reinitiate atrial tachycardia, instead elicited the arrhythmia seen in Fig. 10-25. The atrial activation is concentric now and is coincident with ventricular activation, and SVT started after a long AH interval. All of these features are consistent with AV nodal reentry as a second tachycardia diagnosis.

Ventricular Extrastimuli and Overdrive Pacing in SVT (Figs. 10.26 and 10.27)

Figure 10-26

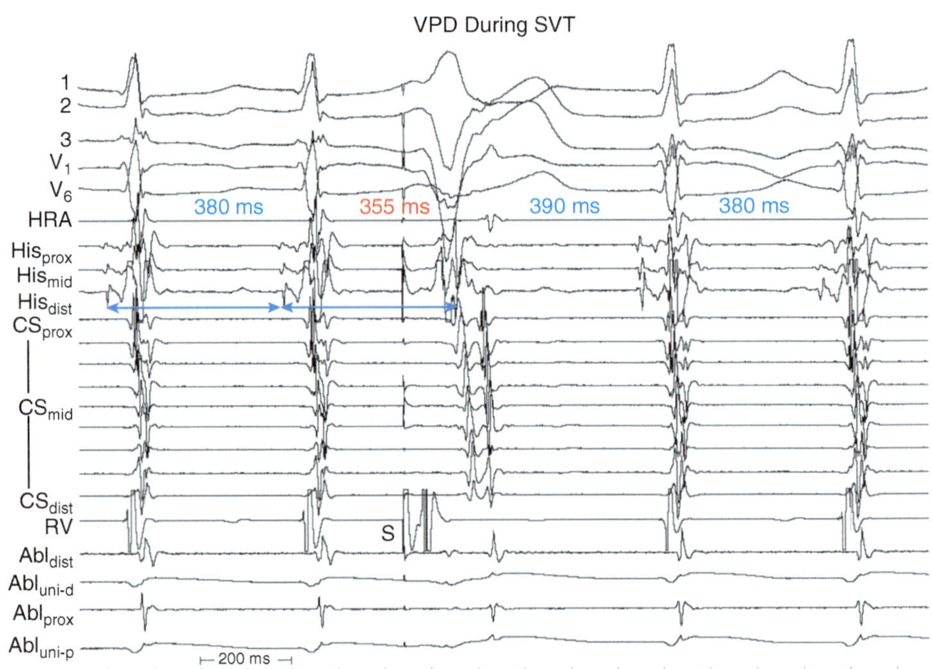

A ventricular extrastimulus (S) introduced during tachycardia advances the timing of atrial activation; however, the extrastimulus occurs at a time when the His bundle is not refractory (Fig. 10-26; *arrows* indicate where next expected His would occur). Thus retrograde conduction could easily have gone through the His bundle and AV node to preexcite the atrium. No inference can be made as to whether a bypass tract is present from this (though almost surely not, because atrial activation occurs within the QRS complex).

Ventricular Overdrive Pacing in SVT

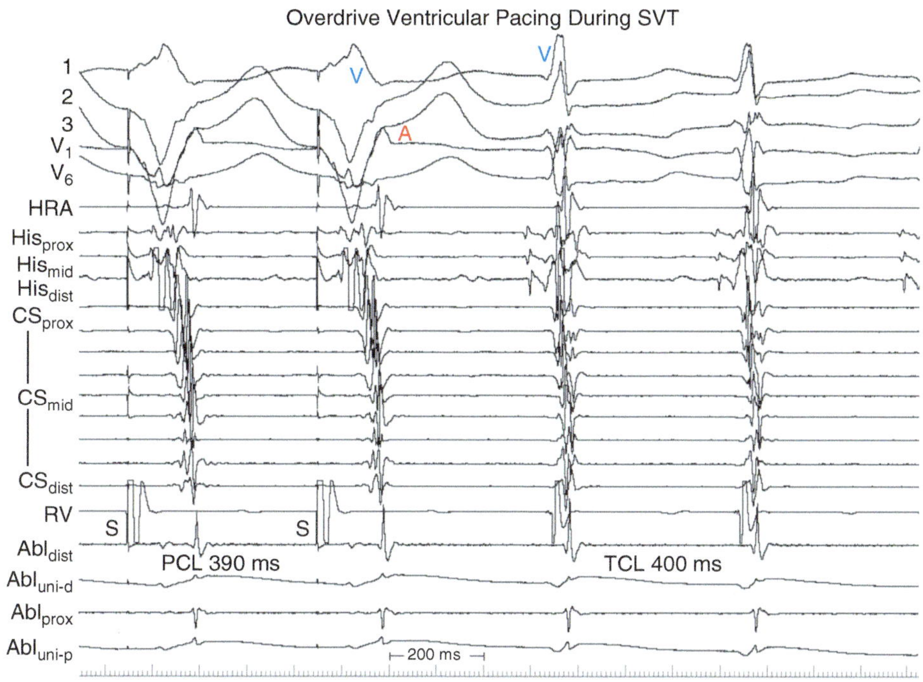

Figure 10-27

A "V-A-V" response seen with ventricular overdrive pacing during SVT excludes atrial tachycardia with a long PR interval and, with all the other data taken together, largely makes a diagnosis of AV nodal reentry (Fig. 10-27). Although this arrhythmia had not been documented clinically, it seemed prudent to undertake ablation at this setting because it was sustained and rather rapid.

Figure 10-28

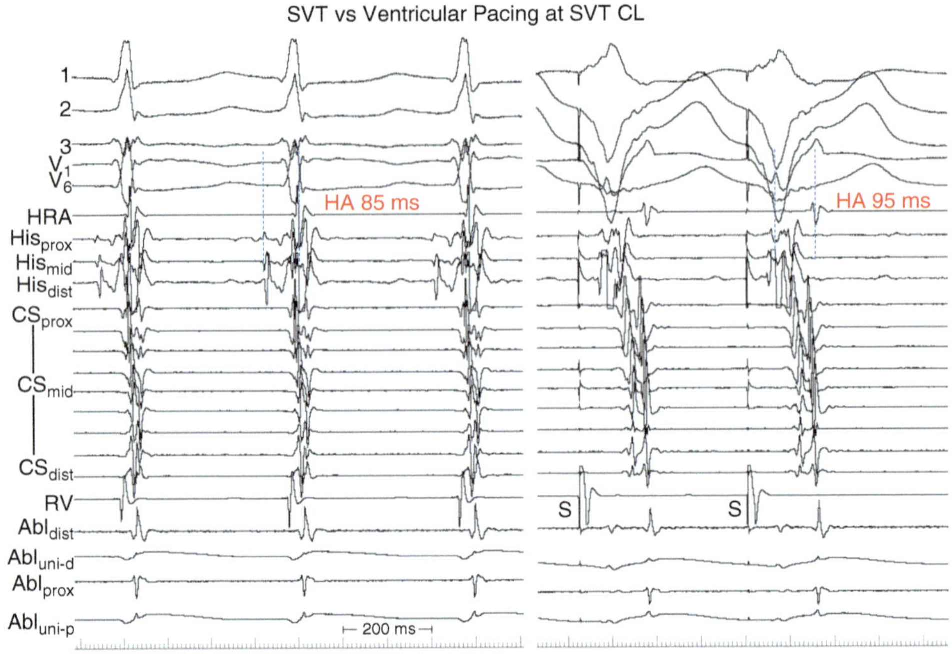

Additional evidence for AV nodal reentry, and against atrial or junctional tachycardias, is the HA interval in SVT vs ventricular pacing at the SVT cycle length. In Fig. 10-28, the HA in SVT (from onset of proximal His potential to HRA atrial recording, *dashed lines*) is 85 ms, slightly less than the HA during ventricular pacing at SVT cycle length (measured from end of proximal His deflection to same HRA atrial recording, *dashed lines*). If this were a junctional/His bundle tachycardia, these intervals should be the same; if atrial tachycardia, there is no reason that they should be similar because retrograde conduction with pacing and AH interval during atrial tachycardia are completely independent occurrences.

Catheter Manipulation at Tricuspid Annulus

Figure 10-29

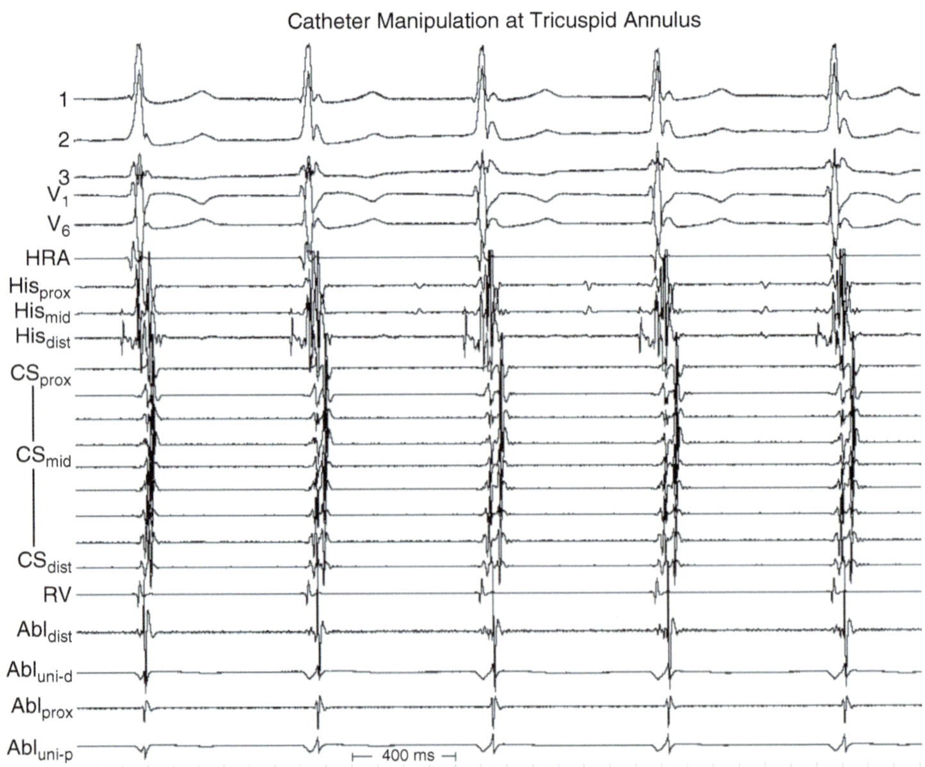

While positioning the ablation catheter for AV nodal slow pathway ablation, the rhythm shown in Fig. 10-29 was recorded. This is irritative junctional rhythm from the catheter rubbing on the slow pathway region, indicative of a good site for ablation. Note that, although this appears to be junctional with retrograde conduction, the P waves in the surface ECG are positive, indicating that this is sinus rhythm at almost the same rate.

Successful catheter ablation of the AV nodal slow pathway was accomplished, resulting in accelerated junctional rhythm; inducible AV node reentry was eliminated and atrial tachycardia likewise did not occur, either in the baseline state or after isoproterenol provocation. Normal AV conduction was present at the end of the procedure. After recovery, the patient did well without recurrence of any form of tachycardia and had normalization of left ventricular systolic function 3 months later.

Summary

- Focal AT can cause tachycardia-mediated cardiomyopathy; it is unusual to have the reverse (cardiomyopathy causing AT).
- Features of tachycardia-mediated cardiomyopathy:
  - No symptoms until HF occurs (no palpitations)
  - Ventricular rate 120–140/min (fast enough to cause HF, slow enough to escape detection/not cause palpitations, etc.)
  - HF can be cured when tachycardia is eliminated.
  - HF can recur if rapid rate recurs.
- Lessons:
  - Before ablating, delineate general mechanism: focal vs macroreentry.
  - Focal tachycardia target site features: <40 ms before P wave; QS unipolar
  - Bump mapping: signifies that the target site occupies a small critical area that is very superficial; but because this often occurs with sudden catheter movement, the catheter tip is rarely still at the "bumped" tissue by the time this is noticed.
  - Patients can have more than one type of tachycardia/cause of symptoms.

11 Focal Left Atrial Tachycardia

Case Presentation

A 73-year-old woman with recent onset renal failure complained of palpitations and near syncope for the last few weeks, with increasing frequency during dialysis. ECG showed non-sustained episodes of wide as well as narrow complex tachycardia, CL ~370 ms. She had a history of hypertension; her renal disease was of unclear cause (normal renal function 6 months prior to being on dialysis [via indwelling subclavian catheter]). She is being considered for living related donor transplant. Her last 10 dialysis sessions were stopped prematurely due to tachycardia episodes. Physical examination findings were normal aside from mild hypertension and the dialysis catheter. Her resting ECG showed a possible old anterior scar. An echocardiogram showed left ventricular hypertrophy, stage 2 diastolic dysfunction and mitral annular calcification. She was referred for electrophysiology (EP) study and possible ablation of narrow and wide QRS tachycardias.

Baseline ECG and Intracardiac Recordings

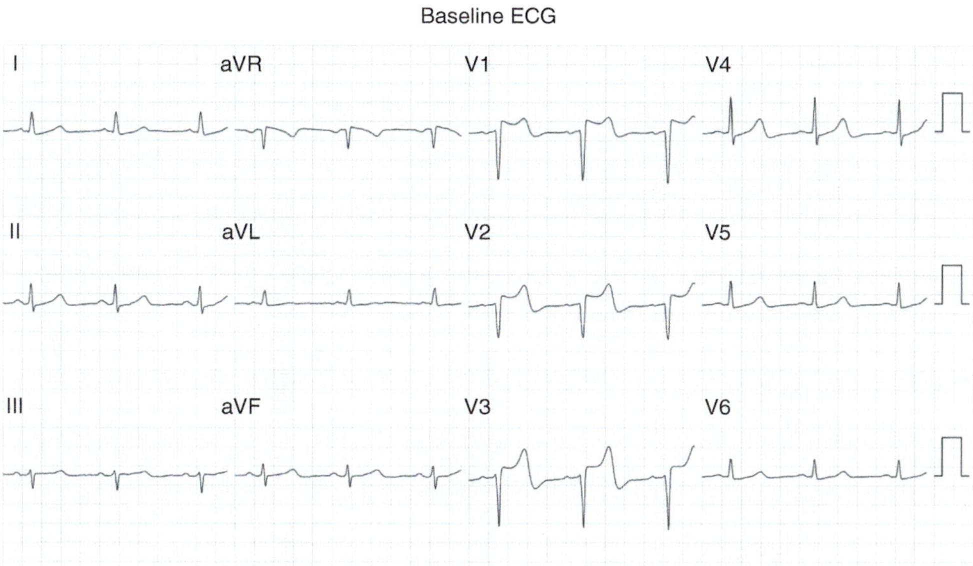

Figure 11-1

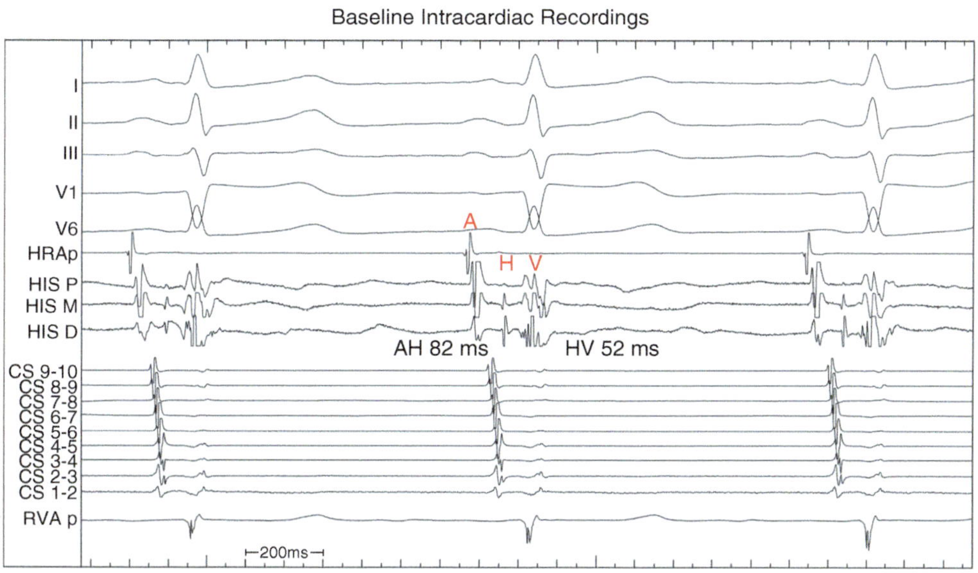

Figure 11-2

In Fig. 11-1 and Fig. 11-2, all intervals are normal. The ST elevation in V1–V3 in Fig. 11-1 is a recording artifact; R-wave progression is delayed but there is no definite infarct pattern. There are no clues from ECG or standard intracardiac recordings as to the nature of the rhythm disturbances.

Ventricular Pacing

What Is the Differential Diagnosis?
Where Is the Block?
[Fig. 11-3]

Figure 11-3

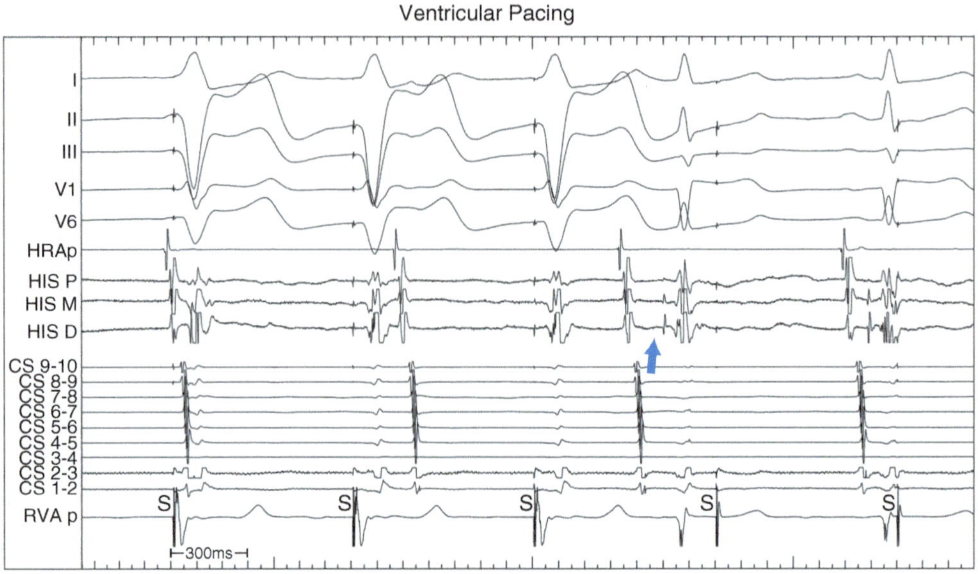

One of the first tests to perform is ventricular pacing to assess retrograde conduction (presence, pattern); in Fig. 11-3, there is no retrograde conduction (sinus complexes continue unaffected by ventricular pacing). This immediately makes orthodromic supraventricular tachycardia (SVT) related to a concealed bypass tract extremely unlikely, and even atrioventricular (AV) nodal reentry usually has retrograde conduction over the fast pathway at rest. In some cases of AV nodal reentry (and rare cases of orthodromic SVT), retrograde conduction may be restored after isoproterenol infusion and SVT can be induced under those conditions. However, the absence of retrograde conduction at this point makes an atrial tachycardia more likely as the cause of the patient's SVT.

The site of retrograde block is identified as the AV node, because the atrio-His interval following a paced complex *(arrow)* is longer than the resting AH (complex at right) because of concealed conduction into the AV node.

What Next?

After some additional testing, we now know that the AH (82 ms) and HV (52 ms) intervals are normal; the AV Wenckebach cycle length is 430 ms; there is no VA conduction; anterograde dual-AV nodal pathways are present, without echoes or inducible tachycardia; and no sustained arrhythmias can be initiated with atrial or ventricular stimulation (bursts, extrastimuli).

Atrial Pacing on Low-Dose Isoproterenol

What Is the Differential Diagnosis? [Fig. 11-4]

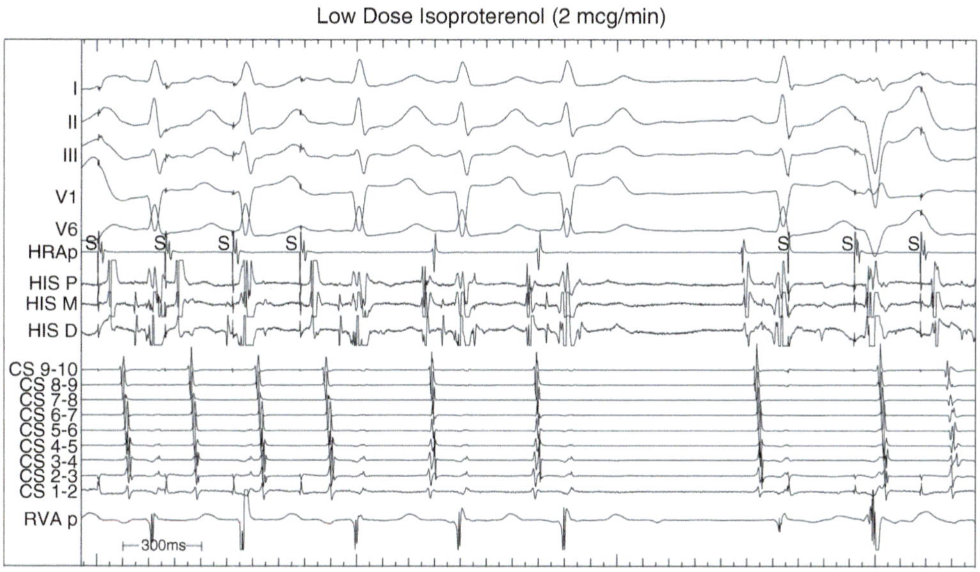

Figure 11-4

In the absence of inducible arrhythmias in the baseline state, isoproterenol infusion is begun. In Fig. 11-4, atrial pacing induces two cycles of tachycardia. This is described as a "long RP" rhythm, the differential diagnosis for which is atrial tachycardia, atypical AV nodal reentry (anterograde fast, retrograde slow pathways), and orthodromic reentry related to a slowly conducting bypass tract. The mode of initiation would be quite unusual for AV nodal reentry, because conduction would have to block in the slow pathway with the last atrial stimulus, conduct over the fast pathway, and yet go back up the slow pathway to form the first beat of tachycardia. The other two possibilities (atrial tachycardia or orthodromic reentry) remain.

Higher Dose Isoproterenol

Spontaneous SVT Onset

What Is the Differential Diagnosis [Fig. 11-5]? What Do You Need to Do to Figure It Out?

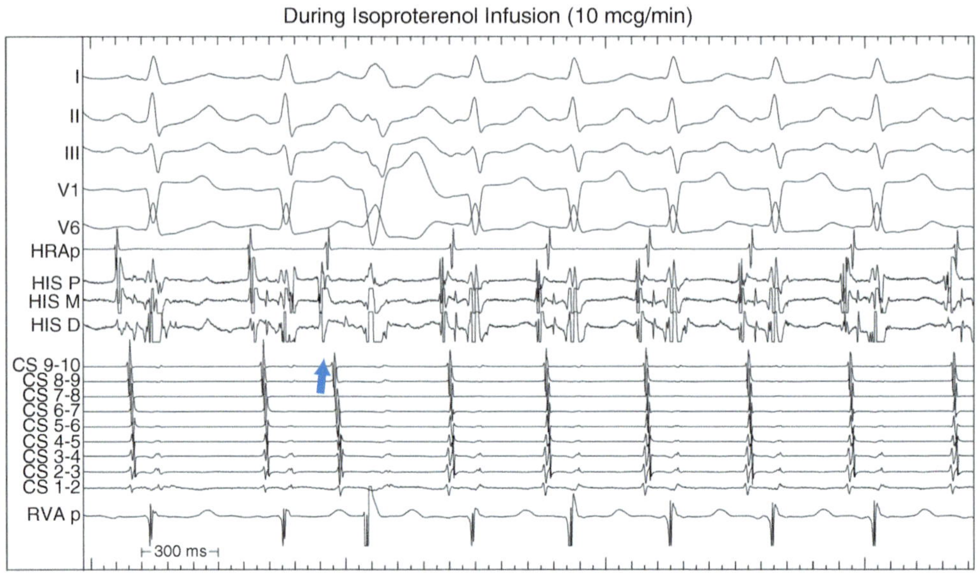

Figure 11-5

With an increase in the dose of isoproterenol, tachycardia occurs spontaneously. A spontaneous atrial premature complex (*arrow*, Fig. 11-5) appears to be conducted with left bundle branch block (LBBB) aberration, after which sustained narrow QRS tachycardia ensues. The atrial activation sequence is the same as in the two cycles of the rhythm seen in the previous figure on a lower dose isoproterenol, and is "concentric." This is consistent with a typical fast pathway exit (less so with slow pathway exit), a septal bypass tract, or a septal (or slightly left-sided) atrial tachycardia. Further testing is needed to distinguish among these possible diagnoses.

ECG and Intracardiac Recordings in SVT

What Is the Differential Diagnosis [Fig. 11-6]?

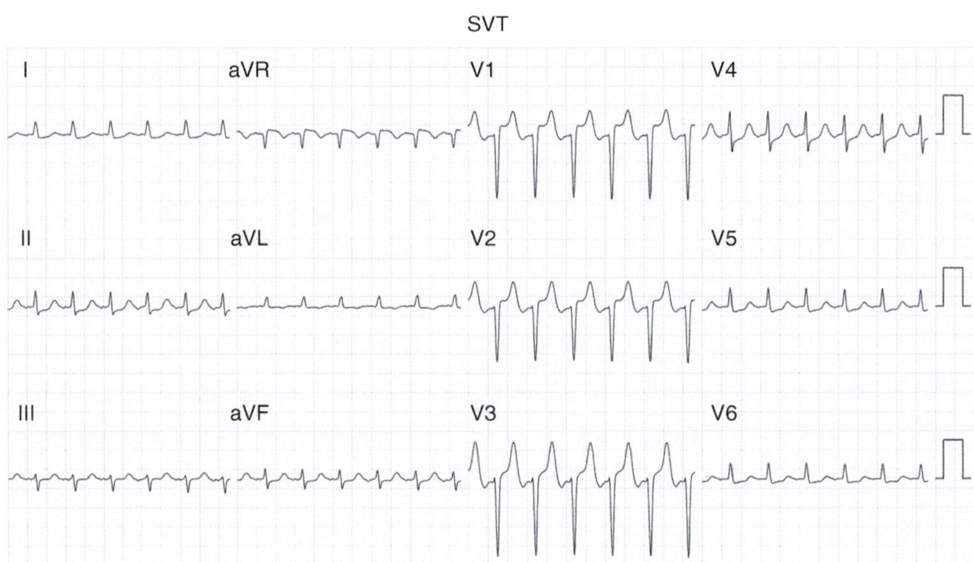

Figure 11-6

A 12-lead ECG of sustained tachycardia is shown in Fig. 11-6. The location and configuration of the P wave is less evident here than on the intracardiac recordings.

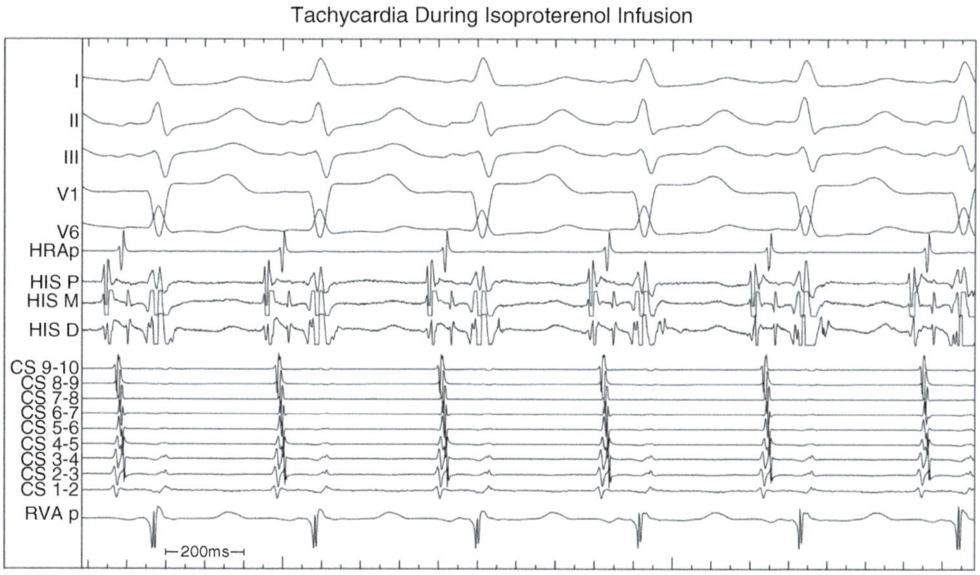

Figure 11-7

Intracardiac recordings of tachycardia are again shown (Fig. 11-7) at a more rapid sweep speed. It is clear that earliest activation among the atrial recordings is at the region of the His bundle.

SVT Termination

What Is the Differential Diagnosis? [Fig. 11-8]

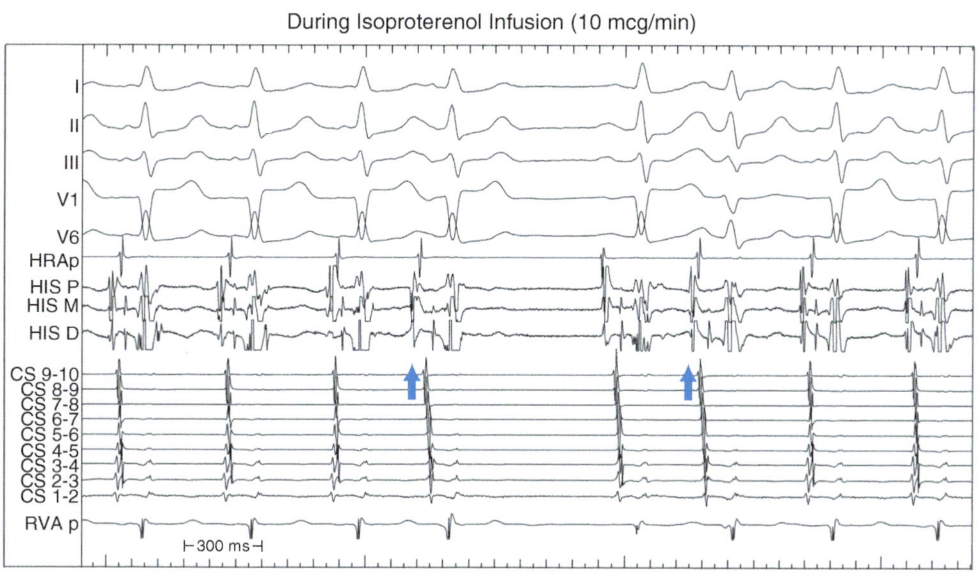

Figure 11-8

In Fig. 11-8, tachycardia suddenly terminates after an atrial premature complex *(arrow)*. A sinus complex follows and then another atrial premature complex *(second arrow)*, and then tachycardia resumes. The fact that sustained tachycardia is terminated as well as initiated by atrial premature complexes that appear to be different from the ongoing tachycardia is suggestive of a reentrant, rather than focal, atrial tachycardia. However, none of the other tachycardia diagnoses have been definitively eliminated as yet.

Ventricular Pacing During Sinus Rhythm

What All Does This Tell? [Fig. 11-9]

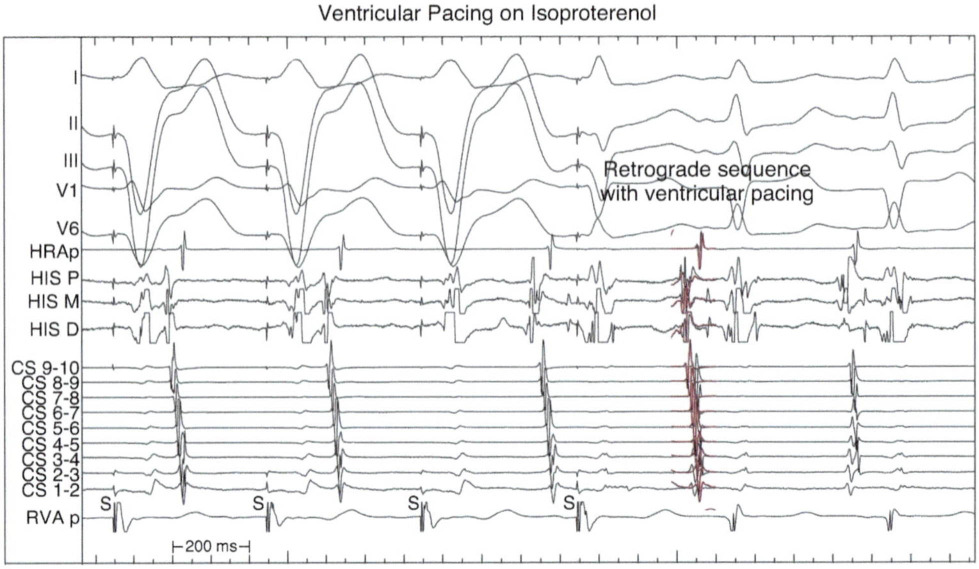

Figure 11-9

Ventricular pacing is now performed during sinus rhythm while on the isoproterenol infusion. As is often the case, retrograde conduction is restored with isoproterenol where it had been absent in the baseline state. On the first two complexes shown in Fig. 11-9, retrograde conduction is concentric with a short retrograde conduction time; on the third complex, a longer retrograde conduction time is seen followed by a His potential and narrow QRS complex despite another stimulus artifact occurring. This is indicative of retrograde dual-AV nodal physiology (retrograde slow pathway, anterograde fast pathway), one of the potential mechanisms of the patient's tachycardia (which starts immediately thereafter). However, the atrial activation sequence of the retrogradely conducted complexes (superimposed in red on an SVT complex) is a little different from that of tachycardia, indicating that the tachycardia diagnosis is probably not, in fact, AV nodal reentry. A slowly conducting bypass tract mediating orthodromic reentry also seems very unlikely because the atrial activation sequence during ventricular pacing is different from tachycardia, but has not been definitively excluded at this point

Wide-QRS Complex Tachycardia ECG and Intracardiac Recordings

What Is the Differential Diagnosis? [Fig. 11-10]

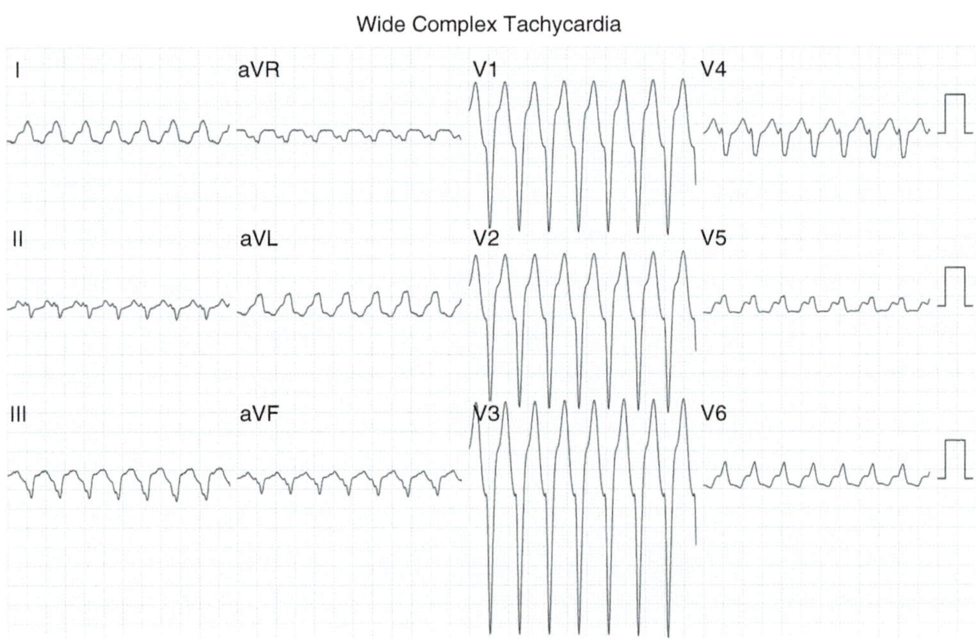

Figure 11-10

A few minutes later, while still on isoproterenol, a wide complex tachycardia occurs (Fig. 11-10). Recall that the patient had both narrow and wide complex tachycardias with similar rates. The tachycardia shown has a rate nearly identical to that of the narrow complex tachycardia encountered minutes earlier, and has a left branch block configuration consistent with SVT with aberration.

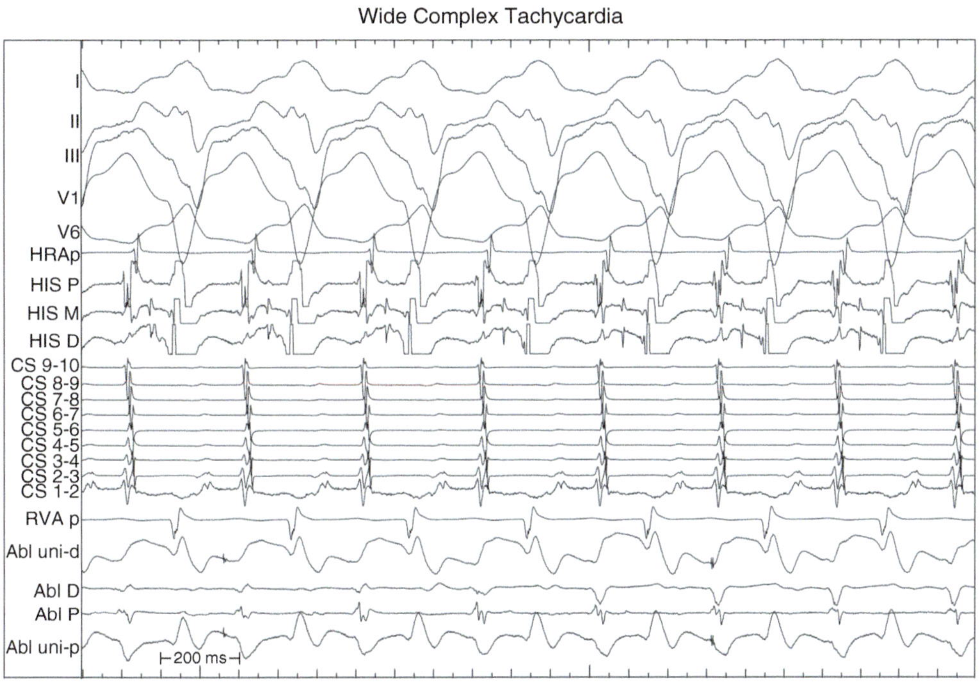

Figure 11-11

Intracardiac recordings from around the same time (Fig. 11-11) show a 1:1 atrioventricular relationship, with an atrial activation sequence identical to that of the narrow complex tachycardia. In addition, a His potential precedes every QRS complex, indicating that the rhythm is supraventricular with aberration.

The coronary sinus catheter has been advanced somewhat, accounting for its change in activation sequence and timing relative to the His bundle atrial activation.

Wide-to-Narrow QRS Tachycardia Transition

Why Did the QRS Narrow? [Fig. 11-12]

Figure 11-12

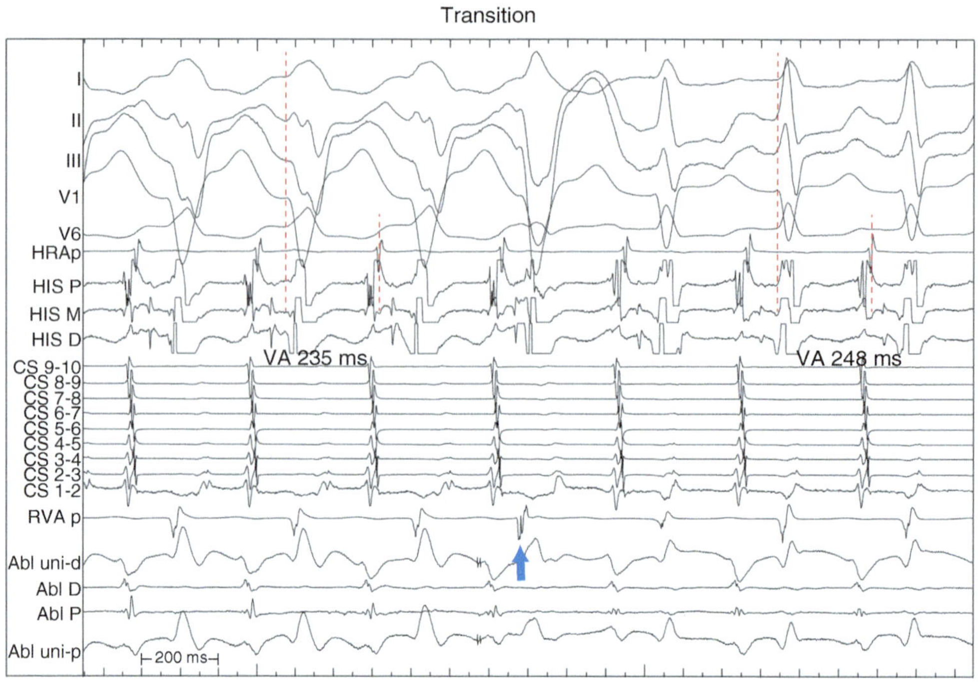

Spontaneous transition from wide to narrow QRS complex is seen in Fig. 11-12. An important measurement to make in this situation is the VA interval (onset of QRS to an atrial electrogram *[dashed lines]*). With orthodromic reentry related to a left-sided bypass tract, the VA interval with LBBB will exceed that during narrow QRS tachycardia by >35 ms. In this example, there is no difference in the VA intervals, excluding participation of a left free wall bypass tract.

The QRS complex narrowed because of a spontaneous premature ventricular complex from the right ventricle *(arrow)* that likely prematurely activated the LBBB, allowing it more time to recover for the subsequent complex, that could then conduct normally.

Ventricular Pacing in SVT to Delineate P-Wave Onset

What's Up with This? [Fig. 11-13]

Figure 11-13

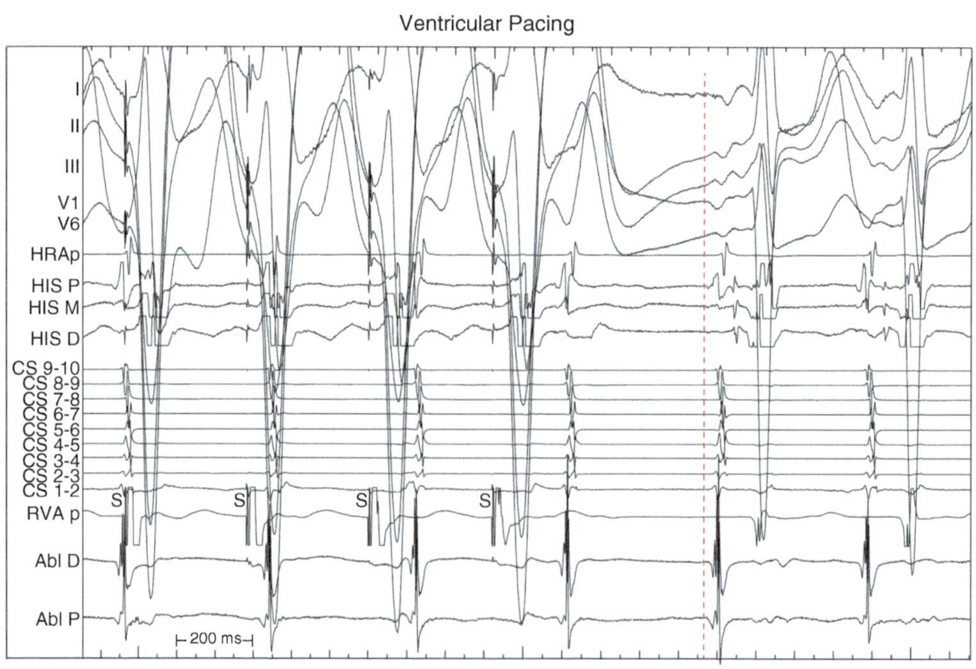

In Fig. 11-13, ventricular pacing is performed during tachycardia; surface ECG leads have increased gain to demonstrate P-wave onset for mapping purposes *(dashed red line)*. Of note, atrial activation continues throughout the figure unaffected by ventricular pacing; this excludes orthodromic reentry, in which atrial activation depends on prior ventricular activation. Because this and AV nodal reentry have now been excluded, the diagnosis is atrial tachycardia. Now that the P wave onset has been clarified, it can be indexed to another more readily seen recording (such as HRA, 50 ms after P wave onset) to compare the timing of mapping sites, without having to guess where the P wave starts or repeat ventricular pacing to discern it.

Right Atrial and then Coronary Sinus Pacing During Tachycardia

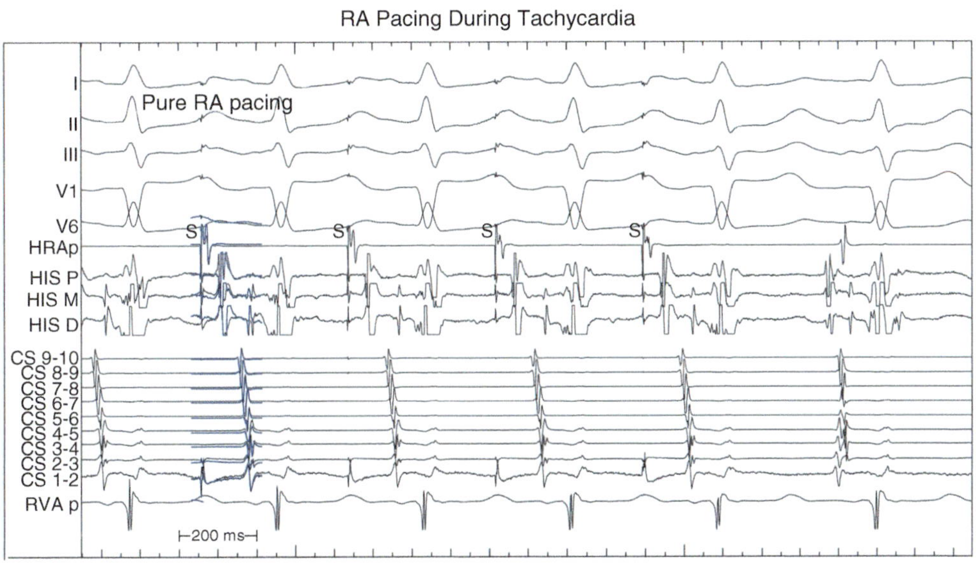

Figure 11-14

Now that a diagnosis of atrial tachycardia has been established, it remains to be determined whether this is because of macroreentry or a focal process. The modes of initiation and termination seen in previous figures are consistent with either. In the example shown in Fig. 11-14, a complex of "pure" right atrial pacing *(blue)* obtained during sinus rhythm is superimposed on a complex of pacing from the same site during tachycardia (a tachycardia beat resumes at right). It is clear that the activation sequence is the same whether pacing during sinus rhythm or tachycardia, indicating absence of fusion. Mere absence of fusion when pacing from one site does not establish a diagnosis of a focal process (however, if macroreentry is present, it is often possible to demonstrate fusion when pacing from a single site).

What Do the Results of Pacing During Tachycardia Tell Us? [Fig. 11-15]

Figure 11-15

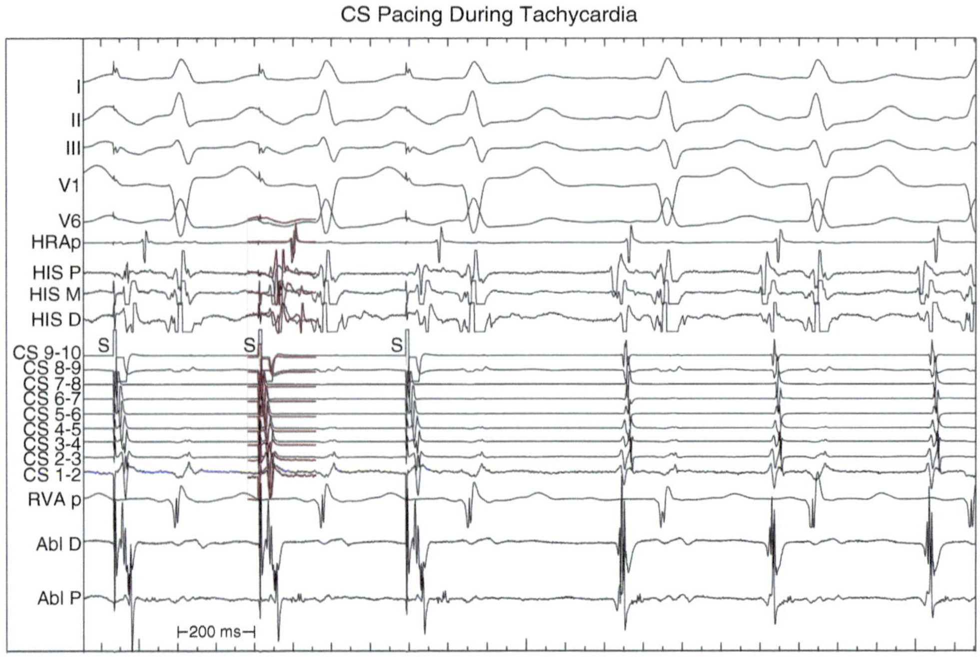

In Fig. 11-15, pacing from the proximal coronary sinus (CS) is shown during tachycardia (that resumes at right) as well as a single complex of "pure" CS pacing during sinus rhythm superimposed *(red)*. Again, there is no difference between these, and thus no fusion. Similar results were obtained when pacing from the distal CS (not shown). Thus absence of fusion when pacing from multiple sites, and ideally at multiple cycle lengths, makes a focal process far more likely. This was the diagnosis in this case.

Activation and Pace Mapping in Right Atrium

Is This a Good Site?

Figure 11-16

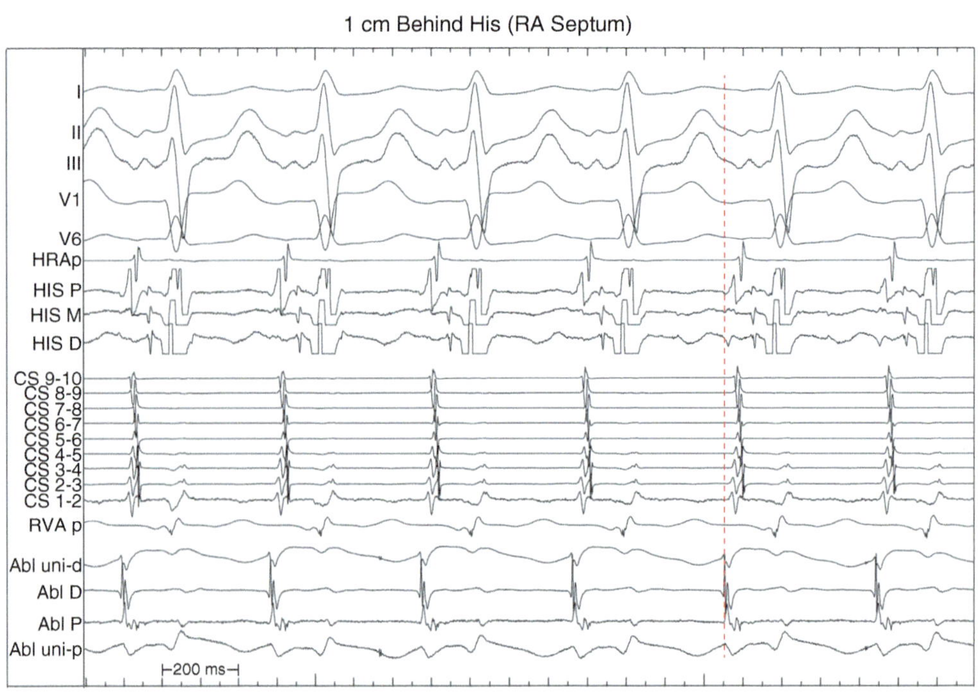

Now that a focal atrial tachycardia has been diagnosed, an electrogram that is 30–40 ms before the P-wave onset may be sought for ablation. Mapping on the right side of the interatrial septum (Fig. 11-16), near the His bundle location, discloses a site about 5 ms before P-wave onset (*dashed red line*, 50 ms before HRA recording as demonstrated in figure). The unipolar recording has a small initial R wave; this, as well as the unimpressive timing of the atrial electrogram, excludes this as a good site for ablation.

Well?

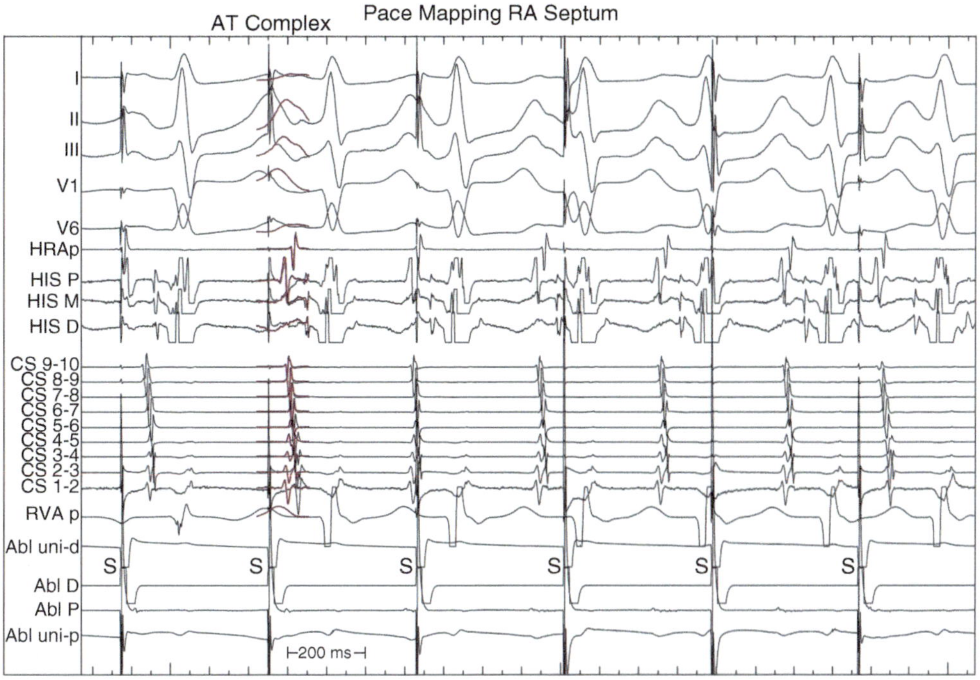

Figure 11-17

Further evidence that this is not a good site for ablation is the fact that pacing from that site yields a very different atrial activation sequence compared with that during tachycardia (Fig. 11-17, in *red*). Pacing from the site of impulse formation of a focal tachycardia should exactly replicate the atrial activation sequence during tachycardia.

Electroanatomic Mapping of Right Atrium

Figure 11-18

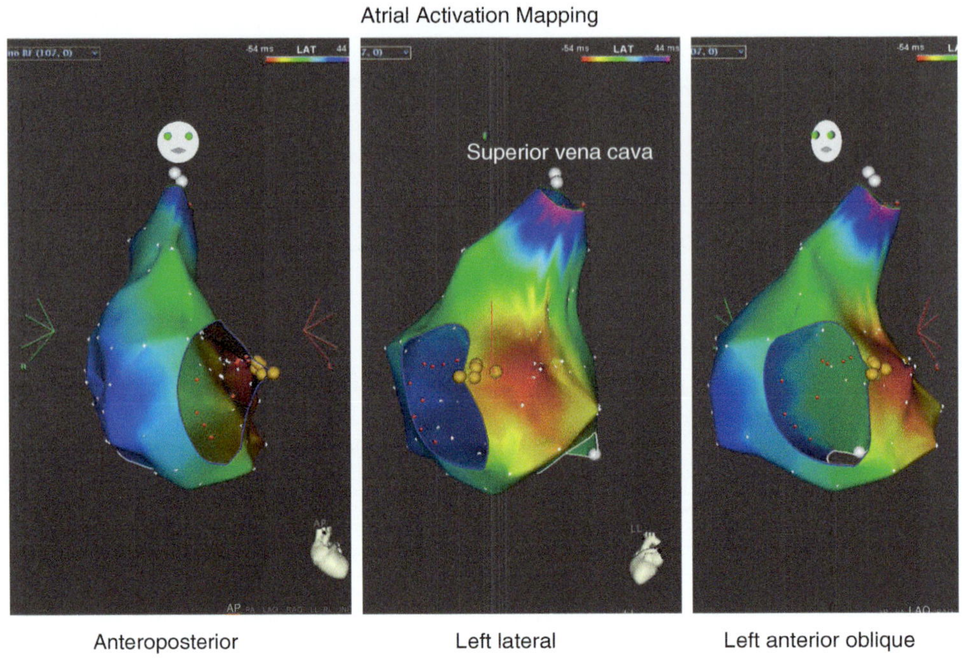

What Next?

Electroanatomic activation mapping of the right atrium during tachycardia (Fig. 11-18) shows a pattern of centrifugal spread from a focus just behind the His bundle location *(orange dots)*. At this time in the procedure, we have diagnosed narrow and wide QRS tachycardia that appear to have the same cause (focal atrial tachycardia); the tachycardia has earliest activation at or just behind the His bundle recording site, but is not very early (5 ms before P-wave onset); the earliest site covers a rather broad area; and the pace-match from there is poor. Isoproterenol is still required to sustain tachycardia for mapping but the patient's blood pressure is 200/120 mm Hg.

Activation and Pace Mapping Left Atrial Site

Figure 11-19

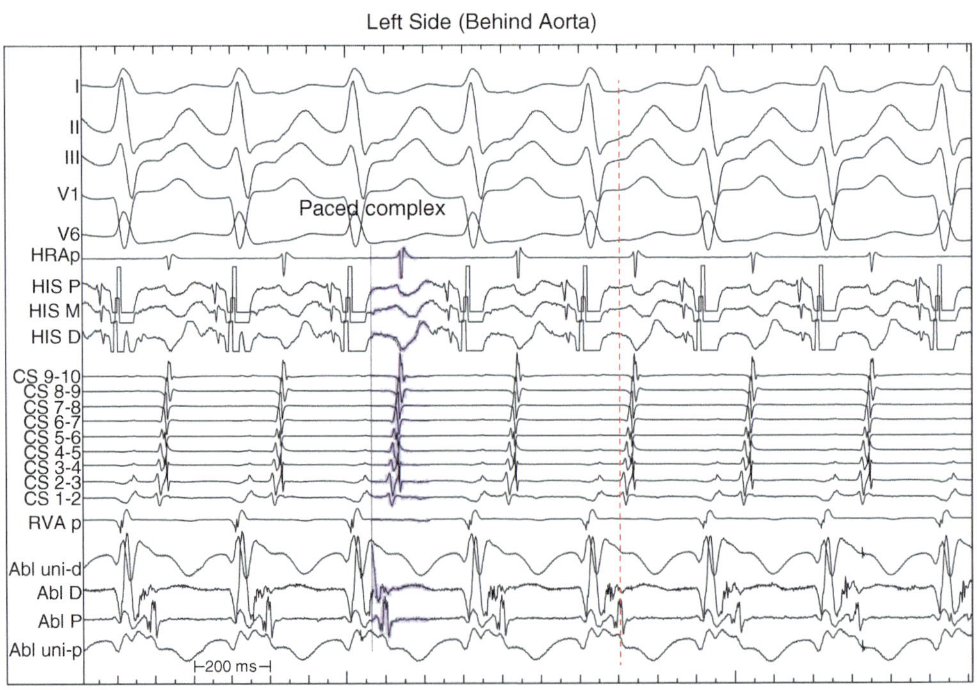

Despite the focal activation pattern on the electroanatomic map, no right atrial site showed reasonable activation times; in such cases, the left side of the septum, right superior pulmonary vein, and aortomitral continuity/mitral annulus should be evaluated before ablating behind the His bundle. After transseptal catheterization, mapping of these structures was accomplished; the site shown in Fig. 11-19 is on the mitral annulus at its junction with the aortic root (large ventricular, small and fractionated atrial electrogram). A single complex of pacing from this site is shown *(purple)* superimposed on tachycardia, yielding a perfect match. The unipolar recording is not as helpful in this situation because a large ventricular electrogram obscures the smaller atrial signal. The electrogram at this site is fragmented and considerably before the P wave onset (*dashed red line*, known from relation to HRA recording as in Fig. 11-13).

Radiofrequency Application at Left Atrial Site

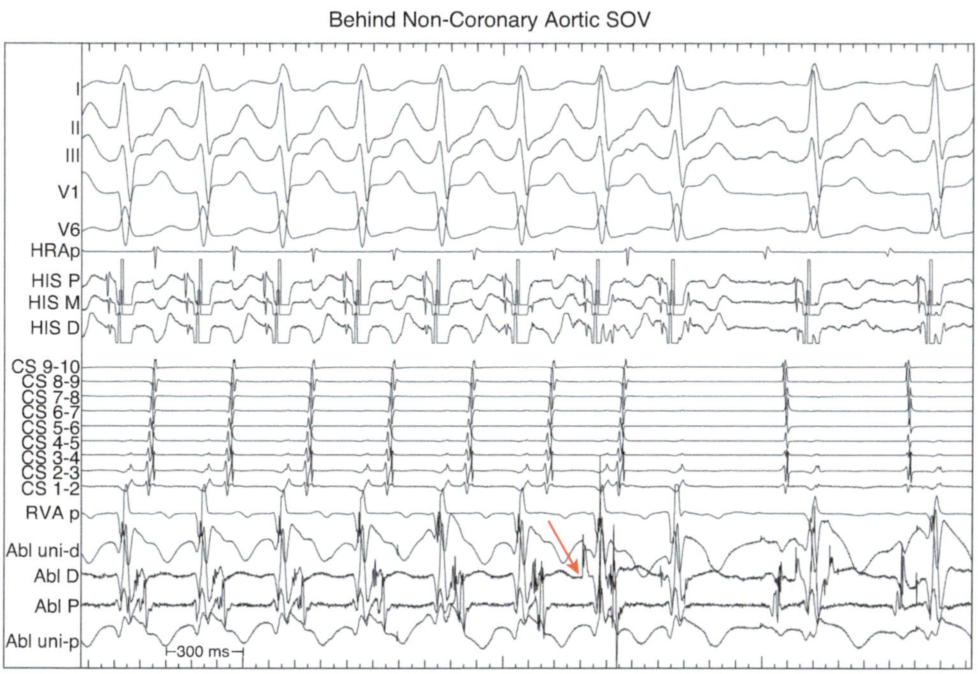

Figure 11-20

Radiofrequency (RF) energy is delivered at the site shown in Fig. 11-20 at the time indicated; tachycardia terminates immediately to sinus rhythm. Additional RF applications were made in this region.

Comparison of Best Right and Left Atrial Sites

Figure 11-21

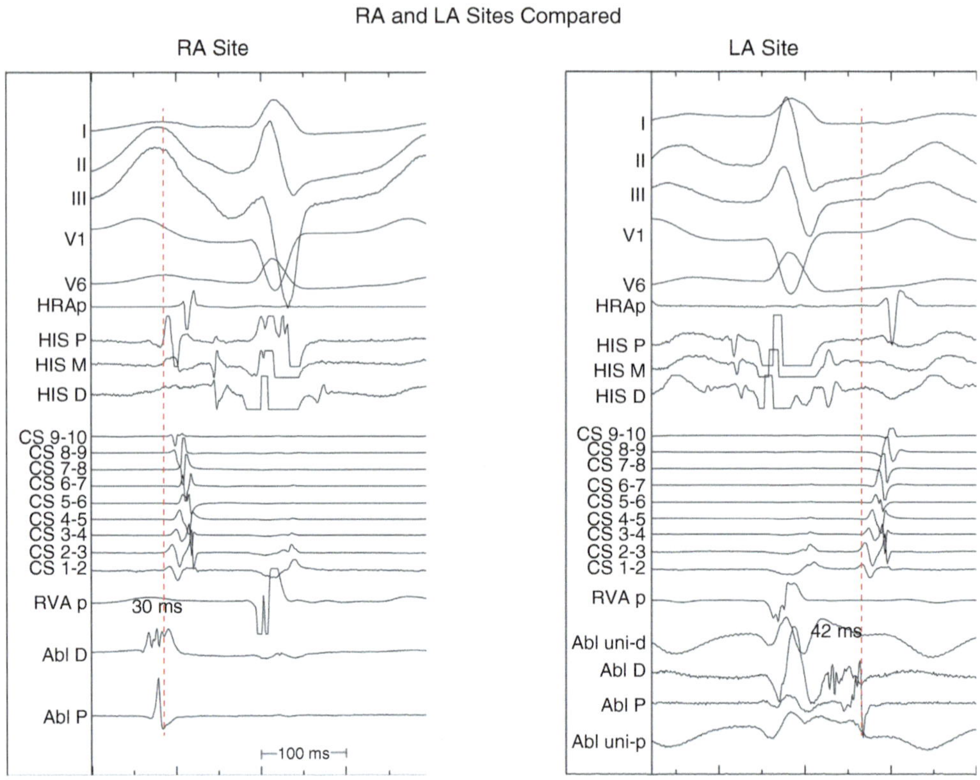

A comparison of mapping sites at rapid sweep speed is shown in Fig. 11-21. The best right atrial site is shown at left, preceding the P-wave onset (*dashed red line*, indexed from the timing of the CS atrial recordings) by 30 ms. In contrast, the successful ablation site on the mitral annulus occurs 42 ms before P-wave onset.

Electroanatomic Map of Left Atrium

Figure 11-22

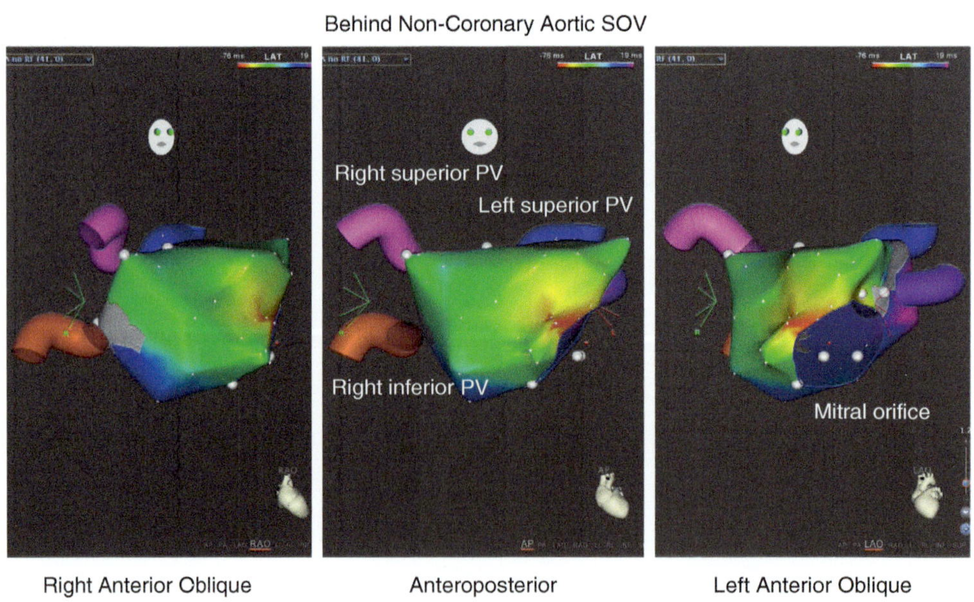

Electroanatomic activation map during tachycardia of the left atrium is shown in Fig. 11-22, with a focal propagation pattern from a site *(red spot)* on the anterior medial mitral annulus.

Fluoroscopic Views of Best Right and Left Atrial Sites

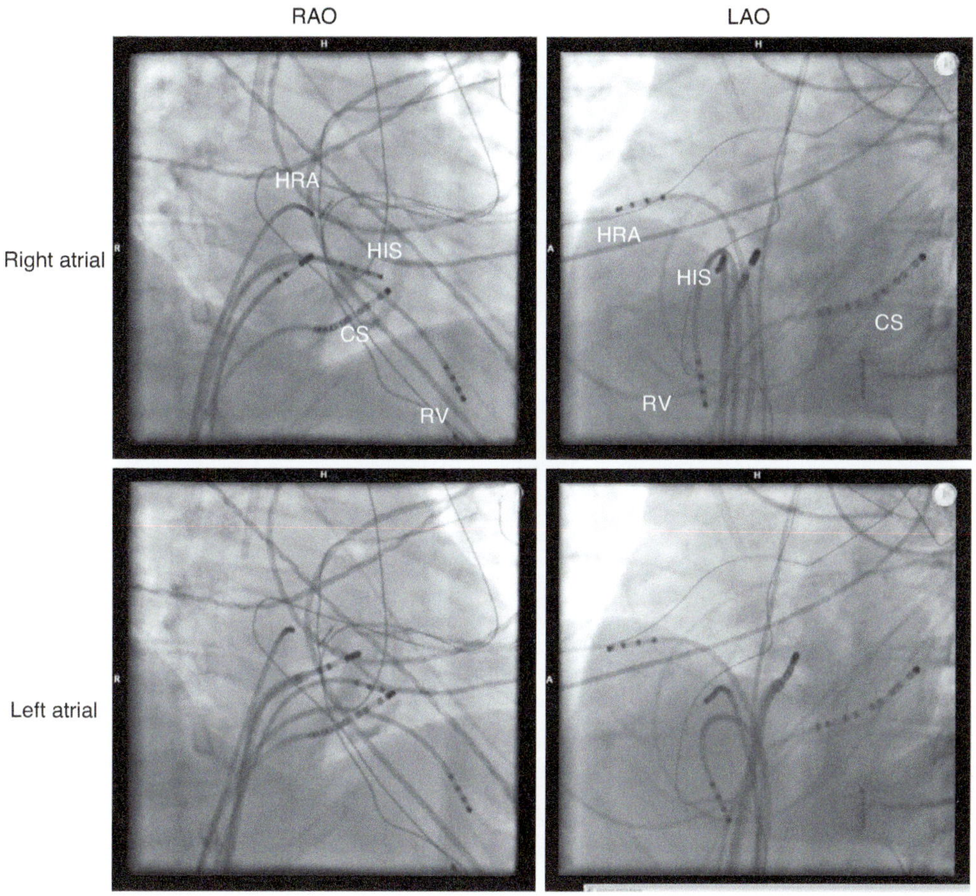

Figure 11-23

Fig. 11-23 displays comparative fluoroscopic views of catheter locations at sites of the earliest right and left atrial activation during SVT (catheter with large electrode at tip). *CS*, coronary sinus; *HRA*, high right atrium; *LAO*, left anterior oblique; *RAO*, right anterior oblique; *RV*, right ventricle.

Cutaway View of Atrioventricular Groove

Figure 11-24

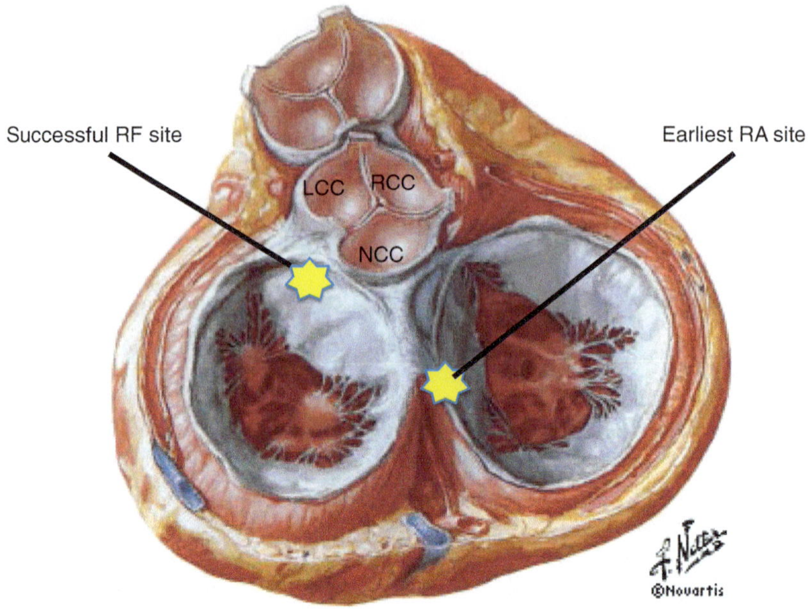

Fig. 11-24 shows atrioventricular valves annuli viewed from above, with both the successful left atrial ablation site and site of the earliest right atrial activation indicated. *LCC*, left coronary cusp; *NCC*, noncoronary cusp; *RCC*, right coronary cusp. (Copyright [2016] Elsevier Inc. All rights reserved. www.netterimages.com.)

Summary

- Atrial tachycardia can strike at any age.
- Know your mechanism (focal vs macroreentry) before mapping (target-site characteristics are determined thereby).
- Focal atrial tachycardia can arise from many places.
- P-wave configuration in SVT provides substantial localization information before and during the procedure.
- "Earliest atrial activation at His" suggests the following:
  - Right superior PV source (His-A after P-wave onset)
  - Left septal source (His-A ~10 ms before P-wave onset)
  - Anterior left atrial source (aortomitral continuity, etc.—His-A ~10 ms before P-wave onset)
  - Para-Hisian source (His-A ~20 ms before P-wave onset)
- Before ablating near the His, check out the left atrium.

Typical Atrial Flutter 12

Case Presentation

A 58-year-old man with a history of palpitations for several years had a diagnosis of atrial arrhythmias as well as bradycardia, but had no treatment for these. One year before his current presentation, he had an unheralded stroke with aphasia and hemiplegia. He underwent successful thrombolytic therapy with no residual neuorologic impairment. At the time of his stroke, he was diagnosed with atrial flutter and soon after, underwent attempted flutter ablation. At the end of an 8-hour procedure, cavotricuspid isthmus block was achieved but flutter was still present (thought to be either lower loop or intraisthmus reentry). He was chronically anticoagulated; he was also treated with propafenone, but without success. He began having palpitations and was referred for another ablation attempt. Left ventricular function was normal on echocardiography.

Baseline ECG and Intracardiac Recordings

Catheter Choices?
[Fig. 12-1]
Strategy?

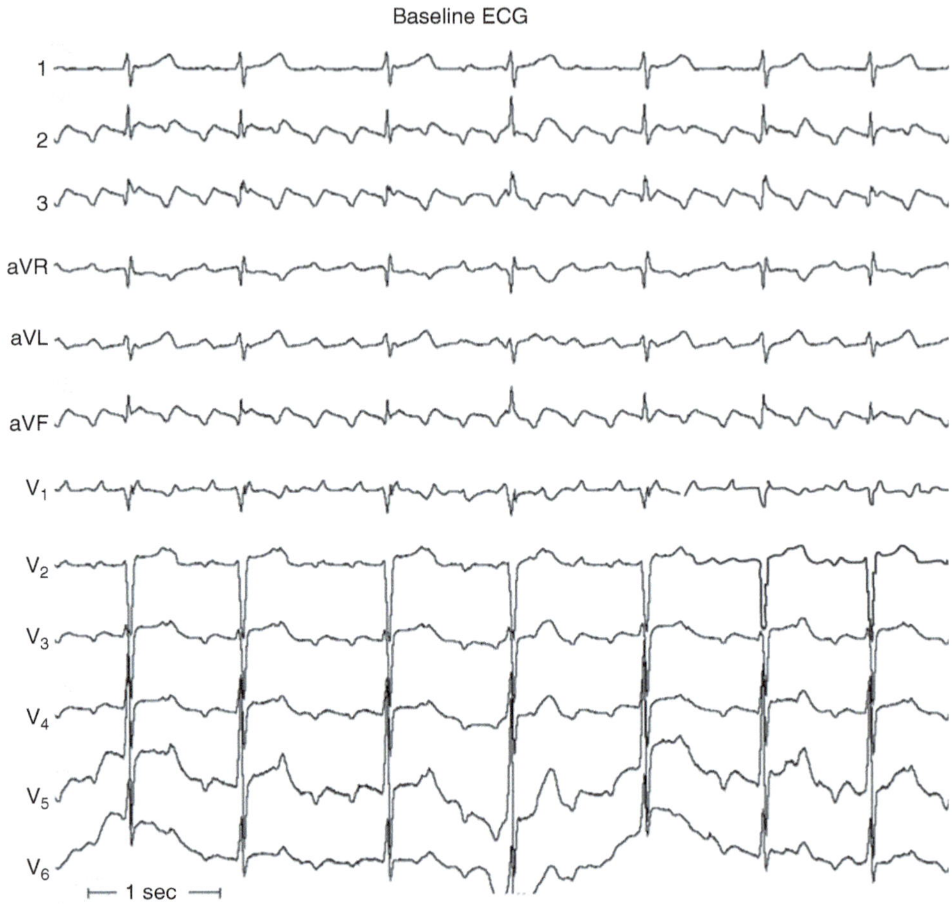

Figure 12-1

The baseline ECG in Fig. 12-1 appears to be consistent with typical right atrial cavotricuspid isthmus-dependent flutter, but that was said to have been ablated at the prior procedure. Reasonable choices for catheters are coronary sinus (with some electrodes near the ostium), tricuspid annular catheter ("halo"), and a His bundle catheter, as well as the ablation catheter.

We Begin with the Differential Diagnosis: [Fig. 12-2 and 12-3]

A. Typical CCW flutter
B. Lower loop reentry
C. Intraisthmus reentry
D. Focal AT near CS os
E. AT from left atrium

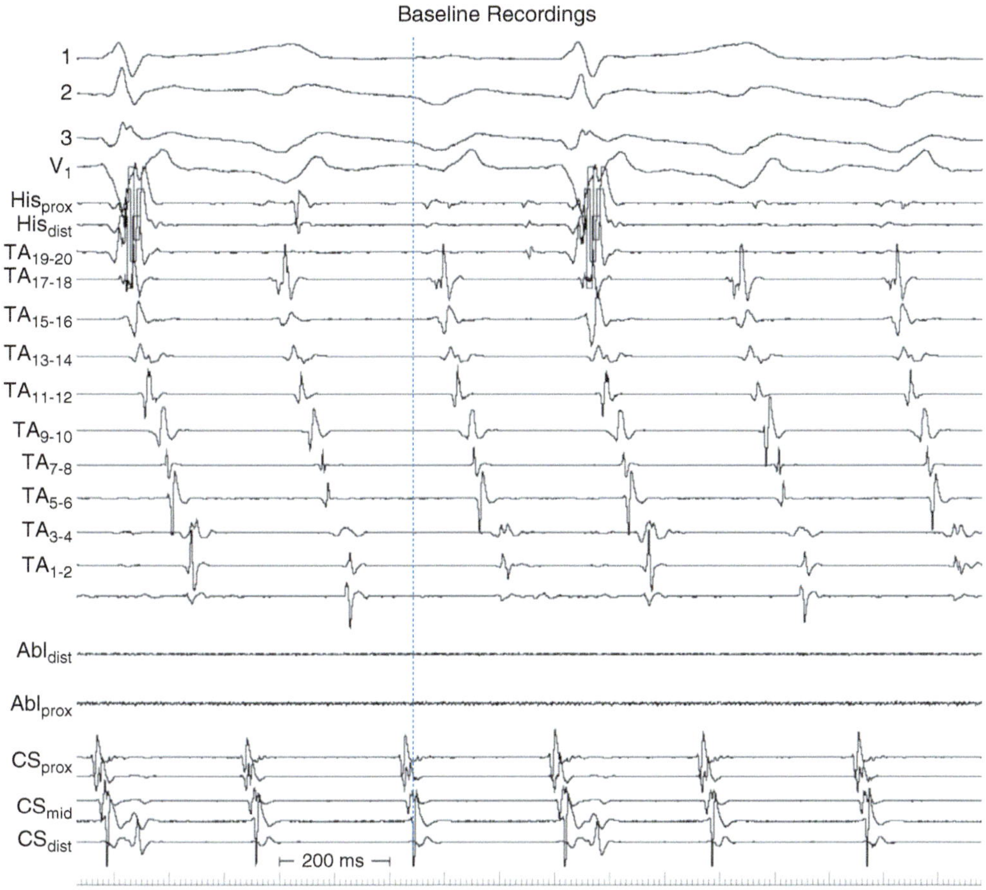

Figure 12-2

Intracardiac recordings of the baseline rhythm are shown in Fig. 12-2. Again, this appears to be entirely compatible with cavotricuspid isthmus reentry—but there are other possible diagnoses that should be eliminated before choosing an ablation target. A broad differential diagnosis includes typical counterclockwise (CCW) cavotricuspid isthmus flutter; lower loop reentry; intraisthmus reentry; focal atrial tachycardia (AT) near the coronary sinus ostium (CS); or atrial tachycardia from the left atrium.

Diagnostic Maneuvers

CS Distal Pacing

Differential diagnosis:
- typical CCW flutter
- lower loop reentry
- intra-isthmus reentry
- focal AT near CS os
- AT from left atrium

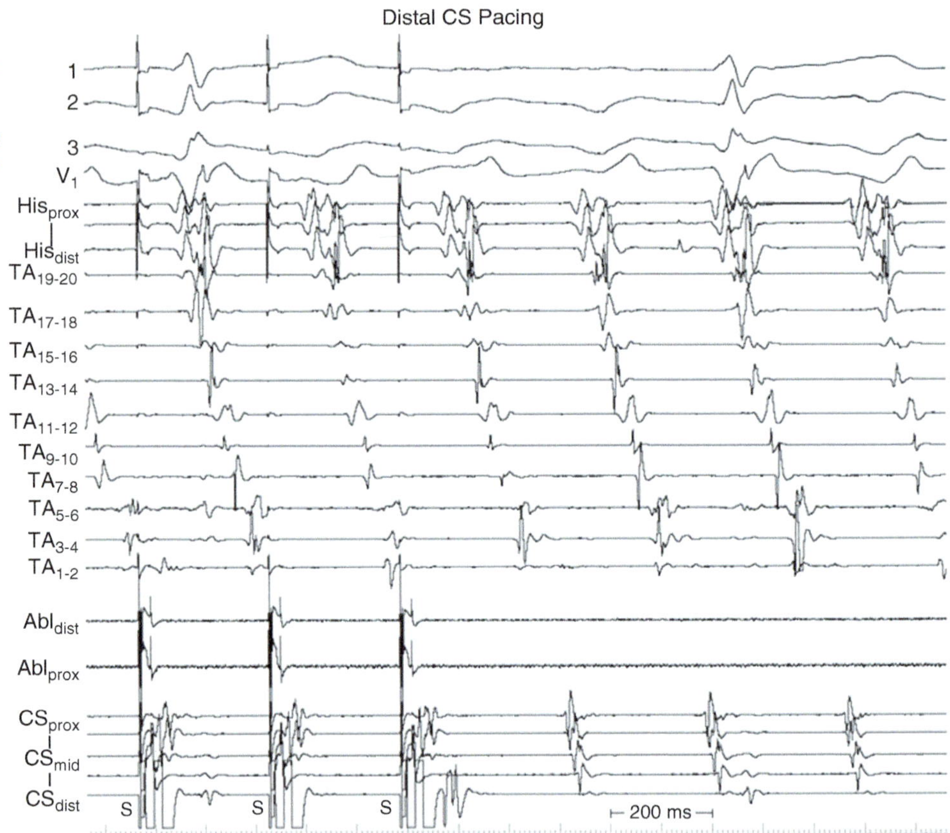

Figure 12-3

Burst pacing from the distal CS, as shown in Fig. 12-3, is a good way to start trying to distinguish among possible diagnoses; in a patient without prior ablation, pacing from this site during sinus rhythm should have a "chevron" appearance to the halo recordings (earlier at TA 1-2 and TA 19-20, latest at lateral right atrium [TA 11-12]). If such a pattern is seen with pacing from the CS during the tachycardia, it is not likely to be typical flutter. The activation pattern in halo recordings shown here looks the same as during tachycardia—suggesting fusion (some contribution from tachycardia, some from pacing). However, it is important to remember that this inference is valid if the patient has not had prior ablation in the right atrium that could disrupt activation patterns. Because this patient has had a previous ablation attempt, we cannot assume what pacing from the distal CS should look like, and thus cannot conclude that entrainment has been demonstrated. Unfortunately, pacing from the distal CS in this case appears to have little diagnostic value, and our differential diagnosis is unchanged.

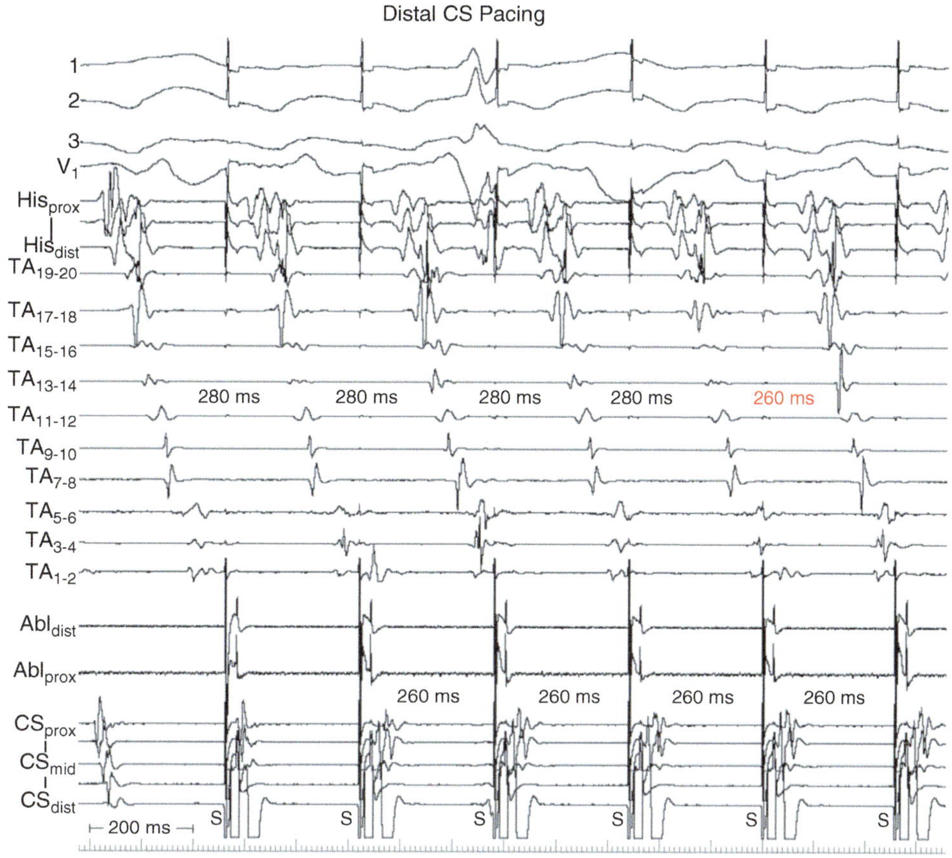

We Can Eliminate AT from Left Atrium from the Differential Diagnosis: [Fig. 12-4]

A. Typical CCW flutter
B. Lower loop reentry
C. Intraisthmus reentry
D. Focal AT near CS os

Figure 12-4

Although most attention is focused on what happens at the end of a pacing attempt, there is also information at the onset of pacing (Fig. 12-4). Here, with the onset of distal CS pacing, the proximal CS electrodes are controlled by the second stimulus and are accelerated to the paced cycle length (260 ms). The halo recordings, by contrast, are not accelerated until the fifth stimulus. If this tachycardia arose in the left atrium, as soon as that chamber is controlled, all other recordings that are passive should be controlled as well. Here, because the right atrial recordings continue unchanged for a few cycles after full left atrial control, the arrhythmia must arise in the right atrium. Thus one choice in the differential diagnosis (atrial tachycardia from the left atrium) has been eliminated.

Differential diagnosis:
- typical CCW flutter
- lower loop reentry
- intra-isthmus reentry

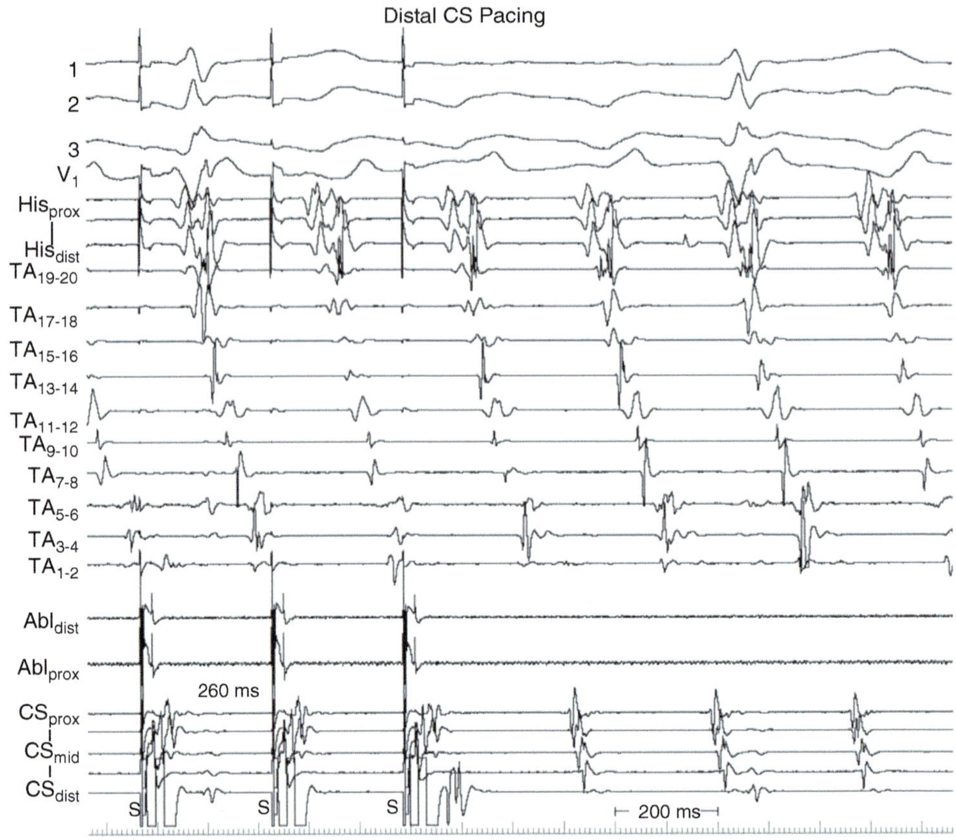

Figure 12-5A

Differential diagnosis:
- typical CCW flutter
- lower loop reentry
- intra-isthmus reentry

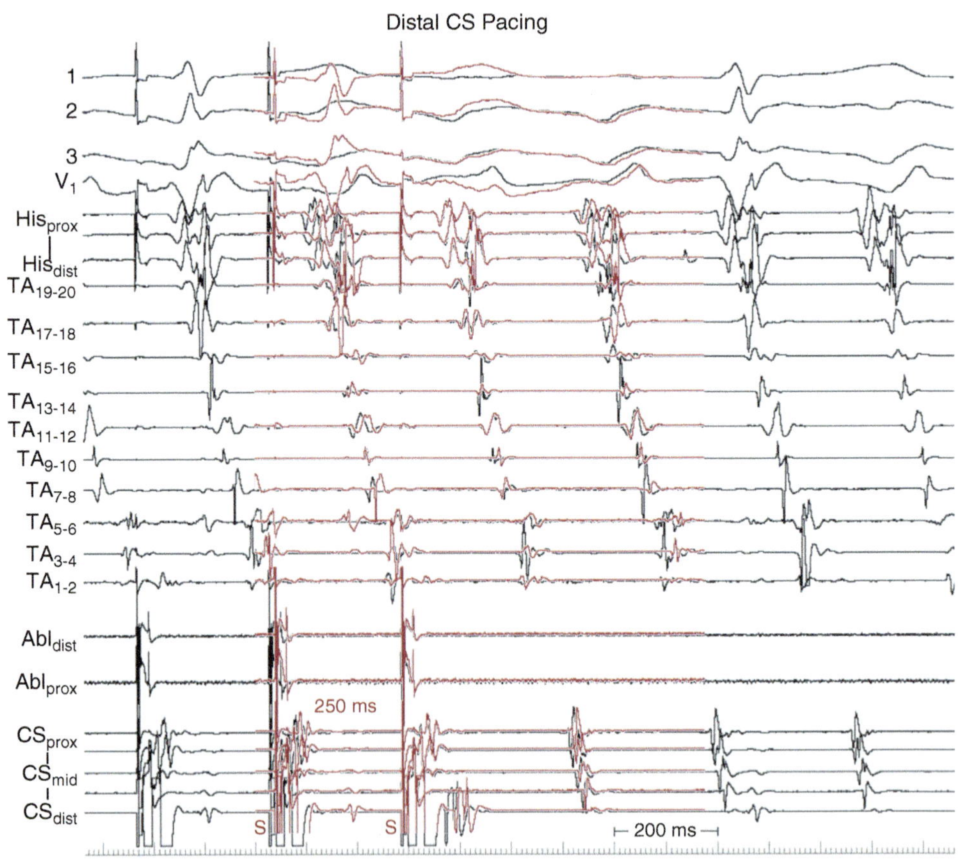

Figure 12-5B

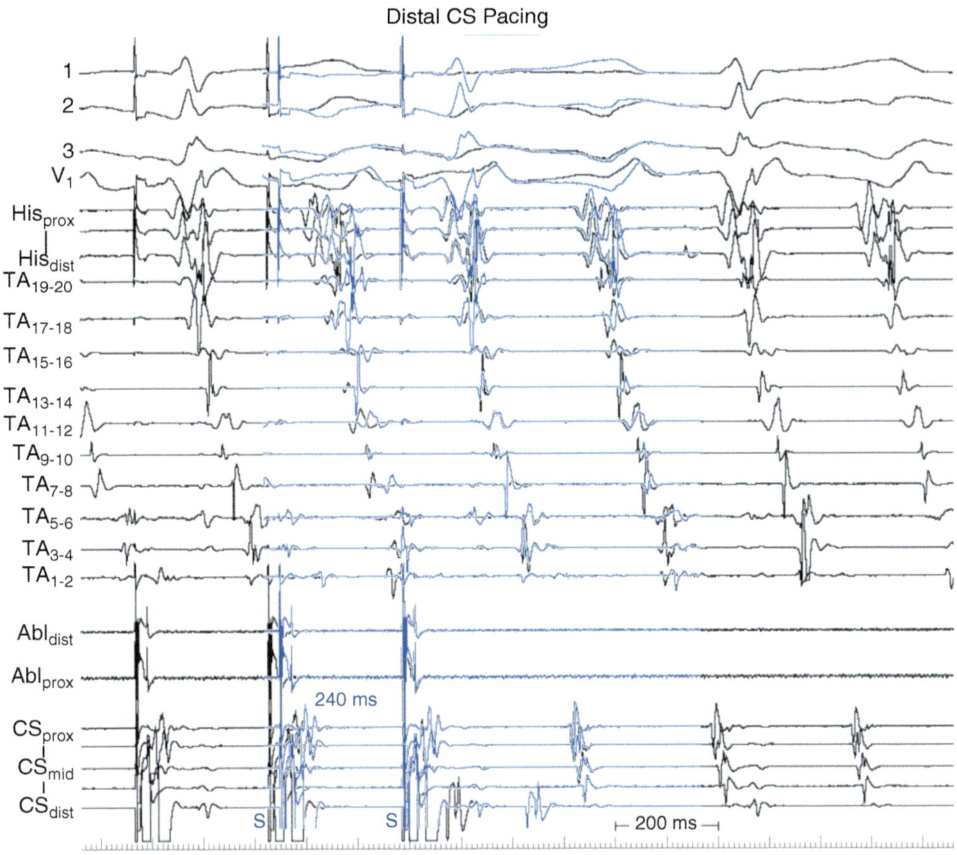

Differential diagnosis:
- typical CCW flutter
- lower loop reentry
- intra-isthmus reentry

Figure 12-5C

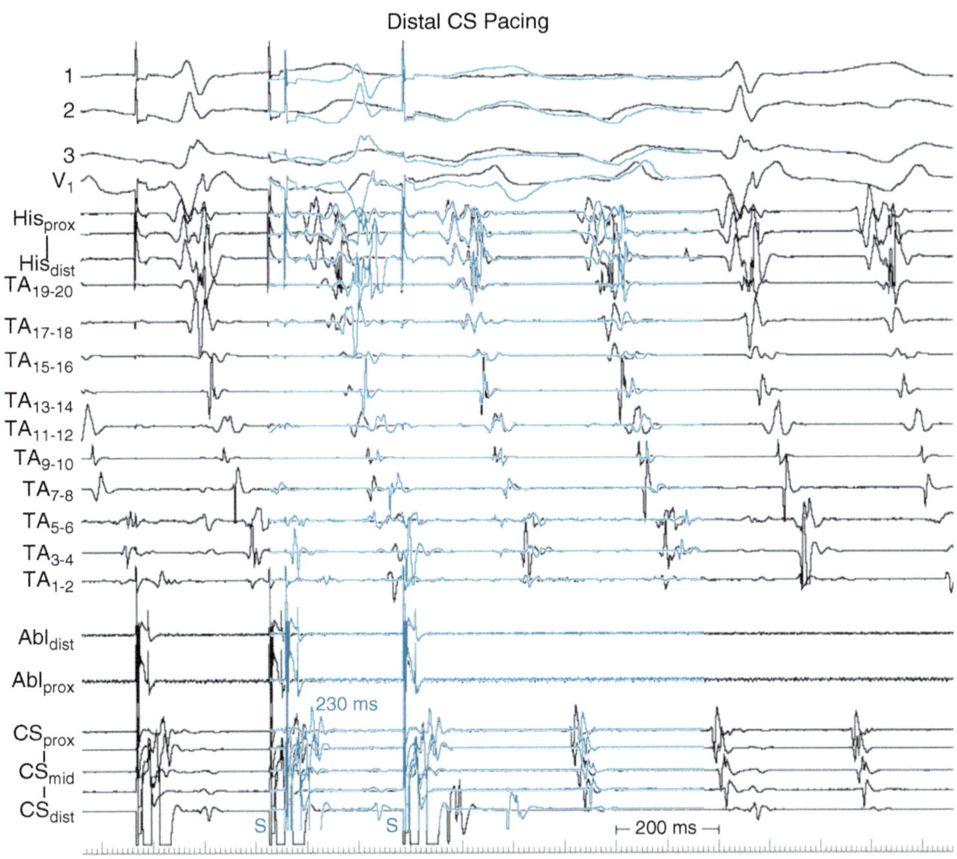

Differential diagnosis:
- typical CCW flutter
- lower loop reentry
- intra-isthmus reentry

Figure 12-5D

Differential diagnosis:
- typical CCW flutter
- lower loop reentry
- intra-isthmus reentry

Figure 12-5E

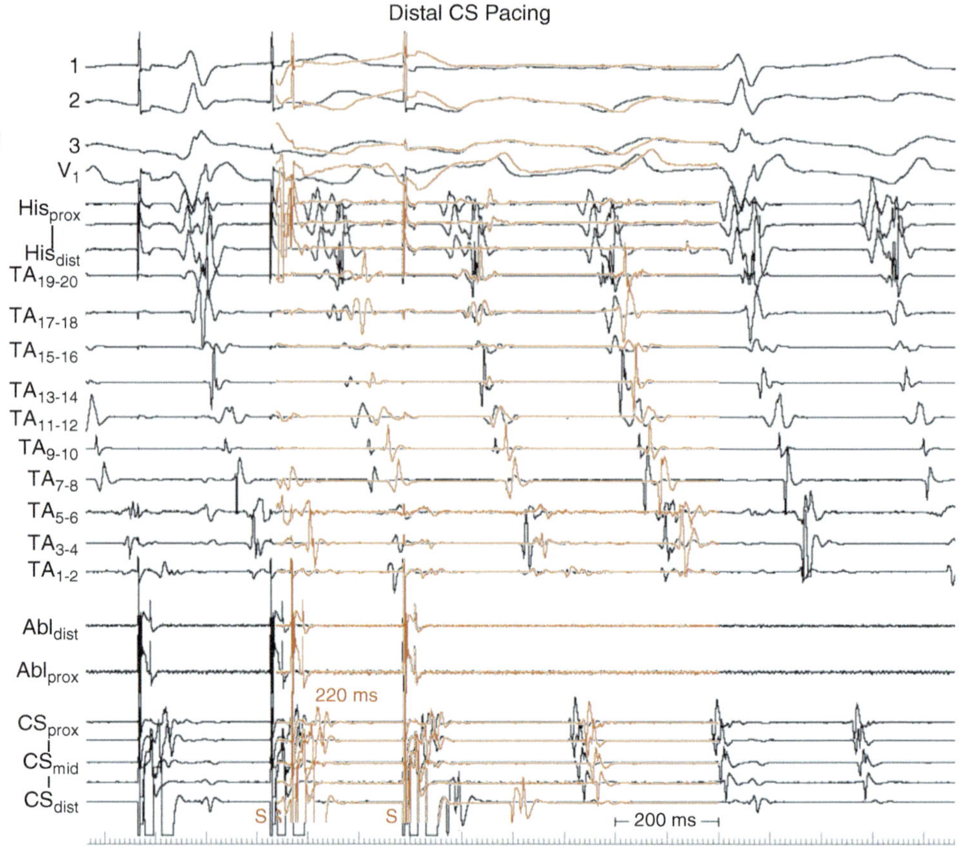

Focal atrial tachycardias often exhibit overdrive suppression; that is, with faster paced rates during tachycardia, the first tachycardia complex after pacing stops will occur after progressively longer delays. In Fig. 12-5 A-E, overdrive pacing at increasingly faster rates (shorter cycle lengths as indicated in different color overlays on Fig. 12-5 B-E) shows no appreciable overdrive suppression. This response is most consistent with a circuit having a fixed path length. Thus a focal tachycardia near the CS ostium (or anywhere else) appears unlikely. Another possible diagnosis has been eliminated.

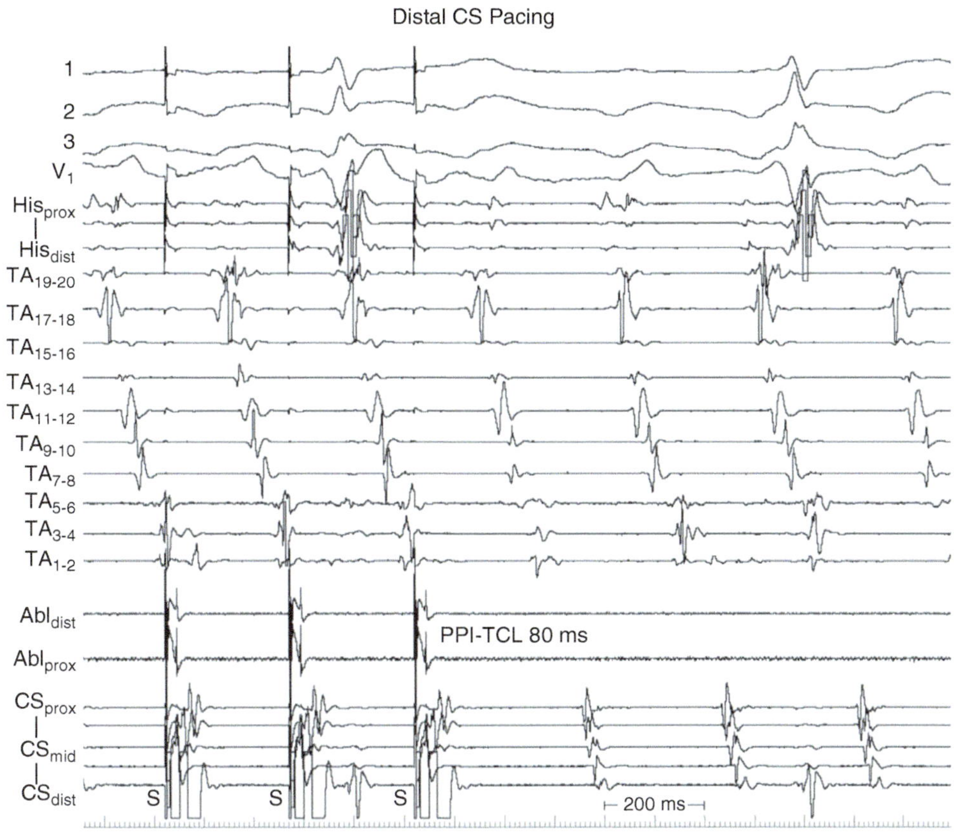

We Can Eliminate Focal AT Near CS os from Our Differential Diagnosis: [Fig. 12-5E and 12-10B]

A. Typical CCW flutter
B. Lower loop reentry
C. Intraisthmus reentry

Figure 12-6

In Fig. 12-6, pacing is again performed from the distal CS, to evaluate relative distance from the pacing site to a suspected circuit. The post-pacing interval (PPI) minus tachycardia cycle length (TCL) difference, 80 ms, suggests a significant distance from the distal CS pacing location to the circuit.

CS Proximal Pacing

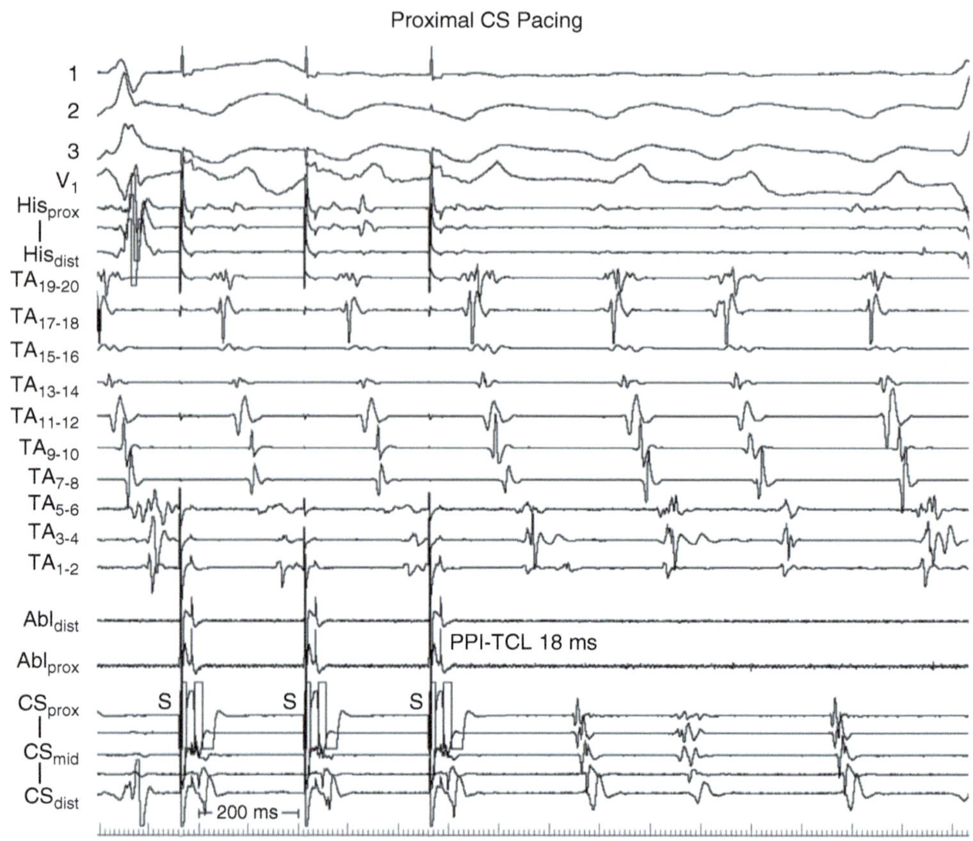

Figure 12-7

Pacing now from the proximal CS electrodes (Fig. 12-7) shows a PPI minus TCL difference of 18 ms, suggesting that it is close to or within the circuit. These electrodes are at the coronary sinus ostium. However, this does not distinguish among the three remaining possibilities—all of which are reentry, and all of which include the region of the CS os in the circuit.

Recording from CTI

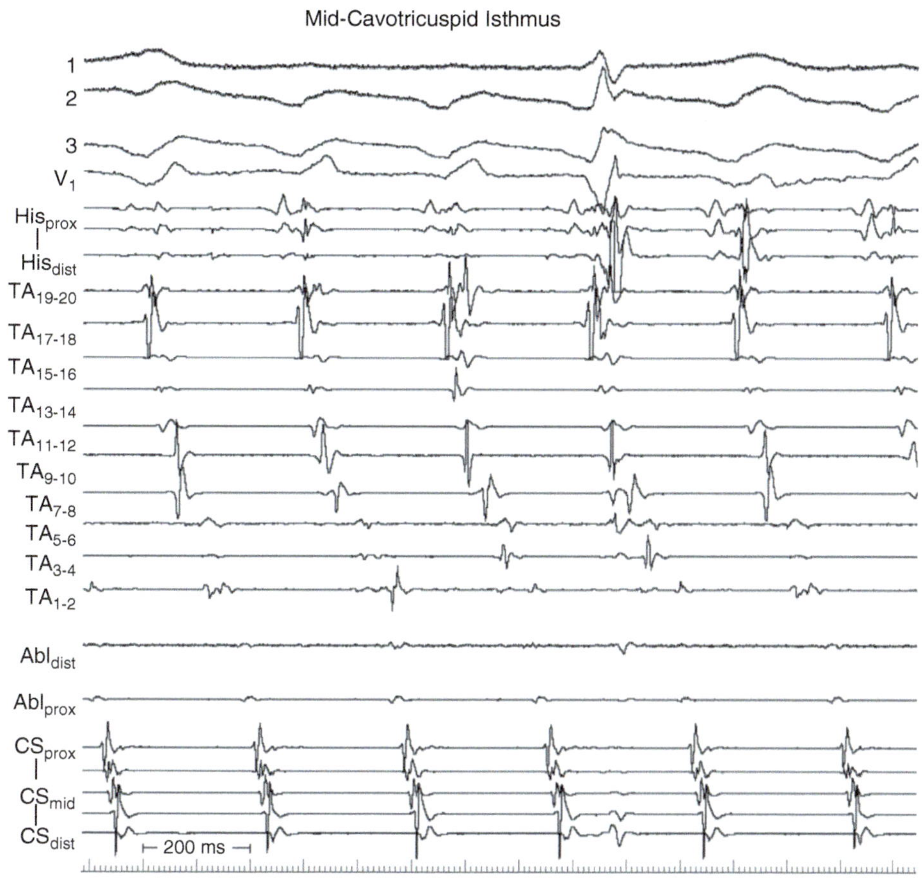

Why Is There No Recording at the Abl_{dist} and Abl_{prox} Leads?

Figure 12-8

In the midcavotricuspid isthmus (Fig. 12-8), there are no remaining electrograms at standard recording gain (Abl recordings). This is anticipated because of the prior extensive ablation.

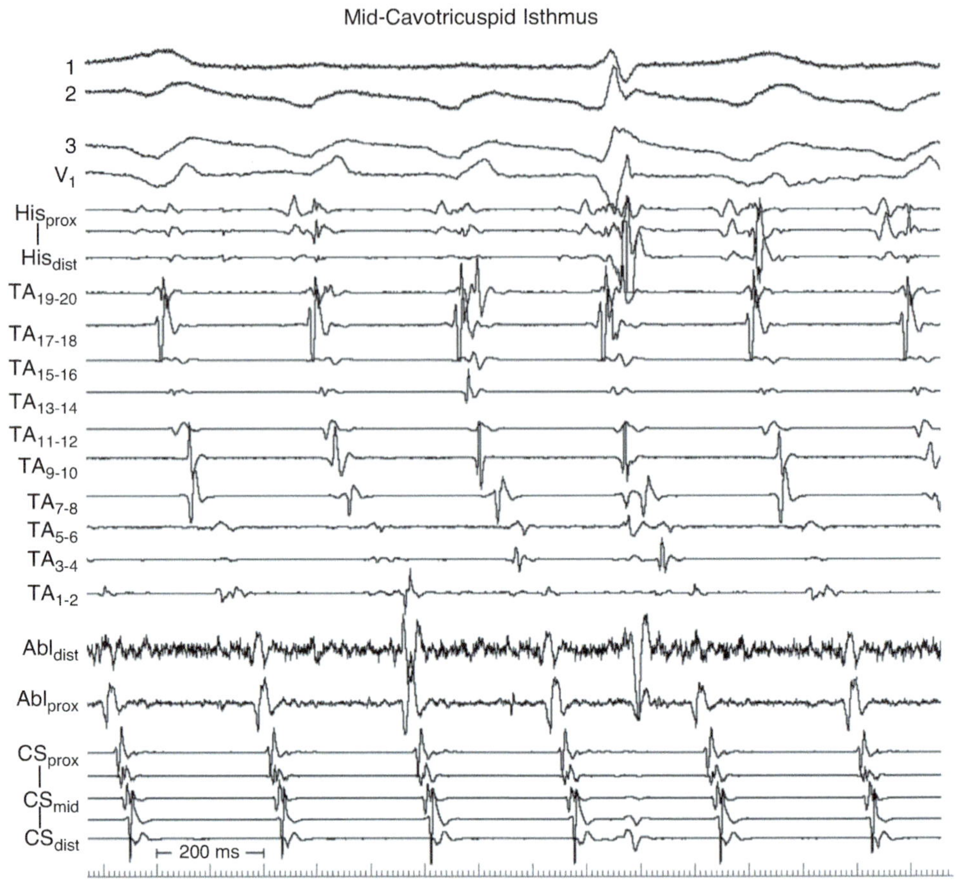

Figure 12-9

However, when the recordings are adequately gained (Fig. 12-9), it is evident that a small but discrete electrogram remains. Two of the three diagnostic possibilities use the cavotricuspid isthmus, but because one does not, it is important to clarify whether this tissue is part of the circuit or not.

Pacing from CTI

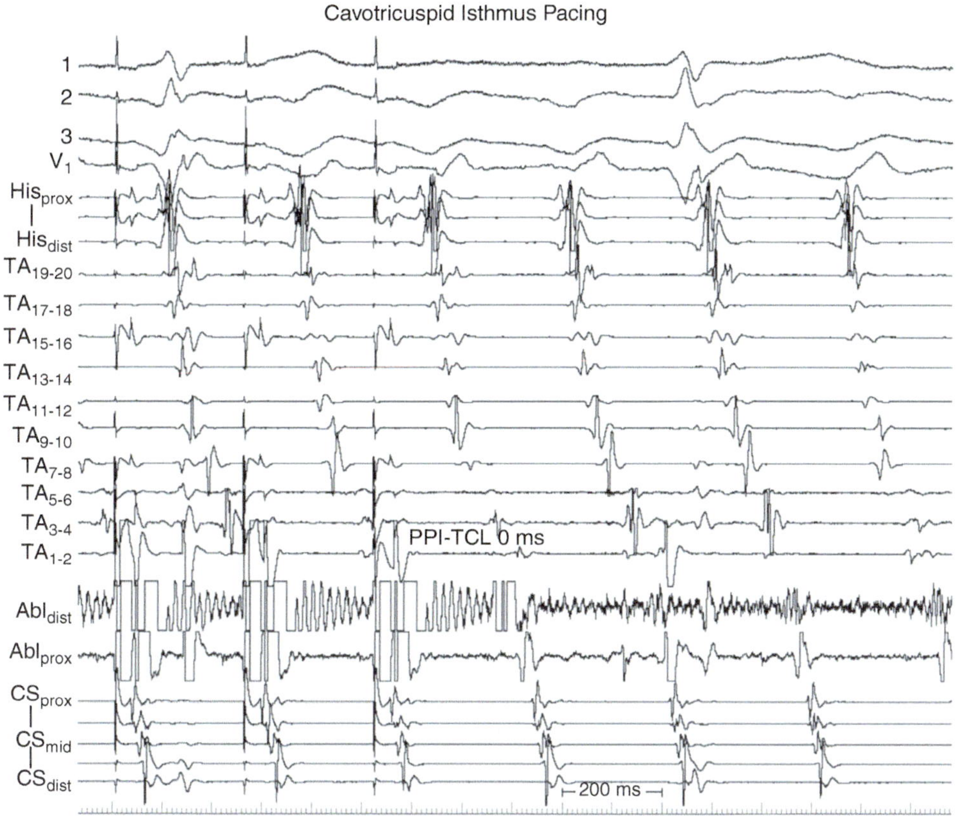

Differential diagnosis:
- typical CCW flutter
- lower loop reentry
- intra-isthmus reentry

Figure 12-10A

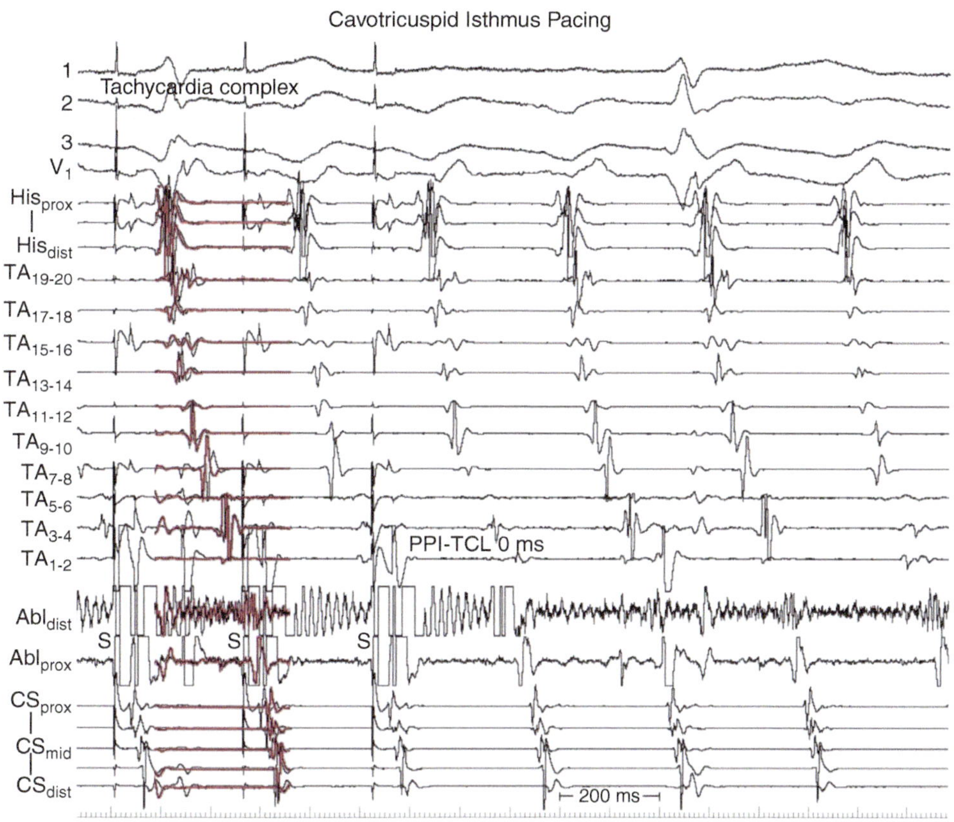

Differential diagnosis:
- typical CCW flutter
- lower loop reentry
- intra-isthmus reentry

Figure 12-10B

Pacing from the cavotricuspid isthmus (Fig. 12-10A) produces a perfect match with the superimposed tachycardia complex (*red*, Fig. 12-10B) as well as the PPI minus TCL difference of zero, indicating that it is part of the circuit. However, this still does not establish a final diagnosis, because two of the remaining possible diagnoses include this tissue in their circuit.

Pacing from Lateral TA

Differential Diagnosis: [Fig. 12-11]

A. Typical CCW flutter

Figure 12-11

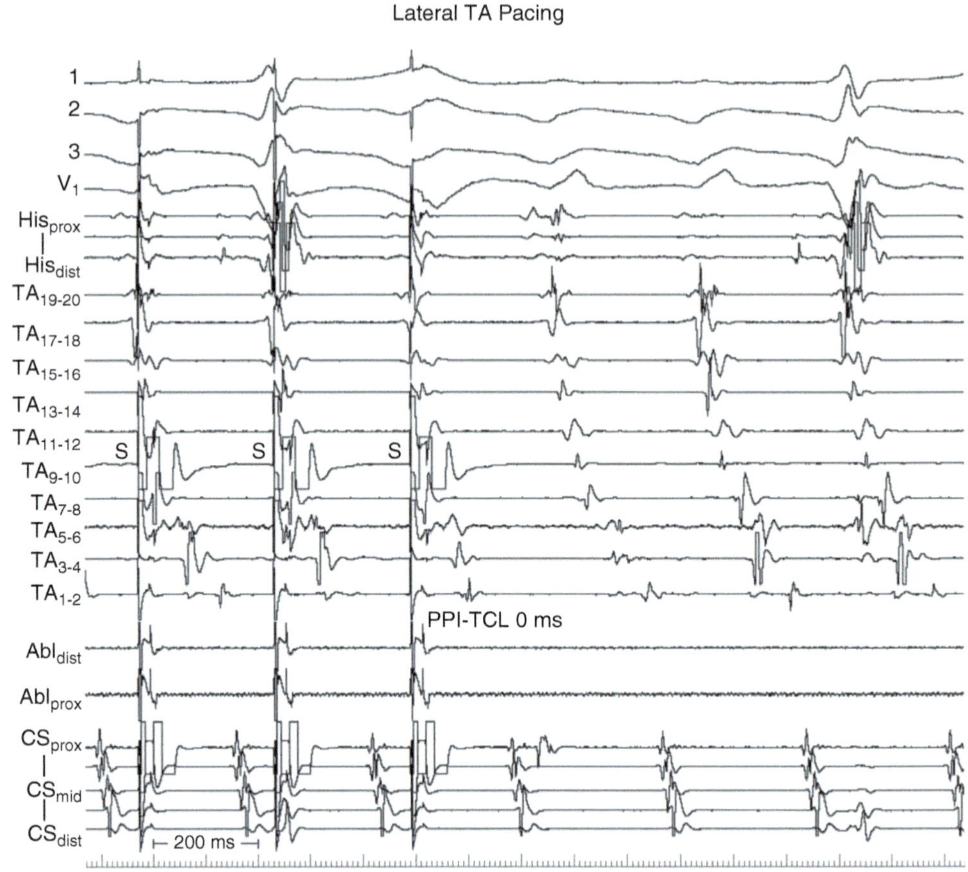

Pacing from the lateral tricuspid annulus as shown in Fig. 12-11 produces a PPI minus TCL difference of zero, indicating that it is part of the tachycardia circuit. Of the remaining diagnostic possibilities, only typical counterclockwise flutter incorporates the lateral tricuspid annulus in the circuit. Thus two more diagnostic possibilities have been eliminated and a definitive diagnosis has finally been established. Of note, macroreentry is established with certainty with this pacing maneuver because the stimulus artifact occurs after the onset of an accelerated flutter wave on the surface ECG and the activation pattern with pacing is unlike what would be expected with pure pacing from the lateral tricuspid annulus—signifying fusion, and diagnosing macroreentry. Ablation in the cavotricuspid isthmus at remaining surviving tissue can commence.

Electroanatomic Mapping

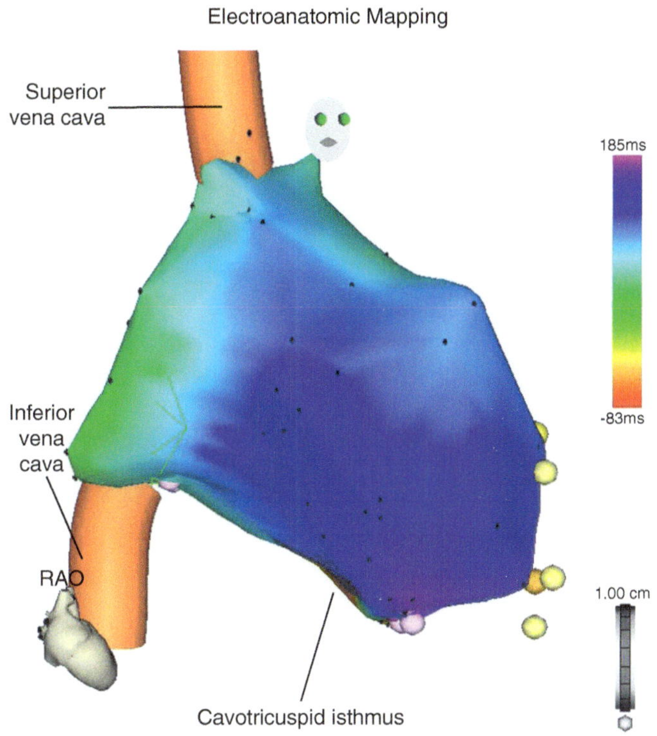

Figure 12-12

In Fig. 12-12, the electroanatomic map of this flutter in the right anterior oblique view is shown; not much useful information can be gathered from this alone.

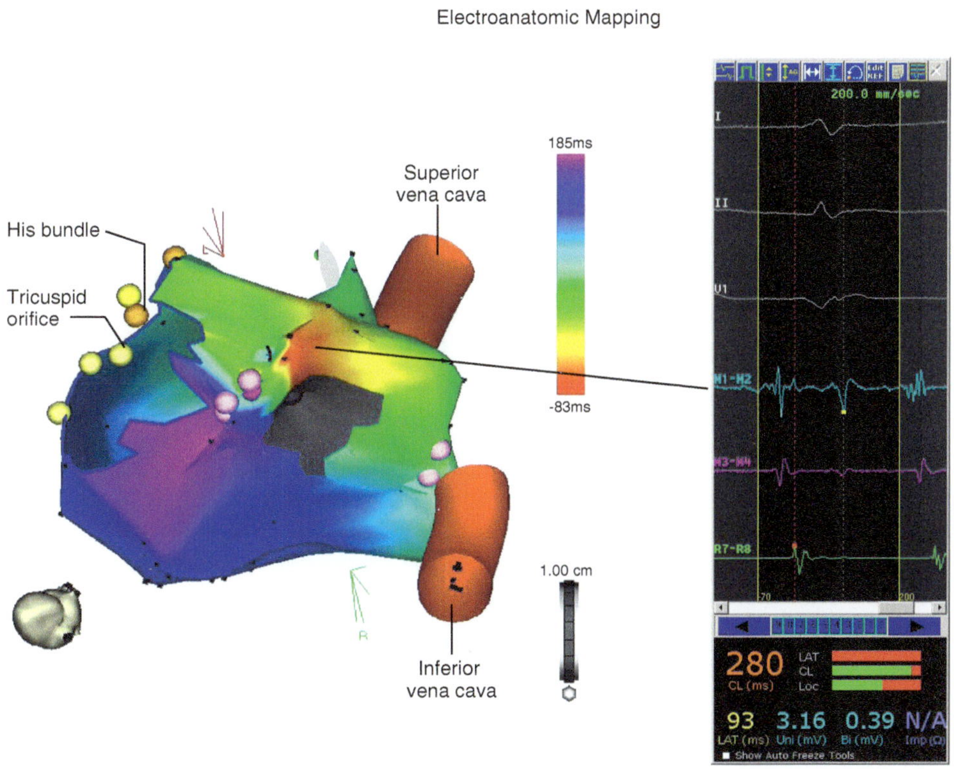

Figure 12-13

In this view from the bottom of the right atrium (Fig. 12-13), the electroanatomic map seems to suggest focal propagation from around the CS os region; the electrogram at the site of earliest activation is shown at right. Unfortunately, the electroanatomic mapping system automatically selected a point on the *ventricular* electrogram as the time of local activation.

Electroanatomic Mapping

Figure 12-14

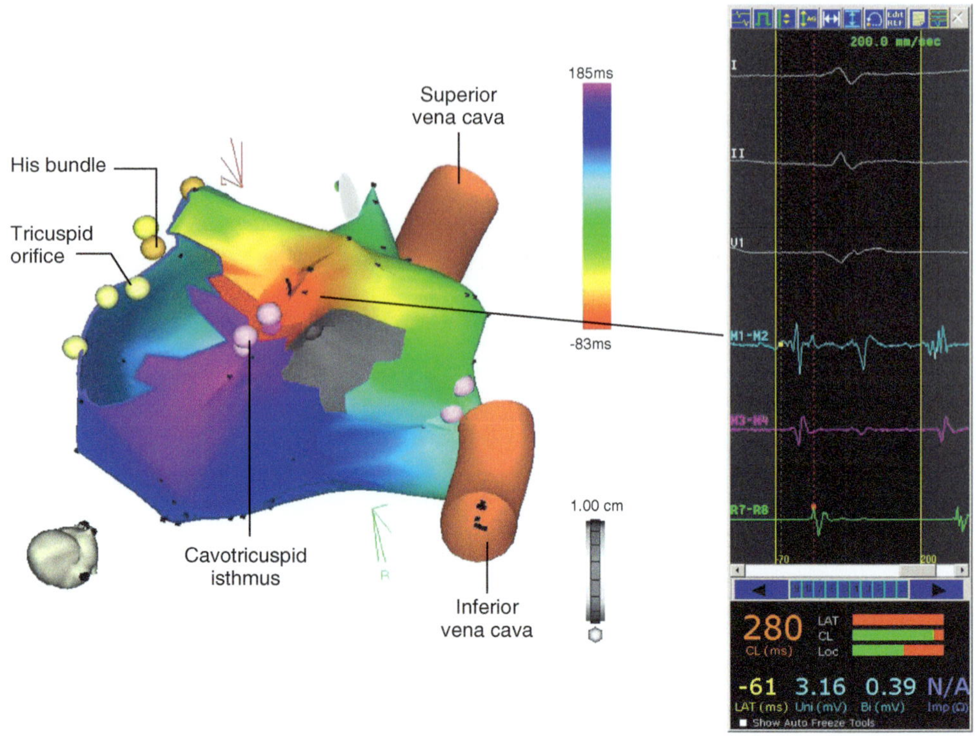

In Fig. 12-14, the same map is shown, however with the atrial electrogram correctly annotated to represent local activation. Now, the appearance of a circuit in a counterclockwise fashion around the tricuspid annulus is evident (colors of red-orange-yellow-green-blue-purple).

Electroanatomic Mapping

Figure 12-15

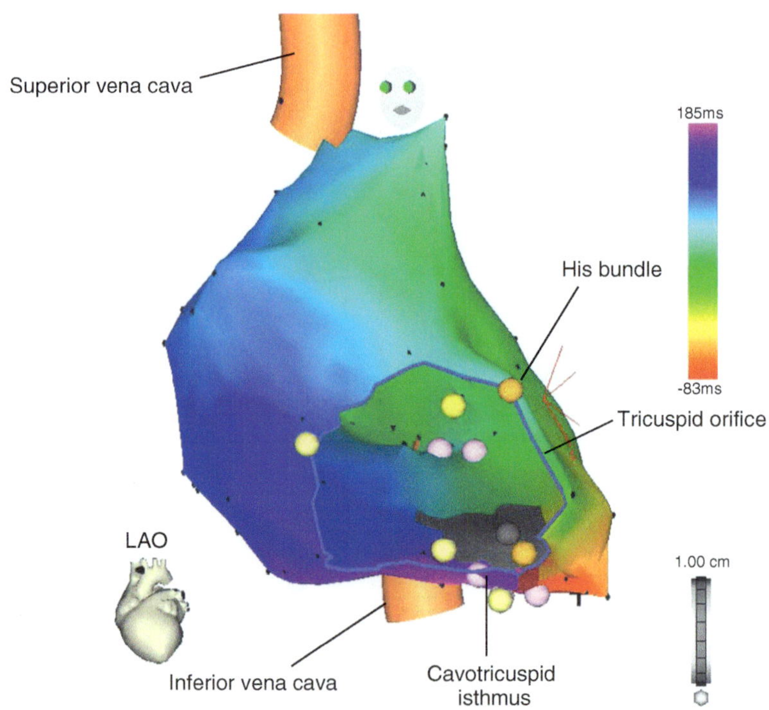

A left anterior oblique view (Fig. 12-15), looking at the tricuspid orifice, shows the propagation around the tricuspid annulus in counterclockwise direction.

Ablation

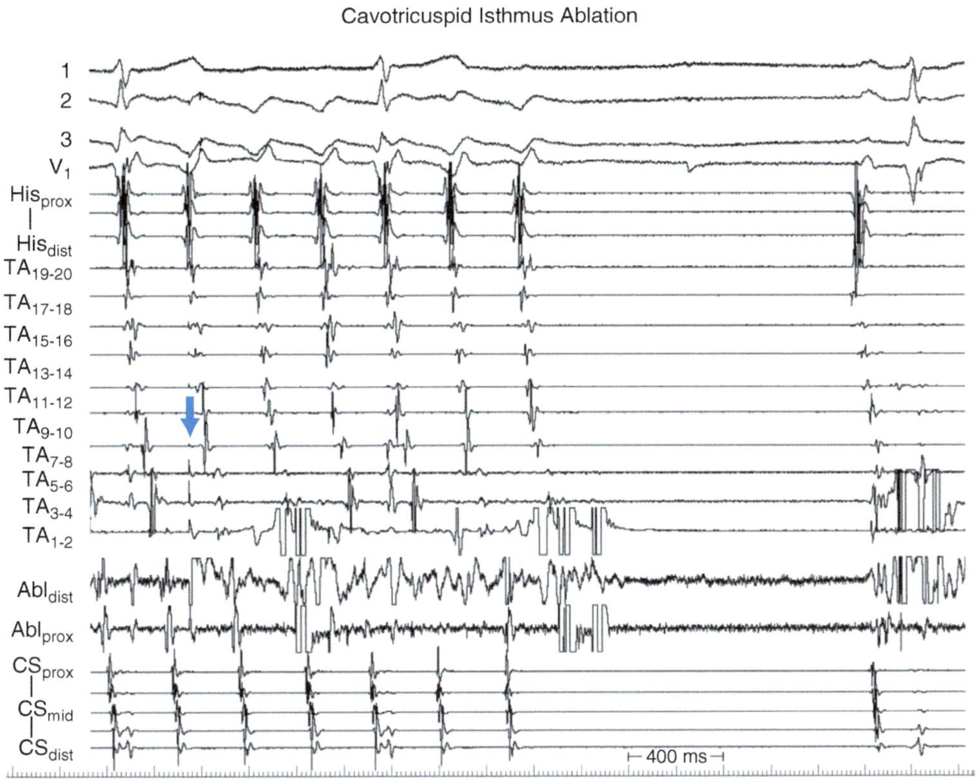

Figure 12-16

The first application of RF energy (onset at *blue arrow*, Fig. 12-16) on the cavotricuspid isthmus at the electrogram shown earlier in Fig. 12-9 results in termination of flutter to sinus rhythm. This corresponded to TA 1-2.

Assessment of Bidirectional Block

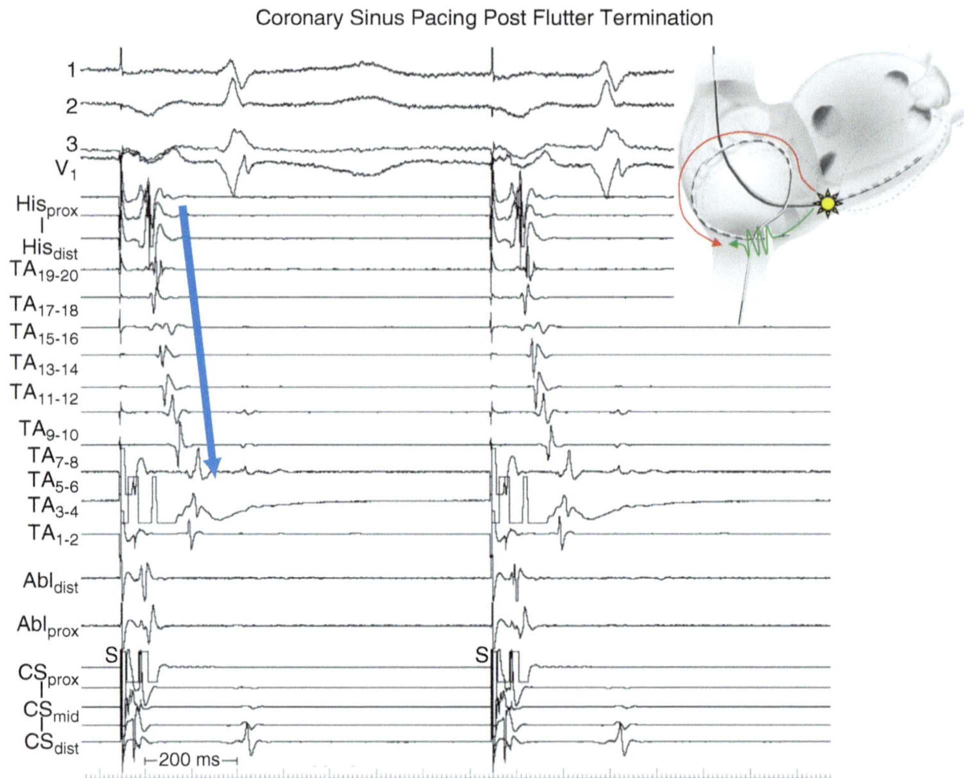

Figure 12-17

In Fig. 12-17, pacing from the CS after flutter termination shows propagation along the tricuspid annulus *(red arrow)* from *top* (TA 19-20) toward the *bottom* (TA 1-2); however, when the wavefront arrives at TA 5-6, it appears to meet a wavefront from the opposite direction (from TA 1-2, *green arrow*). Thus there is still some element of conduction across the isthmus (see diagram at *top*).

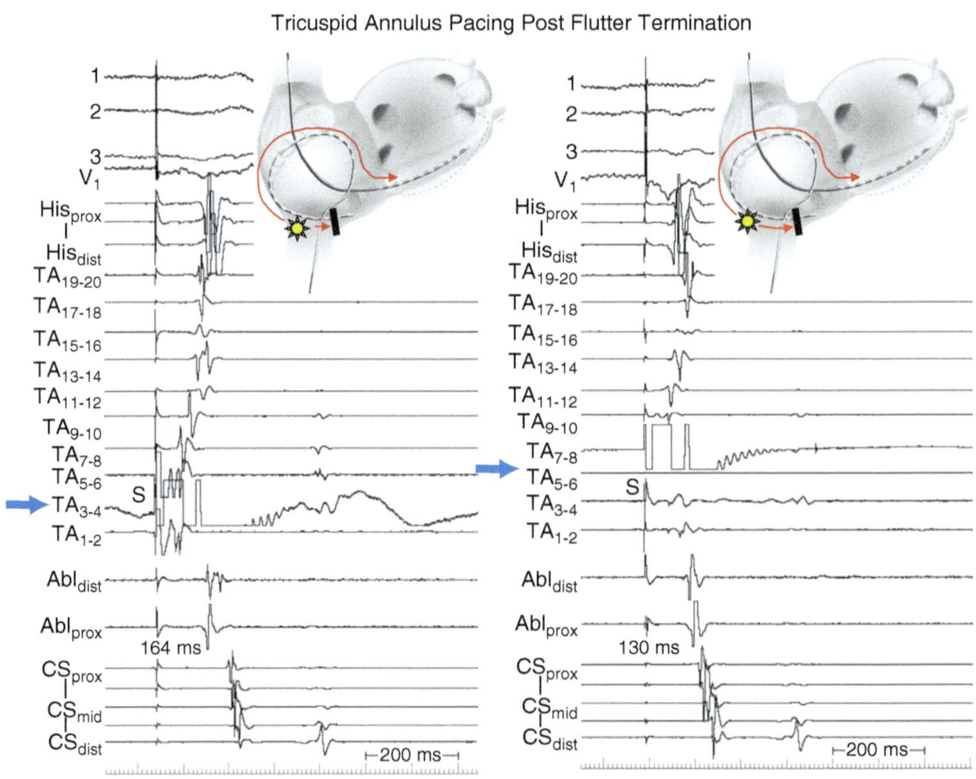

Figure 12-18

Additional ablation was performed at the isthmus (Fig. 12-18). Thereafter, pacing from the indicated electrodes of the halo catheter, lateral to the ablation line, shows a longer interval from stimulus to CS electrodes when pacing from a site closer to the ablation line than when pacing from a site further from the line (see diagrams at top). Though anatomically closer to the CS than TA 5-6 electrodes, the TA 3-4 pacing site is electrically further away. Thus block in the lateral-medial direction is present.

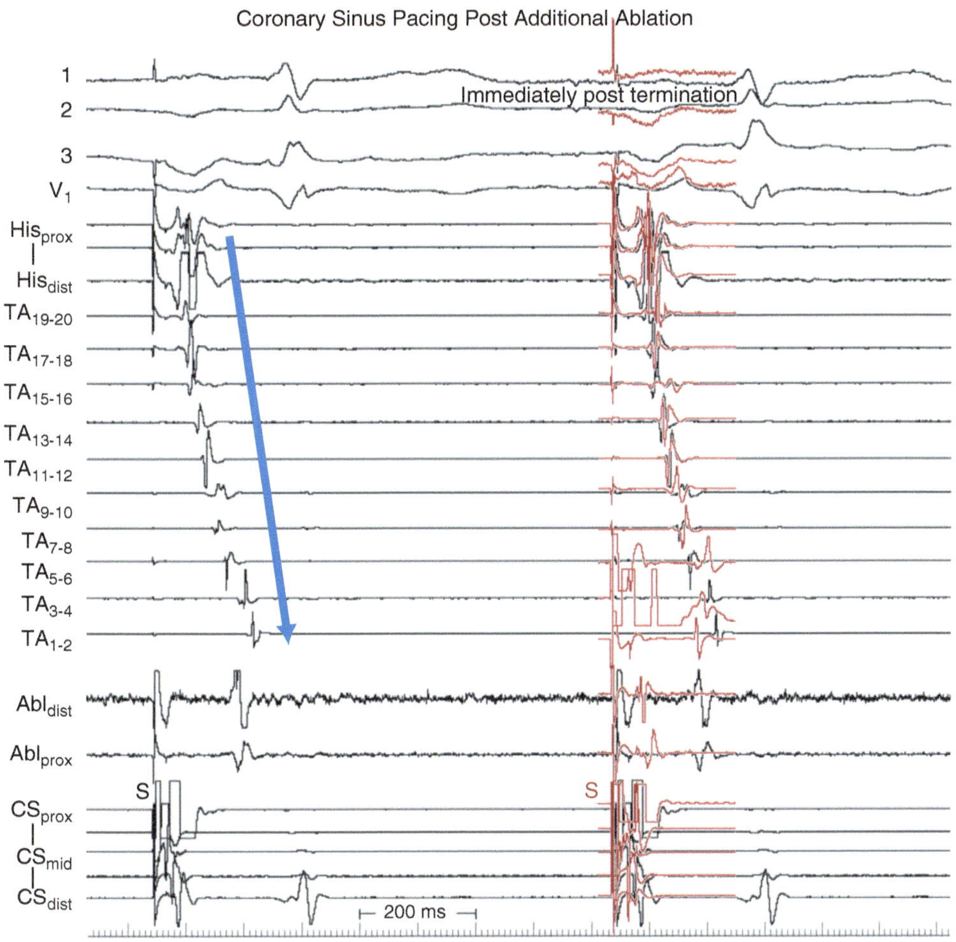

Figure 12-19

After the additional ablation at the isthmus (Fig. 12-19), conduction along the halo catheter is in a straight line (no longer a "chevron"). The activation pattern from immediately after flutter termination is superimposed in *red* (Fig. 12-19) to highlight the difference in activation of atrial electrograms in electrodes TA 1-2 and TA 3-4 in the two settings.

Final ECG

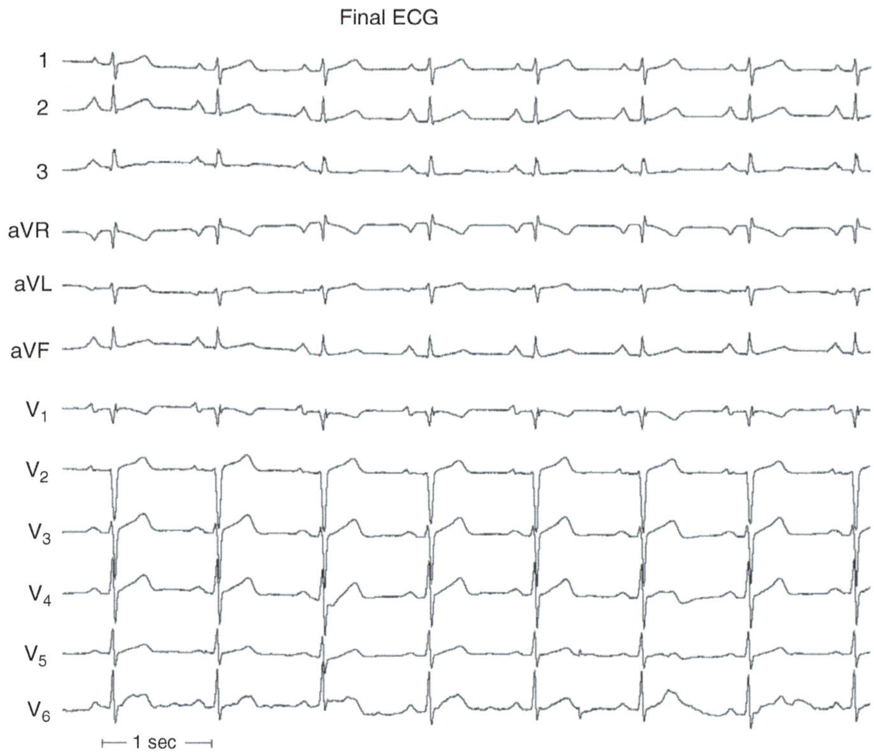

Figure 12-20

At the end of the procedure, sinus rhythm is present (Fig. 12-20), cavotricuspid isthmus block persisted throughout the waiting period and flutter could not be initiated. The procedure took 2 hr, most of which was diagnostic time.

Summary

With recurrent atrial flutter postablation

- Plan for anything (consents, setup, available equipment)
- Prove the nature of the arrhythmia before ablating
- Plan the ablation strategy before ablating (new line, targeting areas of fragmented electrograms, high residual voltage, etc.)
- Terminating flutter during ablation is not an adequate endpoint
- Bidirectional block can be difficult to demonstrate (vs slowing of conduction)
- Electroanatomic mapping is very helpful but
  - Does not make a diagnosis
  - Can be extremely misleading with even one point incorrectly annotated

Atrial Reentry After Valve Surgery

13

Case Presentation

The patient is a 41-year-old woman with rheumatic mitral valve disease. Mitral valve repair was attempted but required replacement in 3/2010, re-replacement was performed in 4/2010 because of dehiscence of valve, and another re-replacement was done in 6/2010 as a result of perivalvular leak. Then she had perioperative atrial fibrillation, and recurrent regular atrial tachycardias were terminated with adenosine injection. Cavotricuspid isthmus (CTI) ablation was performed in 1/2011; in that procedure, flutter terminated during CTI radiofrequency (RF) delivery; bidirectional conduction block was effected across the CTI, and no other arrhythmias were induced. She was referred for ablation because of recurrent episodes of supraventricular tachycardia (SVT) at 145/min. Echocardiographic findings were as follows: LA 4.1 cm, enlarged RA, moderate TR, and normal LV function; estimated right ventricular systolic pressure 30 mm Hg; and normally functioning mechanical mitral valve. Operative reports were as follows: #1 and #2, Waterston's groove left atrium (LA) access; #3, LA dome incised through top of septum to right atrium (RA). There was no mention of atrial septal patching. EP report was as stated previously, and ECG was recorded during SVT.

Approaches to Mitral Surgery

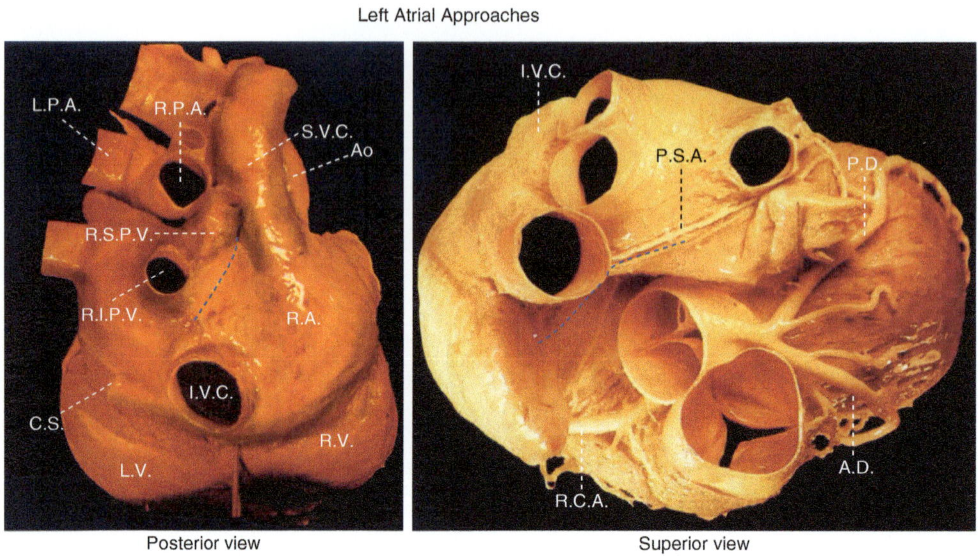

Figure 13-1
(Adapted from McAlpine, WA. *The Heart and Coronary Arteries,* Springer-Verlag, New York, 1975 with permission of Kalyanam Shivkumar, MD, UCLA.)

At left of Fig. 13-1, the heart is viewed from behind. A standard mitral approach incision is through Waterston's groove, just on the left atrial side of the interatrial septum *(dashed blue line)*. This rarely results in macroreentrant arrhythmias. At right, another approach (especially for repeat procedures) is through the atrial roofs; the incision *(dashed blue line)* goes through both atria roughly along Bachmann's bundle, anterior to the superior vena cava and pulmonary veins. *AD*, left anterior descending coronary artery; *Ao*, aorta; *CS*, coronary sinus; *IVC*, inferior vena cava; *LPA*, left pulmonary artery; *LV*, left ventricle; *PD*, posterior descending coronary artery; *PSA*, posterior sinus node artery; *RA*, right atrium; *RCA*, right coronary artery; *RIPV*, right inferior pulmonary vein; *RPA*, right pulmonary artery; *RSPV*, right superior pulmonary vein; *RV*, right ventricle; *SVC*, superior vena cava.

Prior SVT ECG

Any Clues as to SVT Diagnosis? [Fig. 13-2]

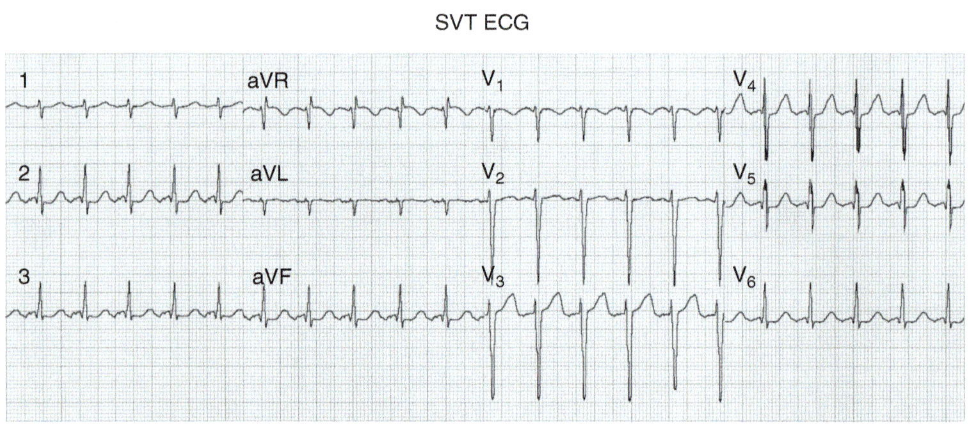

Figure 13-2

In the "long RP" SVT shown in Fig. 13-2, it looks like there is only 1 P wave per QRS, and that is inverted in the inferior leads and positive in aVL; thus a first approximation would be that this indicates a low right atrial focus or exit from a circuit.

Baseline ECG and Intracardiac Recordings

Any Clues as to SVT Diagnosis? [Fig. 13-3]

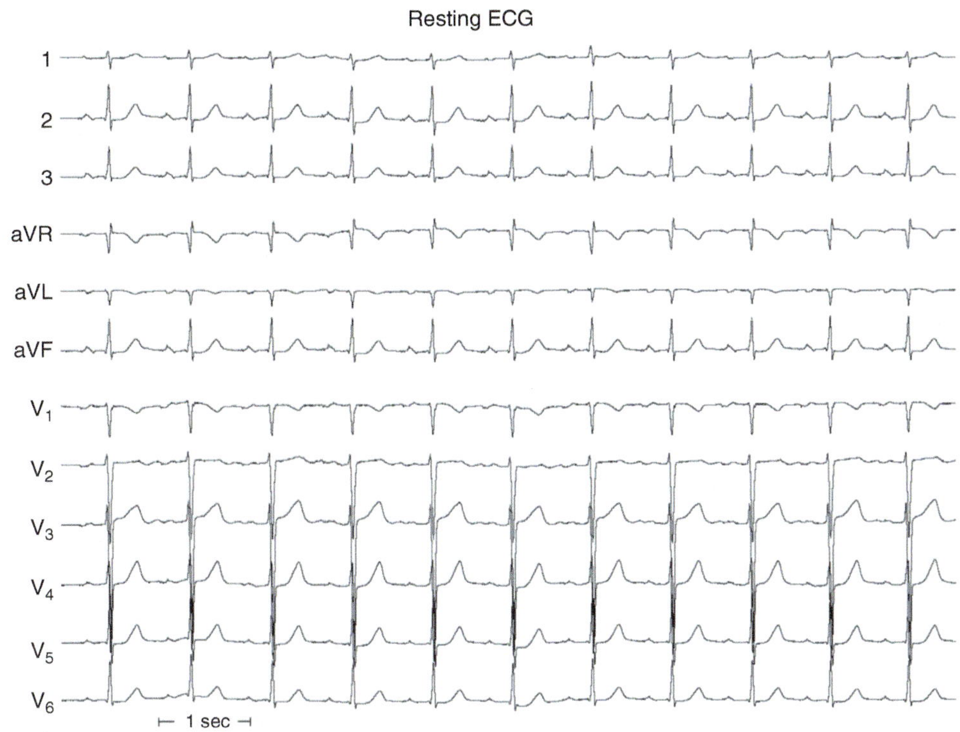

Figure 13-3

The sinus rhythm P wave in Fig. 13-3 is remarkably close to normal despite the history of extensive atrial surgery. In scar-based macroreentry, the P wave in sinus rhythm is often very prolonged and fragmented (more so than is seen here).

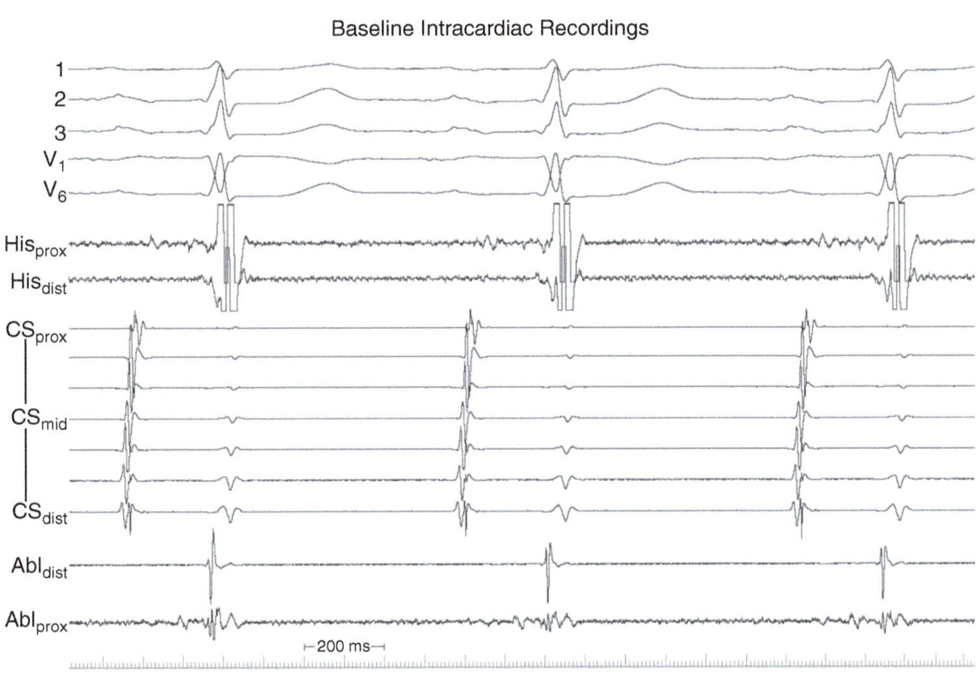

Figure 13-4

Consistent with the relatively normal surface ECG appearance of the P wave, intracardiac activation also appears relatively normal in Fig. 13-4 without much hint of scar that could result in slow conduction, a constituent of macroreentry.

Figure 13-5

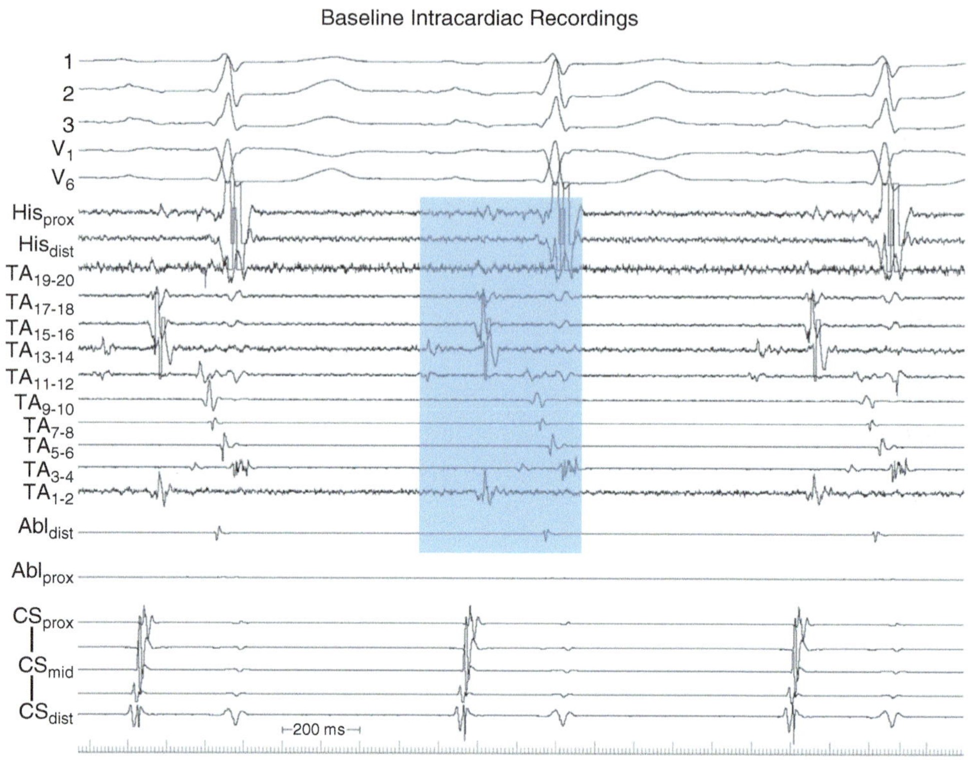

Fig. 13-5 shows the same events as in Fig. 13-4, but with another multielectrode catheter in the right atrium. Now that there are more extensive recordings from the right atrium (RA), dramatically disordered conduction is revealed (duration of RA activation shown in *shaded box* [430 ms]). All of the recordings in the tricuspid annular (TA) catheter are from atrium, despite some of them timing with the QRS complex. With this degree of slow conduction, macroreentry is a real possibility.

Catheter Induction of SVT and ECG and Intracardiac Recordings

Focal or Macroreentry? [Fig. 13-6]

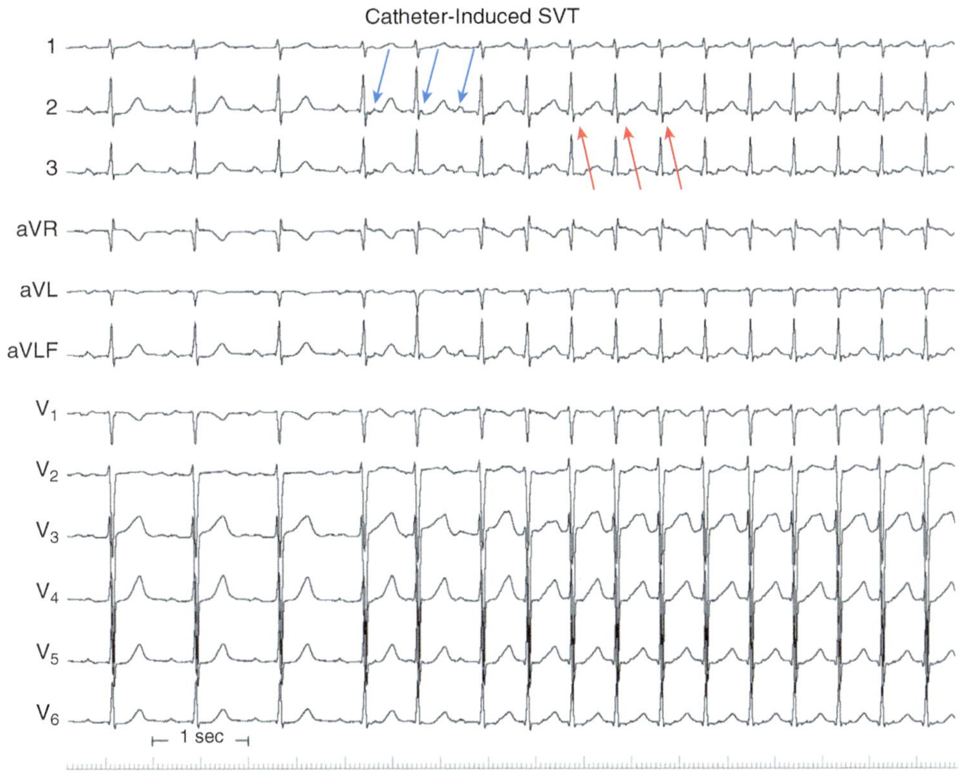

Figure 13-6

Central to achieving a successful ablation outcome is the determination of what the target site of ablation should look like—for focal tachycardias, it is a potential just 30 to 40 ms before the P wave onset, whereas for macroreentry, a middiastolic potential is generally sought. Because the ablation target is very different depending on mechanism, it is important to delineate mechanism (focal vs macroreentry) relatively early in the procedure. A clue to mechanism can sometime be found in how an episode starts (Fig. 13-6); here one or several premature atrial complexes *(blue arrows)*, positive in the inferior leads, seem to start SVT that has inverted P waves in inferior leads *(red arrows)*. A focal tachycardia typically has the same P-wave configuration throughout, whereas in reentrant tachycardias, the initiating P wave is often different from those during tachycardia.

Focal or Macroreentry? [Fig. 13-7]

Figure 13-7

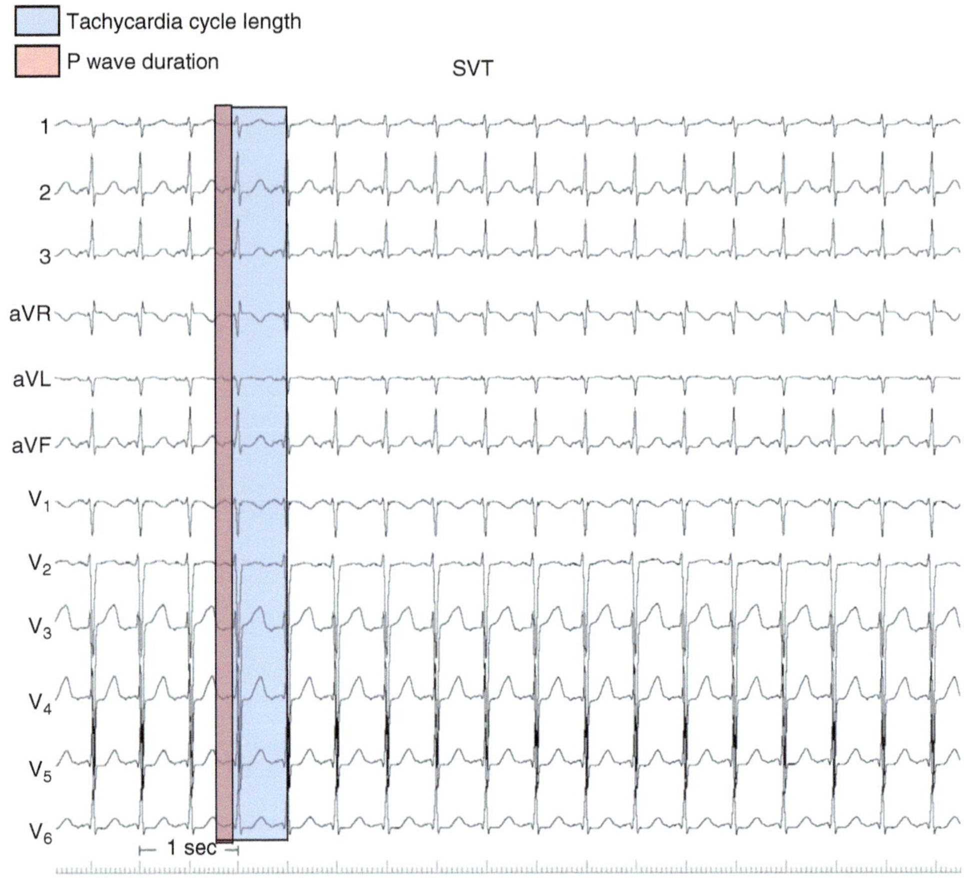

A useful principle for distinguishing a focal process from macroreentry is that, in macroreentry, some of the atrium is always being activated throughout the tachycardia cycle length (TCL) and slow conduction is present (required for tachycardia to continue); this leads to a relatively large portion of the cycle length being occupied by P wave. In focal tachycardias, slow conduction is not needed, and once the focus fires, the atria are depolarized relatively quickly, leading to a P wave that takes up a small portion of the tachycardia cycle length. In Fig. 13-7, it appears that the P wave *(red shading)* is pretty narrow compared to cycle length (*blue shading*, that includes *red shading*). This suggests focality.

Focal or Macroreentry?

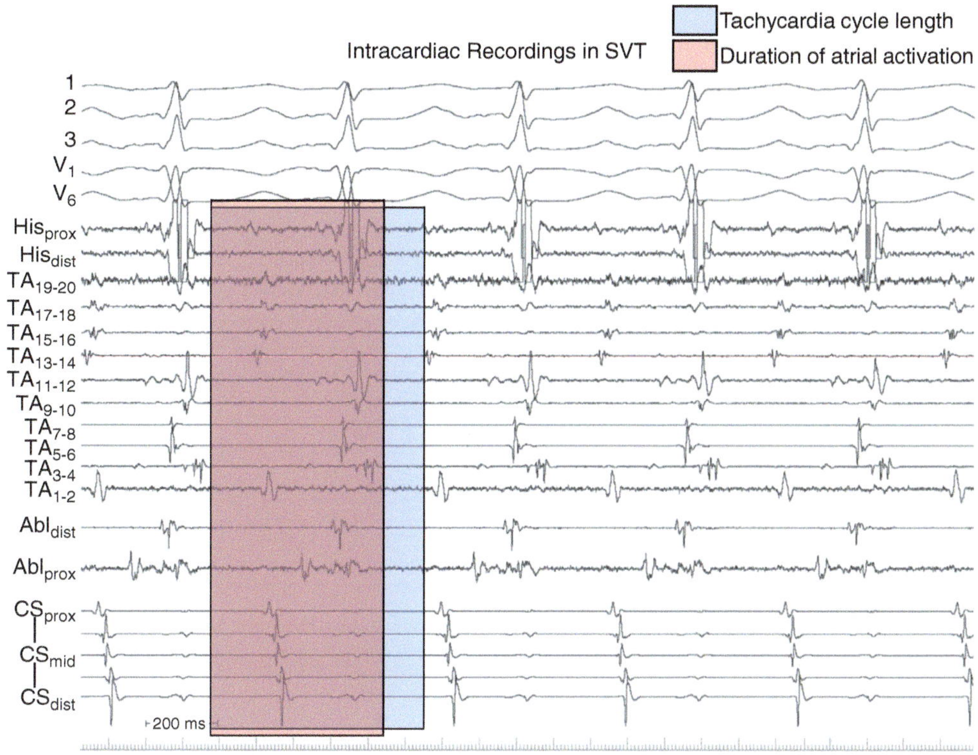

Figure 13-8

With the aid of intracardiac recordings, it becomes clear that atrial activation *(red shading)* takes up much of the TCL (*blue shading*, encompassing *red shading*; Fig. 13-8), now suggesting macroreentry. Specifically, most of the TCL is accounted for in *right atrial* recordings.

Clarifying P-Wave Onset During SVT with Ventricular Pacing

Figure 13-9

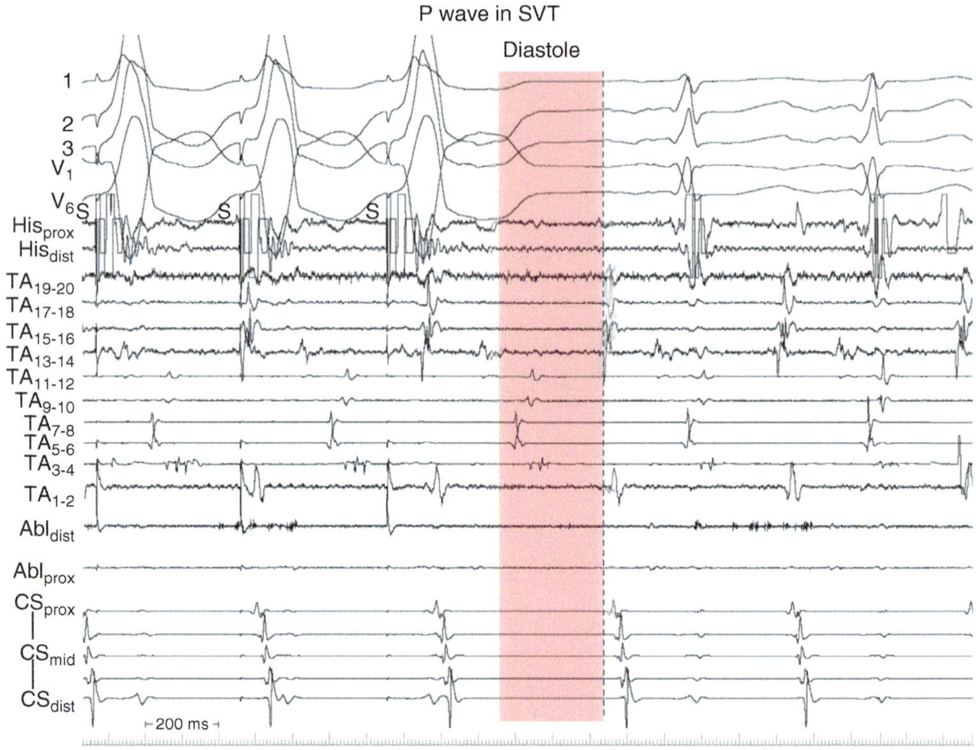

Clarifying the limits of the P wave during SVT helps in mapping, so that the onset of the P wave is clear. However, it may not be evident during ongoing SVT and thus some tricks are needed to reveal a partially obscured P-wave onset, such as introduction of premature ventricular complexes (PVCs) or ventricular pacing during tachycardia. The resulting long diastolic period should provide a P wave standing by itself (Fig. 13-9), allowing clear determination of its onset (as well as end of the prior P wave, for designating window of interest with electroanatomic mapping systems). Atrial diastole (end of 1 P wave to beginning of next P wave) is shown in *red shading*.

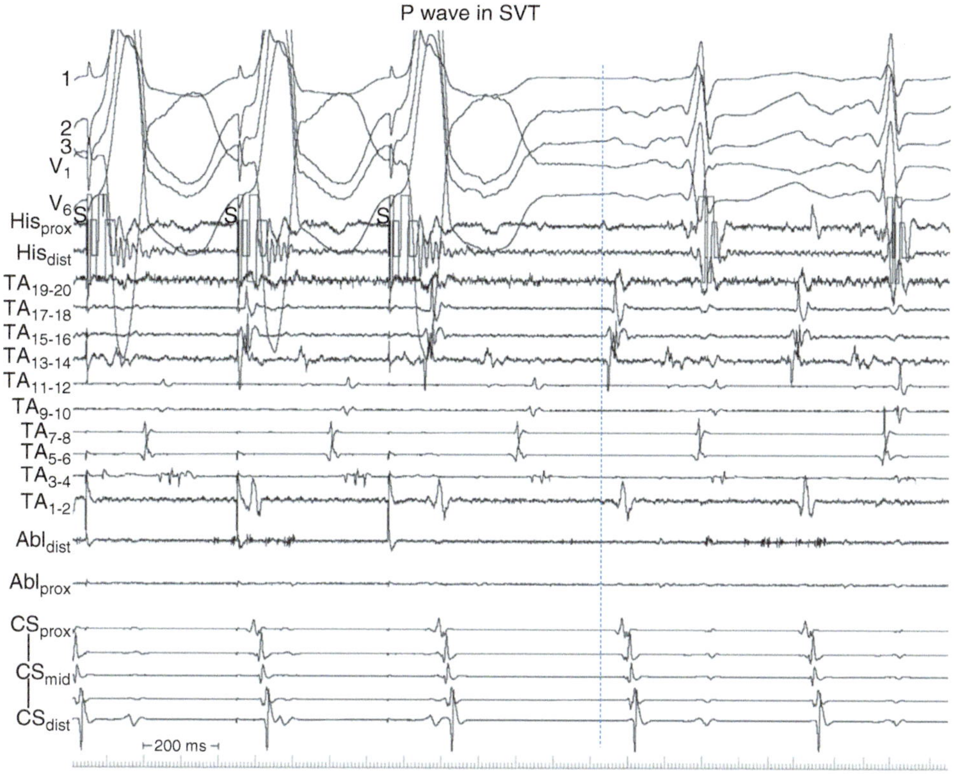

Figure 13-10

Surface ECG leads are shown in Fig. 13-10 with increased gain to better determine P-wave onset *(dashed line)* and morphology. This also shows VA block during SVT, excluding orthodromic SVT as well as almost all cases of AV nodal reentry. The setting (scarred atrium) is perfect for atrial tachycardia.

Overdrive Pacing During SVT

From Distal and Proximal Coronary Sinus

Focal or Macroreentry?

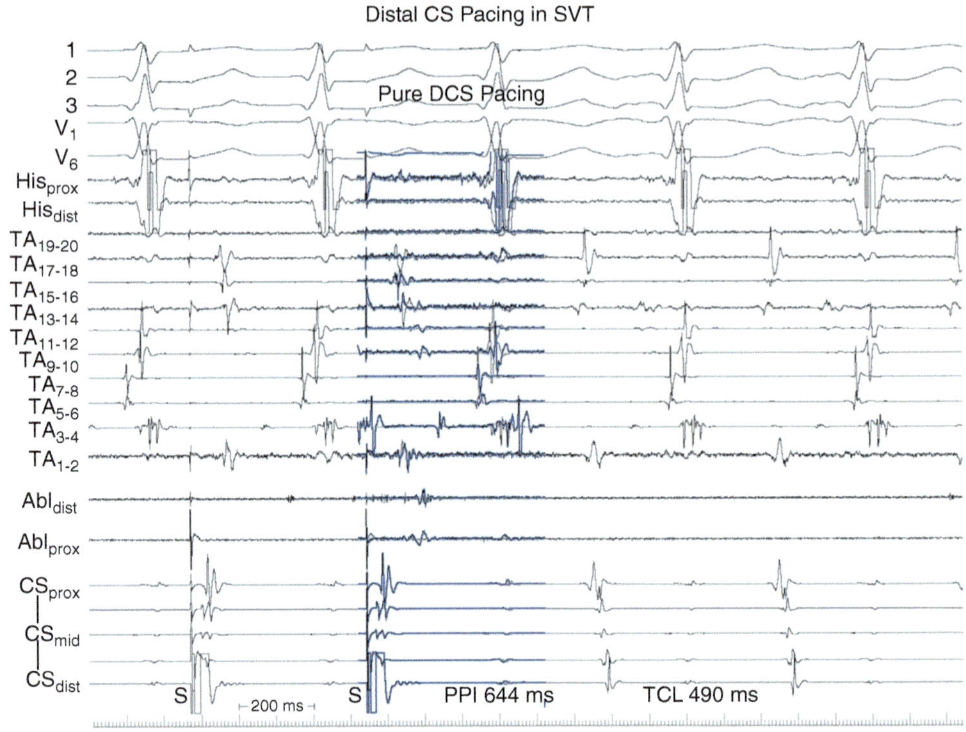

Figure 13-11

To answer the important question of focal versus macroreentry as tachycardia mechanism, overdrive pacing from distal CS—activated late during SVT—is performed, showing a paced sequence during SVT that is a little different from pure CS pacing earlier in the procedure (superimposed in blue) as well as different from SVT (Fig. 13-11). However, the differences are not striking and it is difficult to be definitive that fusion is present. Note also that whatever the mechanism, the distal CS is far from either the focus or exit from a circuit (post-pacing interval [PPI] − TCL = 154).

Focal or Macroreentry?

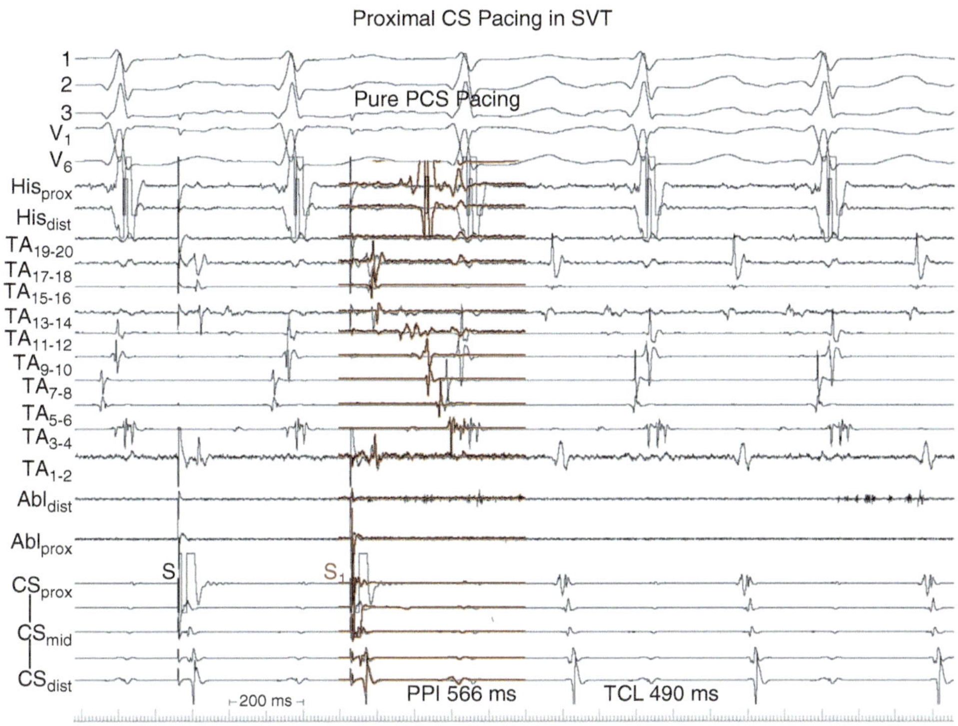

Figure 13-12

Because overdrive pacing from distal CS was equivocal, we should try pacing from a different site, such as the proximal CS. Fig. 13-12 clearly shows a sequence during pacing in SVT that is very different from pure CS pacing earlier in the procedure (superimposed in *orange*), as well as different from SVT. Thus fusion has been demonstrated and macroreentry is diagnosed. The proximal CS pacing site is, like the distal site on the last slide, remote from the circuit but not as far away as the distal CS was (smaller PPI-TCL difference).

From Different Halo Catheter Sites

Figure 13-13

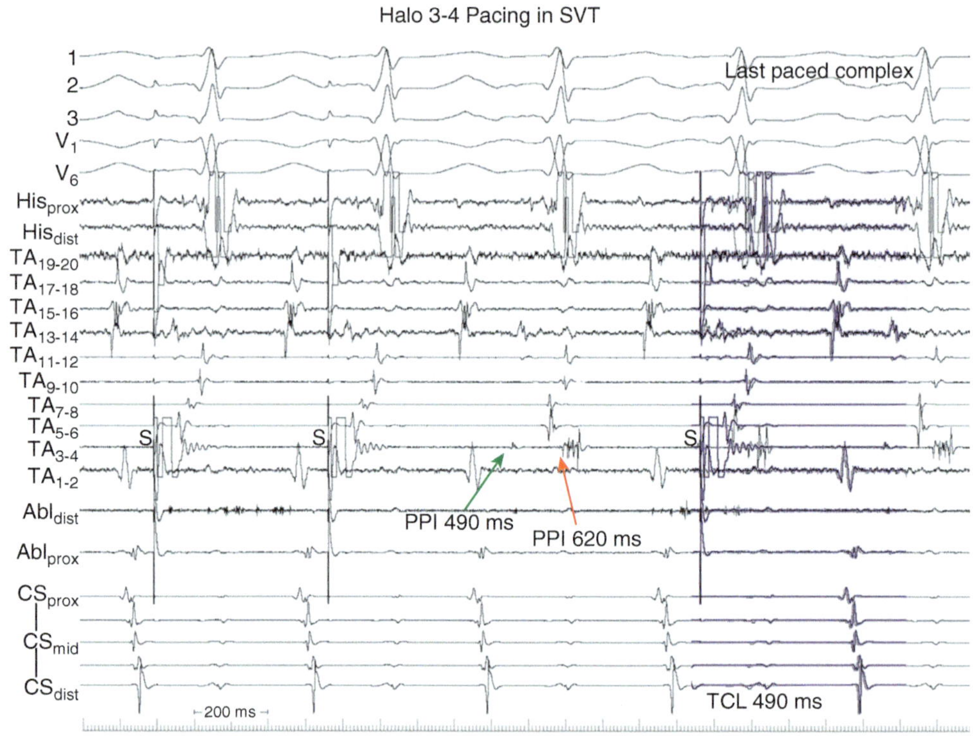

Pacing from a portion of the TA catheter (Fig. 13-13) shows a paced sequence (superimposed in *purple* on a tachycardia complex) that is nearly identical to that during tachycardia (thus almost concealed fusion). The postpacing interval is problematic because the natural place to measure (largest recording) yields a very long PPI (620 ms); however, although that portion is captured, so is the small potential before it, with a PPI identical to TCL. This should be within the circuit; the lack of concealed fusion is likely because of excessive current used in pacing, which captures more than the intended tissue.

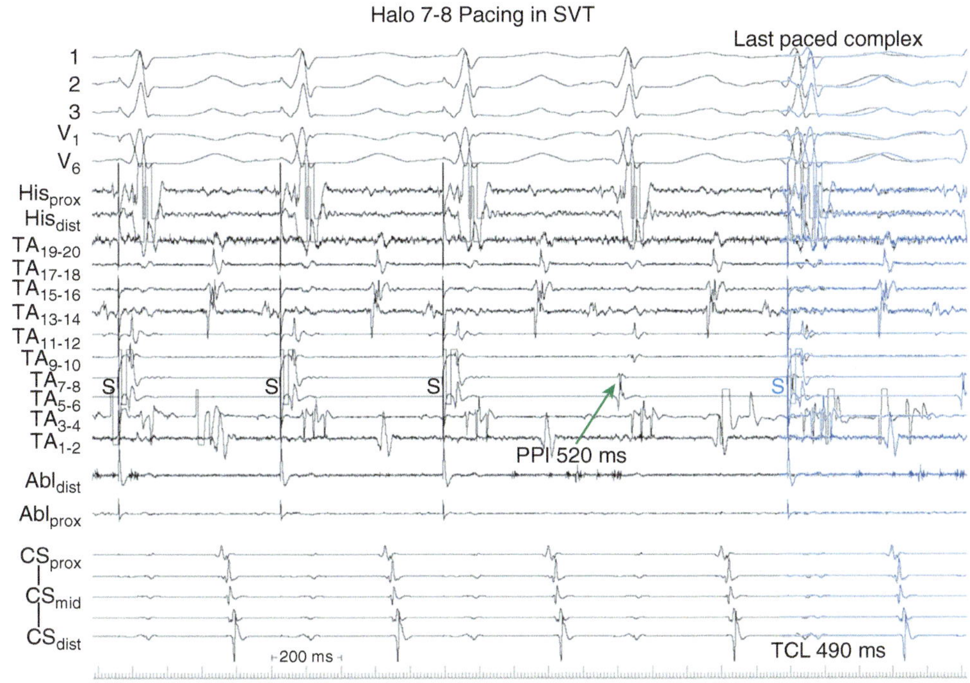

Figure 13-14

Pacing a couple of electrodes away on the TA catheter (Fig. 13-14) shows a less perfect pace match (sequence superimposed on tachycardia complex) and PPI-TCL difference; thus the pacing site is further from the circuit.

From Coronary Sinus Again

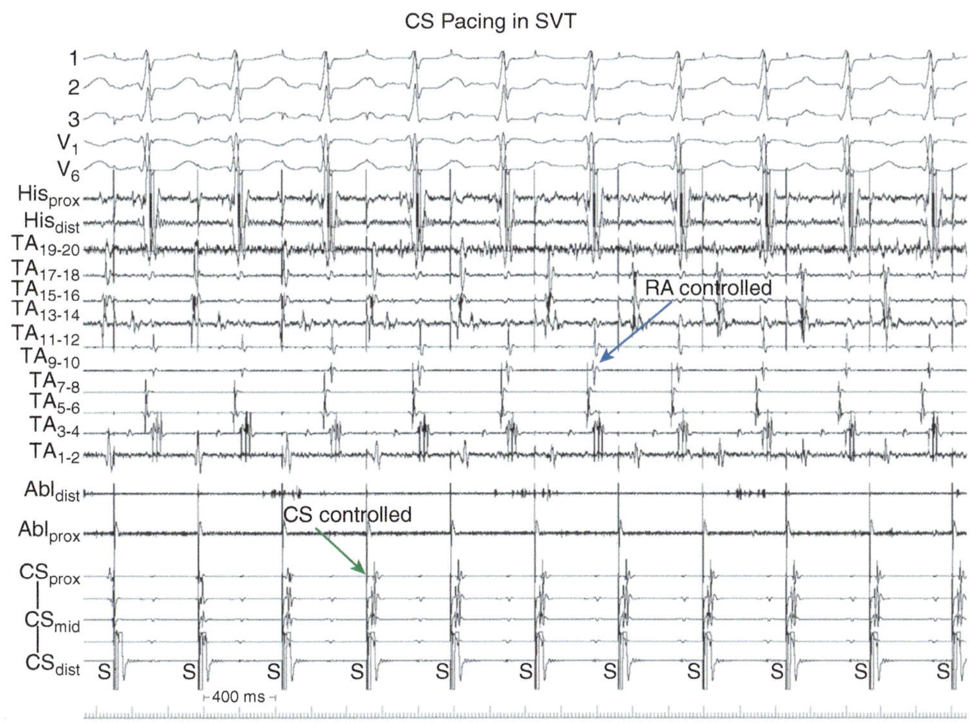

Figure 13-15

In Fig. 13-15, pacing from the distal CS controls all CS recordings long before the TA (RA) is controlled; this signifies that the RA is the chamber of origin (or else it would be controlled coincidently with the control of the LA [CS] if the LA were the chamber of origin).

Spontaneous Change in Atrial Activation Pattern in SVT

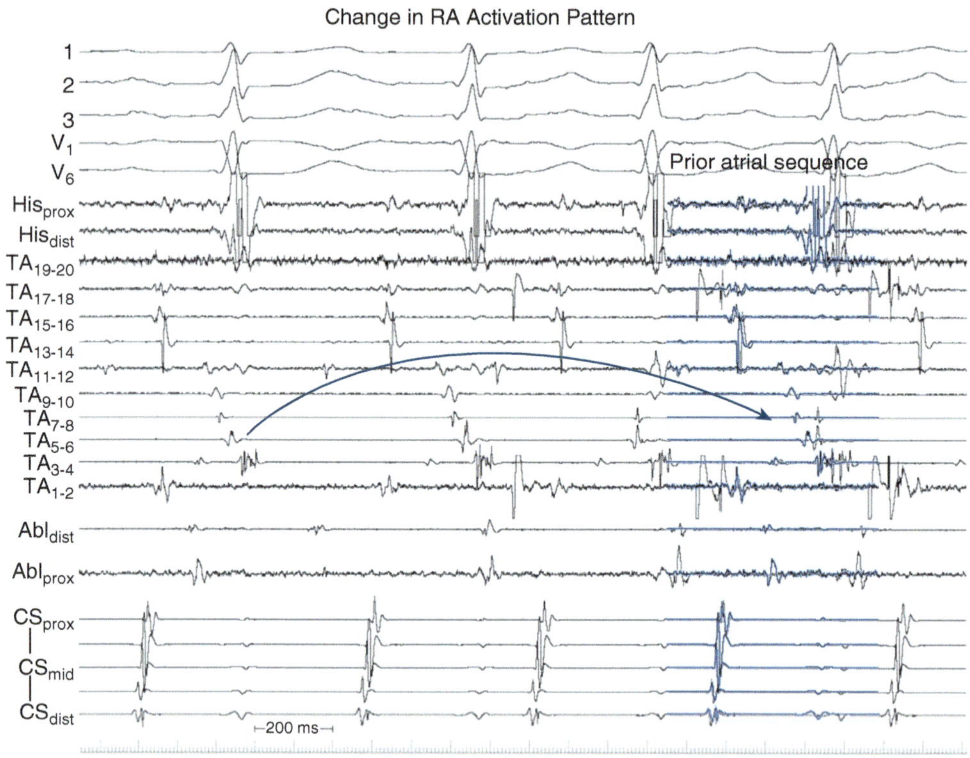

Figure 13-16

Just when we are honing in on the area of interest, the tachycardia changes (Fig. 13-16); the activation sequence on the left half is superimposed in *blue* on the right half to highlight the differences. This may be a change to another circuit, or another path within the same general circuit. It cannot be a sudden reversal of the circuit, as some tissue that had just been activated would have to be activated again too early for its refractory period to have ended (retracing steps during SVT). At some time earlier, another change has occurred: the CS activation was proximal to distal, now reversed.

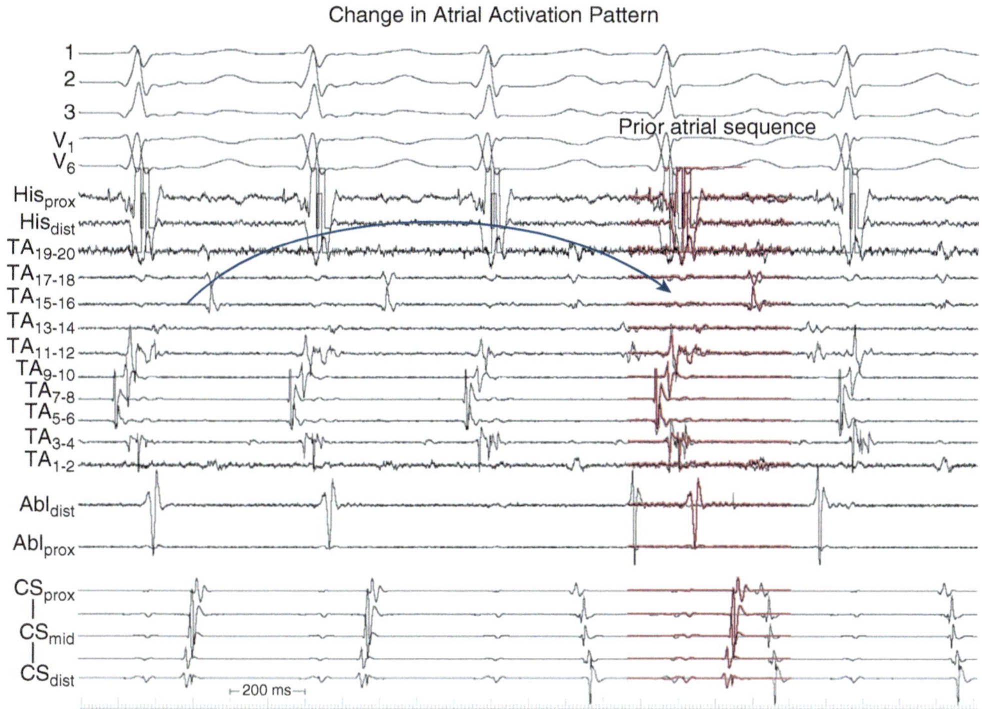

Figure 13-17

A few minutes later, activation changes again (Fig. 13-17). Portions of the TA (RA) are unchanged in both morphology and, largely, cycle length, suggesting that the same basic tachycardia (determined by the diastolic corridor) is continuing, but activation of the rest of the atrium may change (see the CS recordings; although the fundamental tachycardia may not change, the P wave can be altered [not evident here]).

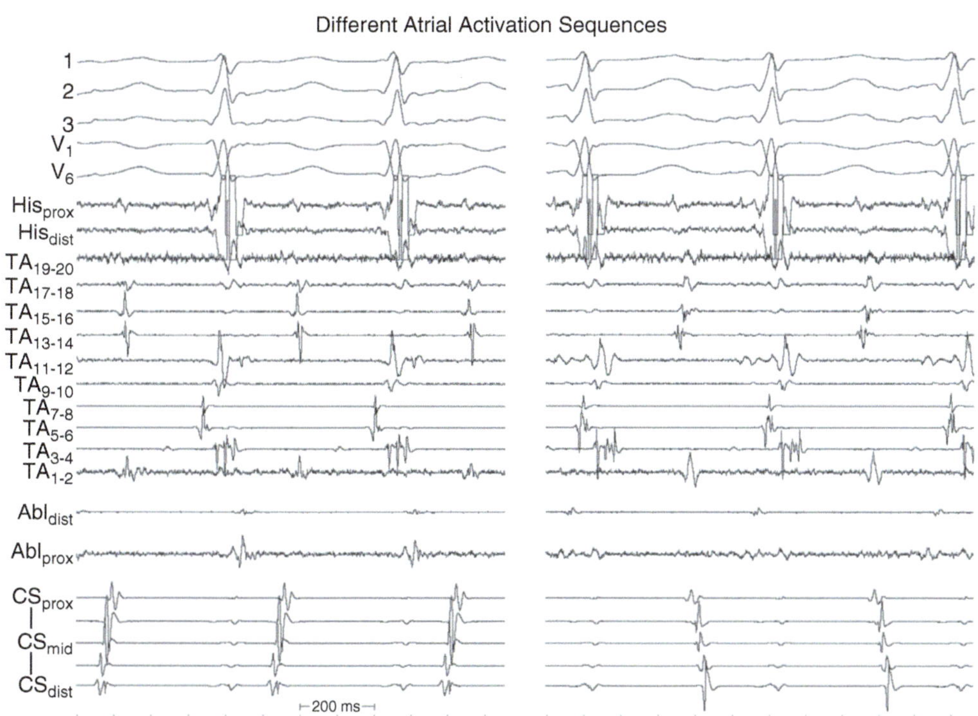

Figure 13-18

Two different atrial activation sequences are compared in Fig. 13-18.

SVT Termination During Catheter Mapping

Figure 13-19

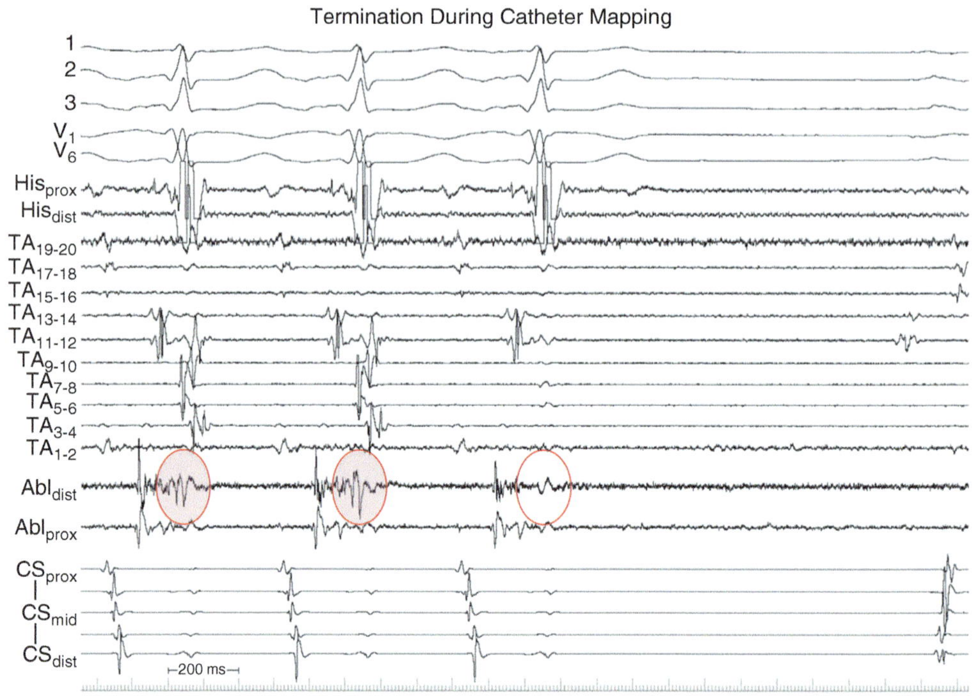

As mapping continues in Fig. 13-19, tachycardia suddenly terminates. Note the change in the electrogram on the ablation distal recording, and the absence of electrograms from TA 9-10 through 1-2 (because of block before they were activated).

Entrainment Mapping: Is It a Good Site?

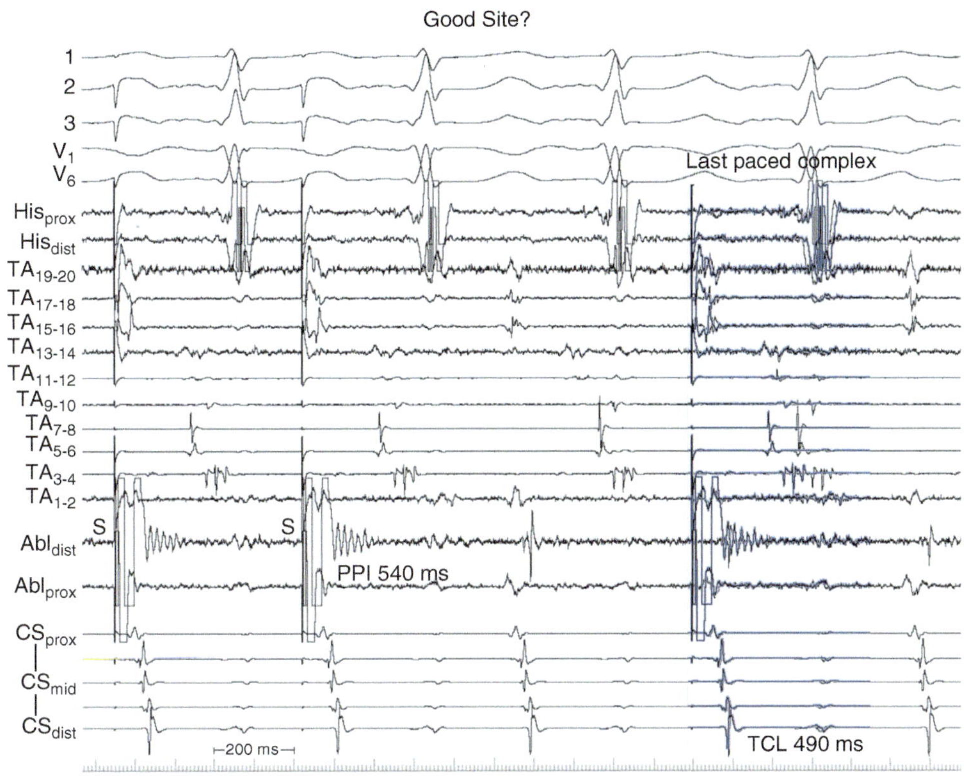

Figure 13-20

Tachycardia was reinitiated and a slightly different site with a diastolic electrogram was chosen for pacing. Fig. 13-20 displays a poor pace match (superimposed on tachycardia) and a long PPI-TCL difference from here—don't ablate at this site.

Figure 13-21

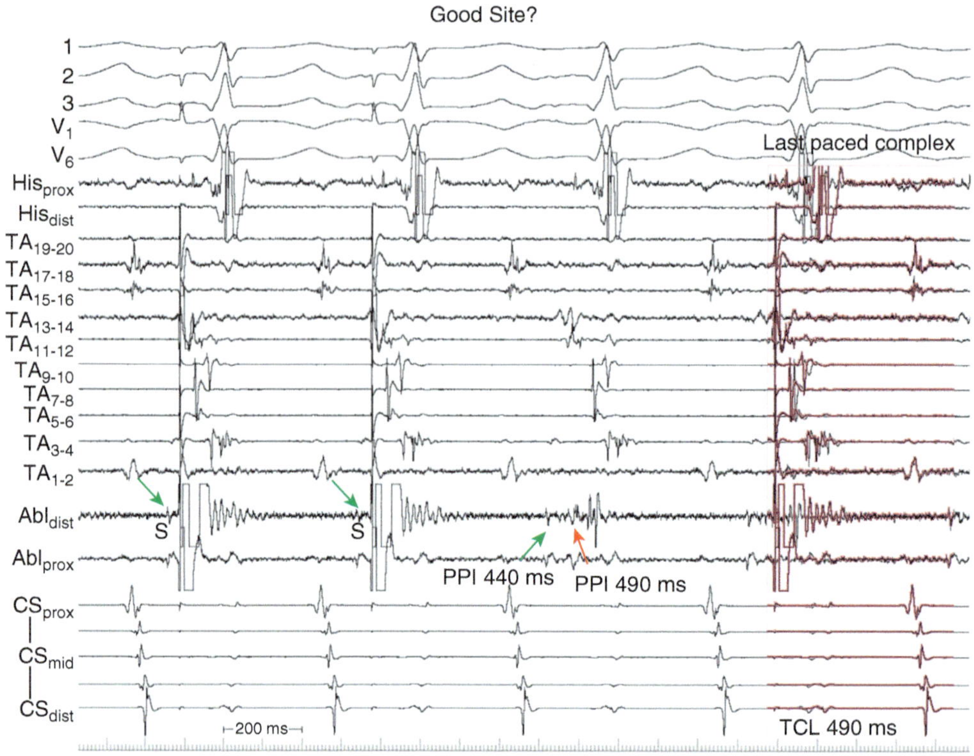

Pacing at a slightly different site—close to TA 13-14—produces a nearly perfect pace match but the PPI is again a problem (Fig. 13-21). If measured to the beginning of the complex electrogram *(orange arrow)*, PPI-TCL is perfect; but if measured to the small diastolic potential as before *(upward green arrow)*, the PPI is too short. The problem with the latter is that the small potential is clearly not captured during pacing because it appears before the stimulus artifact *(downward green arrows)*. The conclusion: this site, with a nearly perfect pacematch and perfect PPI-TCL, is a good site for ablation.

Ablation at Site

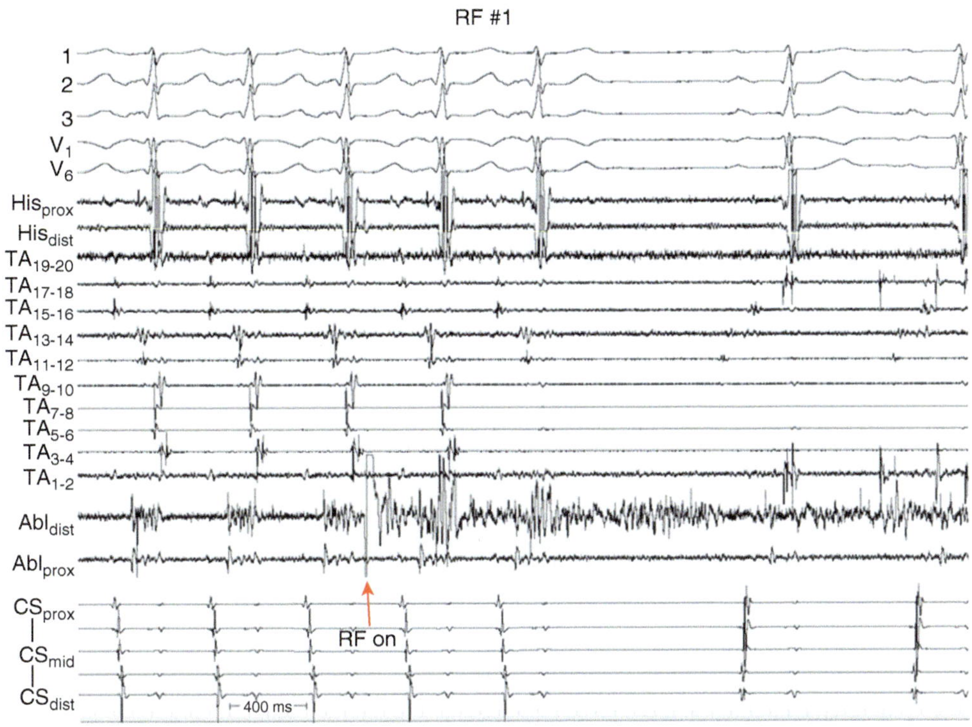

Are We Done Yet?

Figure 13-22

RF delivery (as indicated) at the site predicted to be a good ablation site is rewarded by immediate tachycardia termination (Fig. 13-22).

Electroanatomic Maps

Electroanatomic Mapping - Activation

Figure 13-23A

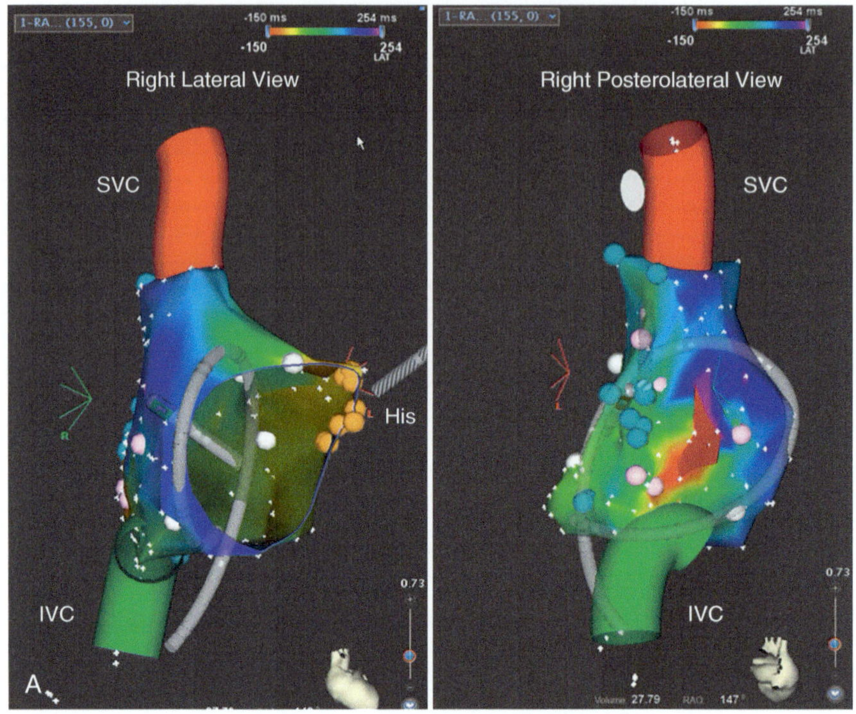

Electroanatomic Mapping - Voltage

Figure 13-23B

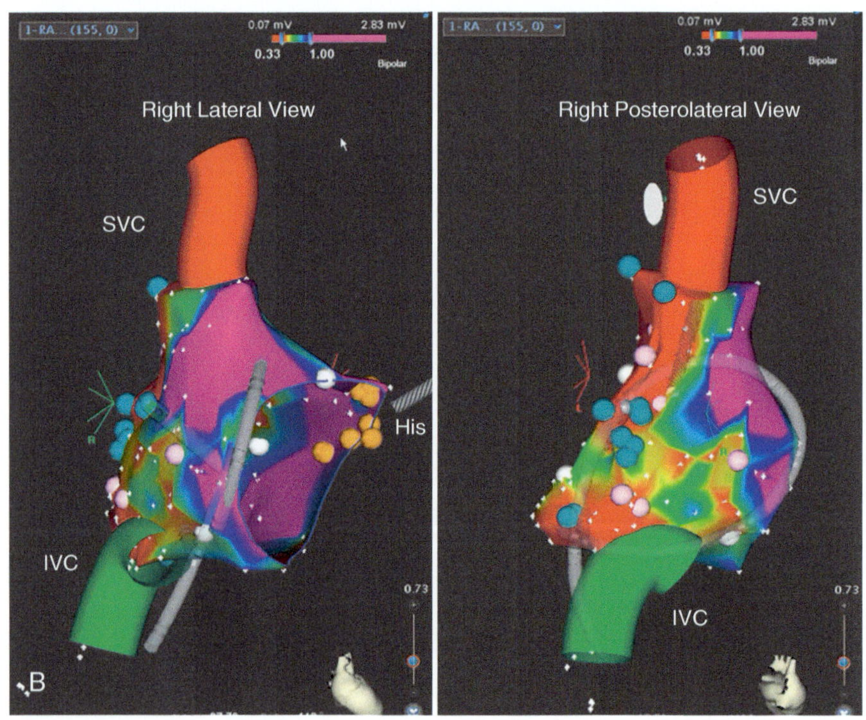

The electroanatomic maps (Fig. 13-23) demonstrate (A) electroanatomic activation mapping of right atrium in tachycardia; (B) electroanatomic voltage map of right atrium; and

Electroanatomic Mapping - Lesion Set

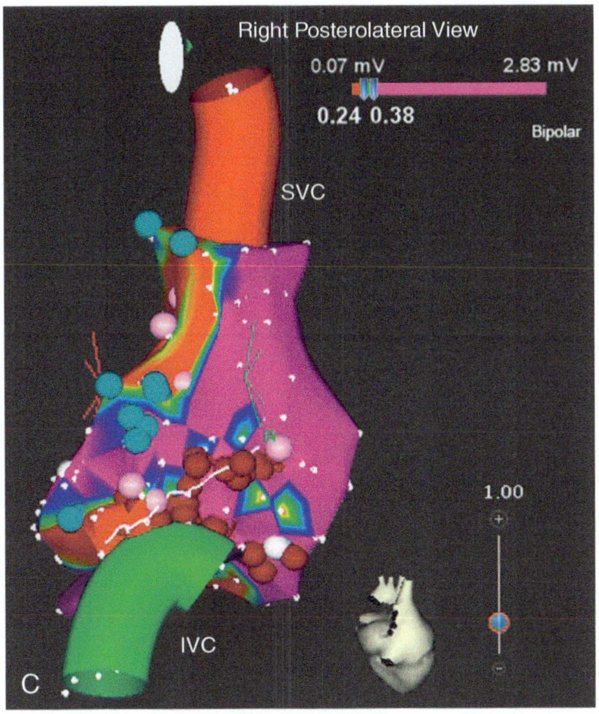

Figure 13-23C

(C) lesion set eventually used to transect the diastolic path and the segment of atrium from this region to the inferior vena cava, to preempt further reentry. In (A), a *red area* corresponding to the diastolic corridor is shown. Representations of the catheters (TA, His, and ablation) are faintly visible.

The prior right atrial cavotricuspid isthmus was evaluated and shown to have persistent bidirectional block from the prior ablation procedure.

Pacing from Various Sites Postablation

Figure 13-24

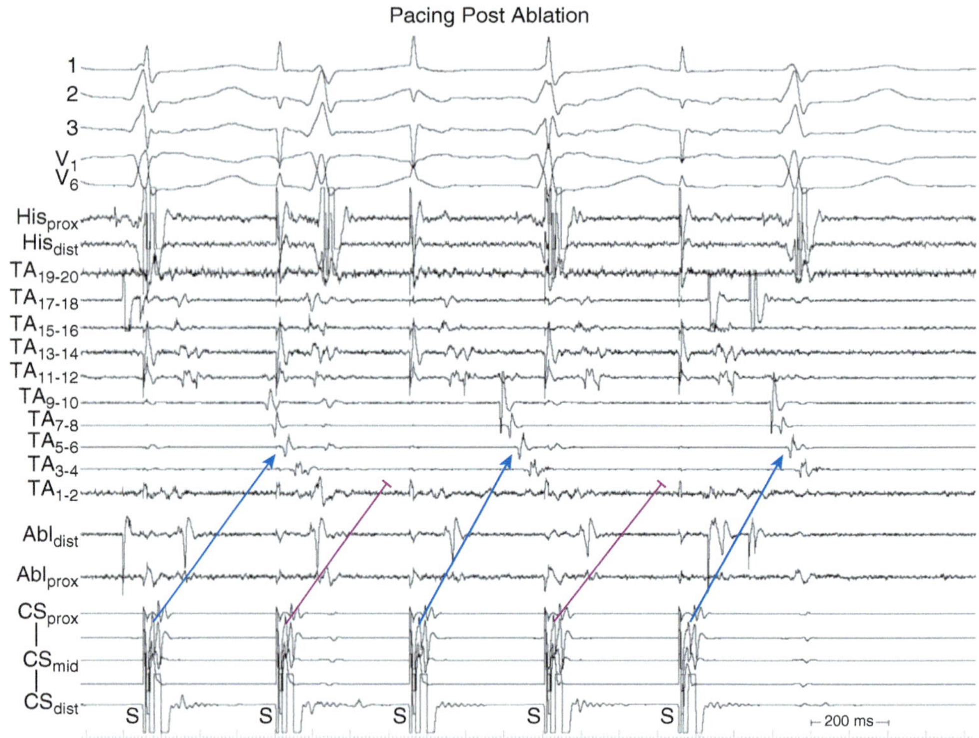

Conduction is so disrupted in Fig. 13-24 that pacing from the CS does not get to the RA each time (indicated by *arrows* and *stopped lines*).

Figure 13-25

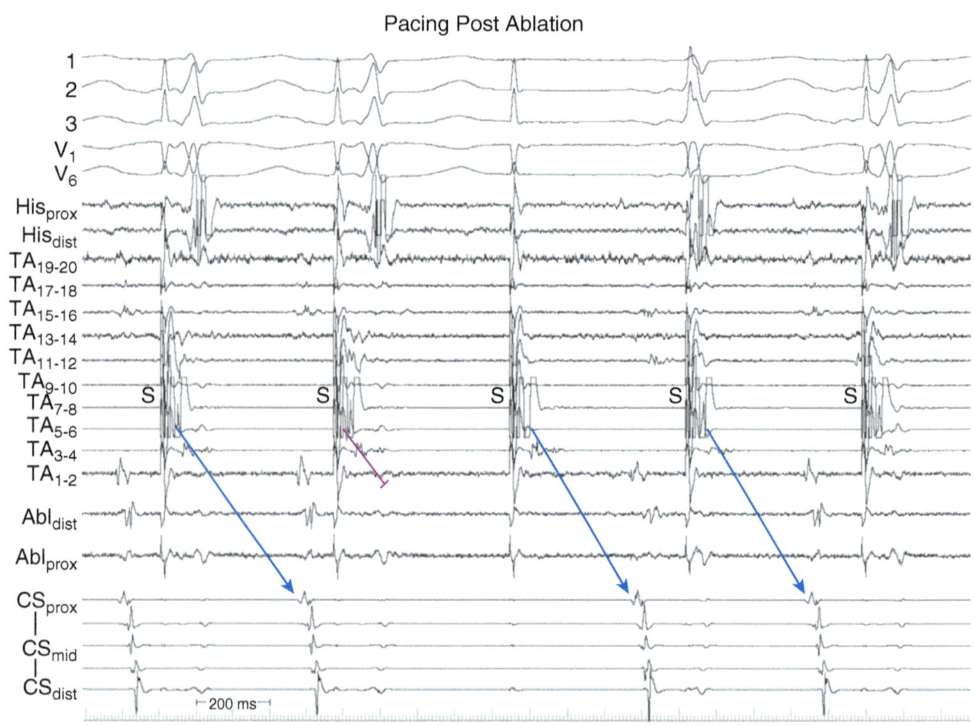

The same is true for pacing from RA (not conducting each time to CS), in Fig. 13-25.

Final ECG

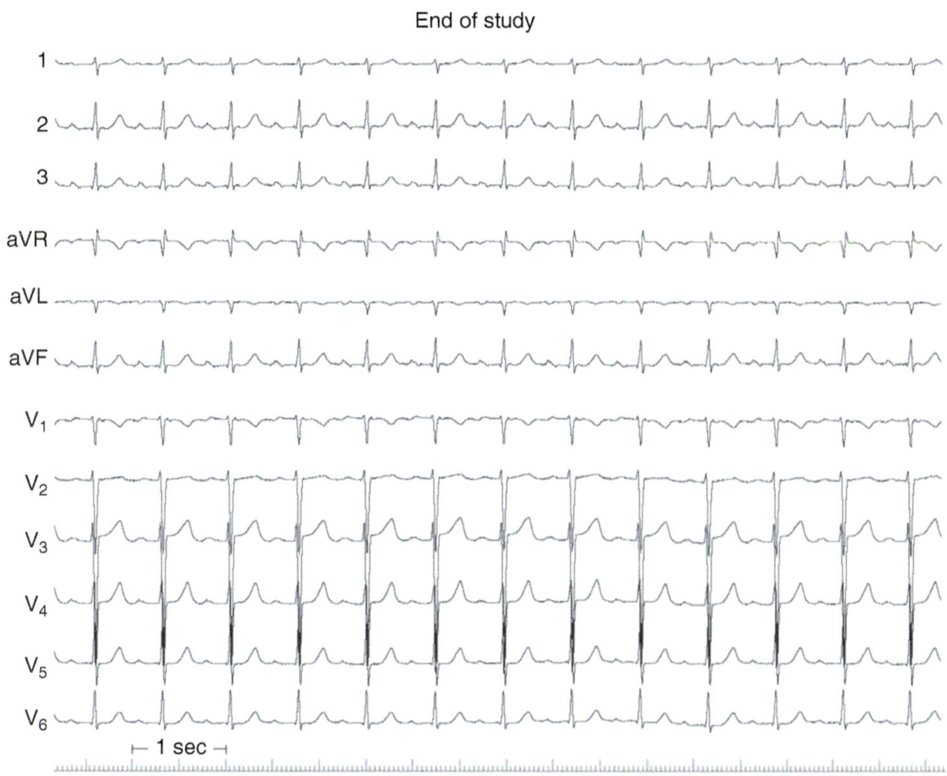

Figure 13-26

The patient's final ECG is shown in Fig. 13-26. She has been free of tachycardia recurrence for several years since the procedure.

Summary

- Atrial tachycardias after (non-maze) atrial surgery are common:
  - Right atrial macroreentry is much more common than left atrial
  - Atrial flutter is as common as (or more than) free wall macroreentrant circuits
  - Right atrial pathology (and circuits) can be present despite absence of prior extensive right atrial incisions
  - Entrain from multiple sites before concluding a focal mechanism
  - Circuits may be "bump-sensitive"—plan your mapping strategy before starting
- In areas of very slow/disrupted conduction, mapping systems:
  - May not be as helpful for tracking activation during AT as they are in other cases
  - May still be very useful for:
    - Delineation of scar/circuit boundaries
    - Designing strategies for ablation (connecting barriers)

14 Atrial Microreentry After Lung Transplantation

Case Presentation

The patient was a 60-year-old man with palpitations, lightheadedness, and dyspnea and referred for catheter ablation of atrial arrhythmias. He had a history of idiopathic pulmonary fibrosis. He underwent bilateral lung transplant in 2002; he had never shown any rejection. Palpitations began in 2013. ECGs showed supraventricular tachycardia ~190/min, and he was treated with metoprolol (failed); diltiazem (failed); flecainide (failed); and flecainide + metoprolol (partially successful?). Dyspnea continued despite "normal" heart rate (~100/min). He stated that his heart rate was constant all day and night unless he tried to exercise, at which point it sped up to twice as fast (200/min). He was referred for EP study and possible ablation.

Differential Diagnosis and Time Course of ATs After Lung Transplantation

What kinds of tachycardias do patients get after lung transplantation?

- Atrial fibrillation
- Atrial flutter/macroreentrant atrial tachycardia
  - Typical right atrial cavotricuspid isthmus-dependent flutter
  - Perimitral reentry
  - Peripulmonary vein cuff reentry
- Pulmonary vein tachycardias with donor–recipient atrial anastomotic electrical connection
- Other SVTs (which anyone may have)
  - AV nodal reentry
  - AV reentry (accessory pathway—WPW)
  - Focal atrial tachycardia

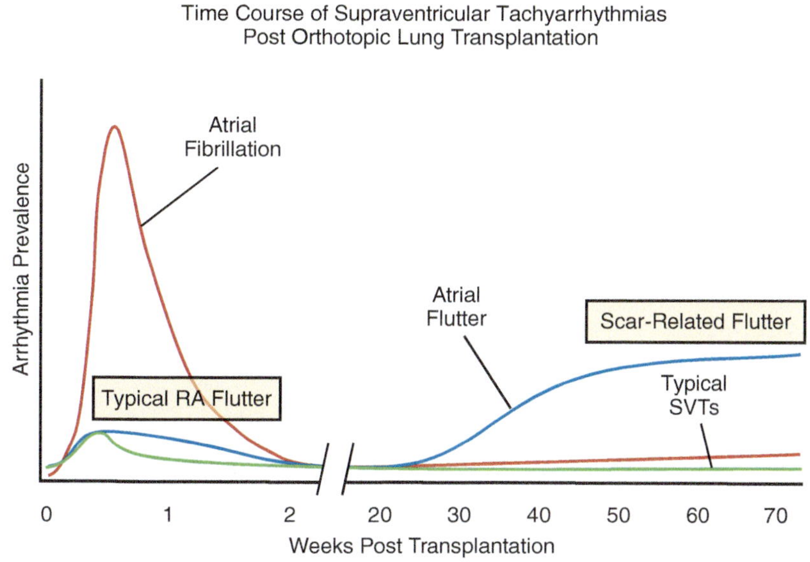

Figure 14-1

Fig. 14-1 demonstrates the time course of supraventricular tachyarrhythmias after lung transplantation. RA, right atrial; SVT, supraventricular tachycardia.

Types of Lung Transplantation Procedures

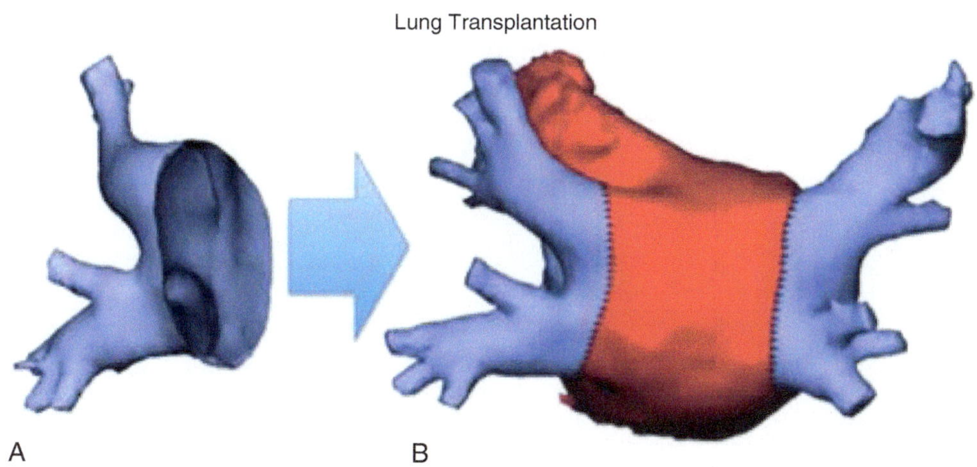

Figure 14-2

(From Lee, G et al. Atrial fibrillation following lung transplantation: double but not single lung transplant is associated with long-term freedom from paroxysmal atrial fibrillation. *Eur Heart J* (2010) 31: 2774-2782.)

A common technique for lung transplantation is to mate the donor lung and pulmonary vein (PV) cuff *(blue)* to the recipient atrium *(red)* (Fig. 14-2).

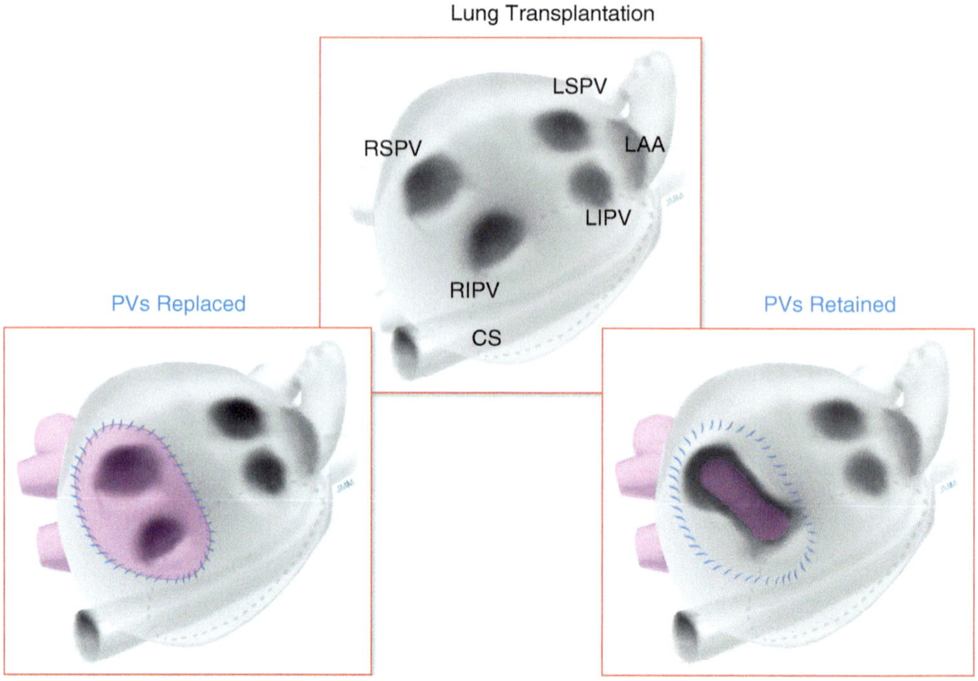

Figure 14-3

Pulmonary veins (PVs) may be replaced as in Fig. 14-2, or retained (with the donor PV cuff sewn around the perimeter of the recipient PVs), as shown in Fig. 14-3. LIPV, left inferior PV; LSPV, left superior PV; RIPV, right inferior PV; RSPV, right superior PV.

Baseline ECG and Intracardiac Recordings

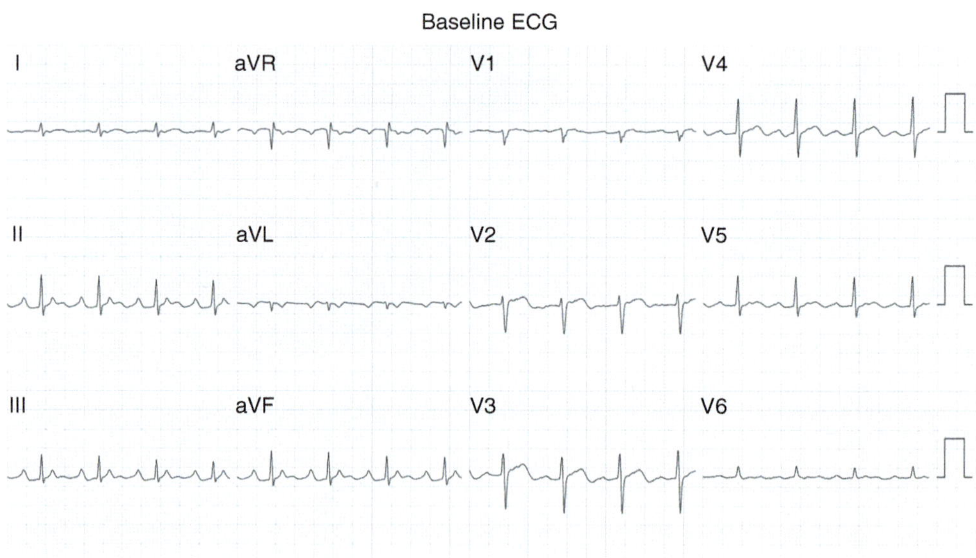

Figure 14-4

Differential diagnosis is only atrial tachycardia; the 2:1 AV relationship excludes orthodromic SVT and the positive P wave excludes AV nodal reentry. What particular kind of atrial tachycardia, however, remains to be diagnosed. The ECG shown in Fig. 14-4 was mistaken as sinus rhythm, which it superficially resembles. However, the rate never varies unless the patient exercises and suddenly conducts 1:1.

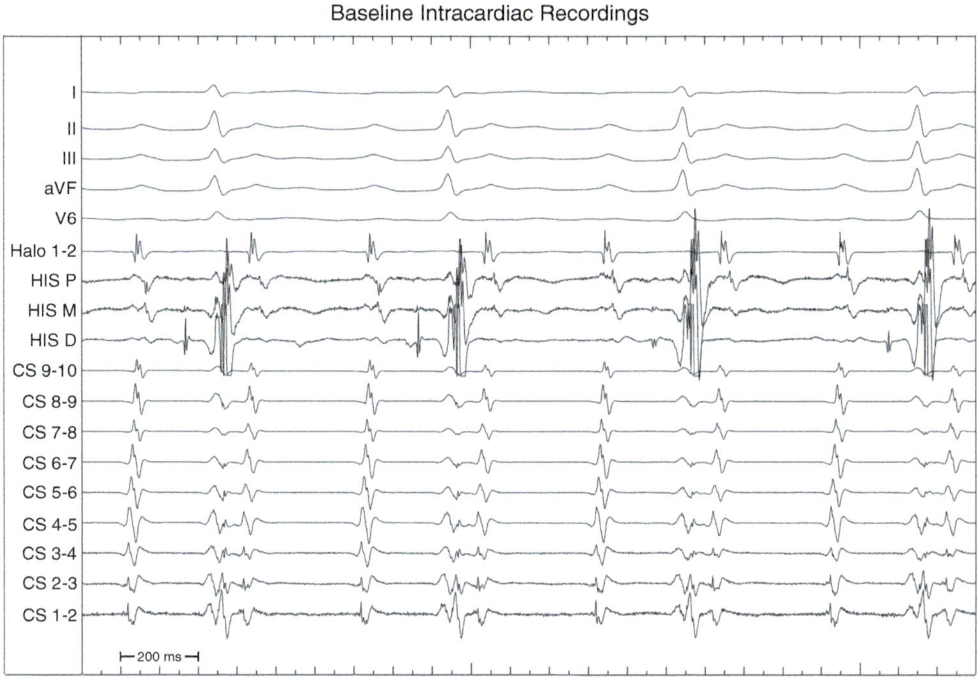

Figure 14-5

In Fig. 14-5, it is hard to tell where the P wave starts because of low-gain ECG channels.

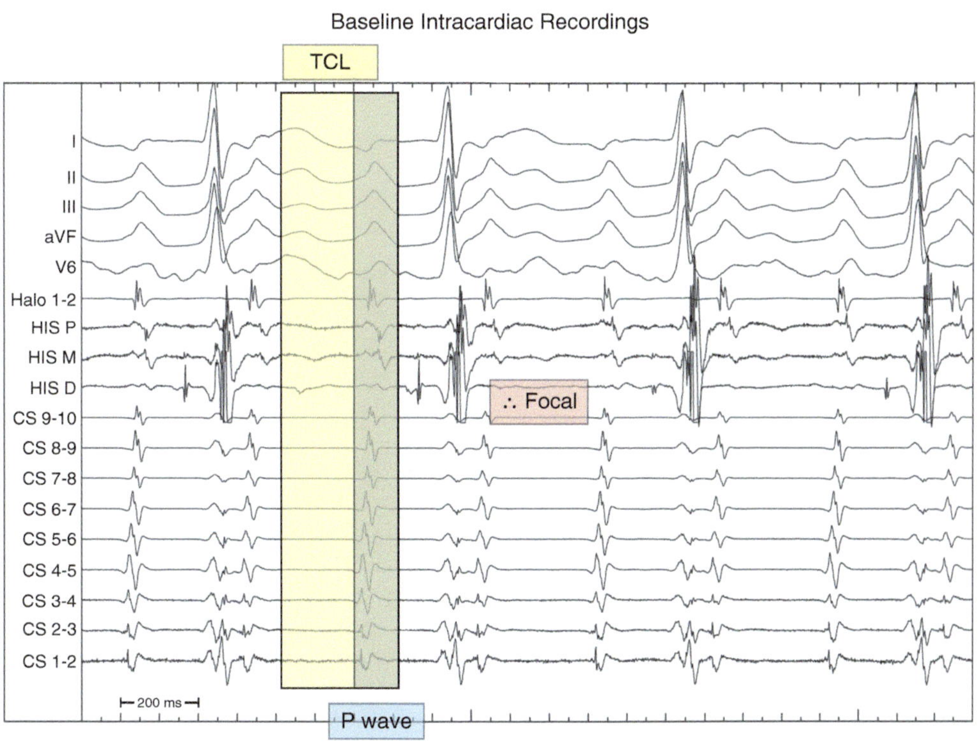

Figure 14-6

One can often infer a mechanism of atrial tachycardia by comparing P-wave duration (and intracardiac electrogram "envelope") to tachycardia cycle length (TCL). The narrower the P wave, especially relative to TCL, the more likely a focal process is involved, but a broader P wave in relation to TCL suggests macroreentry (Fig. 14-6). Specifically, a ratio <0.5 suggests a focal process, because after the focus fires and the atria are activated from that source, there is a pause (diastole) until the next firing of the focus and another P wave begins.

Figure 14-7

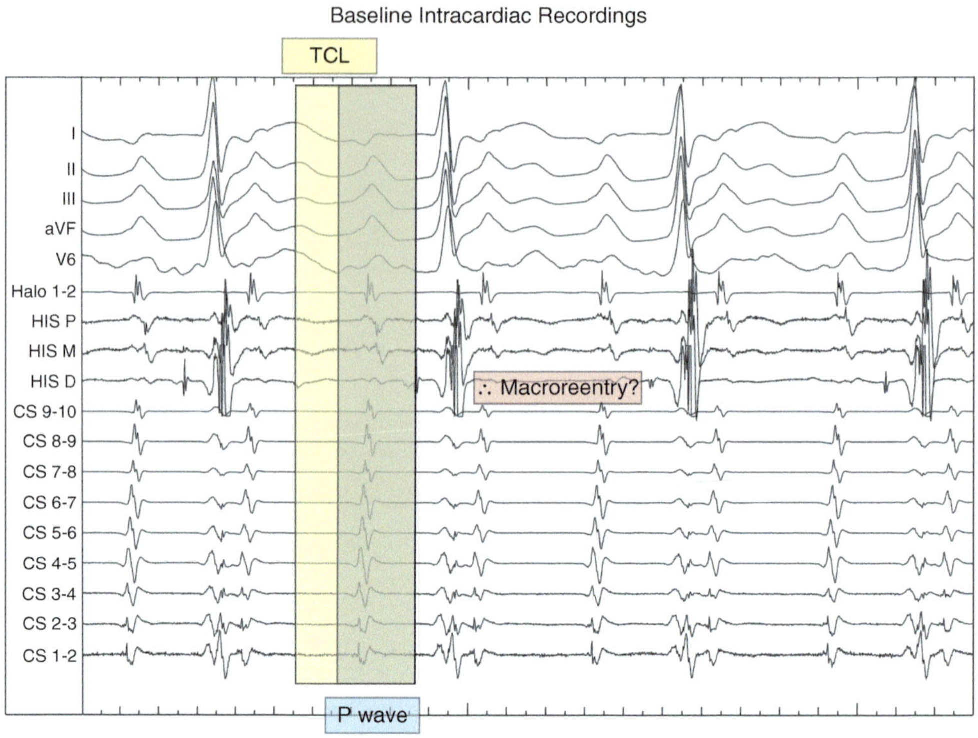

Fig. 14-7 shows a different interpretation of the P-wave duration, while the TCL remains the same. Now, a P-wave duration to TCL ratio >0.7 suggests that atrial activation spreads slowly through large portions of the atrium and thus the mechanism is likely macroreentry. There is considerable overlap with this index (ratio of P duration to TCL) and it is at best suggestive, but not diagnostic, of mechanism.

Figure 14-8

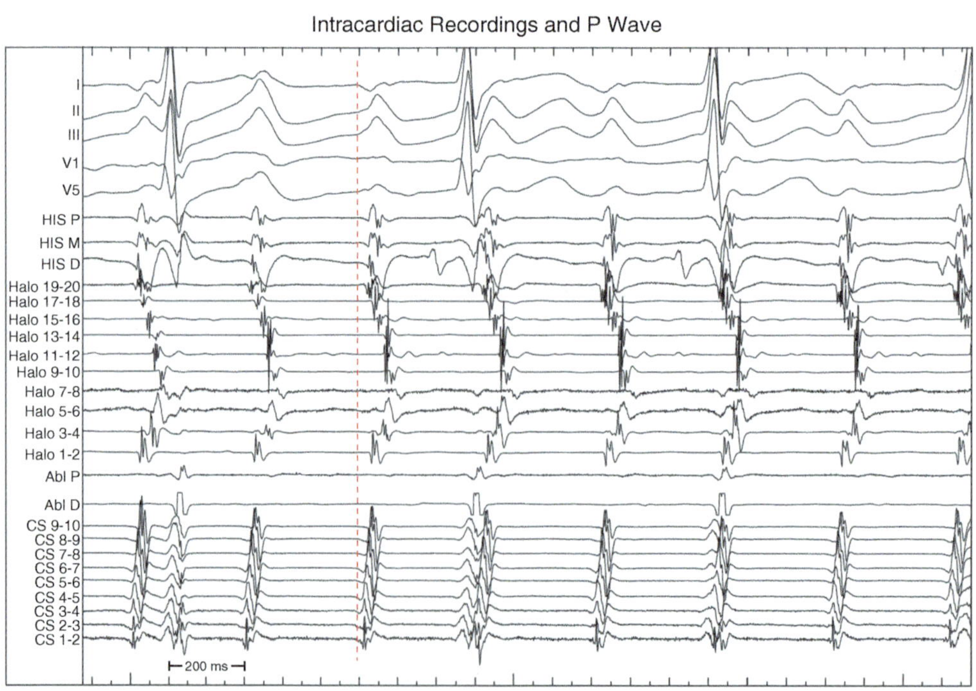

The P-wave morphology (initial negative component) suggests a left atrial origin (Fig. 14-8), as does distal-to-proximal CS activation sequence. None of the recordings show pre–P-wave electrical activity, however (P wave onset denoted by dashed red line).

Status

- Sustained (incessant) SVT is present
- All electrical activity recorded is after P-wave onset
- Recordings suggest left atrial process
  - Initial negative P in lead 1
  - CS activation sequence slightly distal-to-proximal
- Mechanism: unclear
- Choices of strategy at this juncture:
  - Activation mapping
    - Can give idea of where origin/exit is, scar borders
    - Does not designate mechanism
    - Catheter bump-termination can occur
  - Overdrive pacing during tachycardia
    - Can designate mechanism, thus ablation target features
    - Can designate which atrium is involved
    - May terminate tachycardia

Electroanatomic Mapping

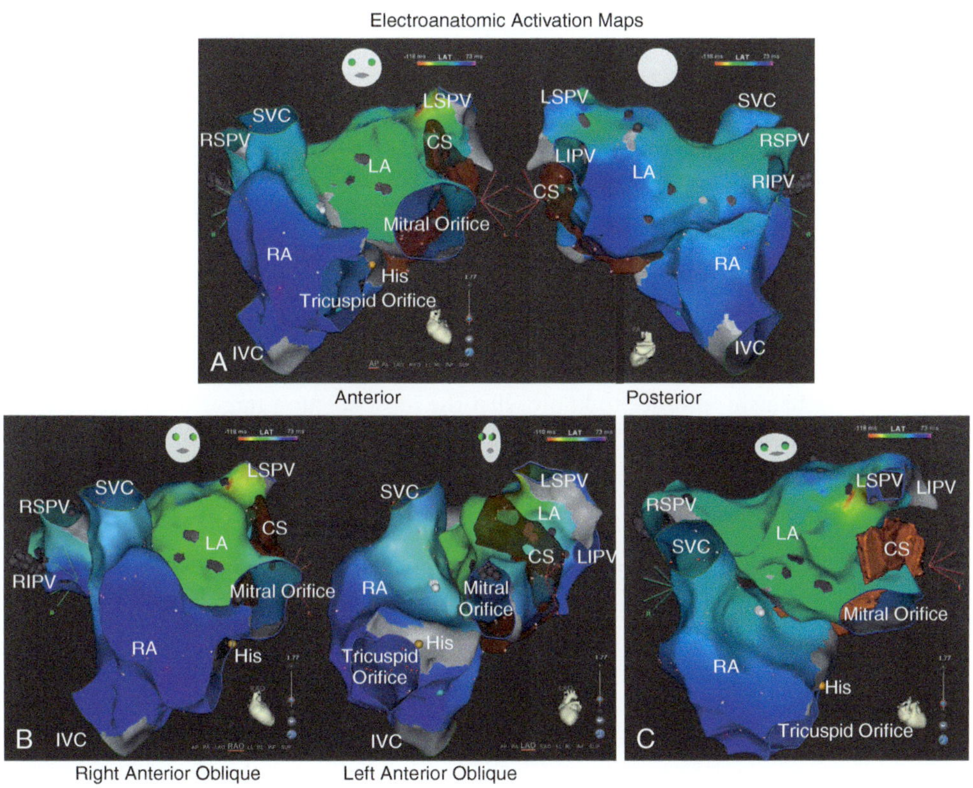

Figure 14-9

We chose activation mapping as the initial strategy, and mapped both atria (Fig. 14-9). The right atrium is clearly activated late in the P wave, but so is everywhere else except for a tiny spot in the top of the left atrium. Note that the span of activation times (−118 to 73 ms, or a total of 291 ms) is almost exactly the TCL (300 ms). This is usually the case with macroreentry but not with focal tachycardias; however, a focus with slow propagation through a scarred atrium can have a total activation time similar to TCL. CS, coronary sinus; IVC, inferior vena cava; LA, left atrium; SVC, superior vena cava.

Mapping

What Does This Mean? [Fig. 14-10]

Recording Near LSPV

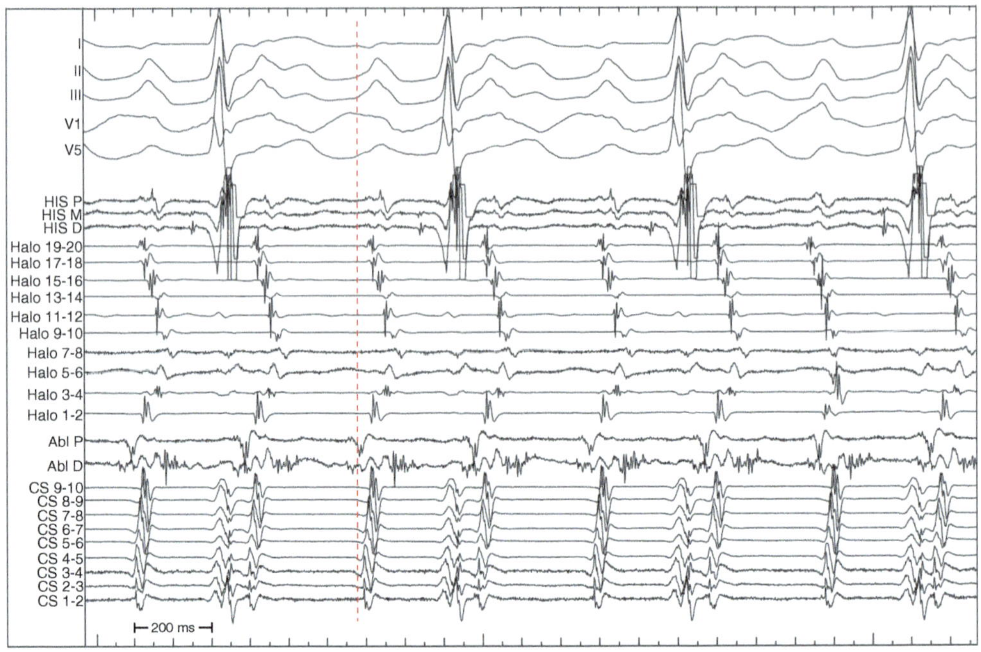

Figure 14-10

A very fractionated electrogram is present near the ostium of the left superior PV, at the site of earliest activation during tachycardia (Fig. 14-10). Although this could still be focal, it raises the question of reentry because the electrogram is so very prolonged and fractionated. At this point, a ring catheter was introduced into the left atrium to interrogate the PVs.

Overdrive Pacing During Tachycardia from Various Sites

Now that we have an idea where the tachycardia exit is (high lateral left atrium), we can clarify the mechanism in order to know what the ideal ablation target site looks like. If a small focus is the cause, a site with minimal pre–P-wave activation (30 to 40 ms) will suffice. If macroreentry, we need a site with middiastolic activation. Responses to overdrive pacing, often from several sites, should provide the answer. In the ablation recording, we already have a middiastolic site near the left superior PV; this could still be a focus there with slow conduction out of it (near a suture line, or conduction from focus in donor PV to recipient LA?), or macroreentry.

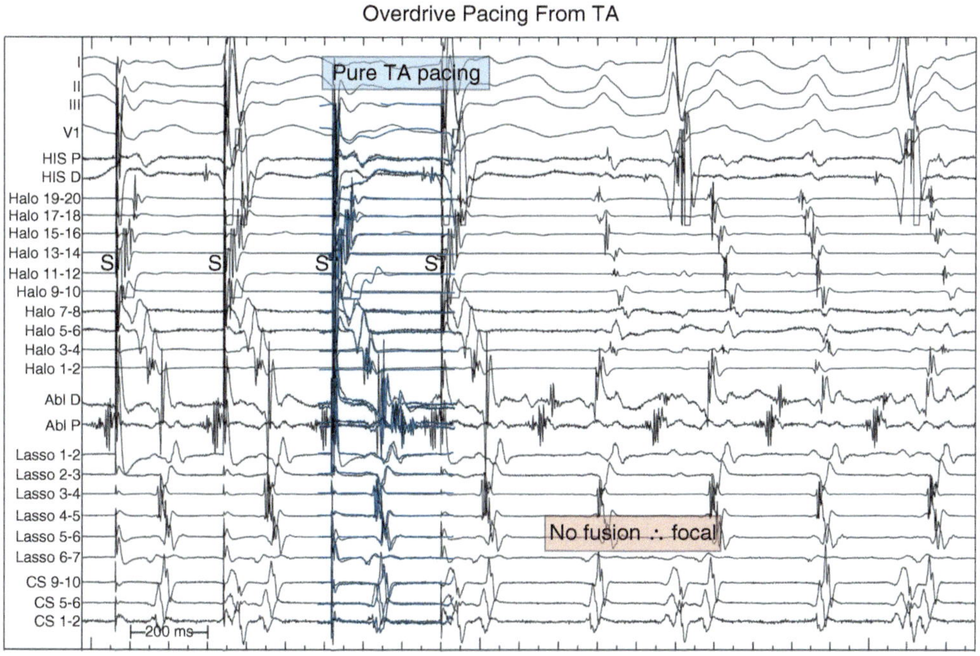

Figure 14-11

In Fig. 14-11, we are overdrive pacing from the lateral right atrium, one of the last places to be activated during tachycardia. Pacing from such a late-activated site makes it easy to see if fusion is present during pacing, because the wavefront caused by pacing and that caused by tachycardia are in theory on opposite sides of the heart. The response to pacing shows that the lateral RA pacing site is indeed among the last to come back on the first beat of resumed tachycardia; superimposition of an example of pure pacing from this site in sinus rhythm shows there to be little, if any, difference between pure pacing and pacing during tachycardia (the ablation catheter position changed between the two recordings and cannot be compared). Thus there is no fusion, further suggesting a focal process.

Figure 14-12

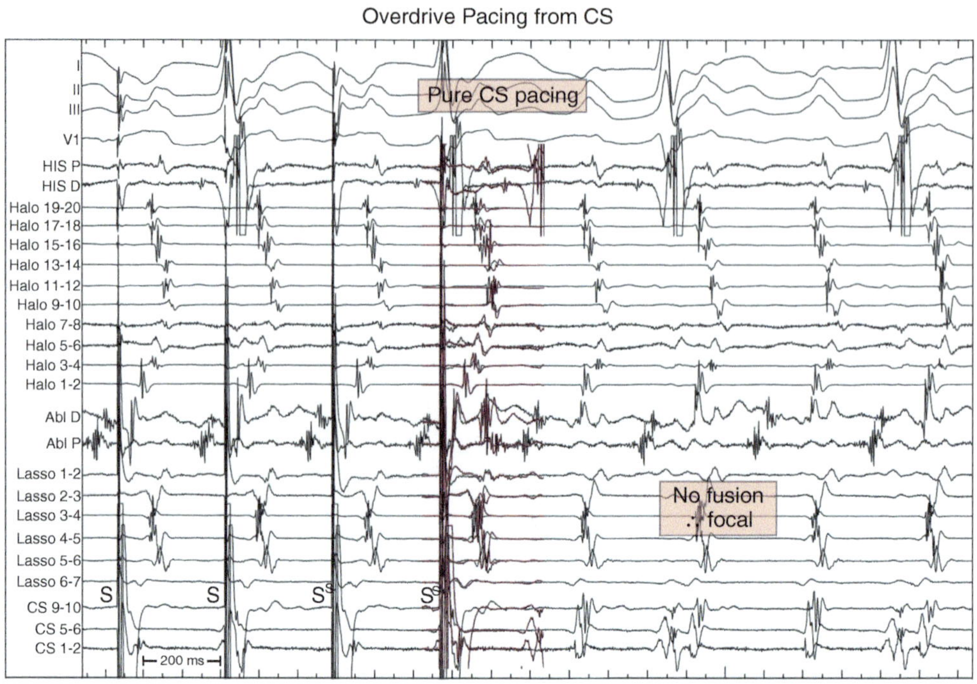

Pacing from another site (Fig. 14-12) yields the same findings as before: no fusion, thus likely a focus (as noted before, the position of the ablation catheter had changed between the two recording times and is thus not comparable). However, we had not seen anything but tachycardia to this point in the procedure; the pure pacing examples were obtained only after tachycardia terminated. Thus the comparison of pure pacing versus pacing during tachycardia was not available at the time pacing during tachycardia was performed (it was before ablation, however).

Figure 14-13

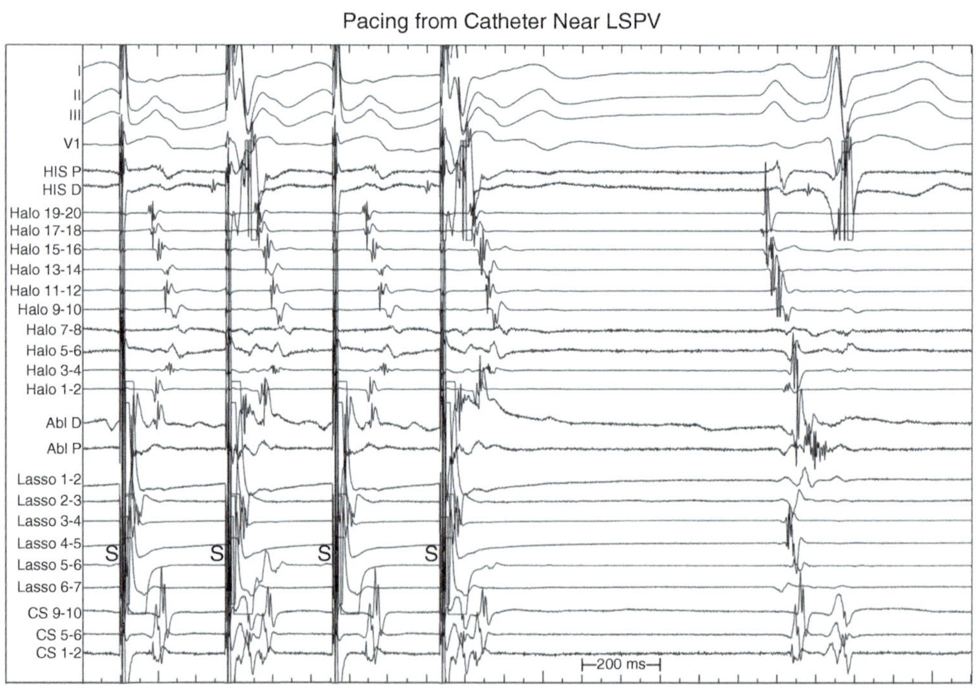

Unfortunately, pacing from the ring catheter in the LSPV, near the earliest site of activation during tachycardia, terminated the arrhythmia to sinus rhythm (Fig. 14-13).

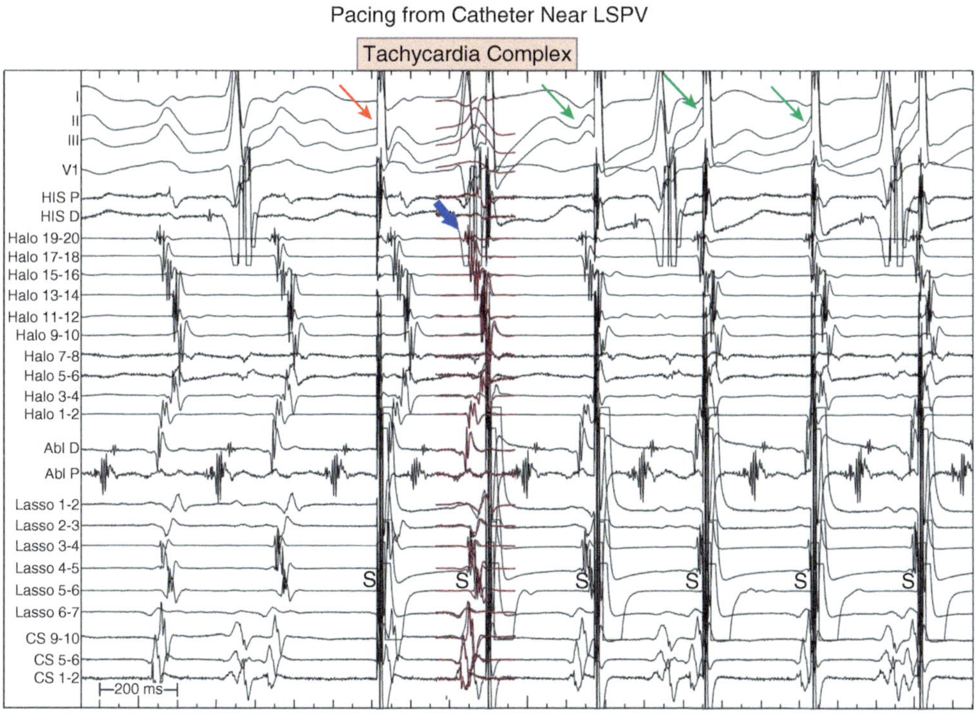

Figure 14-14

All is not lost, however. Looking back at the initiation of pacing at this site in Fig. 14-14 shows some interesting findings. The first complex controlled by pacing, indicated by the *large blue arrow*, appears to have an identical activation sequence to that of tachycardia (superimposed). That in itself is not so unusual; however, the fact that the stimulus artifact occurred at the onset of the P wave that had already been made by the previous tachycardia cycle *(small red arrow)* is suggestive of a circuit with separate entrance and exit locations; this is further exemplified in subsequent complexes, when the stimulus artifact clearly follows the beginning of an accelerated P wave *(green arrows)*. A focus could not do this.

Pacing Donor Left Superior Pulmonary Vein During Sinus Rhythm

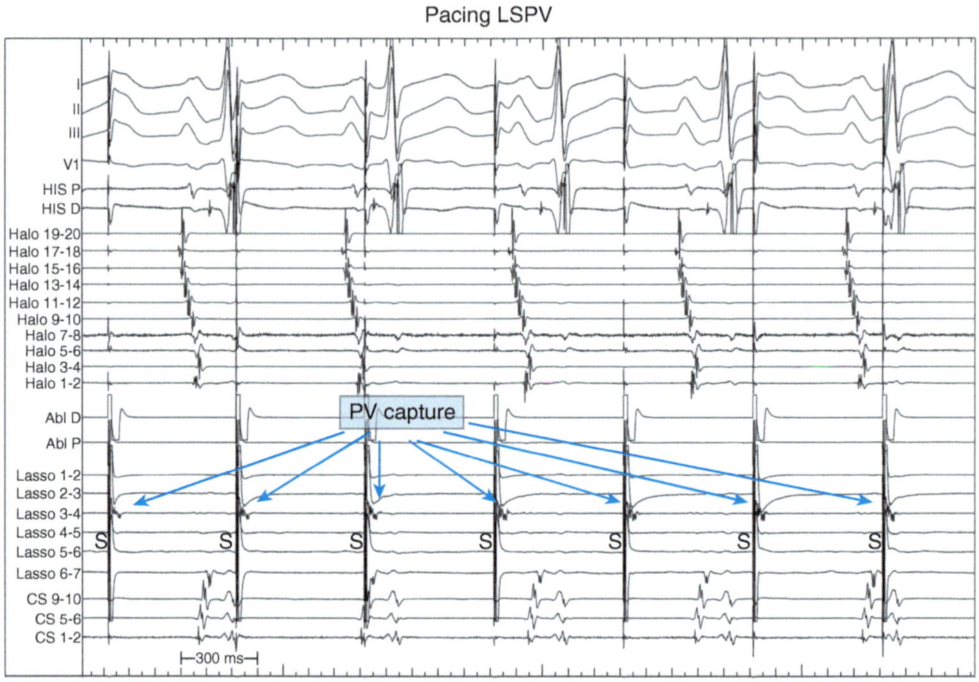

Figure 14-15

Now that tachycardia has accidentally been terminated, we take advantage of the situation. Pacing from the right atrial and coronary sinus sites used in pacing during tachycardia can now be used as examples of "pure" pacing from these sites for comparison. Further, to prove that this was not a pulmonary vein (PV) tachycardia from the donor PV that had made an electrical connection to the recipient atrium, pacing from the left superior PV (Fig. 14-15) showed it to be electrically separate from the rest of the atrium (which is in sinus rhythm at this point).

Pacing from Ablation Catheter Near Ablation Site

Approximates Appearance of SVT

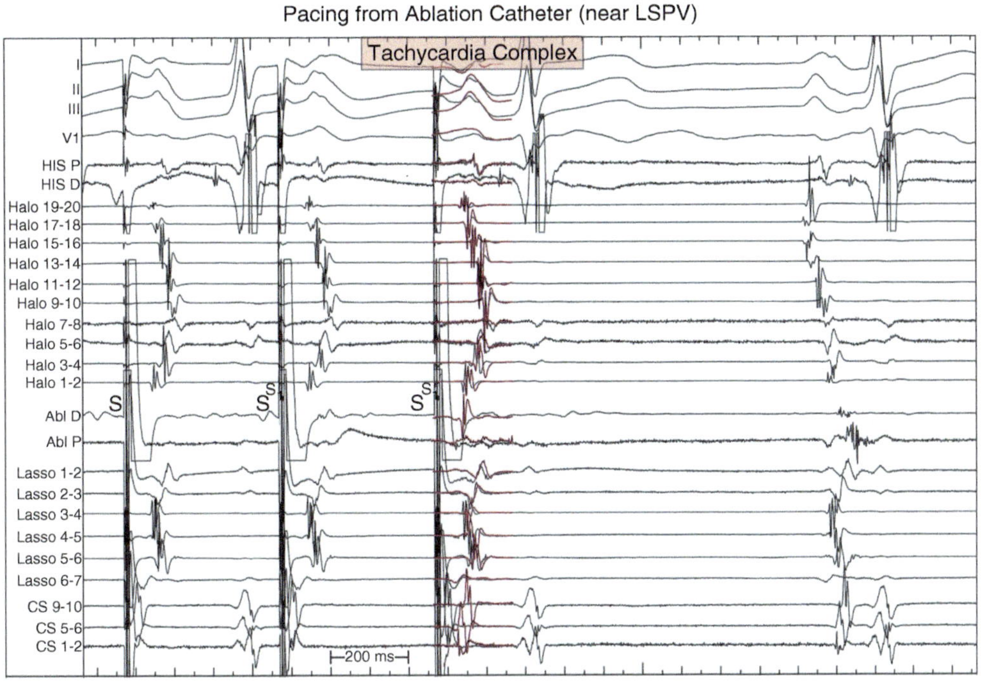

Figure 14-16

In Fig. 14-16, pacing from the ablation catheter (located near the site of the earliest activation during tachycardia) shows an activation sequence almost identical to that of tachycardia—except for the coronary sinus recordings, which are completely different. If this were a focal tachycardia, pacing from the site of the focus should exactly replicate the tachycardia activation sequence and P-wave configuration. The fact is that it does not raise further suspicions about this being a focal firing process.

Initiates SVT

Figure 14-17

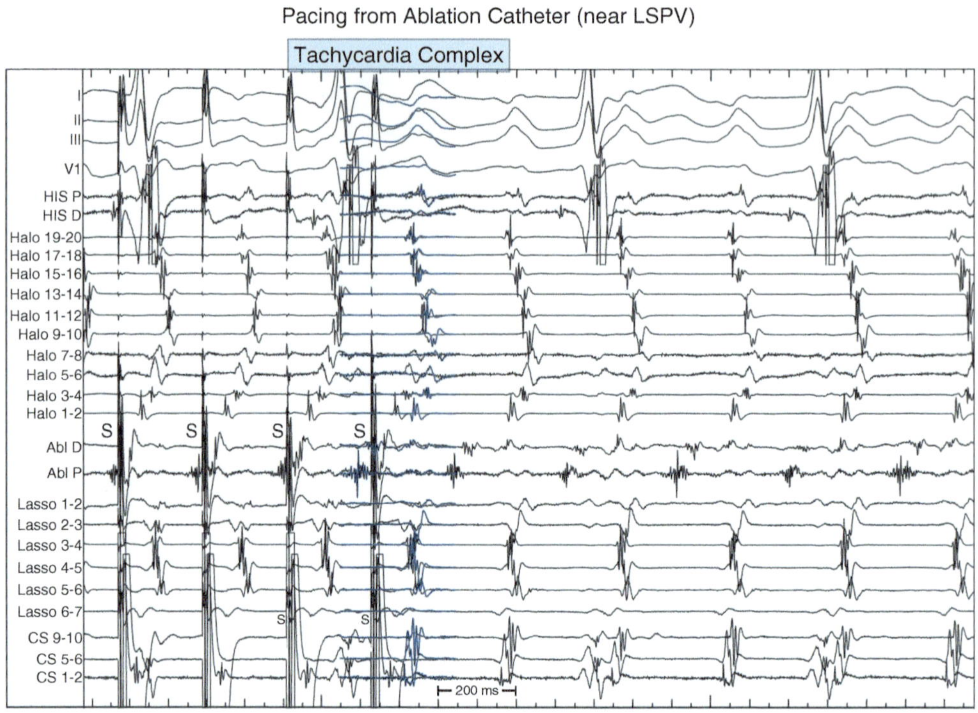

Pacing from near the LSPV initiates tachycardia; this would be unusual for a focal firing process (unless it were related to delayed afterdepolarizations). In Fig. 14-17, a complex of tachycardia is again superimposed on the last paced cycle; once again, if this were a focus, pacing here should look very similar to tachycardia. The fact that it does not further calls into question the focal firing hypothesis.

Replicates SVT Appearance

Figure 14-18

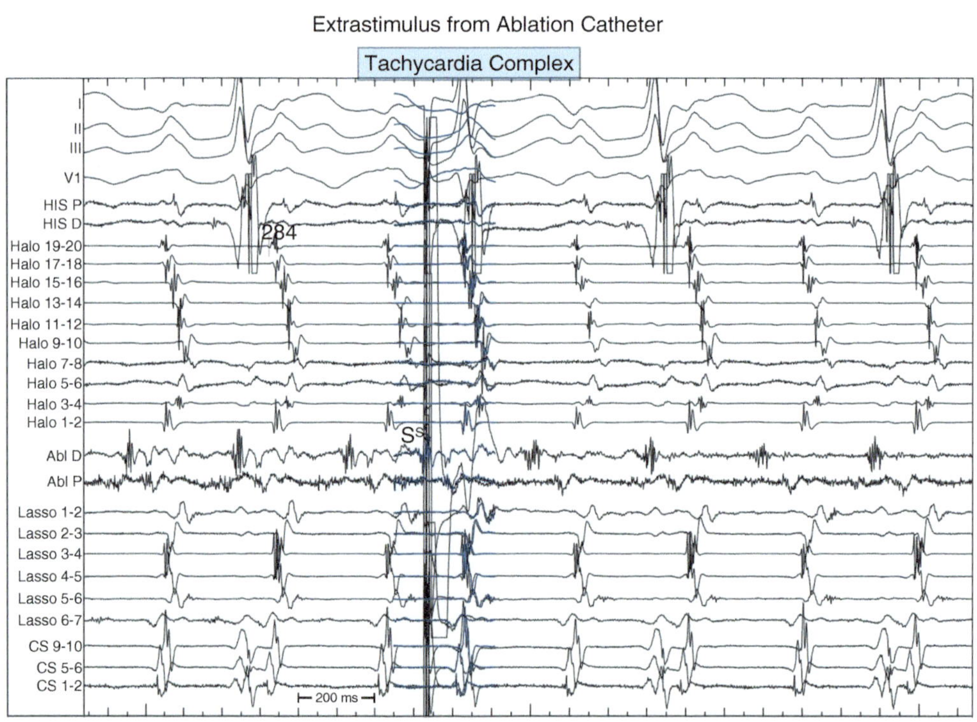

An extrastimulus delivered from ablation catheter (recording of a site of middiastolic ablation) captures, resulting in an atrial activation sequence identical to that of tachycardia (Fig. 14-18). This in itself does not differentiate between a focus and reentrant circuit, as one could stimulate from a focus during tachycardia, depolarize the focus, and have a resulting complex that looks identical to tachycardia, and one can certainly stimulate during a reentrant arrhythmia and have the same result.

Terminates SVT Without Propagation

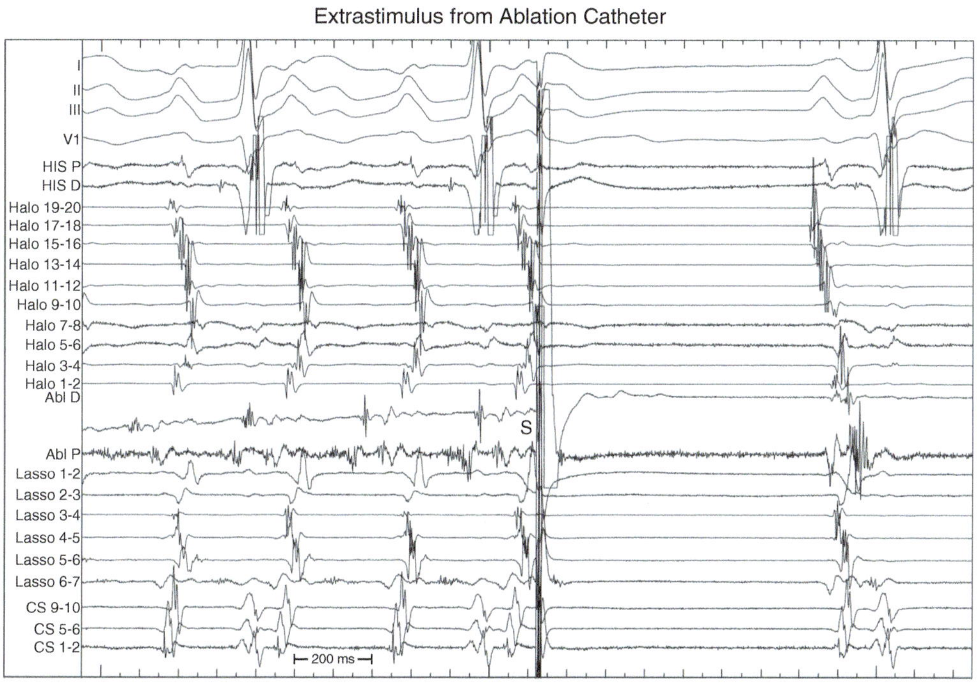

Figure 14-19

As extrastimuli are brought more prematurely (Fig. 14-19), tachycardia terminates, without apparent propagation; this was a reproducible phenomenon during this procedure. This would be extraordinarily unusual behavior for a focus, and strongly suggests reentry (during which this phenomenon is reasonably commonly observed). The very prolonged diastolic electrogram goes along with this. But what kind of reentry? Fusion was never demonstrated, and the activation map did not show an "early-meets-late" juxtaposition of earliest activations to latest activations (in fact, these were on the opposite side of the heart in the right atrium). This could be *micro*reentry, fulfilling all the requirements for reentry (inducible, terminable with pacing, entrainable) but never showing manifest fusion because the circuit is so small. An additional feature of microreentry is an electrogram at the ideal ablation site that nearly spans the tachycardia cycle length. A focus because of delayed afterdepolarizations could conceivably have accounted for most, if not all, of the phenomena encountered before this; however, termination of tachycardia by a nonpropagated stimulus excludes any focal firing process. Instead, this indicates that a reentrant circuit is responsible, and because fusion was not demonstrable from any far-away pacing site, the activation pattern on electroanatomic mapping suggested a small area from which activation emanated simulating a focus, and the electrogram from this site was extremely prolonged, microreentry is the most likely mechanism of tachycardia.

Reinitiates SVT

Figure 14-20

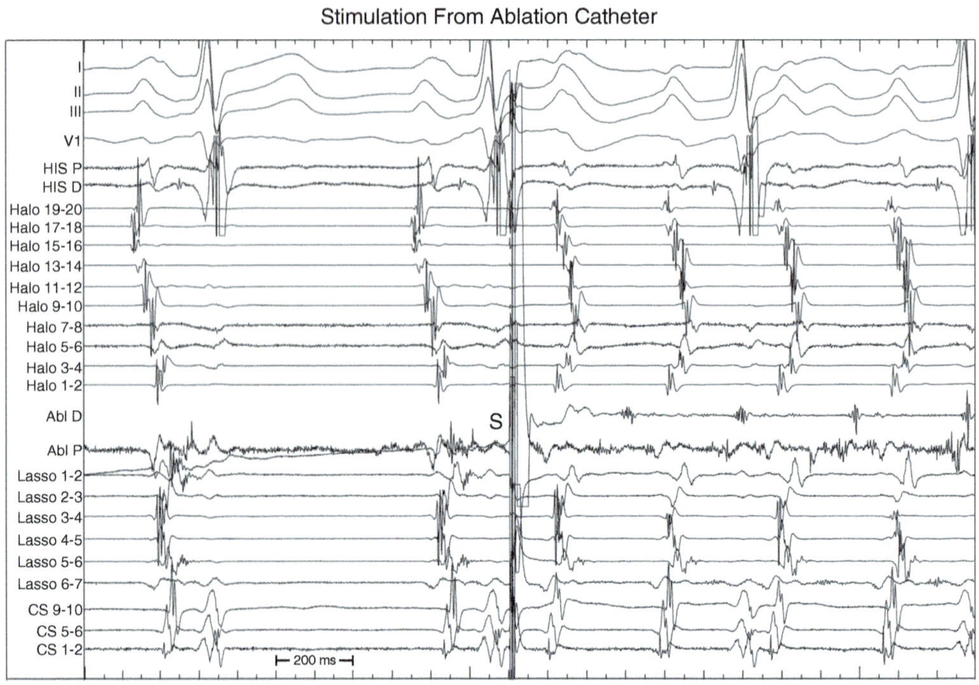

A single extrastimulus (S) delivered from the ablation catheter at the site of the earliest activation during tachycardia easily reinitiates tachycardia (Fig. 14-20). This would again be extremely unusual for a focal-firing process (automaticity), which is typically not inducible.

Recording at Ablation Site

Figure 14-21

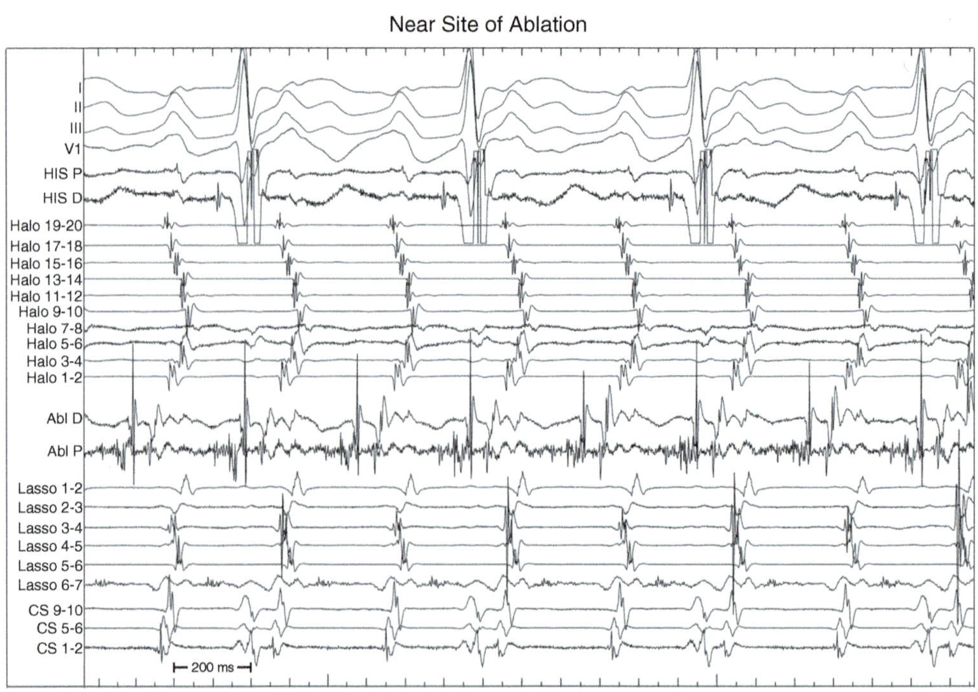

In Fig. 14-21, a nearly continuous electrogram is seen in the proximal recording of the ablation catheter, again consistent with microreentry. Note also a small electrogram recorded from the catheter in the LSPV ("Lasso 6-7"), near this site.

Ablation

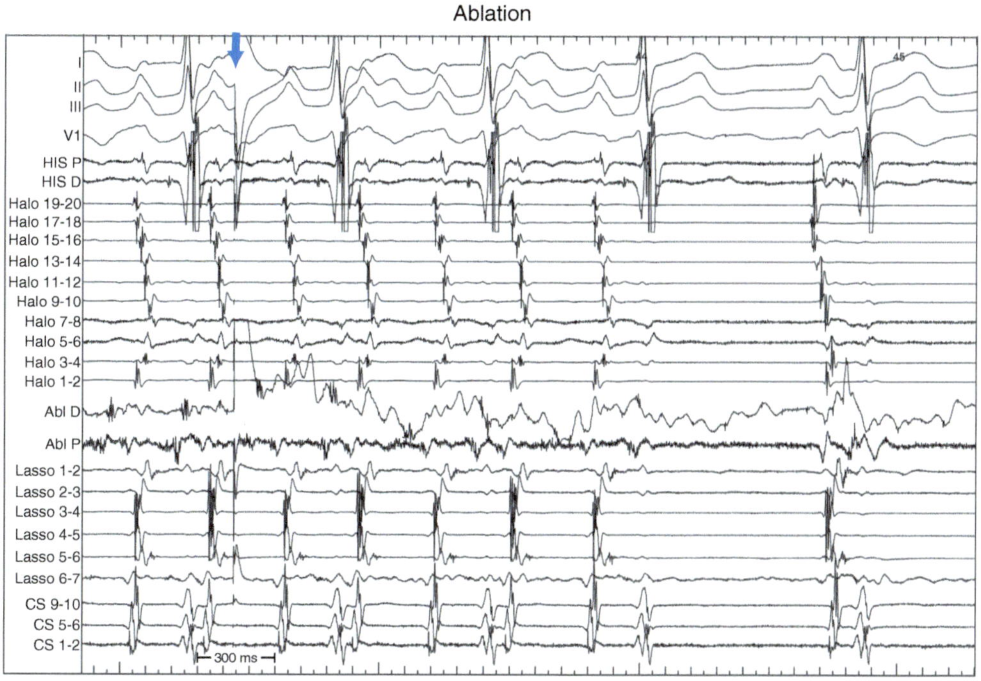

Figure 14-22

After withdrawing the ablation catheter slightly so that the tip was at the site of very prolonged diastolic activation, radiofrequency (RF) energy was applied (Fig. 14-22, *arrow*). Tachycardia terminated in less than 2 seconds. and could not be initiated after this (including with high-dose isoproterenol), whereas it was readily initiated before ablation. A few more RF applications were made in this general area for consolidation of the ablation effect.

Sinus Rhythm at End

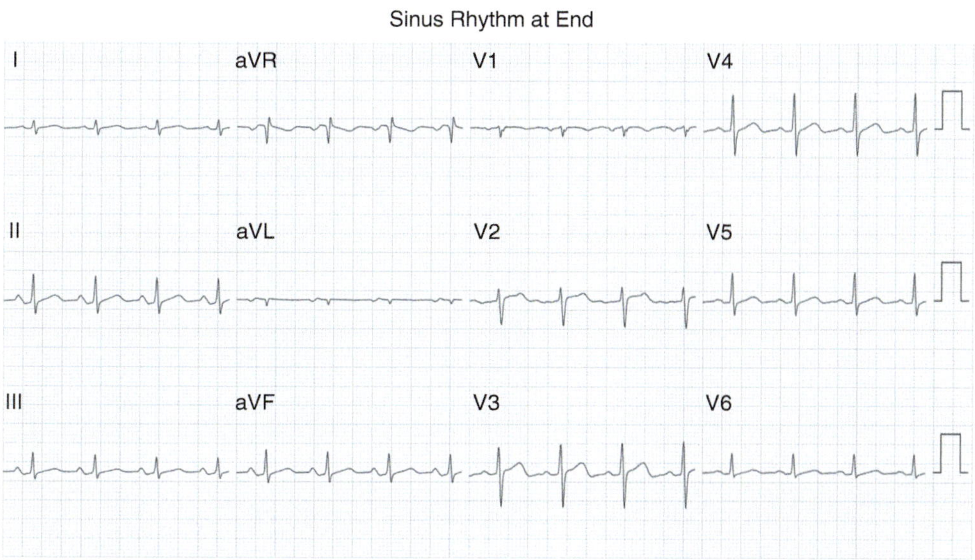

Figure 14-23

The final ECG (sinus rhythm) is shown in Fig. 14-23; the patient has remained free of tachycardia in follow-up and dyspnea is gone.

Summary

- Supraventricular tachyarrhythmias in patients after lung transplantation can have a variety of causes:
  - Atrial fibrillation
  - Atrial flutter/macroreentrant atrial tachycardia
  - Other SVTs (which anyone can have): AV nodal reentry, AV reentry, focal atrial tachycardia
- Successful ablation hinges on correct diagnosis and selection of appropriate target sites
- Microreentry is an unusual but important cause of arrhythmias in patients who have had prior surgery or ablation (practically never occurs in a pristine heart)
  - Overall chamber activation is focal; other features suggest reentry
  - A markedly prolonged diastolic electrogram is a target

15 Atrial Reentry After Pulmonary Vein Isolation for Atrial Fibrillation

Case Presentation

The patient is a 55-year-old man with end-stage renal disease (dialysis, renal allografts + rejection, now on dialysis again), coronary artery disease (CAD) (stents), pericarditis (stripping), pulmonary hypertension, and atrial fibrillation (AF). Longstanding persistent AF was ablated 5 years ago, consisting of pulmonary vein (PV) isolation, left atrial (LA) roof line, mitral isthmus line, complex fragmented atrial electrogram (CFAE) ablation (LA), and cardioverted at the end. He did well initially but then had recurrent atrial tachyarrhythmias despite multiple cardioversions and amiodarone administration. He was very symptomatic despite rate control, and referred for repeat electrophysiologic (EP) study and possible ablation. This is an increasingly common situation, in which ablation either is not completely successful or leads to other arrhythmias.

Baseline ECGs and Intracardiac Recordings

Rhythm Strip at Outpatient Visit

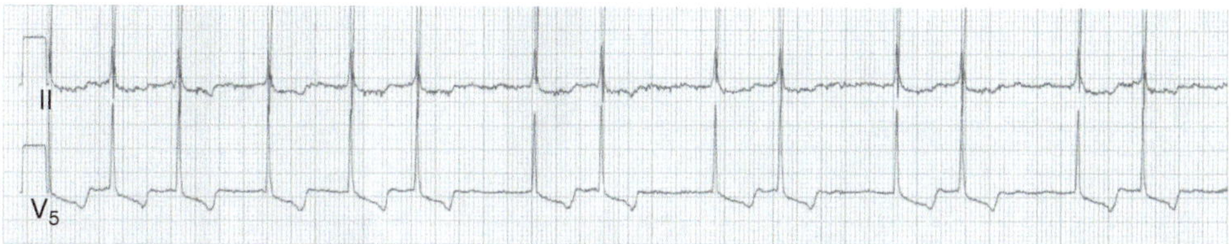

Figure 15-1

The rhythm in Fig. 15-1 appears to be rather irregular (R-R intervals) with no discernible atrial activity and would be appropriately interpreted as atrial fibrillation. However, the last half of the tracing shows QRS complexes that are paired and makes one wonder if there isn't some more organized atrial arrhythmia causing this.

Figure 15-2

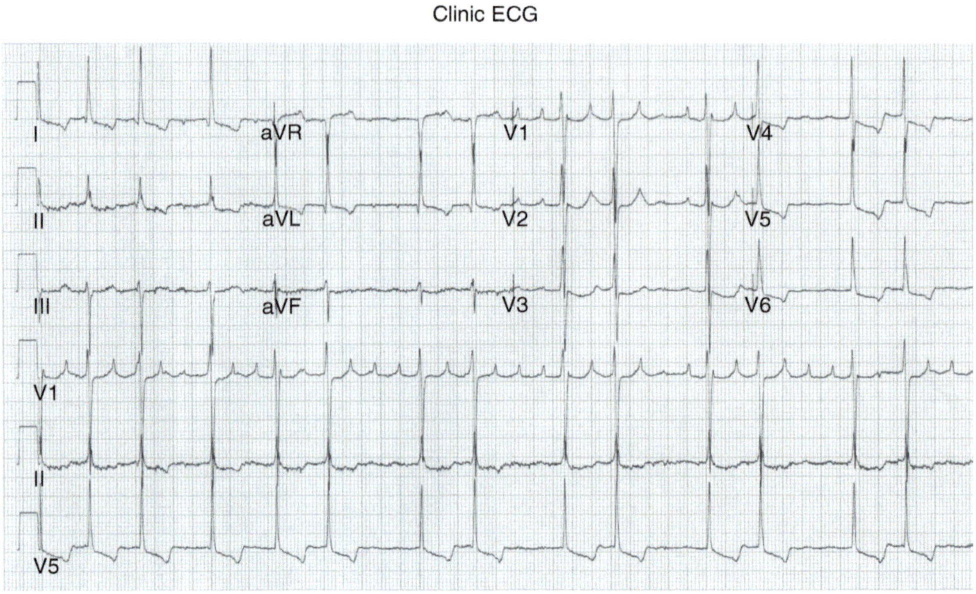

Fig. 15-2 is the rest of that same ECG, showing quite organized activity that is really only evident in lead V1; leads 1 and aVL show very small and narrow P waves.

Figure 15-3

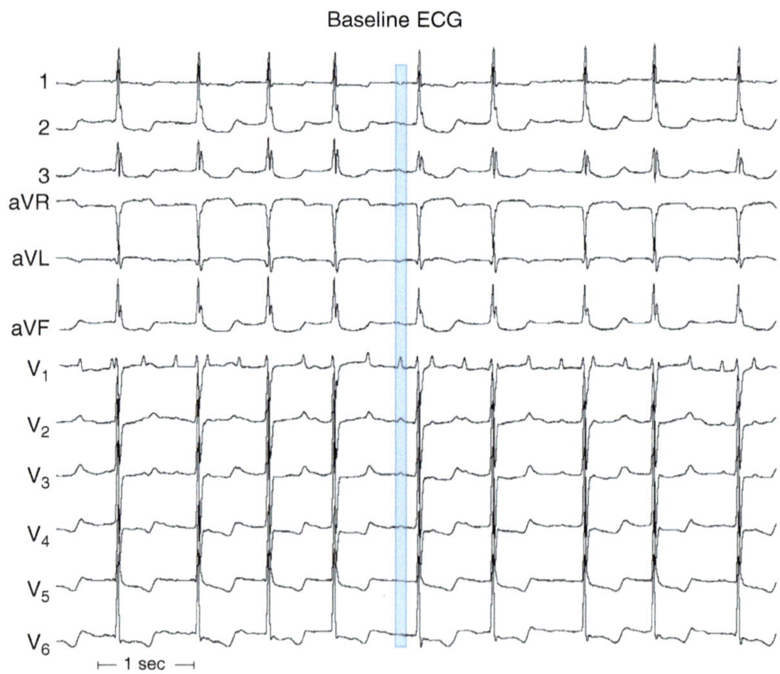

At the beginning of the EP study, the same rhythm was still present. Shown in Fig. 15-3 in 12 simultaneous ECG leads, it is evident that the P wave is quite narrow.

What Is the Likely Mechanism? [Fig. 15-4]

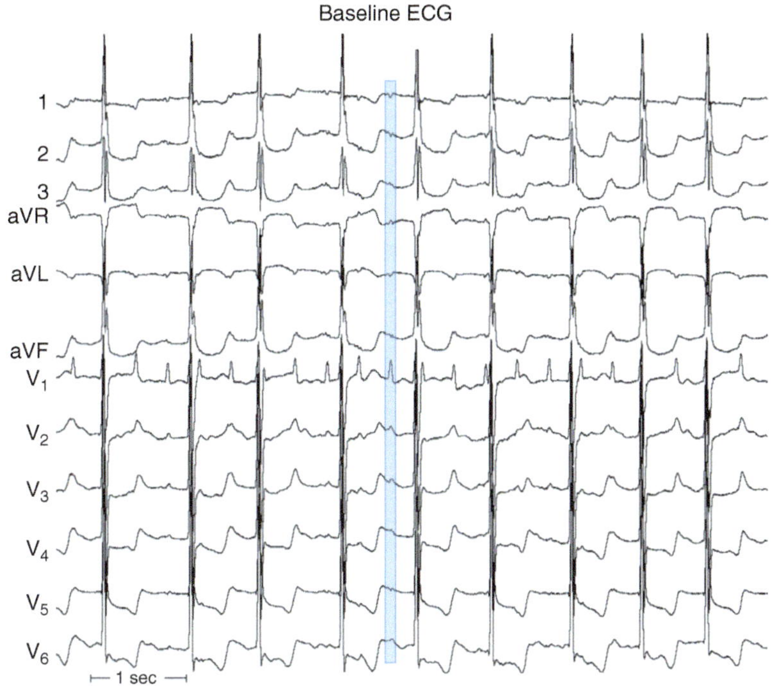

Figure 15-4

Fig. 15-4 is the same ECG, with increased gain on all of the leads. Now, it is evident that there is a very narrow P wave also in lead 1, not readily appreciated on the prior figure. Based on this evidence, the rhythm is clearly not atrial fibrillation, rather an atrial tachycardia (cycle length [CL] 330 ms). But what is the mechanism of the tachycardia? The narrower the P wave relative to tachycardia cycle length, the more likely a focal mechanism is present. If focal, a very late diastolic (ie, just barely presystolic) electrogram will be sought for the ideal ablation target, whereas if it were instead macroreentry, a middiastolic site should be sought. Clearly, it is important to determine whether a focal process or macroreentry is present.

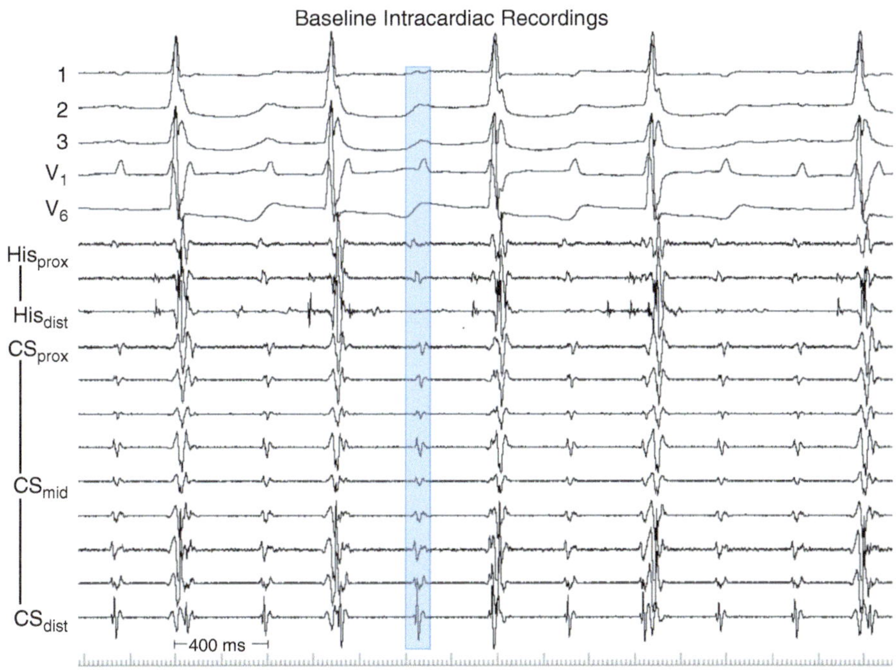

Figure 15-5

After obtaining vascular access and placing electrode catheters in the coronary sinus and His bundle region, the electrograms in Fig. 15-5 are recorded. Again, the "envelope" of atrial activation is very narrow, similar to the P wave during tachycardia.

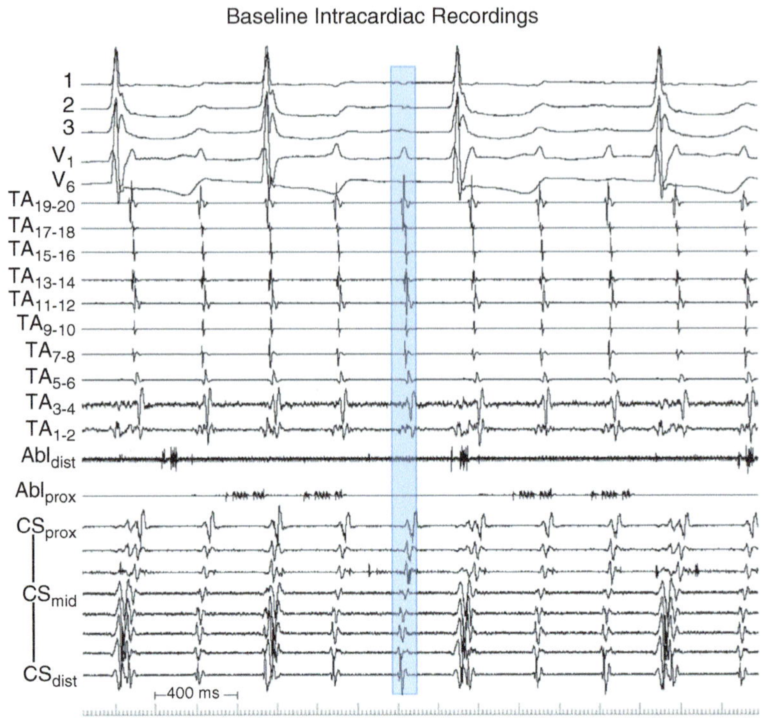

Figure 15-6

Another catheter is placed, this one around the tricuspid annulus (TA), hoping to get more information about atrial activation (Fig. 15-6). All of its electrograms, representing much of right atrial activation, are in the same general "envelope," and all occur within the timing of the surface P wave. This is again suggestive of a focal process. However, this is not certain, and we have to do more to prove or disprove whether it is focal before deciding what our ablation target should look like.

Table 15-1 is a brief comparison of features of different forms of focal propagation from an apparent point source, versus macroreentry.

TABLE 15-1 Atrial Tachycardias

	Focal			
	Automaticity	**Triggered Activity**	**Microreentry**	**Macroreentry**
Onset	Spontaneous	Induced (Burst > PES)	Induced (PES >> Burst)	Induced (PES >> Burst)
Occurrence	Incessant, bursts	Variable	Sporadic, sustained	Sporadic, sustained
P wave vs TCL	Small fraction	Small fraction	Small fraction	Large portion
Atrial envelope vs TCL	Small fraction	Small fraction	Small fraction	Large portion
Isoproterenol effect	Facilitates onset; acceleration	Facilitates onset; acceleration	Minimal effect	Minimal effect
Adenosine effect	Variable effect	Termination	Minimal effect	No affect/acceleration
Response to single premature extrastimuli	Reset or fusion; flat/increasing	Reset or fusion; decreasing	Reset or fusion; flat/increasing	Reset + fusion; flat/increasing
Response to overdrive pacing	Suppression; ↑RC with ↓PCL	Acceleration; ↓RC with ↓PCL	Entrainment; No Δ RC w/↓PCL	Entrainment; No Δ RC w/↓PCL
Ablation target	Late diastolic; unipolar QS	Late diastolic; unipolar QS	Prolonged diastolic	Middiastolic
Response to RF	Accelerate/stop	Accelerate/stop	Slow/stop	Slow/stop

PCL, paced cycle length; PES, programed electrical stimulation; RC, return cycle; TCL, tachycardia cycle length.

Diagnostic Pacing Maneuvers

Pacing from RA at Different Rates

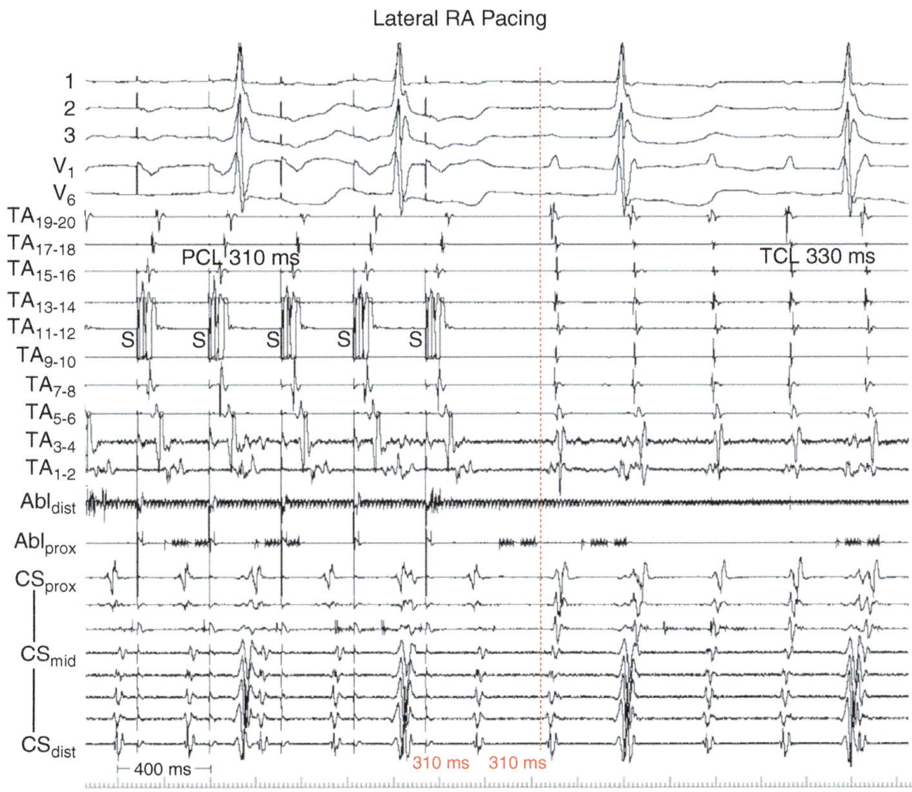

Figure 15-7

In order to try to determine whether a focal process or macroreentry was responsible for the arrhythmia, the first test used was overdrive pacing from the lateral right atrium (RA). We are careful to say "overdrive pacing" rather than "entrainment" at this point, because until we know fusion is present, it is simply "overdrive pacing." In Fig. 15-7, the last five stimuli (S) from the lateral right atrium are shown, after which the same tachycardia resumes. It appears that the right atrium is not part of the process because there is such a long delay until those electrograms are seen again, whereas recordings from the coronary sinus (CS) appear to occur slightly earlier when the tachycardia resumes. However, recordings in the distal half of the coronary sinus catheter are actually controlled by a prior pacing stimulus, because the interval between the first and second CS electrograms after pacing is the same as the paced cycle length. Thus a tremendous amount of slow conduction is present between the stimulation site and the distal coronary sinus, indicating that slow conduction (a necessary constituent of reentry) is certainly present. This in itself does not mean that the arrhythmia is reentrant, however.

Figure 15-8

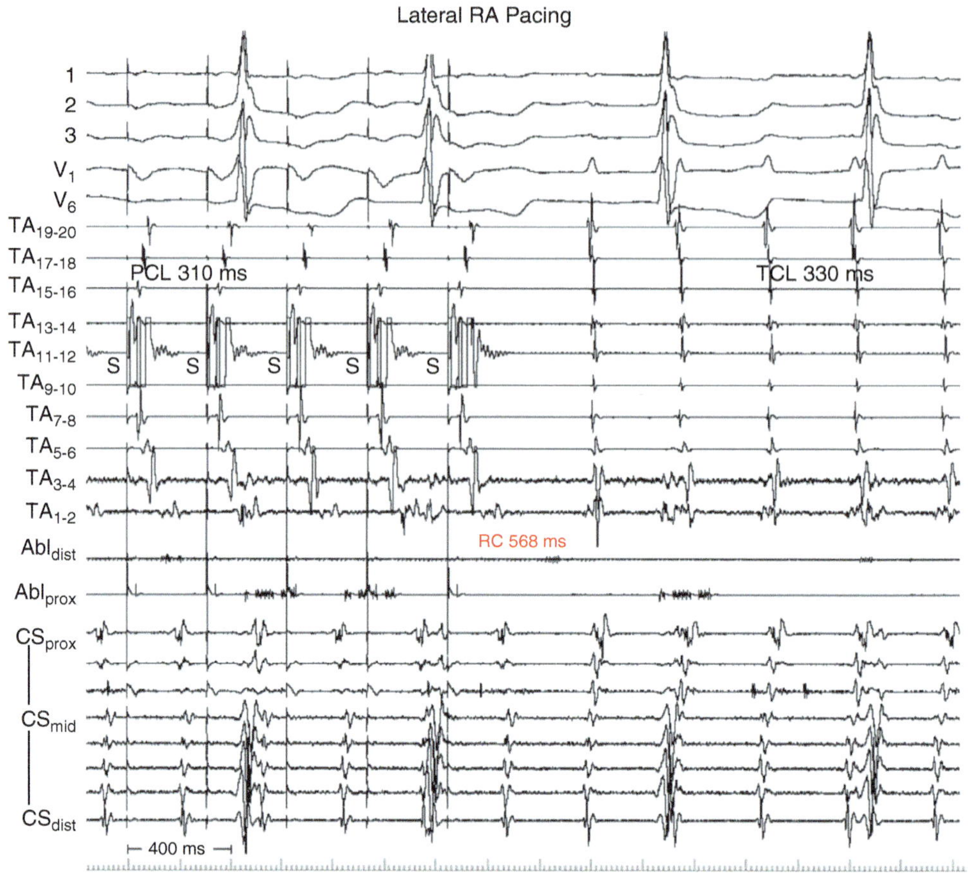

Fig. 15-8 is another burst of pacing at the same cycle length, from the same right atrial site. Here, the "return cycle" (RC) to right atrial recordings is measured at 568 ms, considerably longer than the tachycardia cycle length (TCL). This disparity is not commonly seen in reentry, but may be seen in overdrive suppression of discharge from an automatic focus.

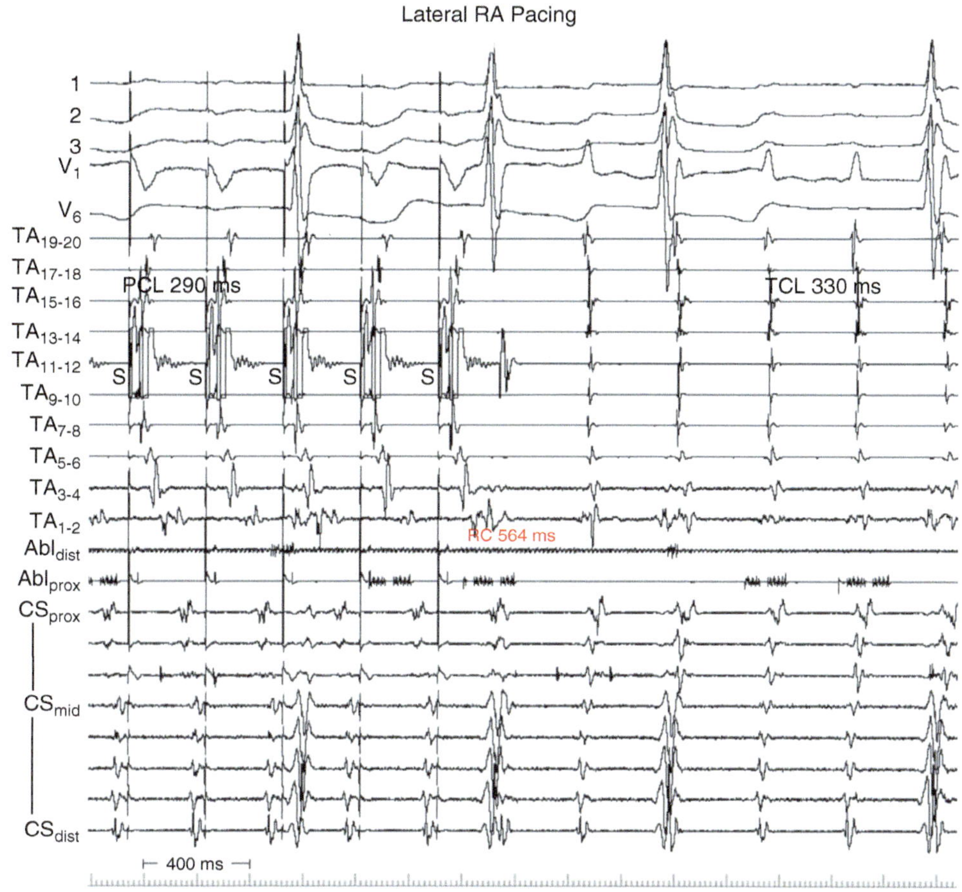

Figure 15-9

In Fig. 15-9, pacing again from the same site, now at a more rapid cycle length, produces a return cycle similar to what was seen earlier. With an automatic focus, more rapid pacing results in more overdrive suppression and a longer return cycle. Thus what is seen here is not entirely keeping an automatic focus.

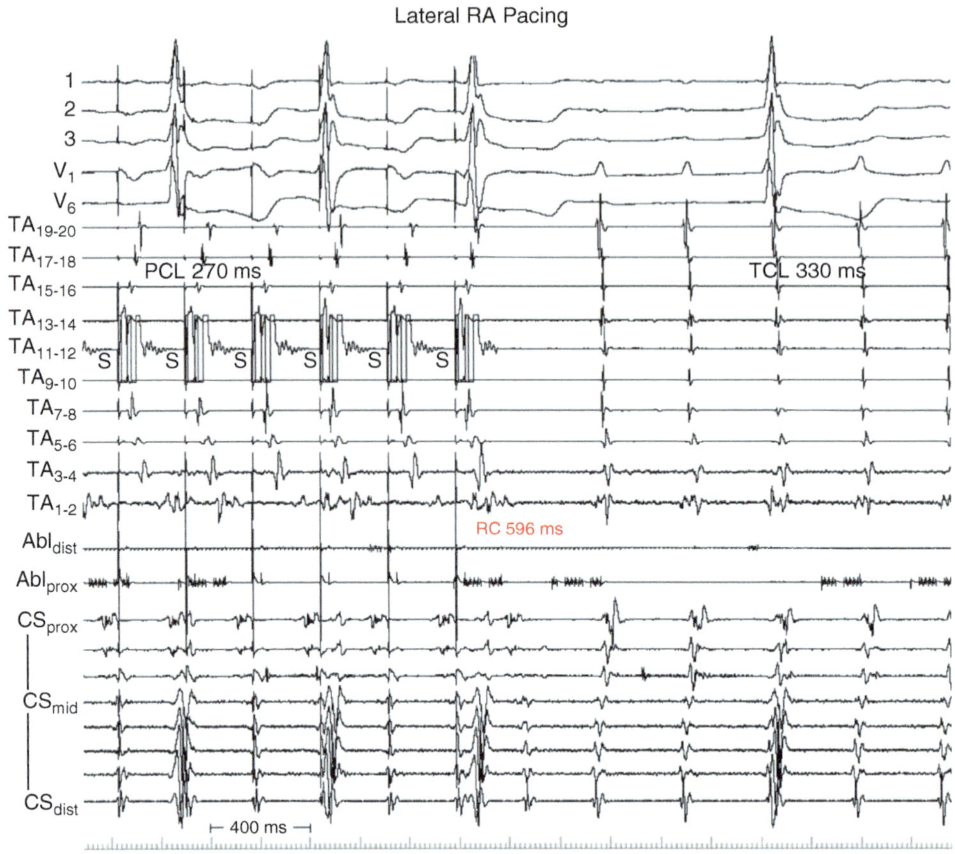

Figure 15-10

However, pacing faster still (270 ms) from the same right atrial site results in a longer return cycle (596 ms), as seen in Fig. 15-10. This *is* consistent with overdrive suppression of an automatic focus.

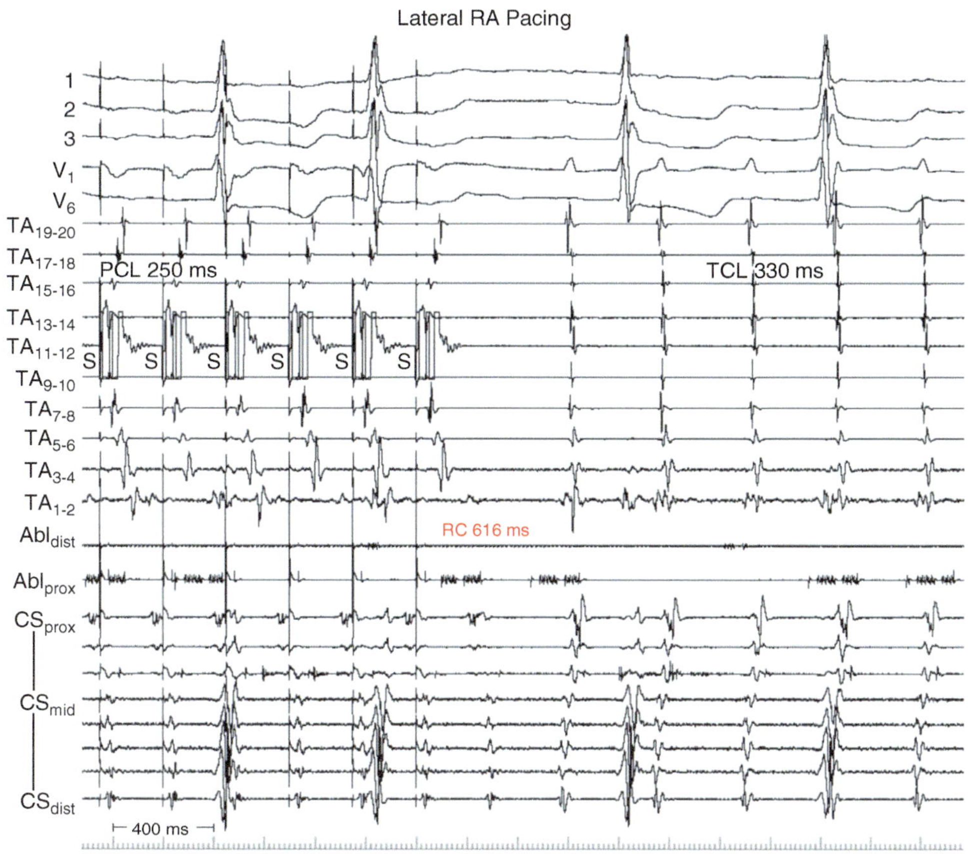

Figure 15-11

Pacing faster still (250 ms), as shown in Fig. 15-11, results in further prolongation of the return cycle to 616 ms, again consistent with overdrive suppression of a focus.

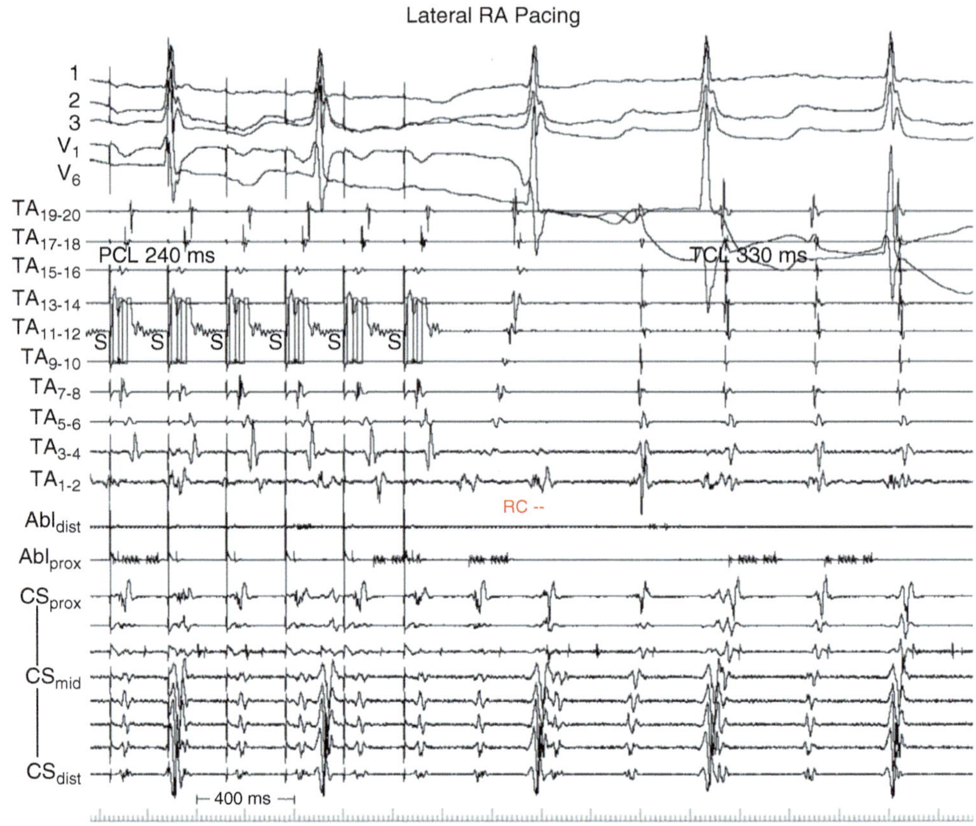

Figure 15-12

Pacing faster still (240 ms) from the same right atrial site (Fig. 15-12) yields uninterpretable results, because the first beat after cessation of pacing is not a tachycardia complex.

Pacing from Different Sites at Same Rate (Figures 15-13 to 15-16)

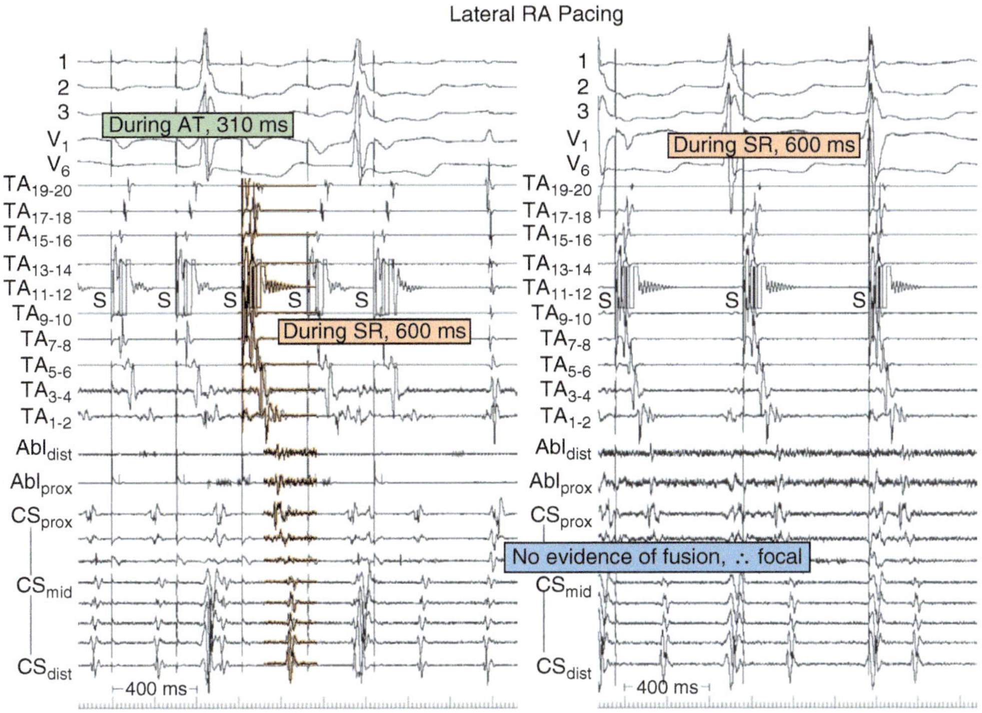

Figure 15-13

So far, there is evidence for and against the presence of an automatic focus. Further information can be obtained by evaluating activation sequences of pacing from different sites during tachycardia; if pacing during tachycardia does not resemble either tachycardia or "pure" pacing from that site during sinus rhythm, fusion is present, and macroreentry is the diagnosis. On the left of Fig. 15-13, pacing from the lateral right atrium at 310 ms (shown previously) is seen, and on the right, pacing from the same site but later in the procedure after tachycardia has terminated ("pure" pacing). A single complex of "pure" pacing from the site is superimposed on pacing during tachycardia (in *brown*). The activation sequences look identical, and thus there is no fusion. This is consistent with, but not diagnostic of, a focal process. If the same results are obtained when pacing from multiple other sites, a diagnosis of a focal process will be more certain.

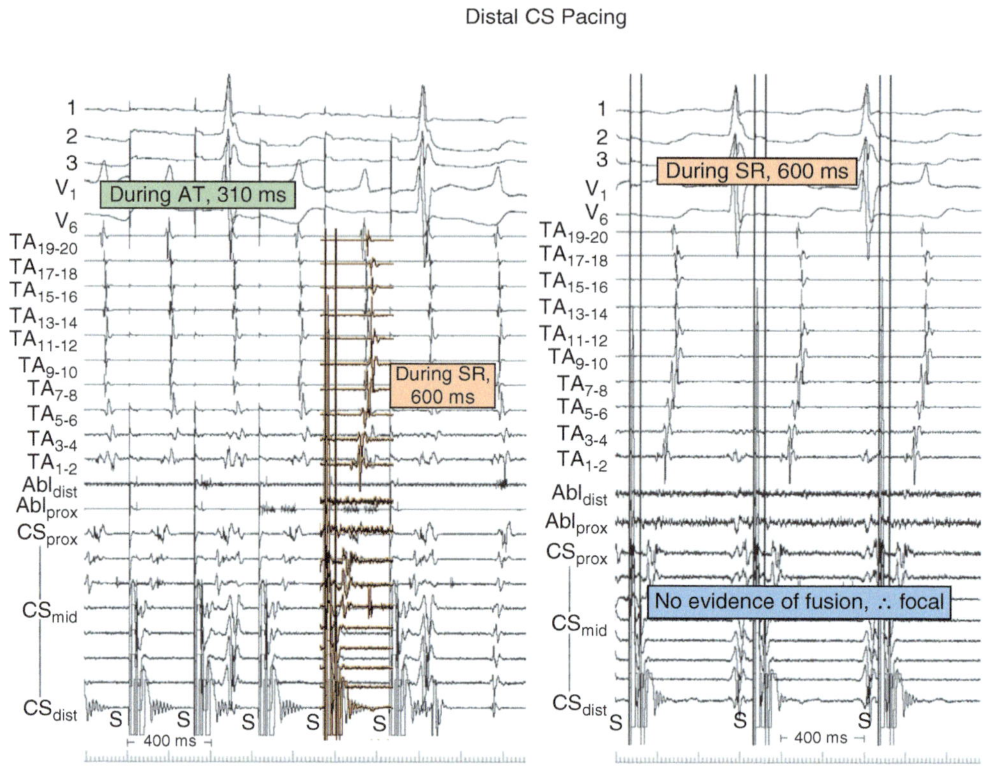

Figure 15-14

In Fig. 15-14, pacing from the distal coronary sinus is shown both during tachycardia at left and during sinus rhythm at right ("pure" pacing). Again, a single complex of "pure" pacing is superimposed on a complex of pacing during tachycardia, which it again very closely resembles. Thus there is again no evidence of fusion, and brings us closer to a diagnosis of a focal process.

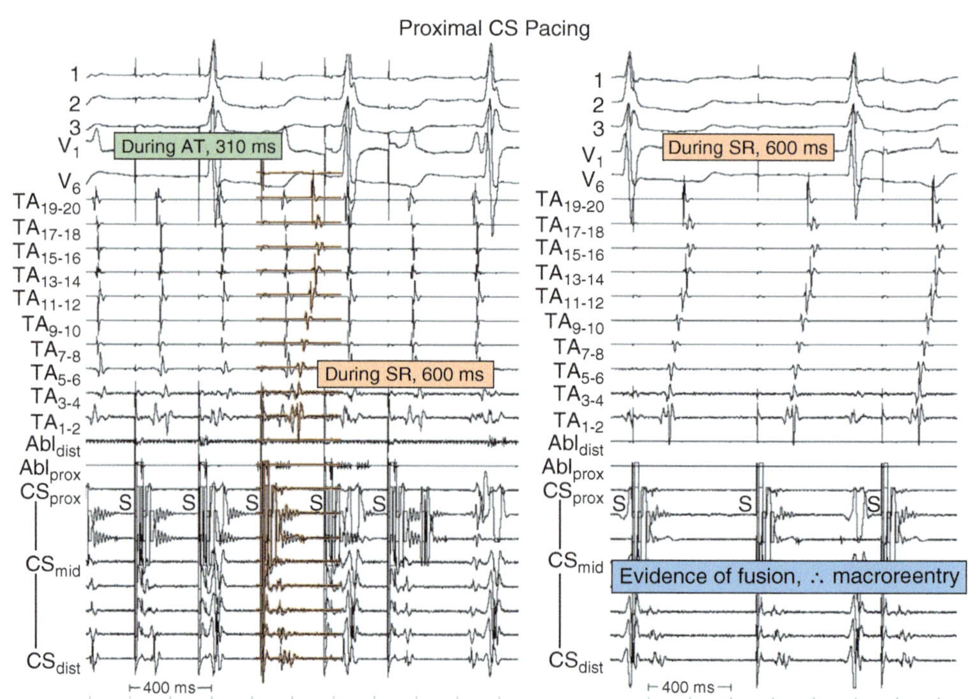

Figure 15-15

Another site is tested, the proximal coronary sinus (Fig. 15-15). As before, pacing during tachycardia is shown at left and pacing during sinus rhythm at right ("pure" pacing). Again, a single complex of "pure" pacing is superimposed on a complex of pacing during tachycardia. In this instance, however, the activation sequences are quite different, indicating the presence of fusion when pacing during tachycardia. This changes everything, and establishes a diagnosis of macroreentry. It is important to note that a single instance of pacing that shows fusion can diagnose macroreentry, whereas it is much more difficult to prove that fusion is *absent,* requiring pacing from multiple sites sometimes at multiple cycle lengths.

Pacing from RA at Different Rates Superimposed

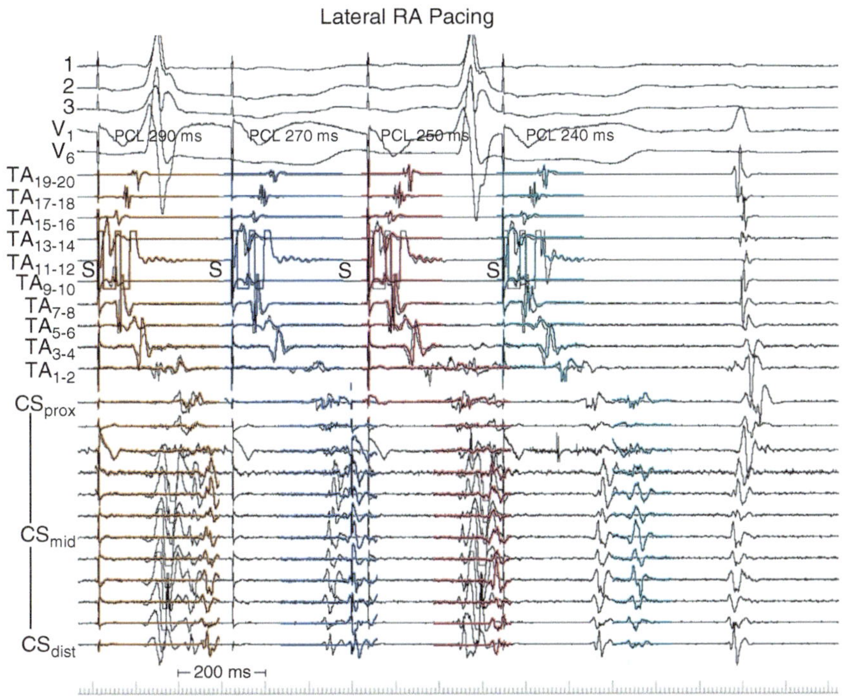

When Looking for Fusion:

A. Pace far away from presumed exit/focus

B. Evaluate signals far away from pacing site

Figure 15-16

Another way in which macroreentry can be diagnosed is the demonstration of *progressive fusion.* This is performed by pacing at the same site, but different cycle lengths. If macroreentry is present, the faster one paces from the same site, more of the chamber will be governed by the wavefront emanating from the pacing site, and less from the circuit. Thus the faster one paces, the more the resultant activation sequence looks like pure pacing and less like tachycardia. In Fig. 15-16, pacing from the lateral tricuspid annulus is shown over five different cycle lengths. The black recordings are at 310 ms, with a single complex of pacing at progressively shorter cycle lengths superimposed on sequential complexes. It is evident that 1) the faster one paces, as stated previously, the more the resultant activation sequence looks like pacing and less like tachycardia, and 2) when evaluating electrograms near the pacing site, they usually look the same, whereas evaluating electrograms more distant from the pacing site shows greater differences at different cycle lengths. Thus to have the greatest chance of demonstrating fusion, one should choose a pacing site far away from the presumed exit of a focus or circuit, and evaluate recordings far from the pacing site.

Mapping in Left Atrium

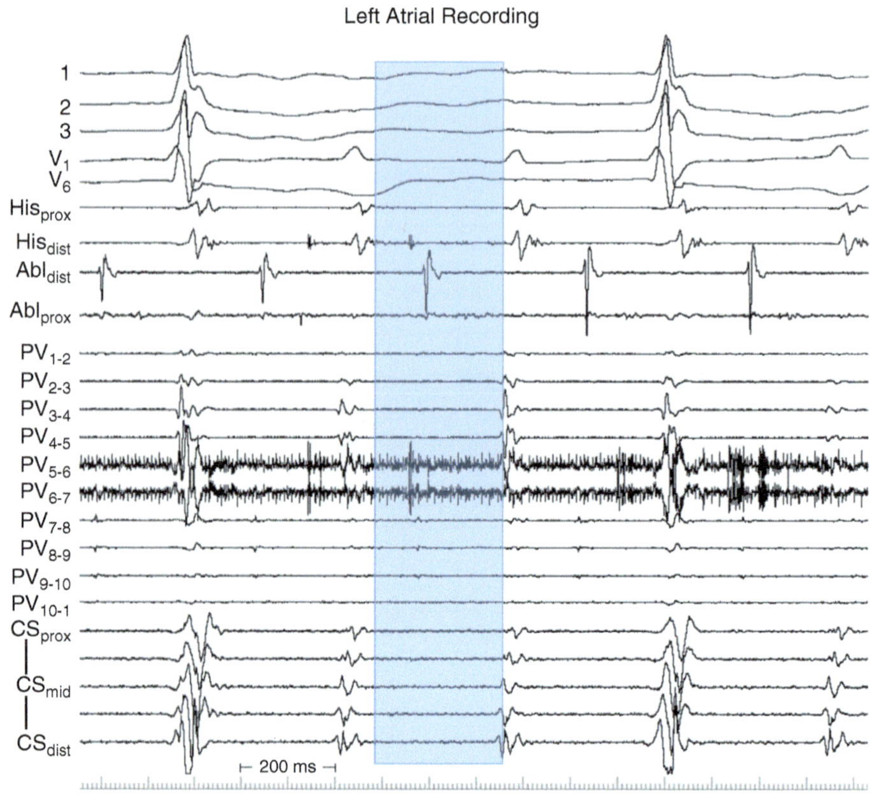

Figure 15-17

Now that a firm diagnosis of macroreentry has been established by a couple of methods, the ablation target becomes a middiastolic potential that can now be sought. Before establishing whether a focal process or macroreentry is present, great caution must be exercised in performing activation mapping because results may be misleading especially in instances in which the focal process is actually present, but substantial slow conduction is also present (such as after a previous ablation procedure). In Fig. 15-17, the ablation catheter records a sharp, isolated potential almost exactly in the middle of diastole (*blue shaded box* from the end of one P wave to the beginning of the next). It appears that we have a good ablation target already.

Electroanatomic Mapping

Left Atrial Activation Mapping

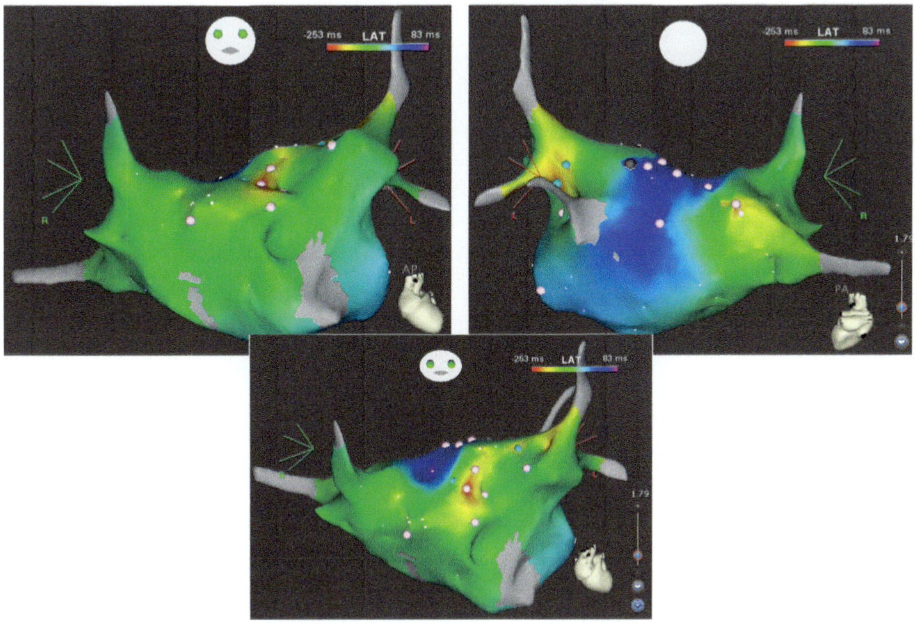

Figure 15-18

Fig. 15-18 is an activation map of the left atrium in several attitudes. This is somewhat disturbing because although a diagnosis of macroreentry has been established, the activation map suggests a focus on the roof of the left atrium *(red area)*, or perhaps a second focus in the region of the left upper pulmonary vein (also *red*). How can this be resolved with the diagnosis of macroreentry?

Mapping and Touch-up Ablation in Pulmonary Veins

Figure 15-19

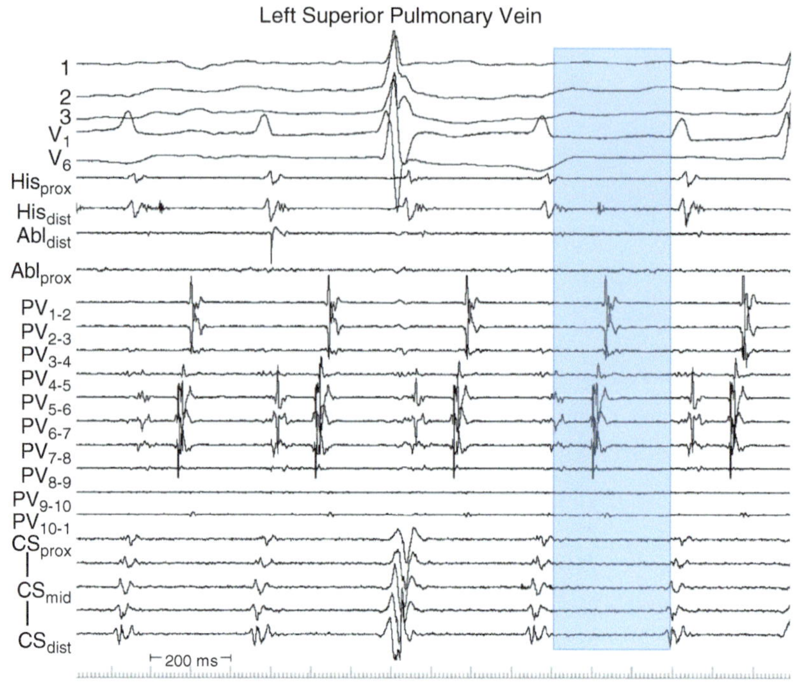

The problem with the prior middiastolic potential and the electroanatomic activation map was that pulmonary vein potentials were "contaminating" the activation map, and the middiastolic signal was actually a pulmonary vein recording (Fig. 15-19). Could this be a focus in a pulmonary vein? No, because it has been established as being macroreentry rather than a focus. However, the pulmonary vein potentials are quite large, and it is difficult to know how they should be incorporated into an electroanatomic activation map. One strategy that can be quite useful is to proceed with pulmonary vein isolation at this point; if tachycardia terminates, perhaps pulmonary veins were involved. If tachycardia persists, the PVs were obviously not involved, and the confusing signals they harbored will no longer be problematic.

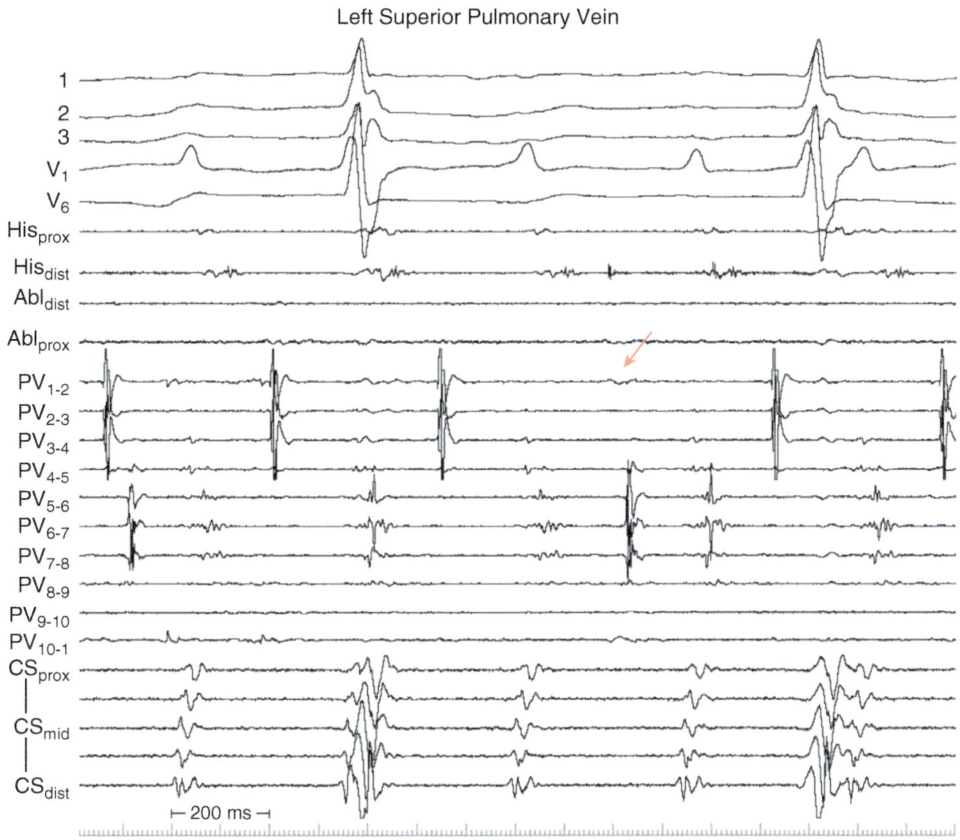

Figure 15-20

Immediately before attempts at isolating the left pulmonary veins, the recordings in Fig. 15-20 were made. Clearly, because the tachycardia persists despite the absence of the signal in PV 1-2 through PV 3-4 on one of the cycles *(orange arrow)*, this pulmonary vein cannot be responsible for the ongoing arrhythmia.

Figure 15-21

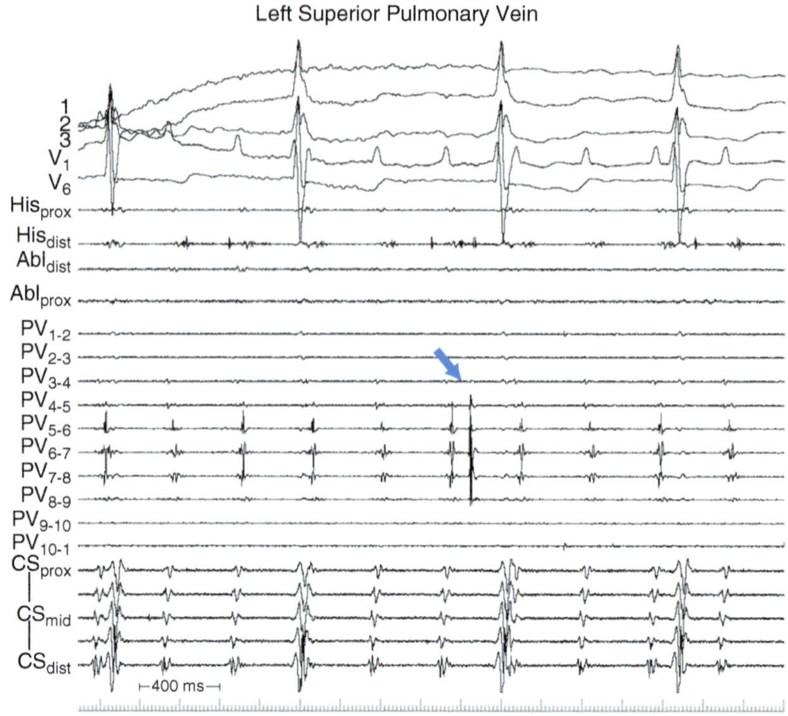

After ablation to encircle the left pulmonary veins, they have been isolated (Fig. 15-21). The *blue arrow* points to a random, dissociated potential spontaneously firing from the PV. Other signals noted in PV 5-6 through PV 7-8 were proven to be "far-field" recordings from the adjacent left atrial appendage. Clearly, the left pulmonary veins were not responsible for the ongoing arrhythmia.

Figure 15-22

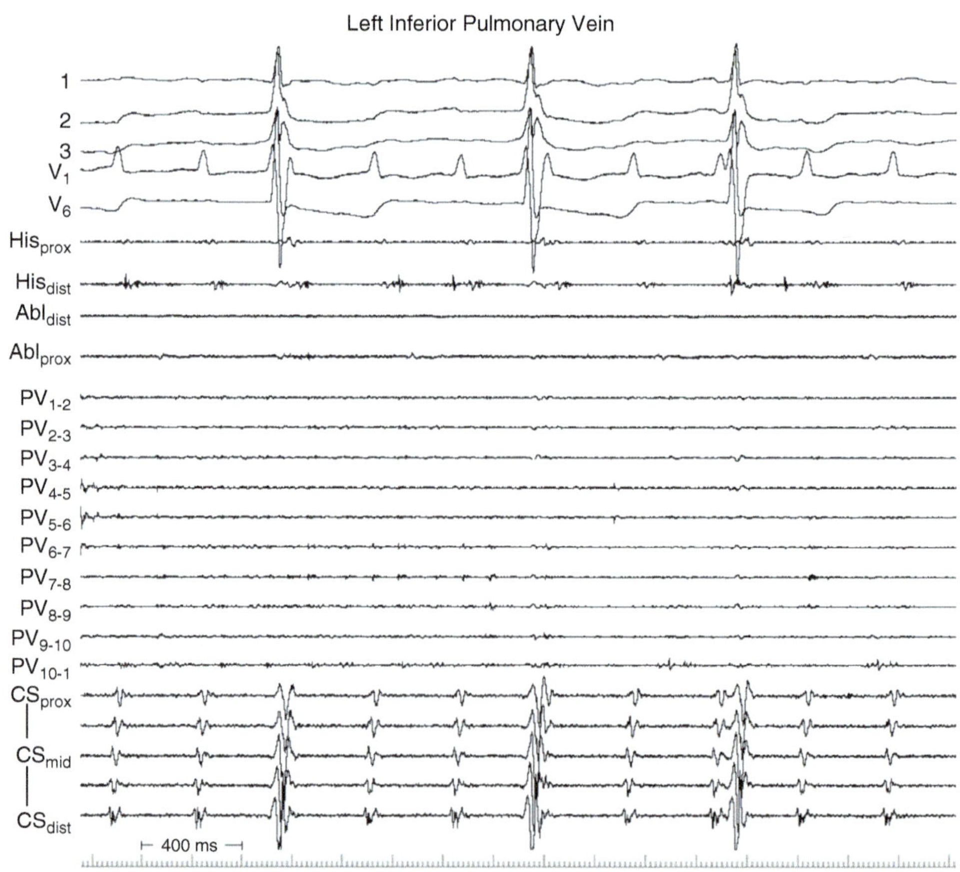

Recording from the left inferior pulmonary vein after wide area catheter ablation (Fig. 15-22) reveals no potentials whatsoever.

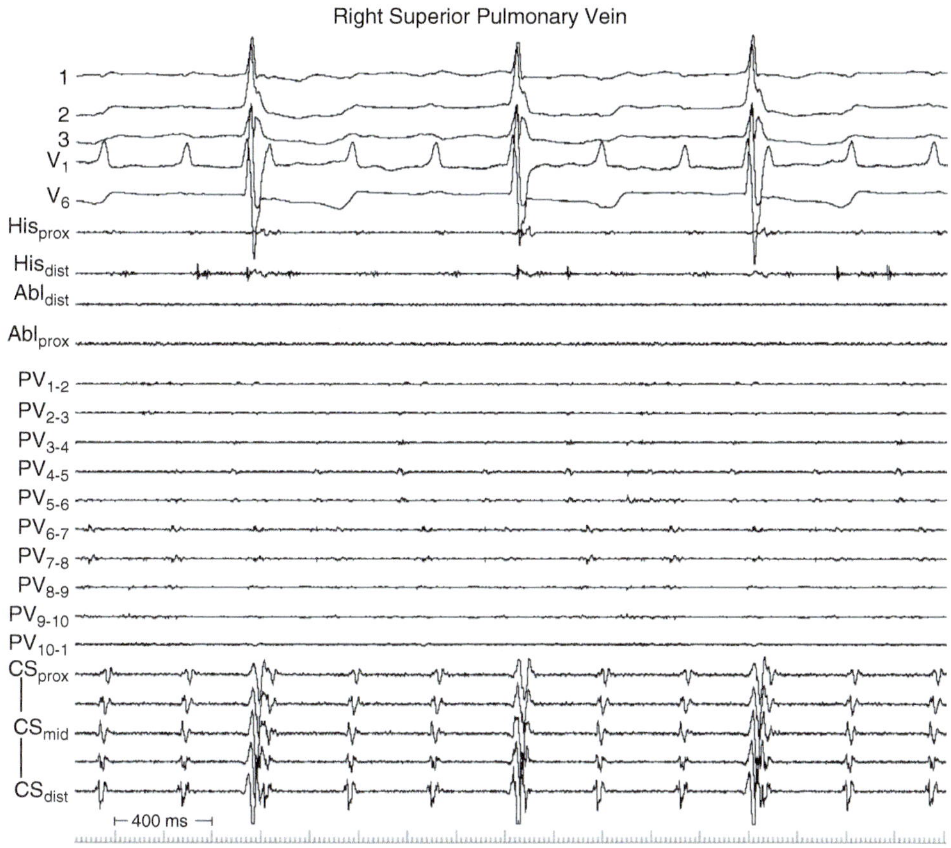

Figure 15-23

Similarly, as shown in Fig. 15-23, the right superior pulmonary vein showed no potentials, having been permanently isolated at the time of the prior procedure.

Figure 15-24

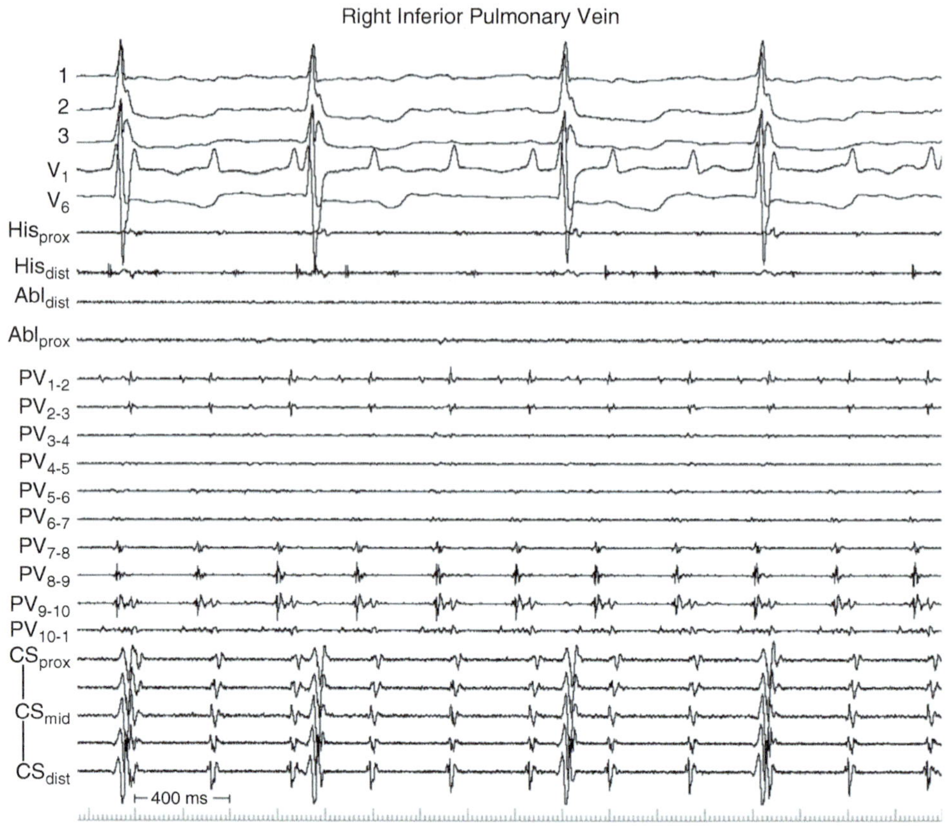

The right inferior pulmonary vein showed residual potentials of some interest (Fig. 15-24), because they were quite prolonged.

Figure 15-25

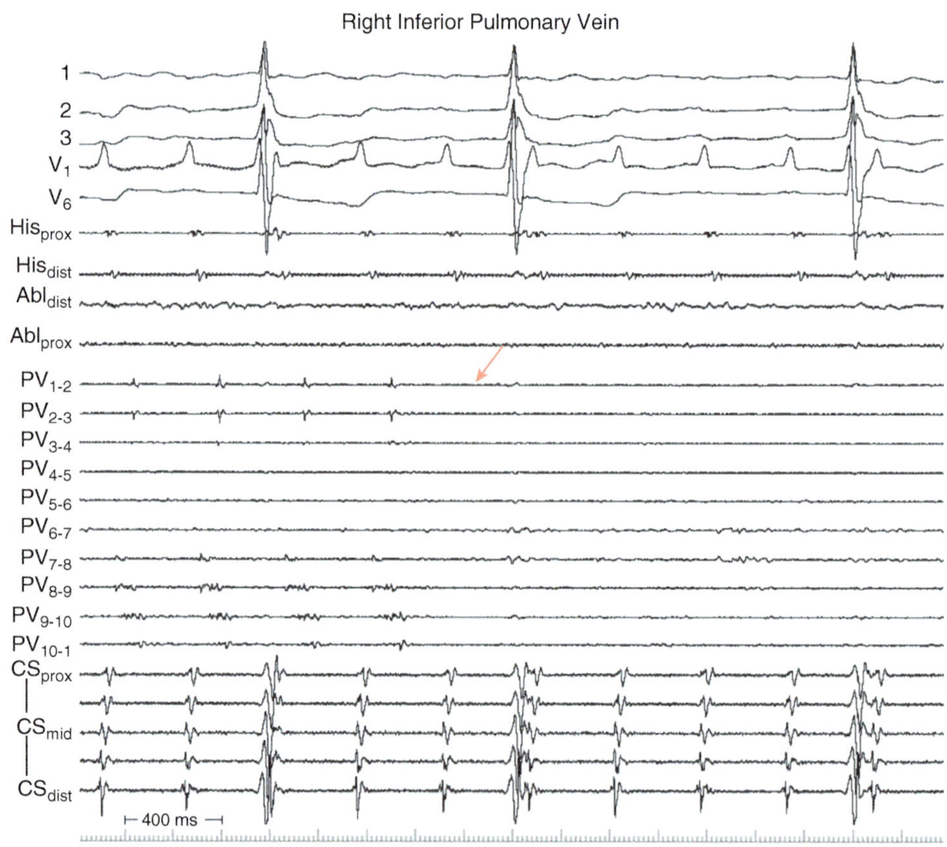

Isolation of this pulmonary vein occurs midway through the recordings in Fig. 15-25 *(orange arrow)*, again indicating that it is not responsible for the ongoing arrhythmia.

Electroanatomic Mapping Before and After PV Isolation

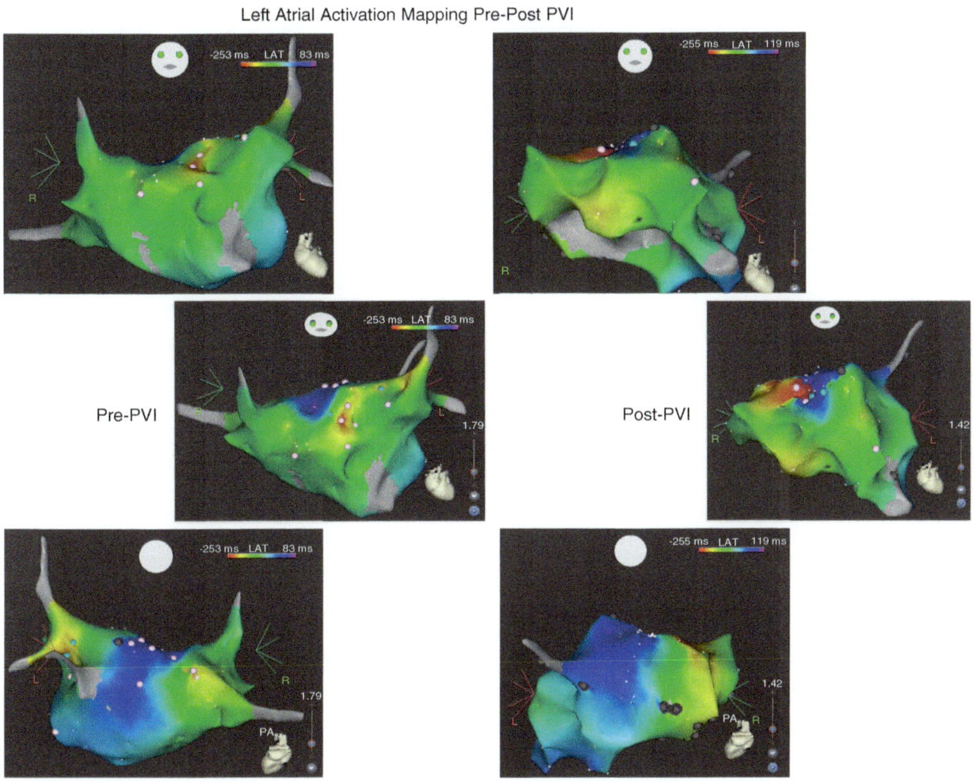

Figure 15-26

The prior electroanatomic map is shown on the left in Fig. 15-26, and on the right when repeated after PV isolation. Now that confusing pulmonary vein potentials have been removed from the activation map, a large reentrant circuit is more readily evident, involving the left atrial roof.

Mapping and Pacing at Left Atrial Roof

Figure 15-27

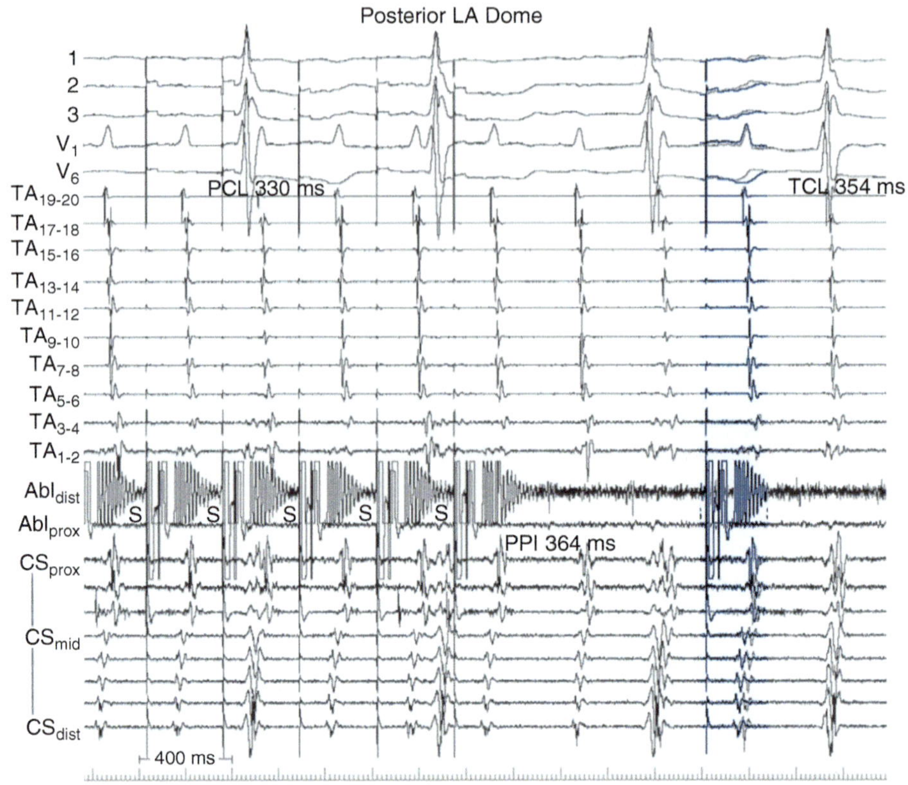

Candidate sites for ablation can be tested by overdrive pacing, to ascertain whether they are actually good target sites or not. In Fig. 15-27, pacing from a site on the roof of the left atrium (showing a middiastolic recording during tachycardia, not readily evident here because of distortion after pacing) yields a postpacing interval (PPI) slightly longer than tachycardia cycle length (TCL); a single complex of pacing on the left side has been superimposed on a single beat of tachycardia on the right side, showing strong similarity (though not an exact match). This could be a reasonable site for ablation.

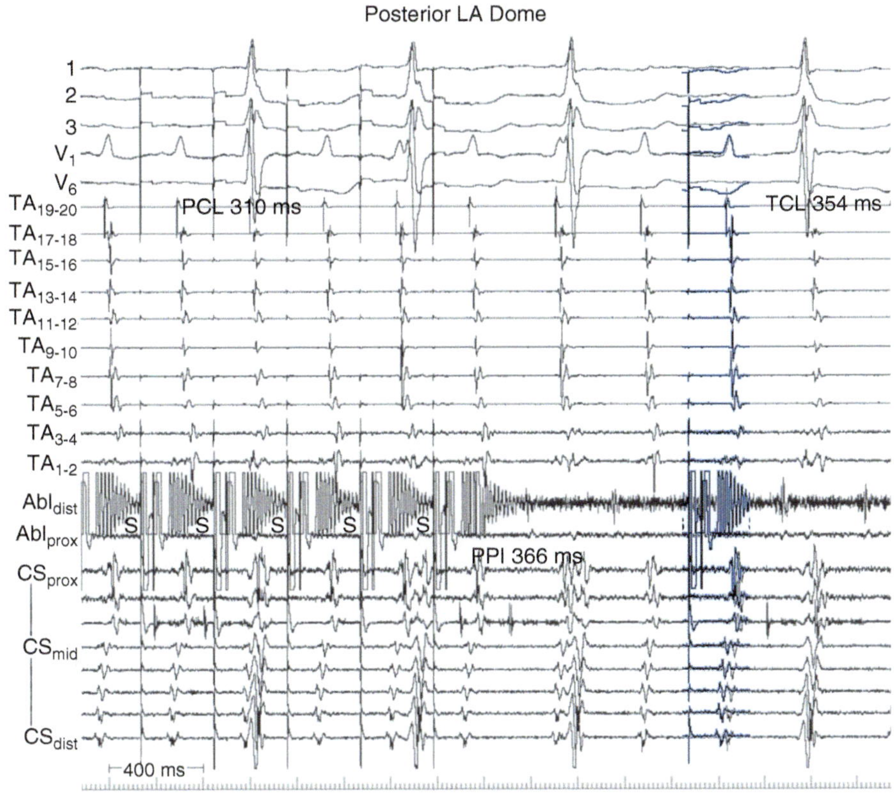

Figure 15-28

Earlier in the procedure, pacing at progressively rapid cycle lengths showed progressive lengthening in the return cycle, leading to suspicion of suppression of an automatic focus. Those data are still valid, and must be explained. In Fig. 15-28, pacing from the same site at a more rapid cycle length yields a similar return cycle to that of the previous figure. This amount of similarity was also seen at relatively slow pacing rates earlier in the procedure.

Figure 15-29

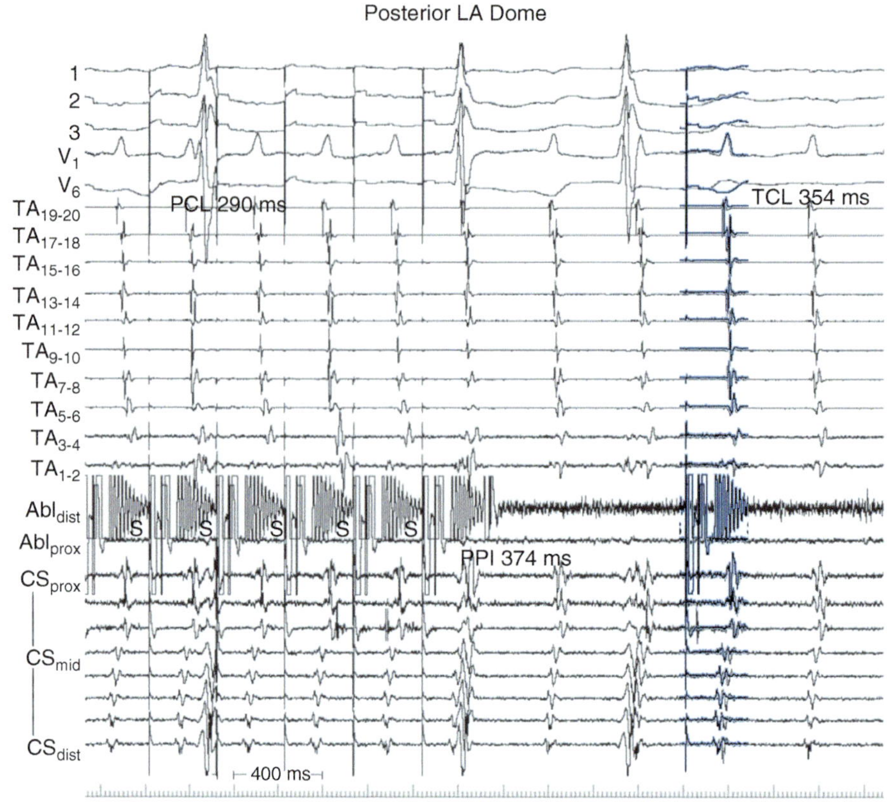

Pacing more rapidly from the same site in the left atrium now yields a longer postpacing interval (Fig. 15-29).

Figure 15-30

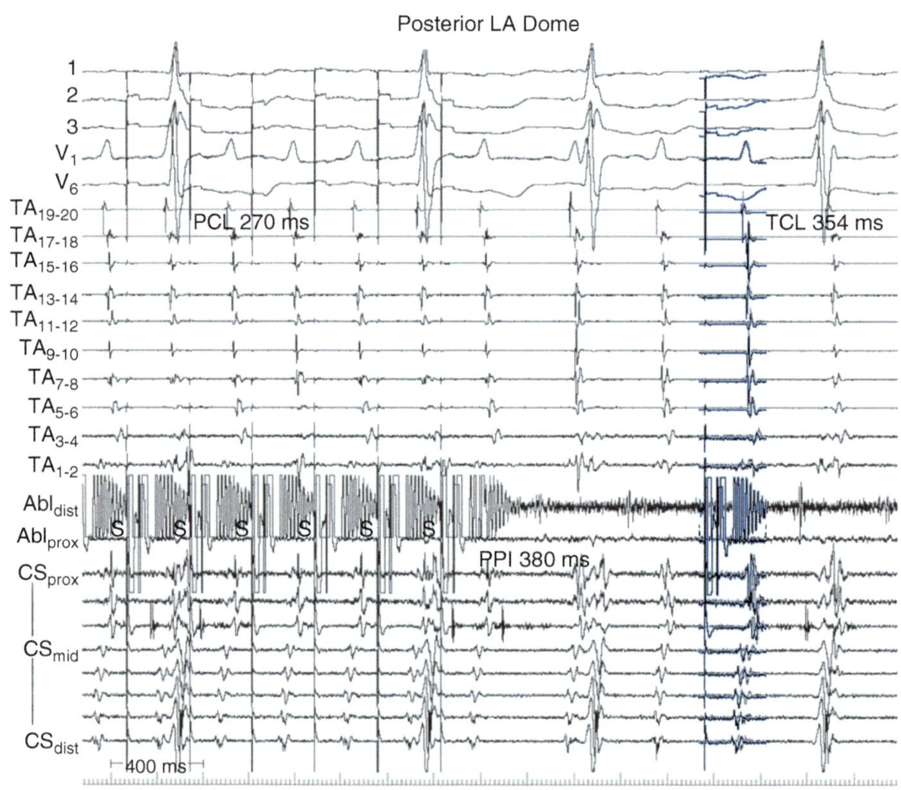

Pacing more rapidly still again yields a longer postpacing interval, as shown in Fig. 15-30. This is more than likely because of cycle length–dependent slowing of conduction ("decremental conduction"), not commonly observed in macroreentrant circuits because of their fixed length and conduction properties. However, in the presence of extensive scar, or medications that exhibit use dependence (sodium channel blockers), this phenomenon may be observed. The main significance is that one may never achieve a good "match" between postpacing interval and tachycardia cycle length (the desired result when pacing from the ideal ablation target site), because cycle length–dependent slowing of conduction will always artificially lengthen the postpacing interval.

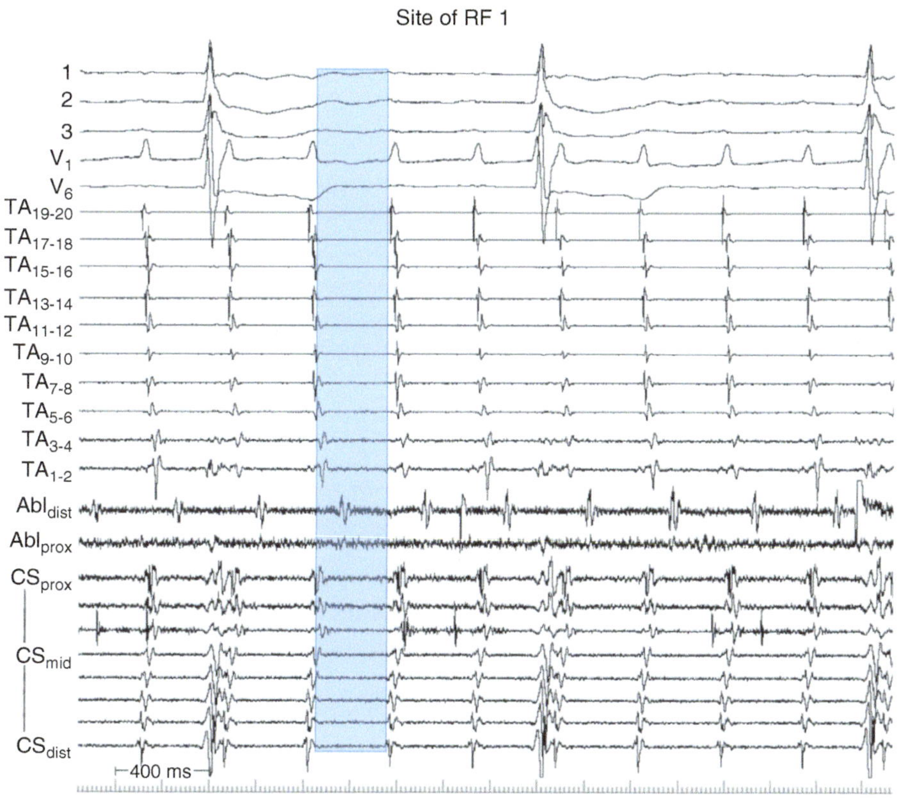

Figure 15-31

A site on the left atrial roof with an early-to-middiastolic recording (Fig. 15-31, diastole shown in *blue shading*) that had good responses to overdrive pacing (PPI similar to TCL, near-perfect pace match with tachycardia activation sequence) was chosen for ablation.

Ablation at Left Atrial Roof

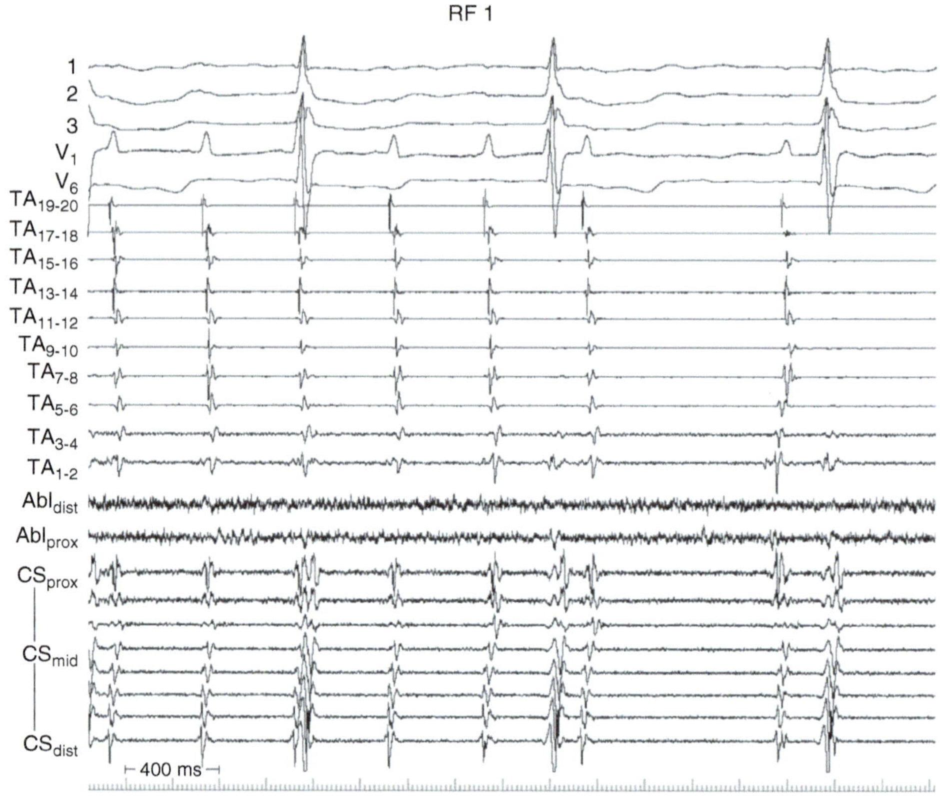

Figure 15-32

After several seconds of the first energy application, tachycardia slows and terminates to sinus rhythm (Fig. 15-32). A line of RF applications on the left atrial roof connecting the two lines encircling the pulmonary veins was made to complete the lesion set. Tachycardia was not inducible thereafter.

Right Atrial Cavotricuspid Isthmus Ablation and Assessment

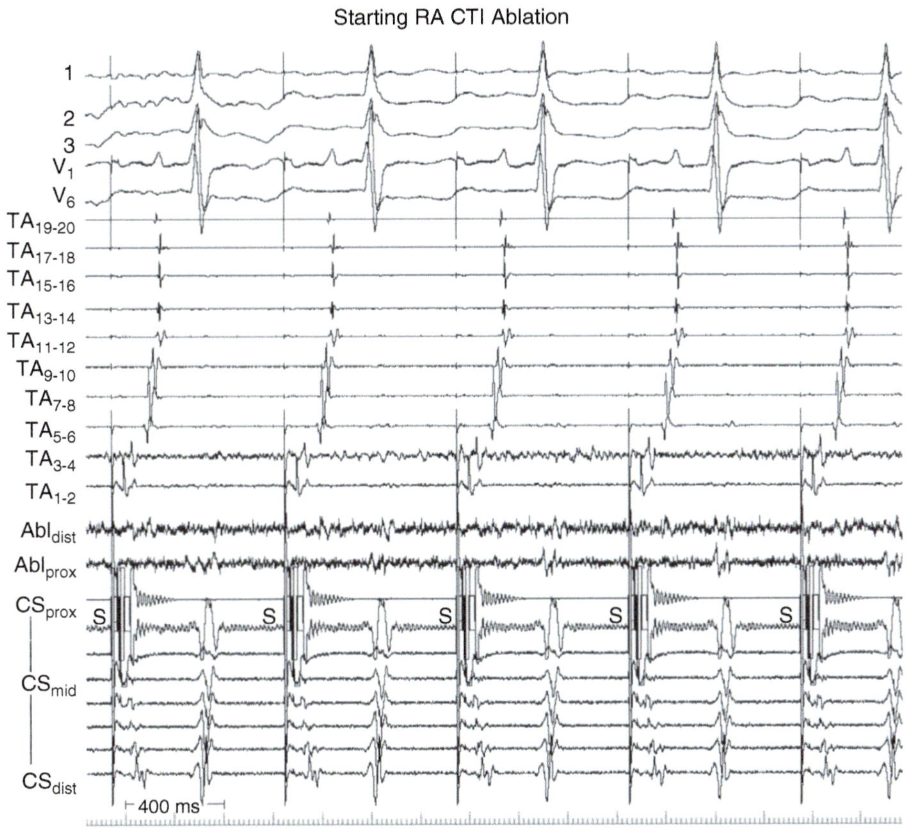

Figure 15-33

Because the patient had some ECGs from 2 yr previously that were compatible with right atrial cavotricuspid isthmus-dependent reentry, this area was also targeted for ablation. In Fig. 15-33, at the beginning of isthmus ablation, pacing from the proximal coronary sinus shows a uniform activation wavefront along the tricuspid annulus (TA).

Figure 15-34

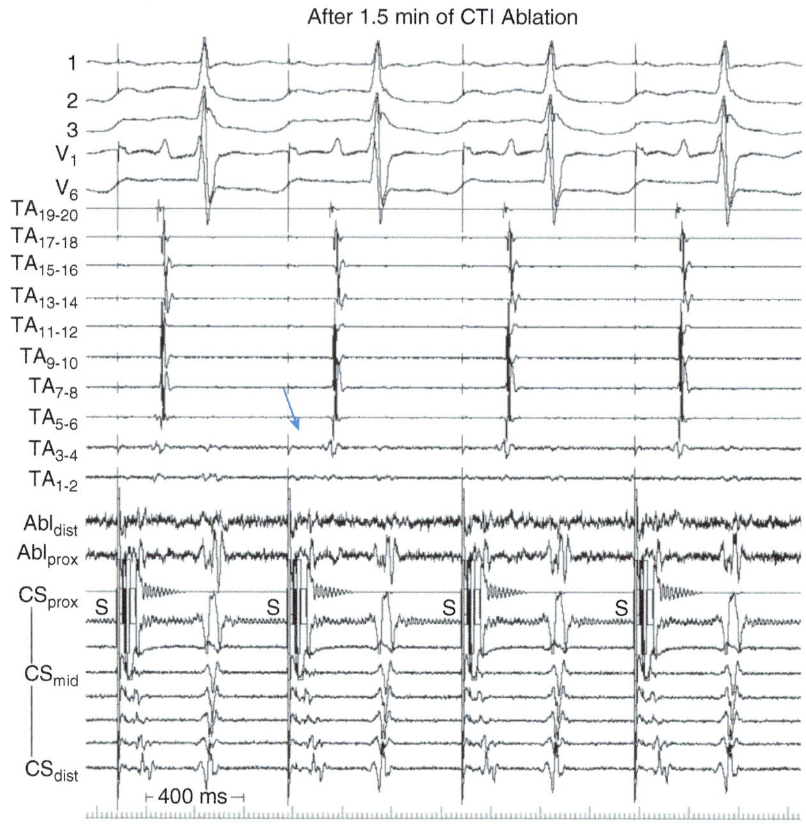

After just one and a half minutes of ablation, electrograms in the cavotricuspid isthmus have already shown substantial delay (Fig. 15-34, *blue arrow*).

Figure 15-35

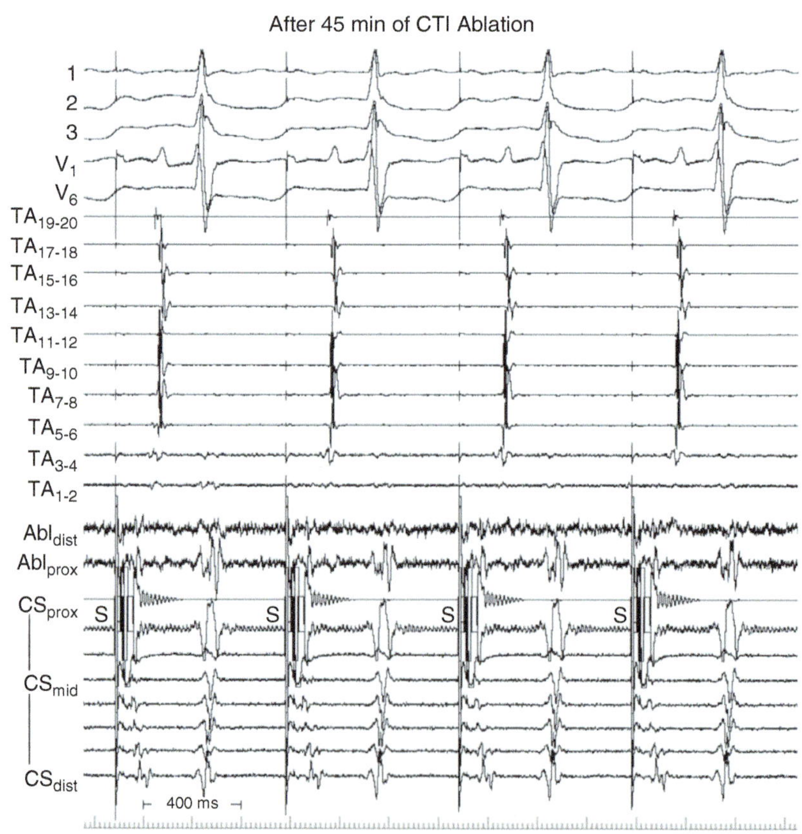

Although Fig. 15-35 is actually exactly the same figure as shown previously (Fig. 15-34), it serves to illustrate that after 45 minutes of further ablation in the cavotricuspid isthmus, there has been no substantial change beyond what was seen very early during ablation. This can be because of difficult anatomy ("pouch"), very large bundles of muscle that are difficult to ablate, or incorrect positioning of the tricuspid annulus catheter. Note the absence of any ventricular electrograms on any recording from this catheter, suggesting that it may be too posterior.

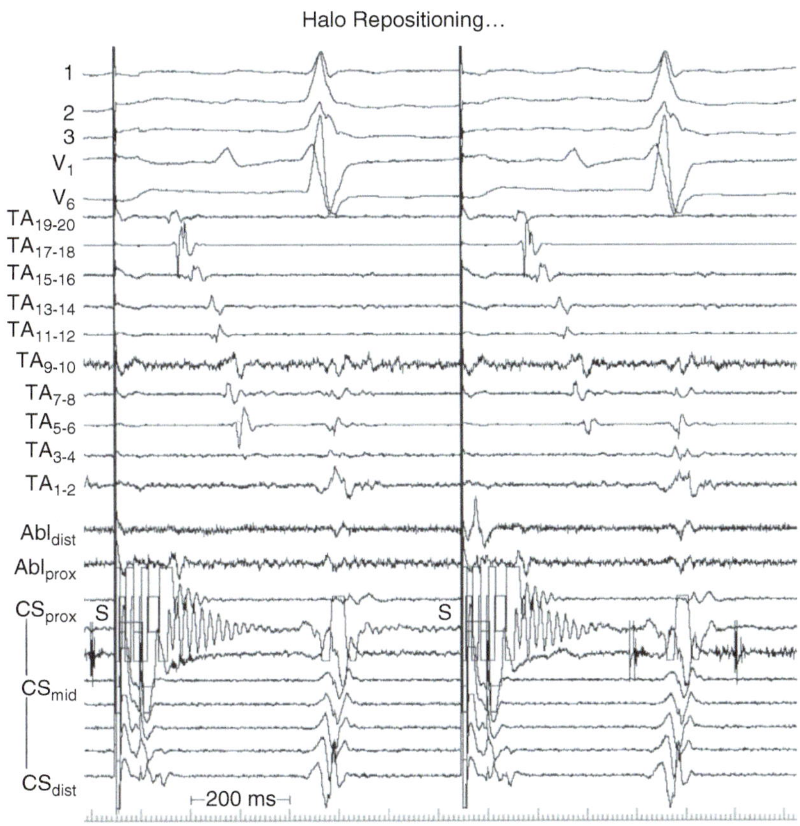

Figure 15-36

After repositioning the tricuspid annulus/"halo" catheter (note at least far-field ventricular signals on electrodes 1 to 10), the paced activation sequence seen in Fig. 15-36 is concordant with what would be expected when block is present in the cavotricuspid isthmus.

Figure 15-37

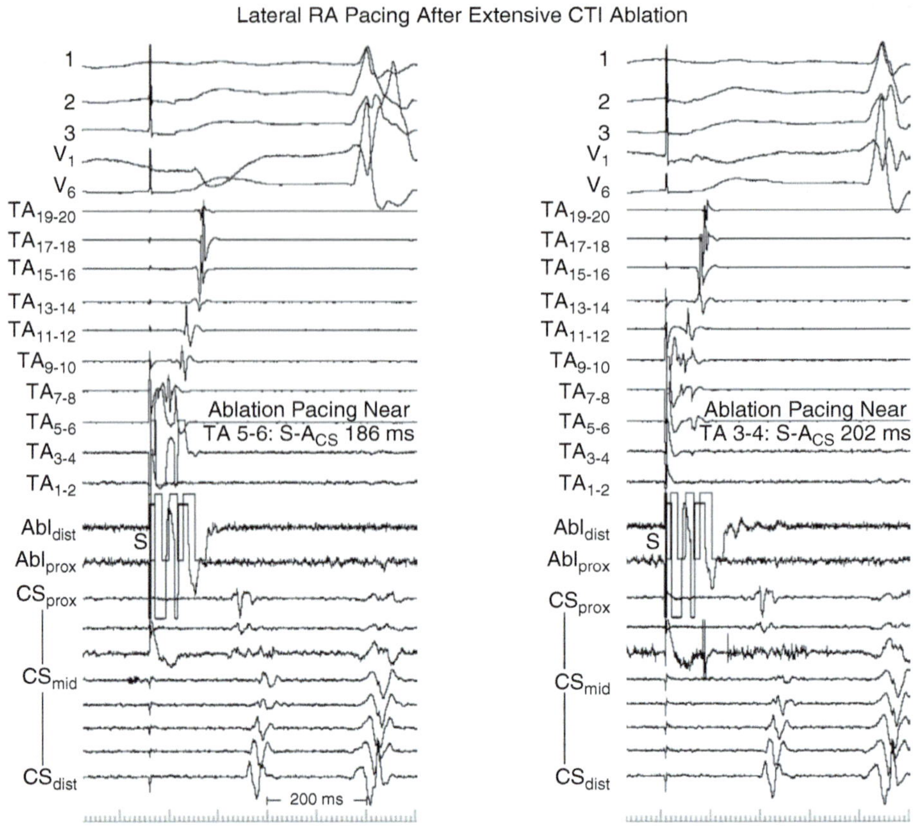

Pacing from the tricuspid annulus close to the ablation line (Fig. 15-37) demonstrates block in the lateral-medial direction, because electrodes that are anatomically closer to the ablation line (at right) are electrically further from the opposite side of the ablation line (CS recordings), and sites that are anatomically further away (at left) are electrically closer.

Final ECG

Figure 15-38

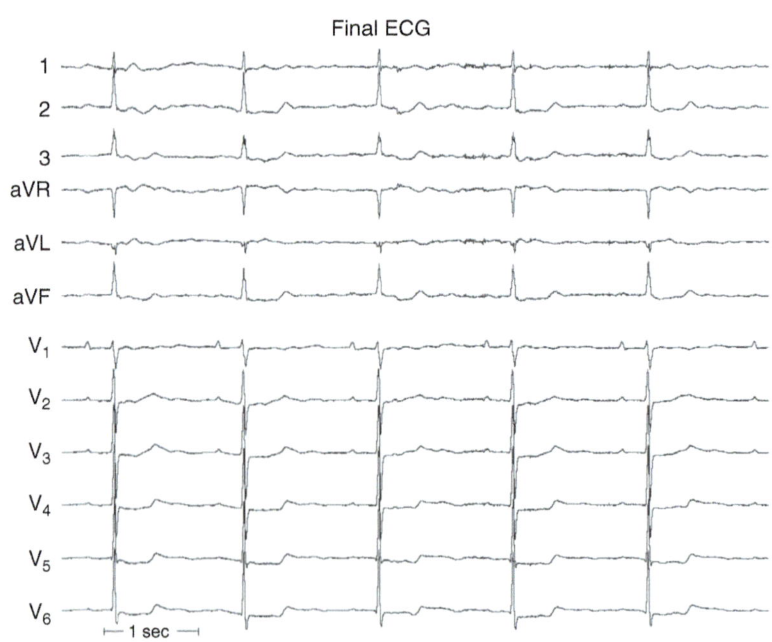

At the end of the procedure, sinus rhythm prevailed as shown in Fig. 15-38.

Summary

- Atrial tachycardias in the setting of extensive atrial disease (postsurgical, postablation, postirradiation, etc.) can be focal or reentrant (micro or macro)
- P-wave duration, P-wave duration relative to TCL, and intracardiac activation "envelope" relative to TCL can suggest focality versus macroreentry
- Overdrive pacing techniques are invaluable in diagnosis, revealing:
  - Whether the pattern is focal or macroreentry (and thus the ablation site characteristics)
  - Whether "decremental conduction" is present
- Maintaining correct catheter position (halo) may be critical
- PV potentials can cause confusion during activation mapping

16 Pulmonary Vein Isolation for Atrial Fibrillation

Case Presentation

The patient was a 57-year-old man with paroxysmal atrial fibrillation (AF) present for 3 years. Symptoms were palpitations, lightheadedness, and marked exertional fatigue during episodes 1 to 2 times weekly. His AF was refractory to antiarrhythmic drugs (sotalol, dronedarone), and atrial flutter was observed on some ECGs. Noninvasive evaluation findings were left atrial size 4.1 cm; normal left ventricular systolic function; and no valvular disease. He was referred for electrophysiology (EP) study and possible ablation because of drug-refractory symptomatic AF.

Baseline ECG

Figure 16-1

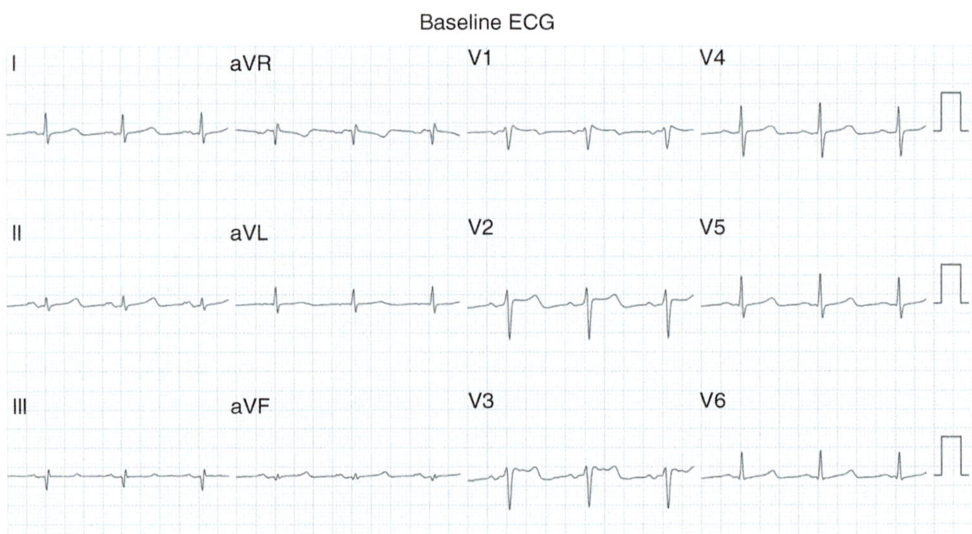

Baseline ECG (Fig. 16-1) is pretty normal; the P wave is slightly broad in lead 2.

Recordings from Right Inferior Pulmonary Vein

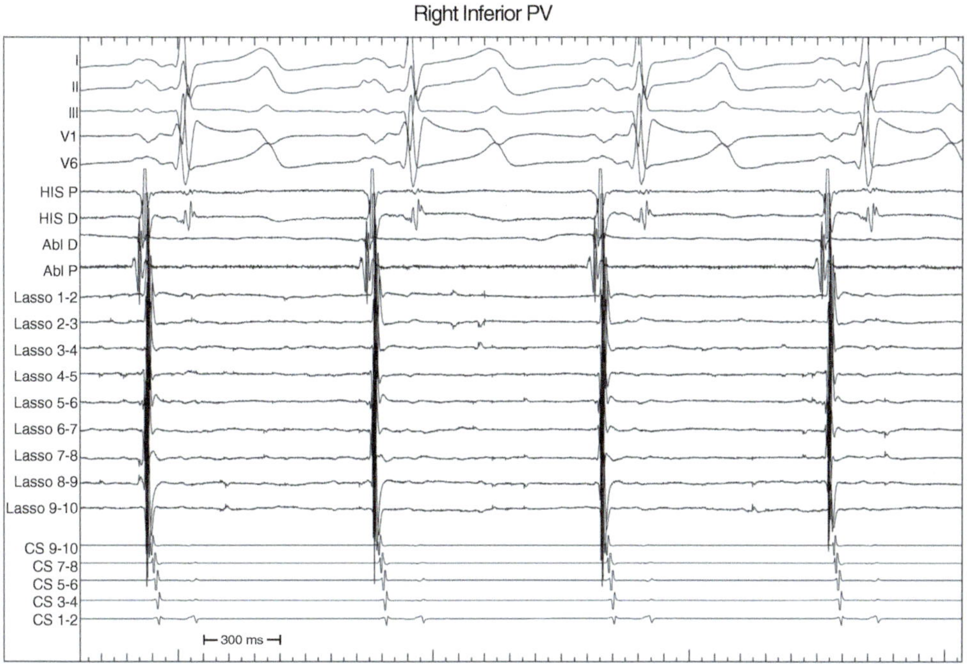

Figure 16-2

After obtaining left atrial access with transseptal catheterization, the left atrial anatomy is delineated by moving a catheter around the chamber. In addition, pulmonary veins (PVs) are interrogated using a ring catheter ("Lasso"). In Fig. 16-2, the catheter is in the right inferior PV and shows very large-amplitude PV recordings. They appear to be atrial recordings, and only by knowing where the catheter was when the recordings were made can we know their nature.

Recording and Pacing from Left Superior PV

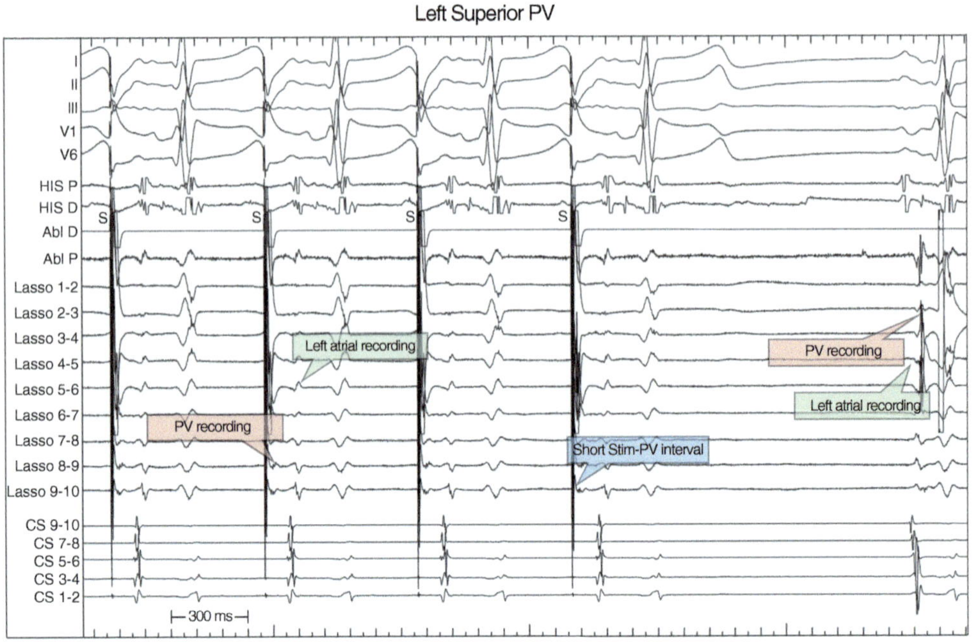

Figure 16-3

With the ring catheter in the left superior PV, pacing from a site more distally in the vein is performed (Fig. 16-3); this location is "tagged" on the electroanatomic mapping system. This will provide a means for checking exit block from the vein after isolation: if pacing from this site captured the PV reliably before isolation, and pacing from the same site does not conduct to the atrium after attempted isolation, one can be assured that exit block is present (even if the ring catheter is no longer recording in the vein). There is a very short interval from stimulus to captured PV potentials, after which conduction to the left atrium occurs (as indicated by *blue arrow*).

Recording from Left Superior PV, Pacing from Left Inferior PV

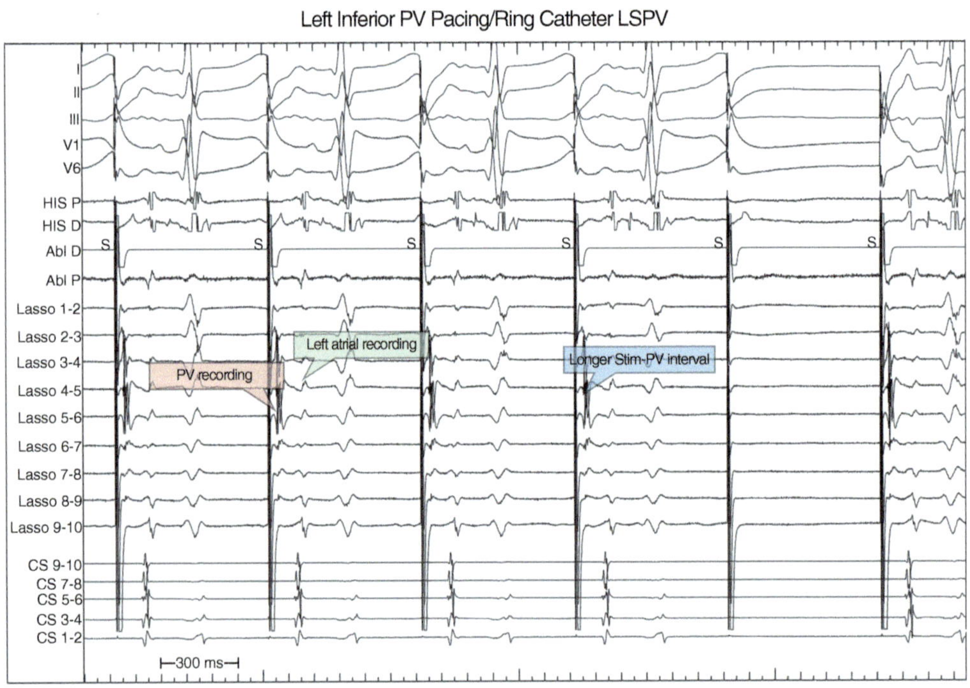

Figure 16-4

In Fig. 16-4, the ring catheter remains in the left superior PV but the ablation catheter has been moved to the inferior vein. Note the slight increase in stimulus-PV potential interval because the impulse must travel from inferior to superior vein before activating these cells.

Recording and Pacing from Right Superior PV

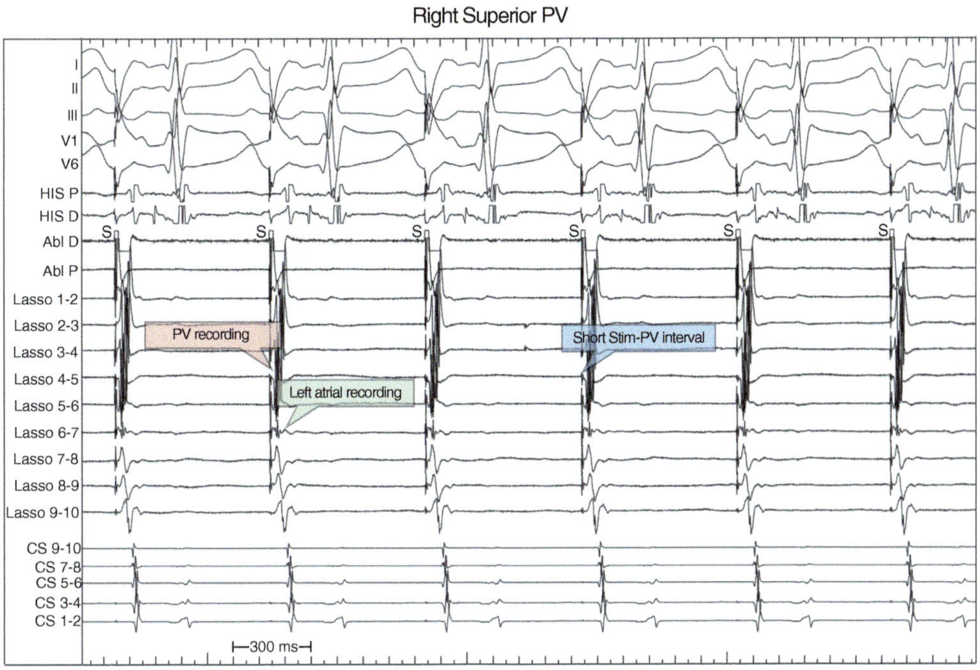

Figure 16-5

Similarly, with the ring catheter in the right superior PV, pacing from a site more distally in the vein is performed (Fig. 16-5); this location is "tagged" on the electroanatomic mapping system. This will provide a means for checking exit block from the vein after isolation.

Recording from Right Superior PV, Pacing from Right Inferior PV

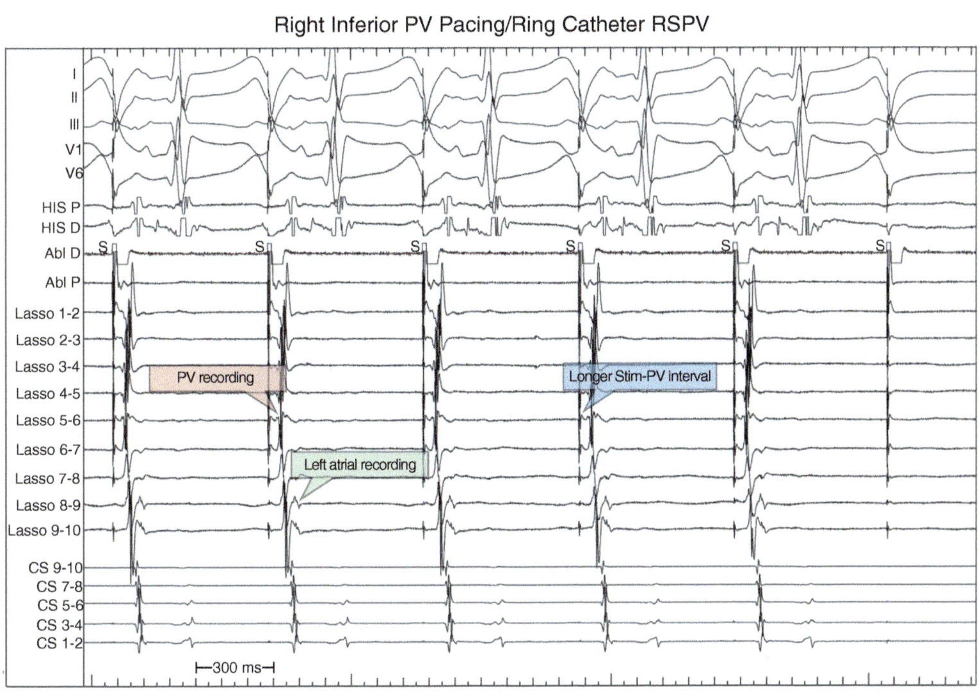

Figure 16-6

In Fig. 16-6, the ring catheter remains in the right superior PV but the ablation catheter has been moved to the inferior vein. Note the slight increase in stimulus-PV potential interval because the impulse must travel from inferior to superior vein before activating these cells.

Atrial Anatomy on Electroanatomic Maps

Figure 16-7

Atrial Anatomy

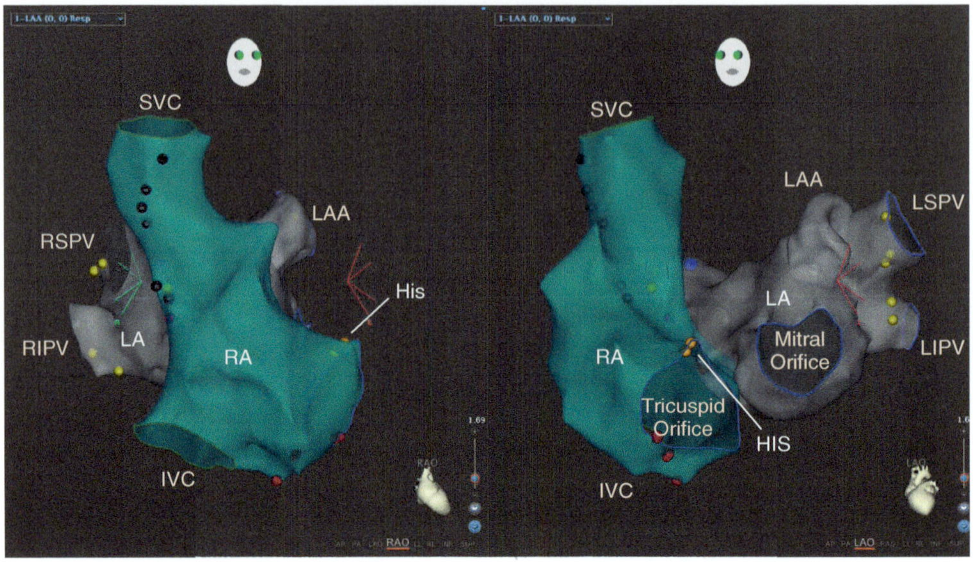

Right Anterior Oblique
Black dots: phrenic nerve capture

Left Anterior Oblique
Yellow dots: pulmonary vein capture

Figure 16-8

Atrial Anatomy

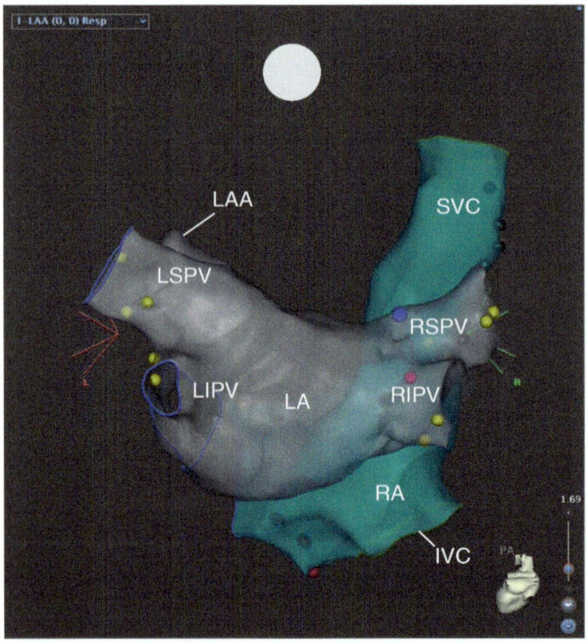

Figs. 16-7 and 16-8 display the posterior views of fast anatomic map (FAM) generated by manipulating catheters in the atria. *His*, His bundle location; *IVC*, inferior vena cava; *LA*, left atrium; *LAA*, left atrial appendage; *LIPV*, left inferior pulmonary vein; *LSPV*, left superior pulmonary vein; *RA*, right atrium; *RIPV*, right inferior pulmonary vein; *RSPV*, right superior pulmonary vein; *SVC*, superior vena cava. *Black dots* denote locations at which pacing resulted in phrenic nerve capture; *yellow dots* indicate sites at which pacing captured PV sleeves.

Progressive Left PV Isolation

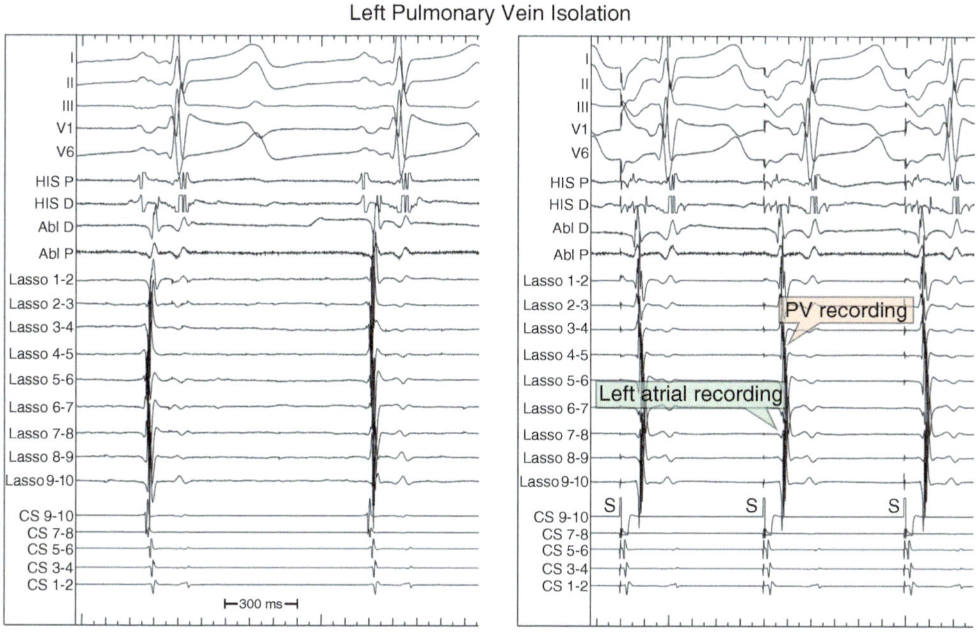

Figure 16-9

The left PVs were isolated as a unit with wide-area catheter ablation (WACA). At left of Fig. 16-9, during sinus rhythm, it is difficult to distinguish PV potentials from nearby left atrial signals; at right, during coronary sinus pacing, high-amplitude, high-frequency PV potentials are slightly more readily distinguished from lower-amplitude, lower-frequency left atrial recordings.

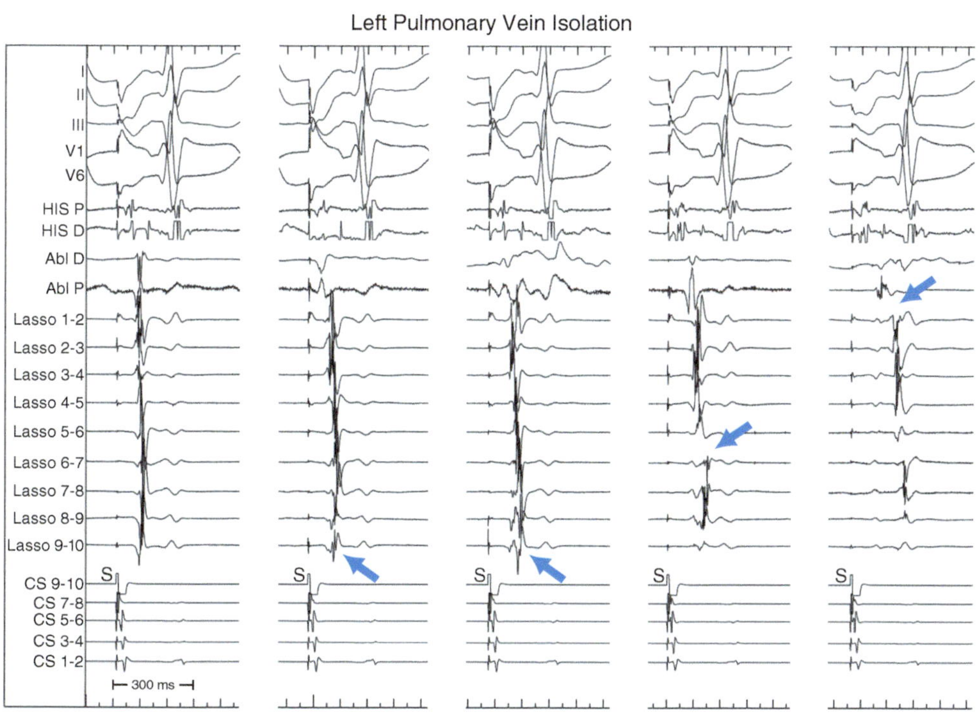

Figure 16-10

Over the span of several minutes, ablation around the left PV antrum results in progressive delay of PV potentials (Fig. 16-10, *arrows*).

Figure 16-11

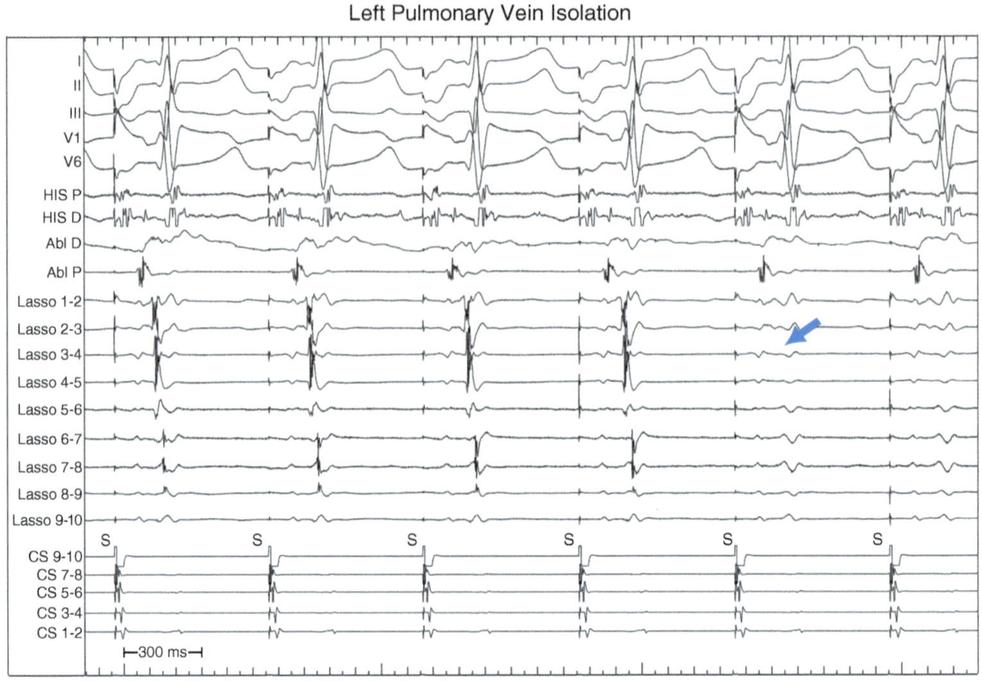

Finally, after nearly completely circumscribing the left PV antrum with RF applications, progressive delay of PV potentials is followed by complete loss of PV potentials (Fig. 16-11, *arrow*). Entrance block is now present in the left superior PV.

Figure 16-12

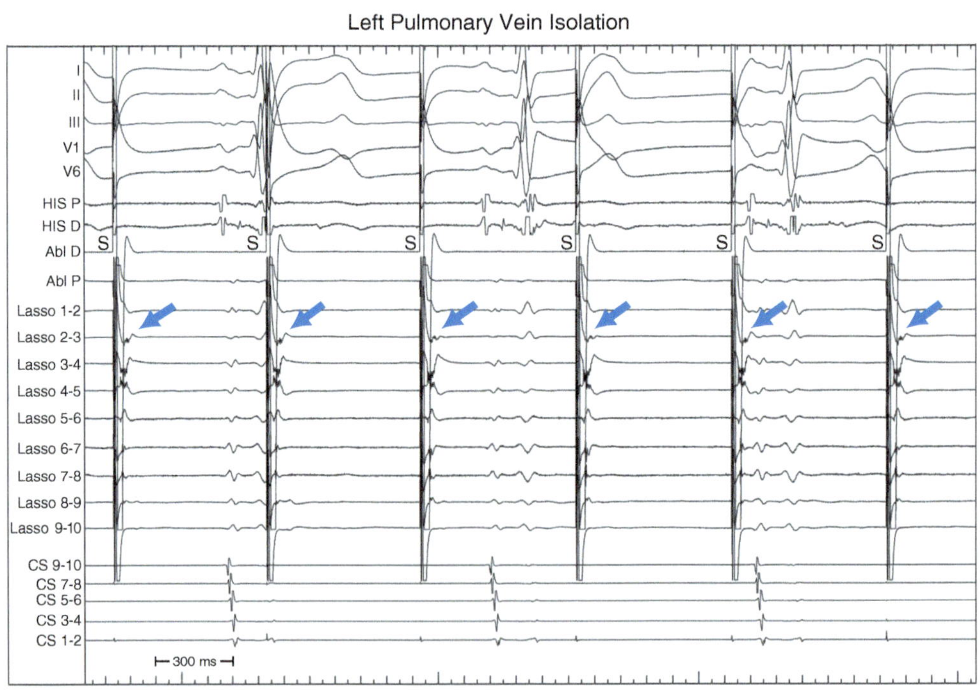

After demonstrating entrance block in the left superior PV, the ablation catheter is moved into the PV to a location tagged before ablation as a site at which pacing captured the PV. Pacing at this site (Fig. 16-12, *arrows*) now shows capture of potentials but no conduction to the adjacent left atrium, which remains in sinus rhythm. Exit block has now been demonstrated in the left superior PV. The same maneuver was performed in the left inferior PV with the same findings.

Progressive Right PV Isolation

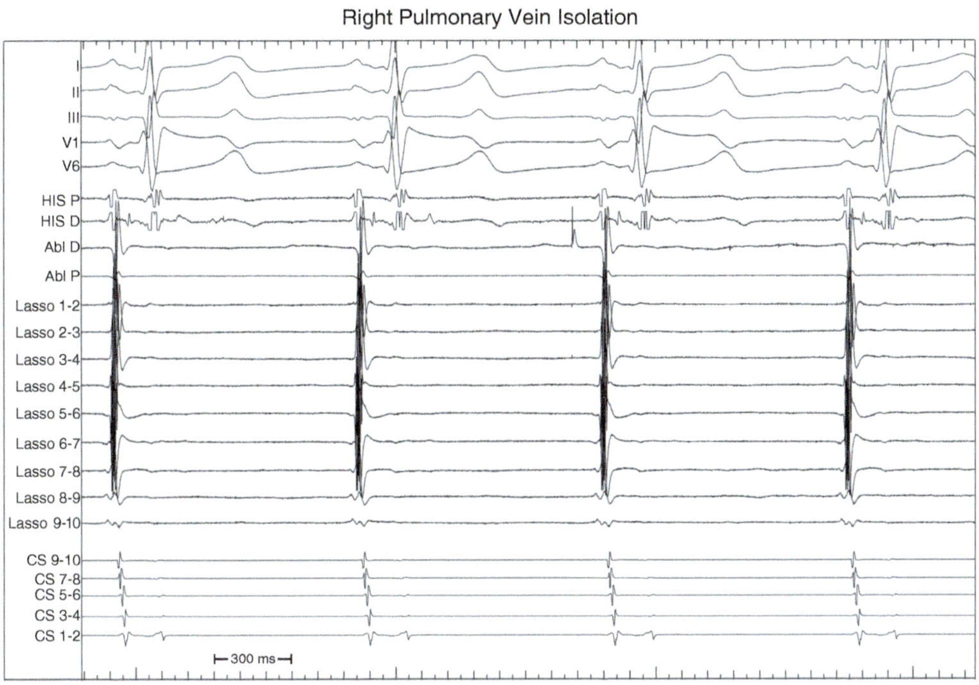

Figure 16-13

Attention is now turned to the right PVs. In Fig. 16-13, the ring catheter is in the right superior PV. Pacing rarely separates PV potentials (large, sharp signals in Lasso recordings) from nearby left atrium, so ablation is performed during sinus rhythm.

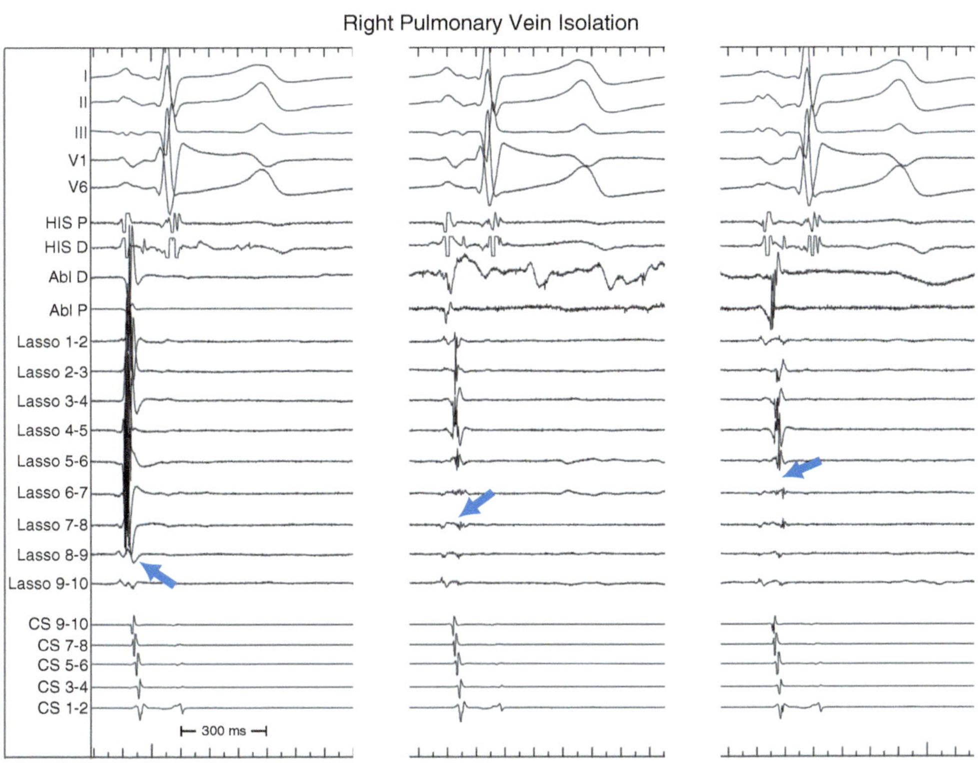

Figure 16-14

With progressive encirclement around the right PVs, PV potentials become more delayed in Fig. 16-14; the ring catheter has shifted slightly in the PV over the course of ablation, and thus the recordings are not identical in morphology.

Figure 16-15

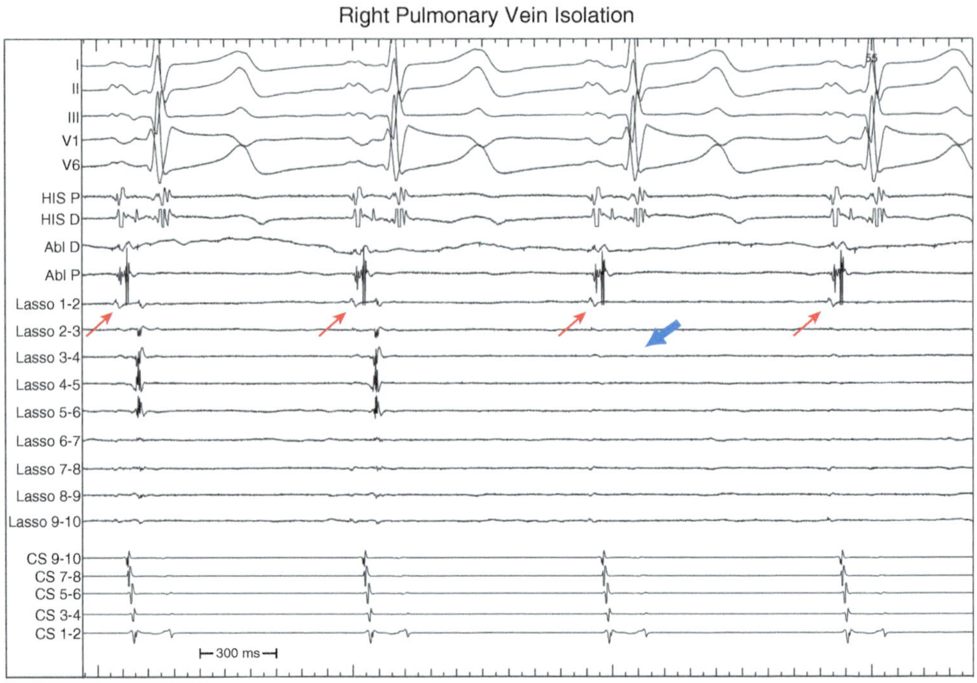

With still further encirclement around the right PVs, PV potentials cease (Fig. 16-15, *blue arrow*); this could be because the ring catheter had suddenly become displaced deeper in the PV or into the left atrial cavity, but far-field left atrial potentials are unchanged *(red arrows)*; thus the catheter has not moved and the loss of PV potentials means that this PV has entrance block.

Figure 16-16

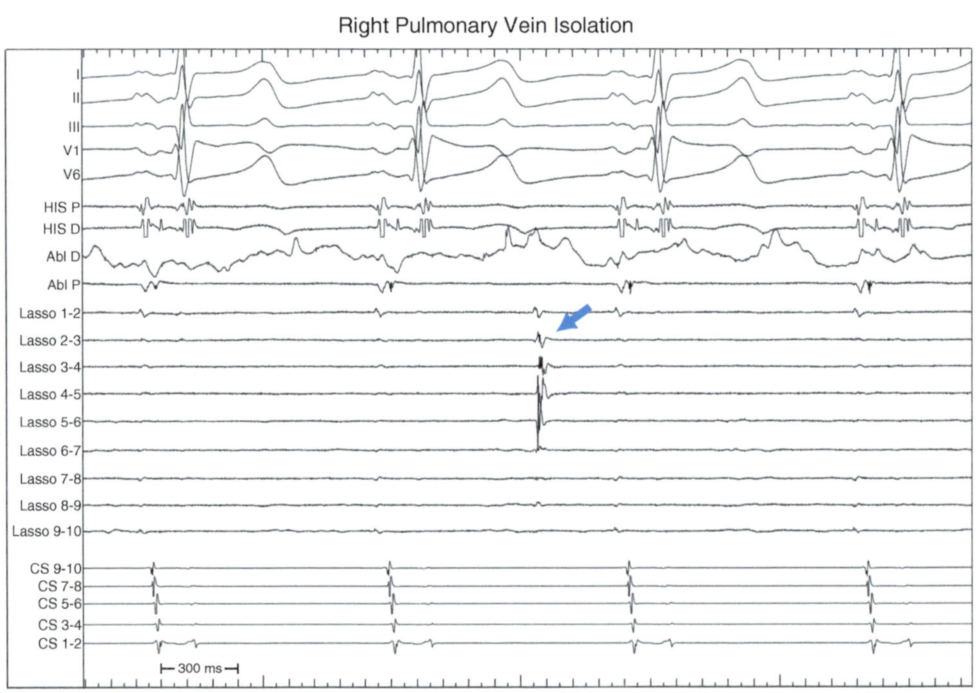

After encirclement and establishing entrance block into the right superior PV, a dissociated potential is observed in Fig. 16-16 (unaffected by the prevailing atrial rhythm, nor affecting the atrial rhythm).

RIPV Pacing/RSPV Recording

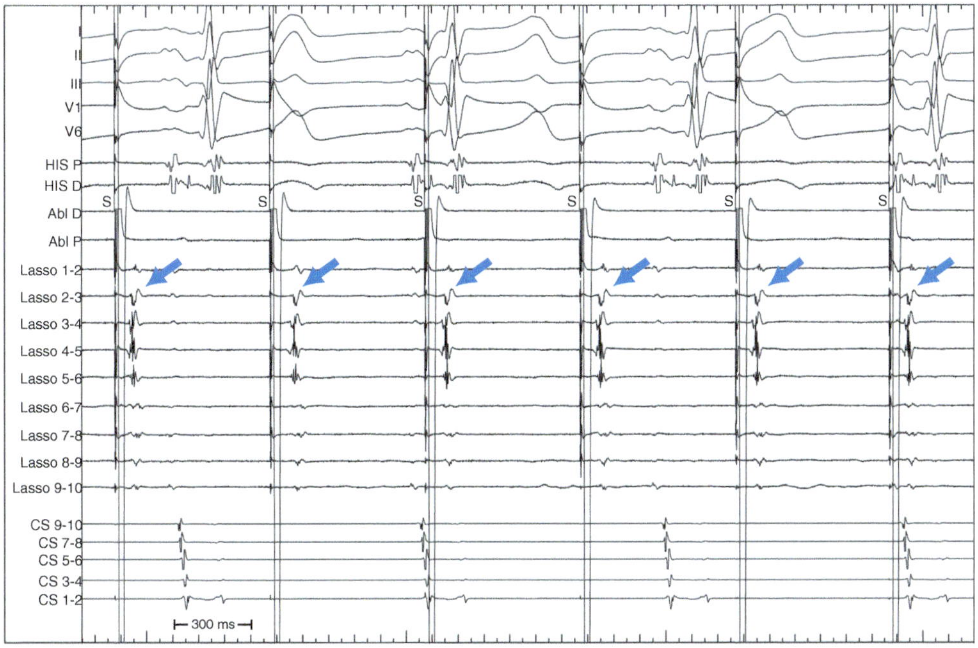

Figure 16-17

Pacing is performed in the right inferior PV with the ring catheter in the right superior PV; this shows PV potentials after each stimulus artifact without conduction to the atrium (Fig. 16-17). Capture of the right inferior PV is inferred, because it conducts to the right superior PV. This shows exit block of *both* PVs.

RSPV Recording

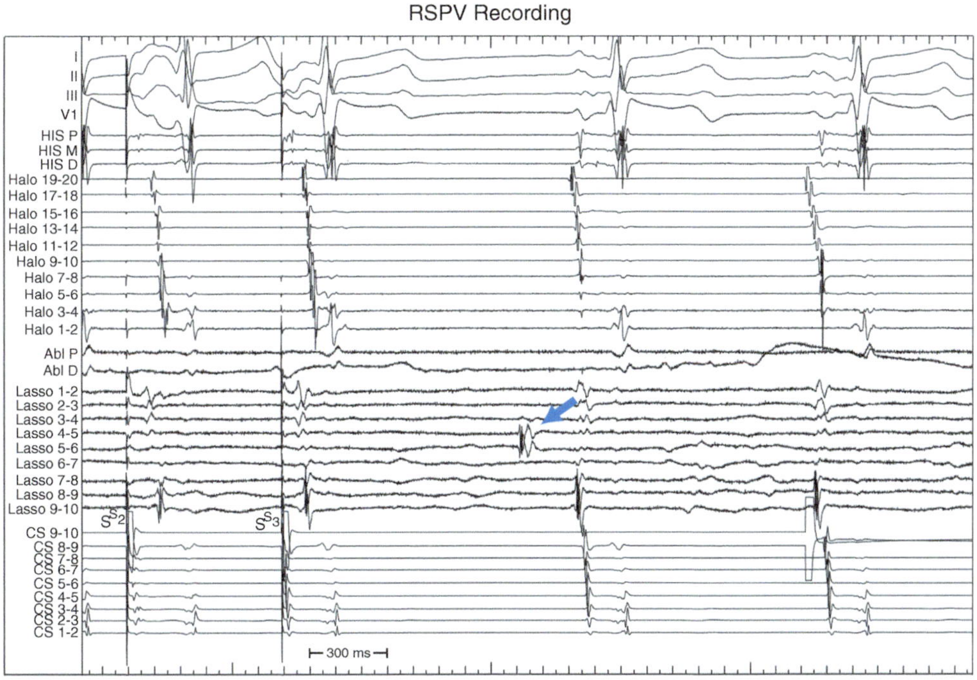

Figure 16-18

A dissociated PV potential is recorded with the ring catheter in the right superior PV (Fig. 16-18, *arrow*). A "halo" catheter has been placed around the tricuspid annulus in preparation for flutter ablation (because of his history of this arrhythmia). Cavotricuspid isthmus ablation was performed resulting in bidirectional conduction block (not shown).

Adenosine Administration

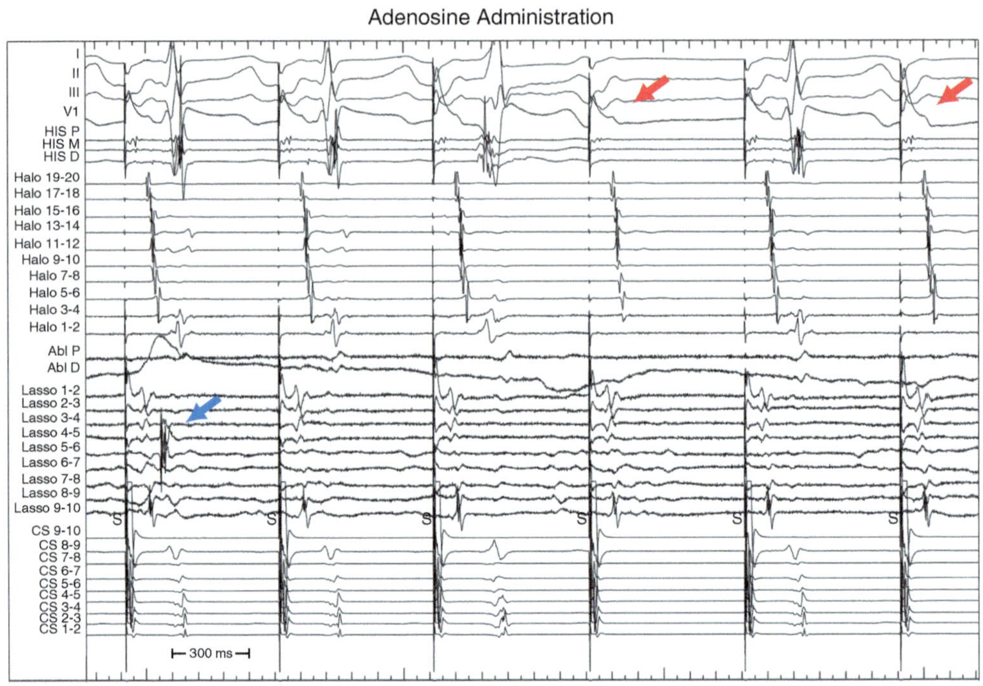

Figure 16-19

After cavotricuspid isthmus ablation, adenosine is administered (12 mg IV bolus). Its effect on the AV node is manifest by heart block (Fig. 16-19, *red arrows*) but cavotricuspid isthmus block persists as does right superior PV isolation; a dissociated PV potential is seen in the ring catheter recordings from this PV *(blue arrow)*.

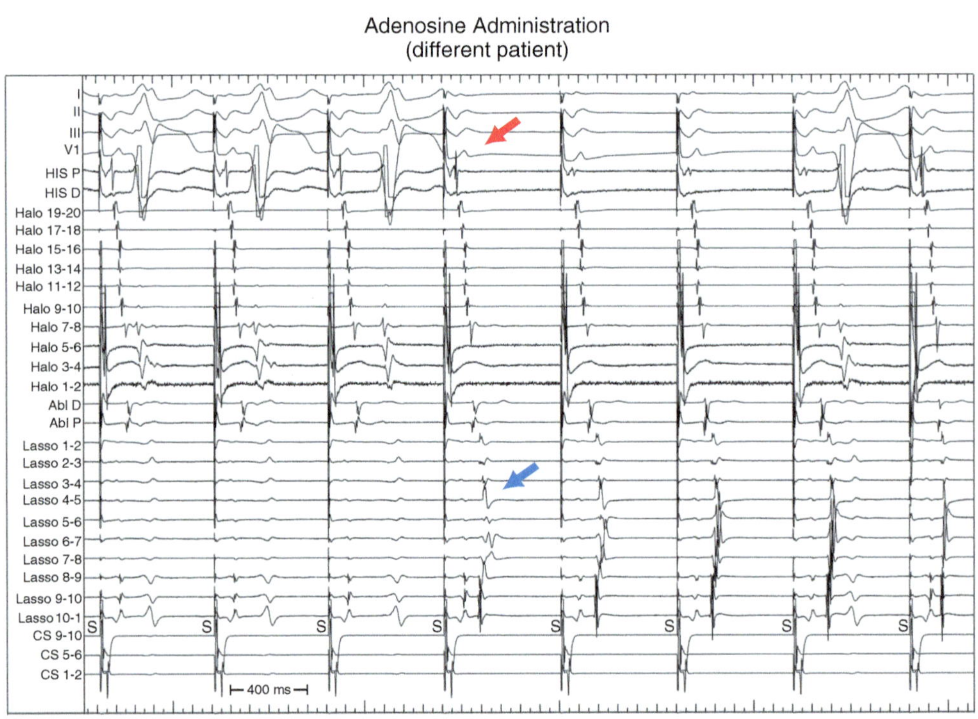

Figure 16-20

Adenosine administration is a different case (12 mg IV bolus). Its effect on the AV node is again manifest by heart block (Fig. 16-20, *red arrow*), and though cavotricuspid isthmus block persists, potentials are seen again in the left superior PV *(blue arrow)*. Additional ablation around this PV eliminated this response.

Electroanatomic Maps with RF Sites

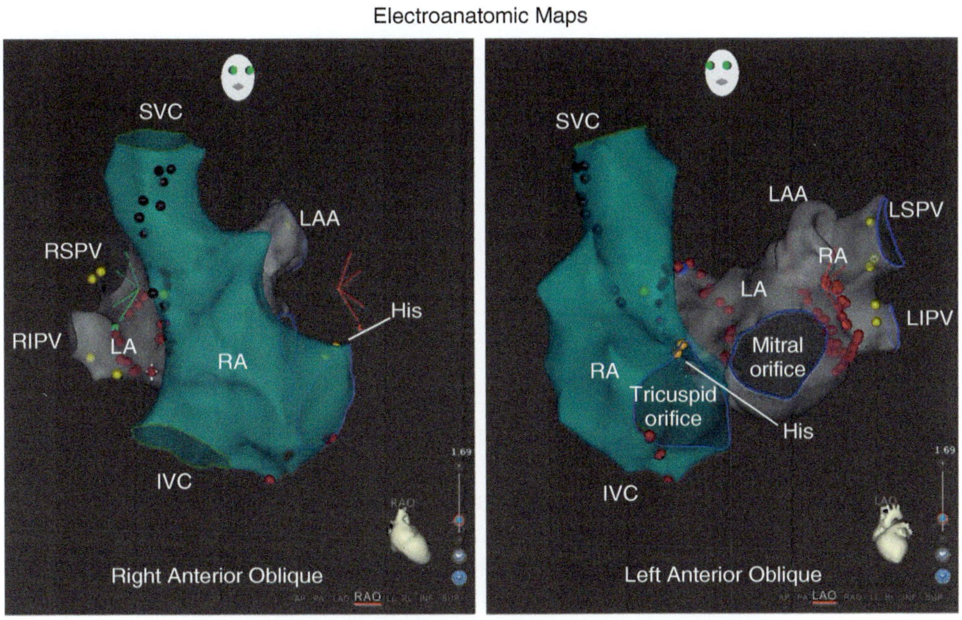

Figure 16-21

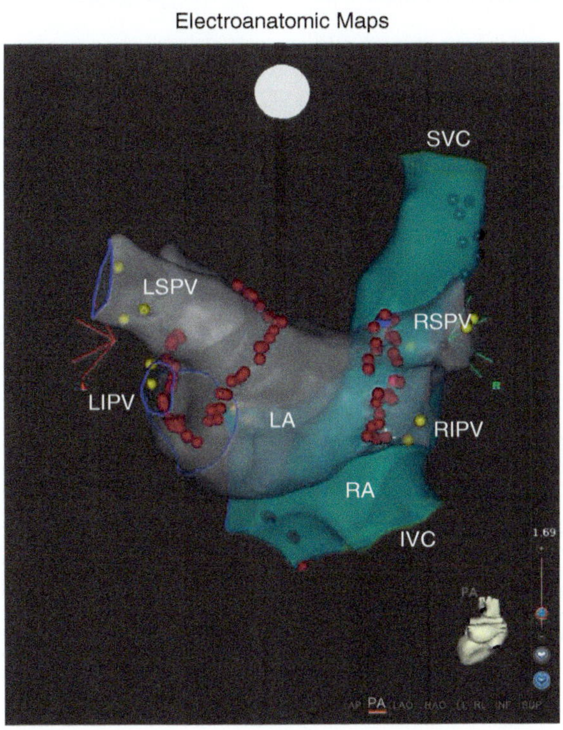

Figure 16-22

In Figs. 16-21 and 16-22, *red dots* show points at which radiofrequency energy was delivered (around PVs).

Summary

- PV isolation remains the standard for catheter-based therapy of atrial fibrillation
- Entrance and exit block should be demonstrated
- Additional means of assuring durable PV isolation may be used, including
  - Voltage mapping (not very sensitive or specific)
  - Adenosine (showing lack of resurgence of conduction)
  - Pacing along ablation line (showing inexcitability)

17 Pulmonary Vein Isolation, Rotor Mapping and Ablation, and Flutter Ablation for AF/Flutter

Case Presentation

The patient was a 67-year-old man with atrial fibrillation (AF) for the past 4 years or more; episodes were paroxysmal but arrhythmia is now persistent. His symptoms included lightheadedness, fatigue, and palpitations. Medical therapy with Metoprolol and then with diltiazem had no effect on his symptoms. Cardioversion without and with amiodarone failed to maintain sinus rhythm. He was referred for electrophysiology (EP) study and possible ablation; amiodarone was discontinued 1 month before the procedure. He was anticoagulated with dabigatran until 1 day before the procedure.

Baseline ECGs and Intracardiac Recordings

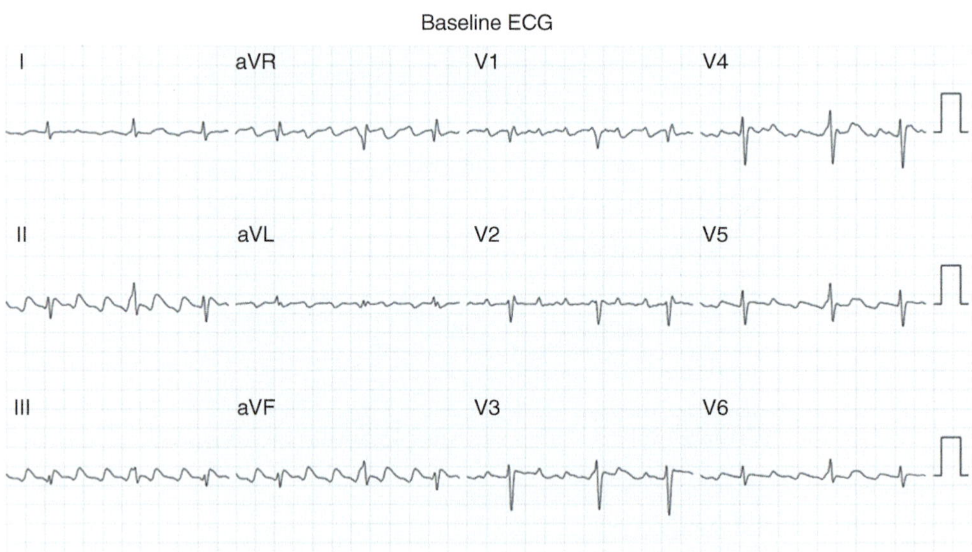

Figure 17-1

Fig. 17-1 was the baseline ECG at the start of the procedure. It is consistent with clockwise right atrial flutter, though slower than usual (300 ms atrial cycle length), and is the first recorded ECG of this arrhythmia (all others had been fibrillation). This may be an effect of residual amiodarone, or just another manifestation of his atrial arrhythmias independent of drug effect.

What Does This Mean? [Fig. 17-2]

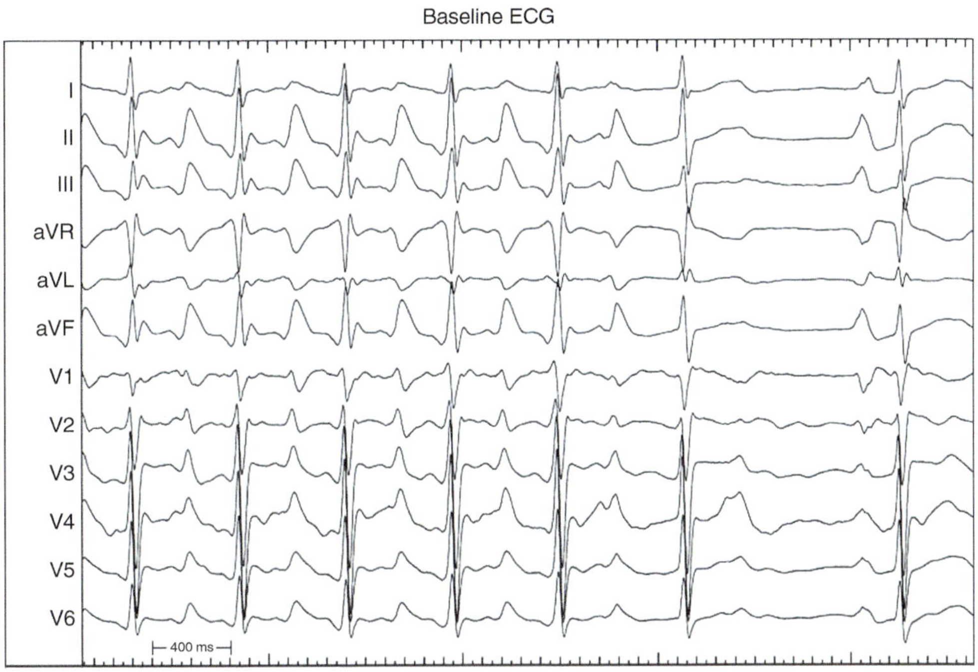

Figure 17-2

Shortly after obtaining the baseline ECG, the presenting arrhythmia terminated spontaneously to sinus as shown in Fig. 17-2. This occurred shortly after placement of the coronary sinus catheter and did not appear to result from catheter-mediated trauma or ectopy. This would be very unusual behavior for typical right atrial flutter and is perhaps more suggestive of a focal process. In addition, the morphology of the P wave in the inferior leads is less consistent with typical right atrial flutter.

What Does This Mean? [Fig. 17-3]

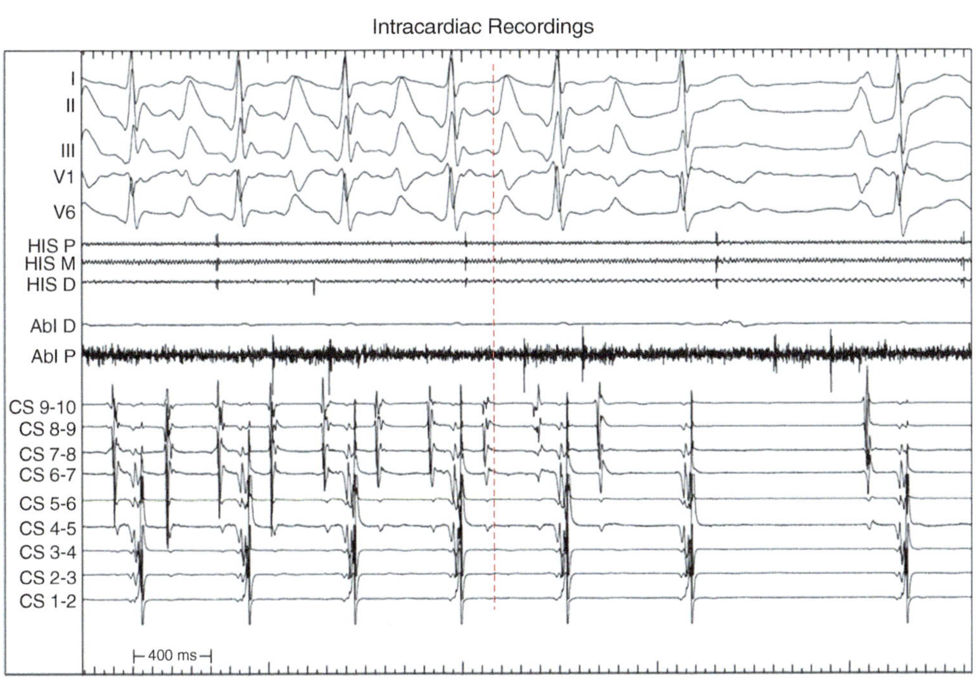

Figure 17-3

Fig. 17-3 are surface ECG and intracardiac recordings from the coronary sinus (CS) catheter (the only catheter in the heart then) at the time of termination of the presenting arrhythmia. It is clear that there was no catheter-induced ectopy or cycle length change before termination. It also appears that the CS catheter electrodes are activated before the apparent onset of the surface P wave *(dashed line)*, as well as in a proximal-distal direction.

Figure 17-4

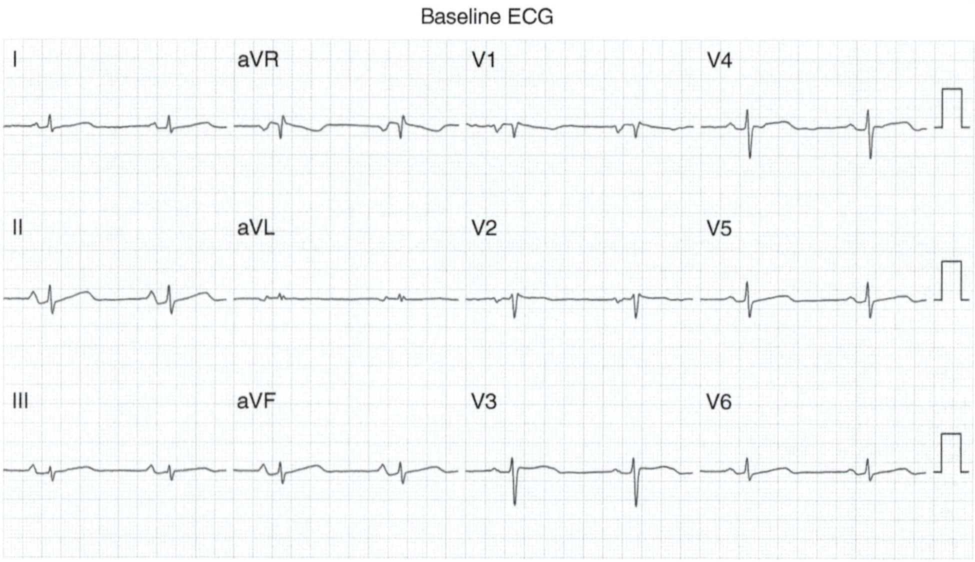

Fig. 17-4 shows sinus rhythm immediately after termination of the presenting arrhythmia. Terminal negativity of the P wave in V1 is consistent with left atrial hypertrophy but there are no other abnormalities.

What Does This Mean? [Fig. 17-5]

Figure 17-5

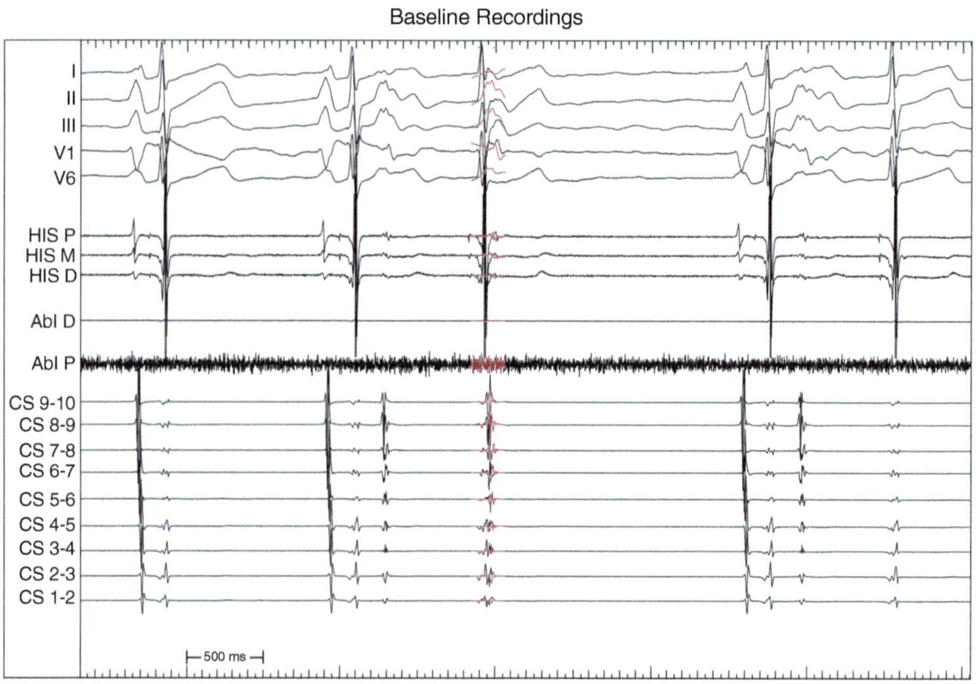

Seen in Fig. 17-5, premature atrial complexes (PACs) can certainly initiate AF episodes; in addition, PACs can emanate from the "culprit pulmonary vein (PV)," the one that is responsible for AF (either as a trigger or driver). Thus targeting consistent, repetitive PACs may be a useful adjunctive strategy in treating AF. The middle QRS complex has an atrial activation associated with it, the timing of which suggests a typical atrioventricular (AV) nodal echo; however, the P wave appears to be positive in the inferior leads (unlike AV nodal echoes) and has a configuration similar to the PAC when that complex is superimposed on it *(red)*.

Right Superior Pulmonary Vein Recordings

Is the PAC Coming from Here? [Fig. 17-6]

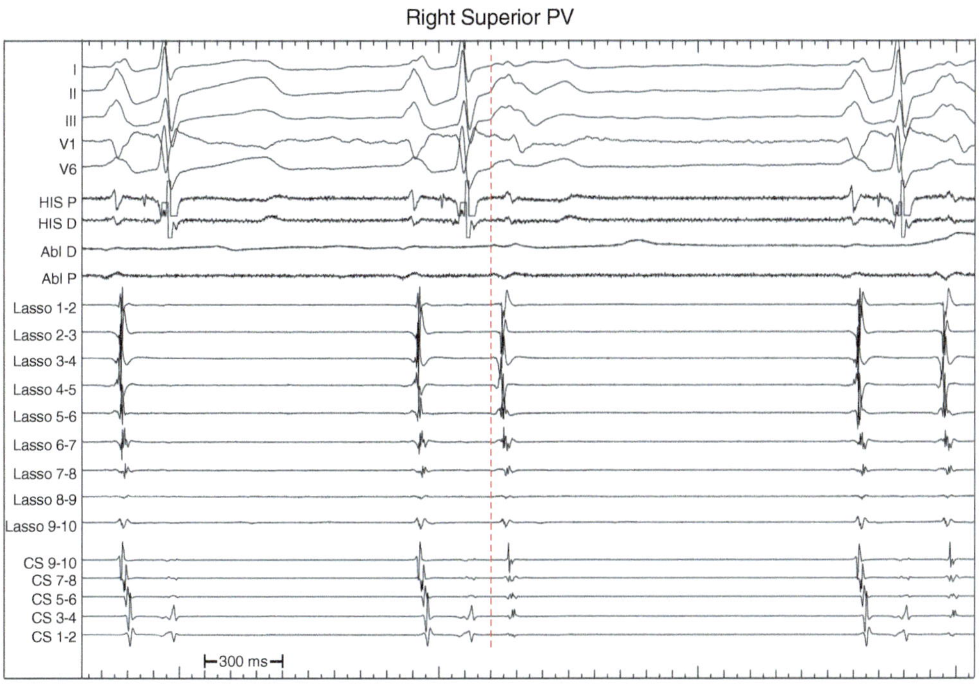

Figure 17-6

Left atrial access was obtained with transseptal catheterization, and a ring catheter ("Lasso") was used to record within PVs. When recording from the PV of origin of PACs (Fig. 17-6), the PV potentials always occur >50 ms before the P-wave origin because of slow conduction when exiting the PV. In this case because the PV potentials in the right superior PV occur after the P-wave onset *(red dotted line)*, the PAC cannot be originating here.

Left Inferior PV Recordings

Is the PAC Coming from Here? [Fig. 17-7]

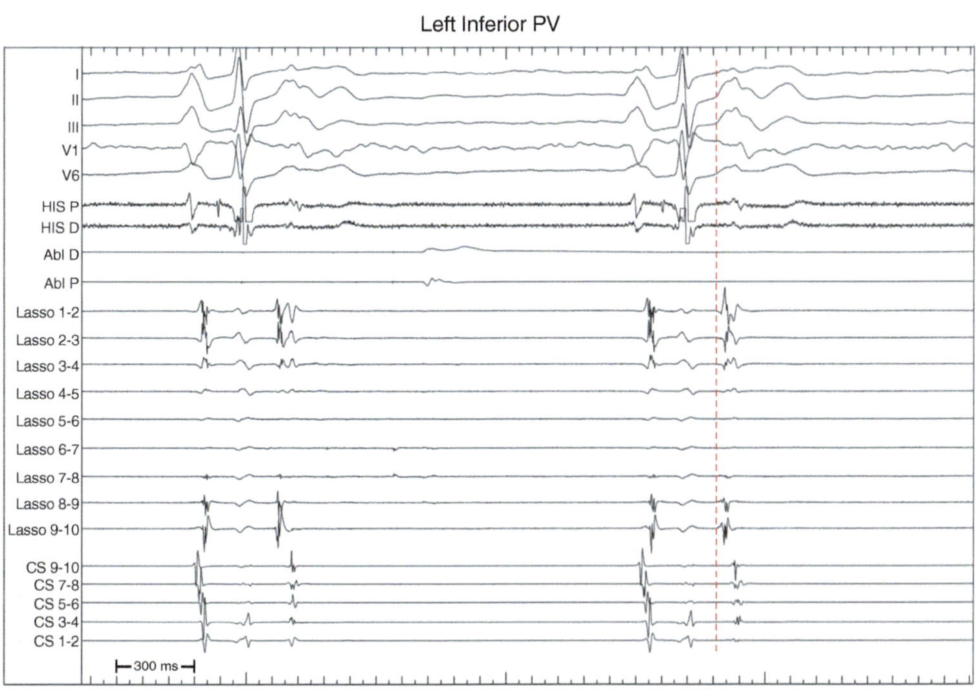

Figure 17-7

Using the same reasoning as in the prior figure, because the P wave of the PAC starts before the electrograms in the left inferior PV occur *(red dotted line)*, the PAC cannot be originating from this PV (Fig. 17-7).

Left Pulmonary Vein Wide-Area Circumferential Ablation

Baseline Pacing

Figure 17-8

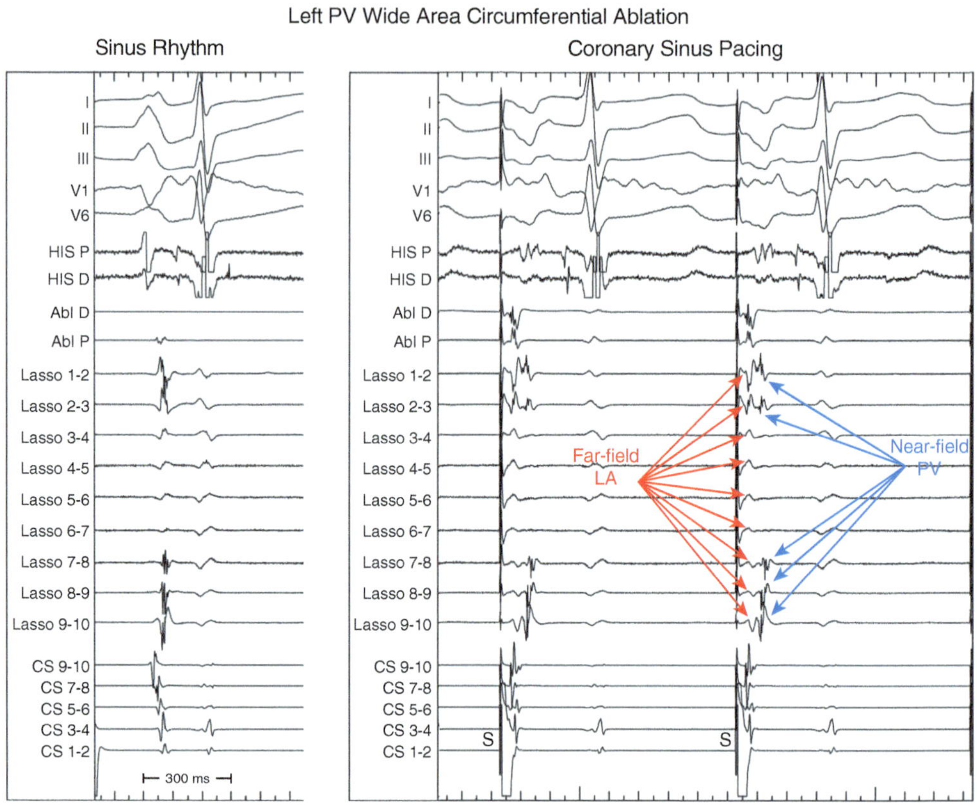

In Fig. 17-8, the left superior PV could not be easily engaged with the ring catheter but was the suspected source of the PACs. Circumferential wide-area catheter ablation was begun around the left PVs while the ring catheter was in the left inferior PV. During sinus rhythm, it is not clear which of the recordings represents atrial versus PV potentials; with coronary sinus pacing as shown, PV potentials *(blue arrows)* are clearly separated from far-field left atrial recordings *(red arrows)*.

Start of Ablation

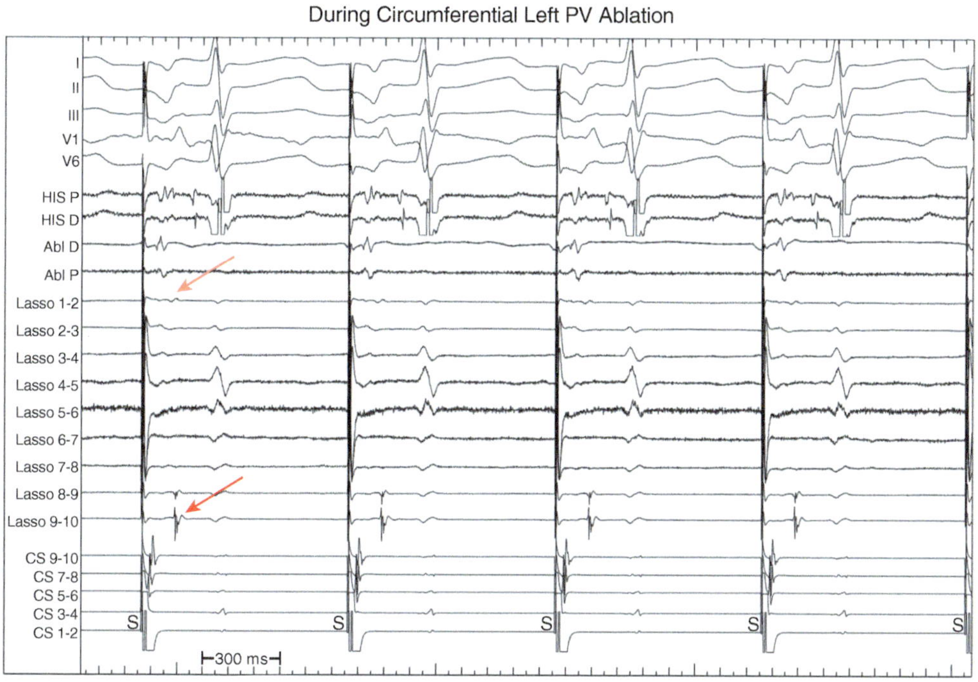

Figure 17-9

In Fig. 17-9, as circumferential ablation around the left PVs continues, some of the PV potentials have been eliminated *(pink arrow)*, whereas others are substantially delayed from their prior timing *(red arrow)*. Of note, the ring catheter has moved slightly within the PV (judging by the appearance of the far-field LA potentials compared with the prior figure), but the fact remains that PV potentials have been dramatically delayed from some, as well as eliminated from other recordings. Additionally, the PACs (which had occurred several per minute before) ceased at this time, signifying that their source was likely along the line of ablation, rather than in a PV; if it had been in a PV, most likely isolated, dissociated firing of PV potentials from the PAC focus would persist (but did not).

Isolation Occurs

Figure 17-10

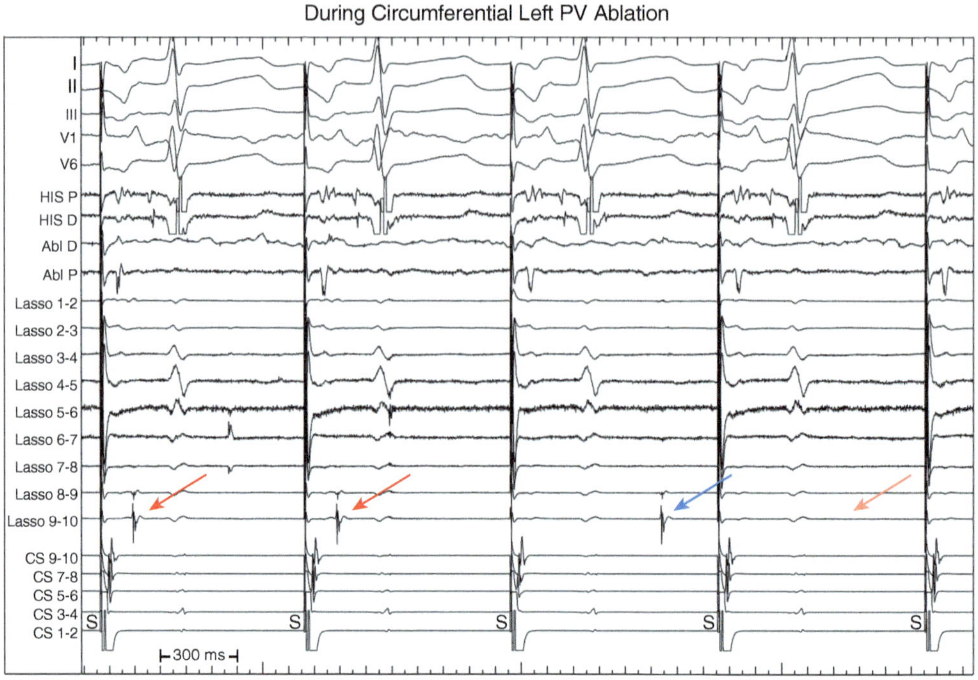

As circumferential ablation around the left PVs nears completion in Fig. 17-10, PV potentials *(red arrows)* show further delay after the third stimulus *(blue arrow)*, and then are finally eliminated *(pink arrow)*.

Sinus Rhythm After Isolation

Figure 17-11

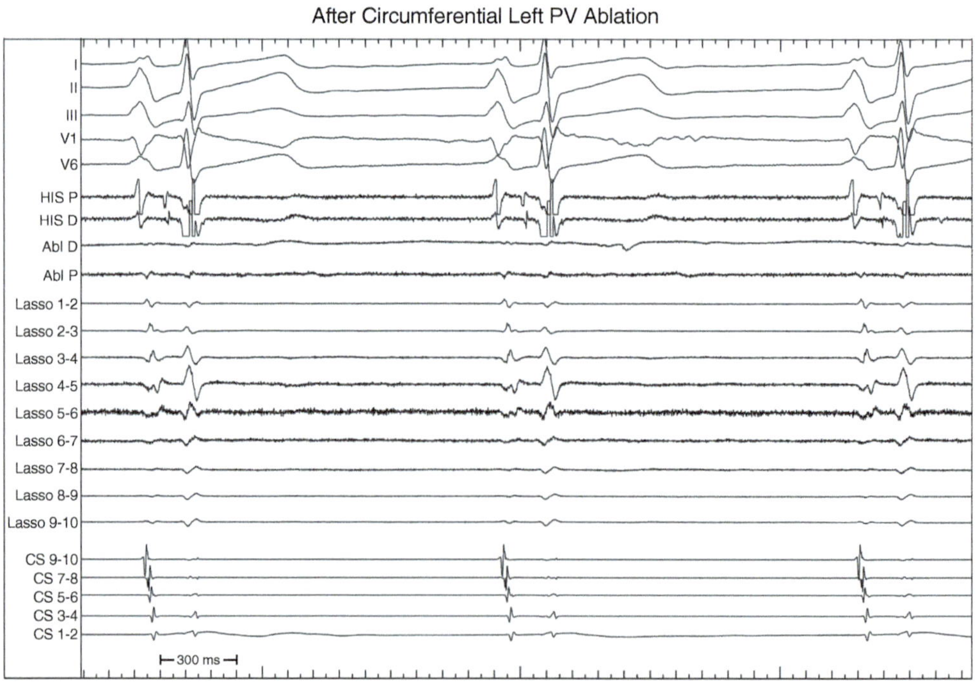

After circumferential ablation around the left PVs (Fig. 17-11), no PV potentials are seen during sinus rhythm; PACs are also absent at this time.

Exit Block After Isolation

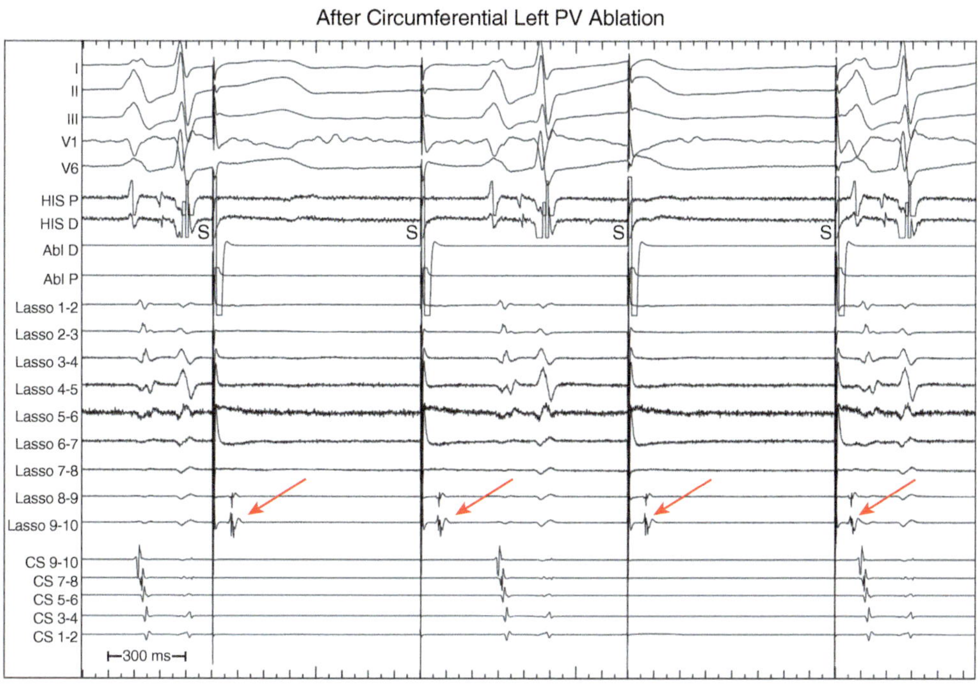

Figure 17-12

Entrance block (propagation into the PV) has been demonstrated, but it is important to show exit block (from PV to atrium) after circumferential ablation around the left PVs. Pacing from the left superior PV, while recording from a ring catheter in the left inferior PV (Fig. 17-12), shows inferred capture of PV potentials in the left superior PV, with conduction to the left inferior PV where potentials are recorded *(red arrows)*, but no conduction to the left atrium (which remains in sinus rhythm, unaffected by PV pacing). Thus both left PVs have been isolated (both entrance and exit block) as a unit.

Right PV Wide-Area Circumferential Ablation

Start of Ablation

Figure 17-13

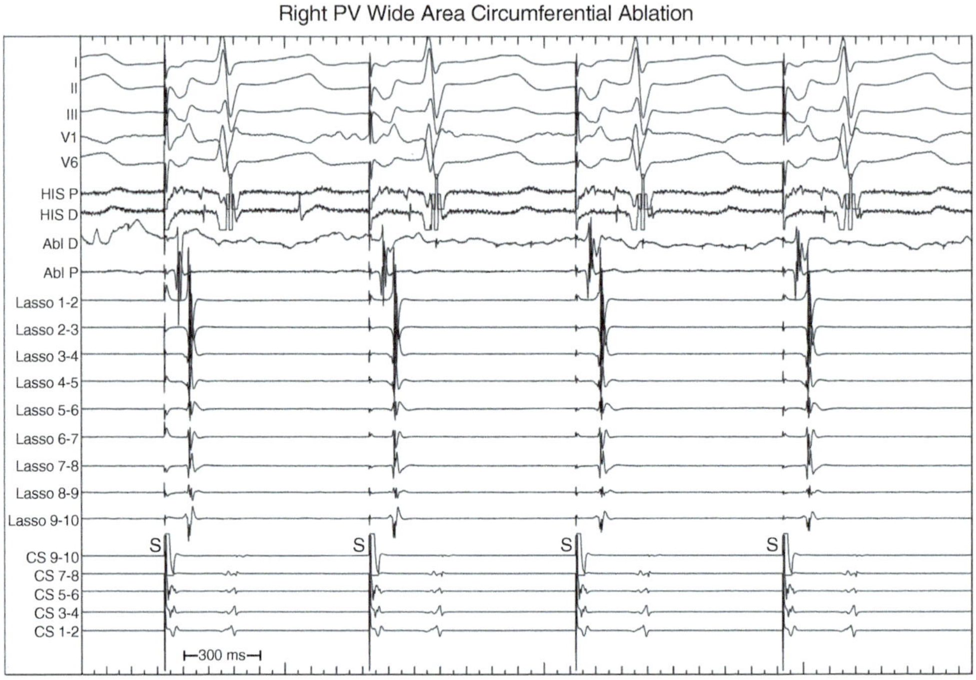

After completion of left PV isolation, attention is turned to the right PVs (Fig. 17-13). Here, the ring catheter is in the right superior PV, again during coronary sinus pacing. With right PVs, coronary sinus pacing usually does not separate left atrial and PV potentials nearly as well as it does with left PVs; pacing was done in this instance because of bradycardia.

Flutter Initiates

Figure 17-14

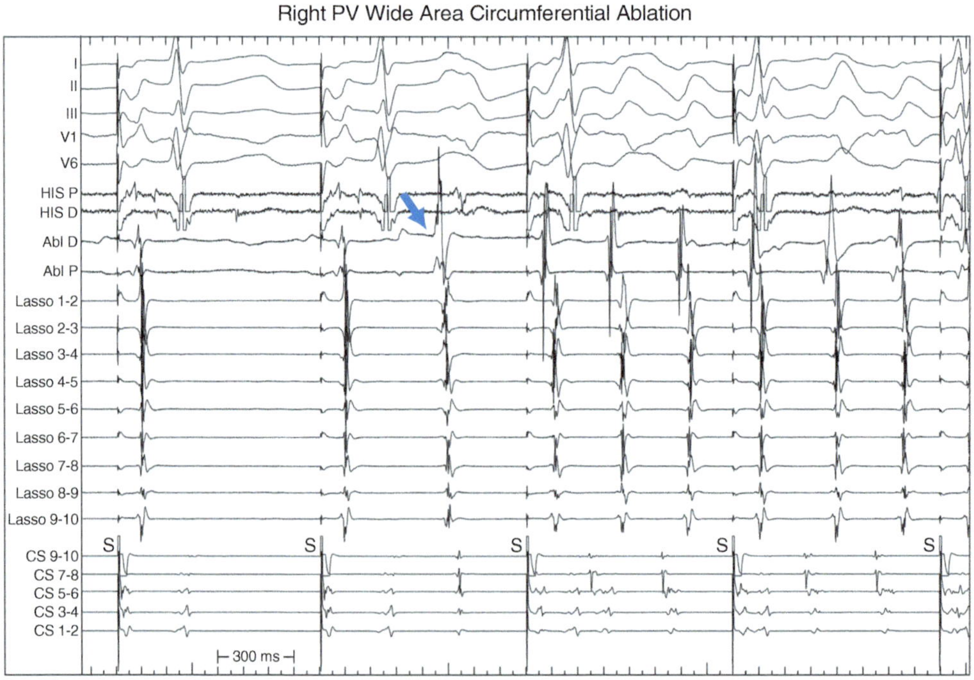

During attempted right PV isolation (Fig. 17-14), a PAC *(blue arrow)* occurs (perhaps due to irritation from the ablation catheter) that initiates what appears to be atrial flutter, with upright flutter waves in the inferior leads. This is reminiscent of the arrhythmia that was present at the beginning of the procedure when catheters were first being placed.

Flutter Terminates in Right Atrium

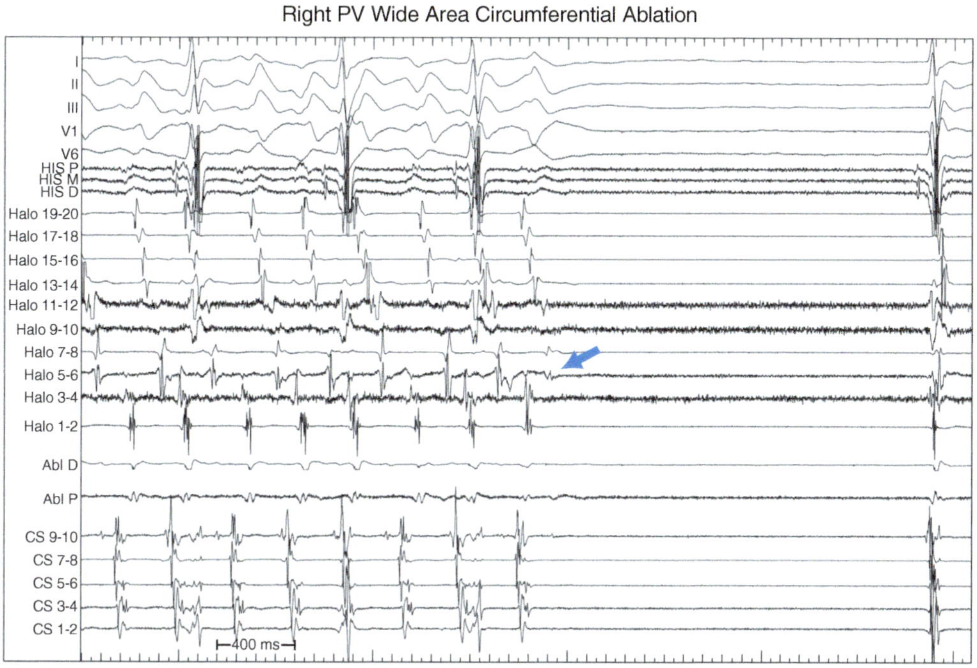

Figure 17-15

Since the last figure, a 20-pole catheter ("Halo") has been placed in the right atrium to record around the tricuspid annulus (Fig. 17-15). Here, a spontaneous termination of the arrhythmia is shown. The last electrograms that are seen are from the tricuspid annulus *(arrow)*, suggesting that the rhythm originates in the left atrium (because, when the arrhythmia ceased, the last cycle was transmitted to the right atrium and no further activity is seen until a junctional escape complex at the far right). It is also possible that the arrhythmia is actual right-atrial, peritricuspid reentry that terminated because of tenuous conduction properties in the tissue between electrodes 5-6 and 3-4 on the tricuspid annular catheter; there is clearly poor conduction in this area, indicated by the prolonged interval between these adjacent electrode pairs compared with others.

Partial Isolation

Right PV Wide Area Circumferential Ablation

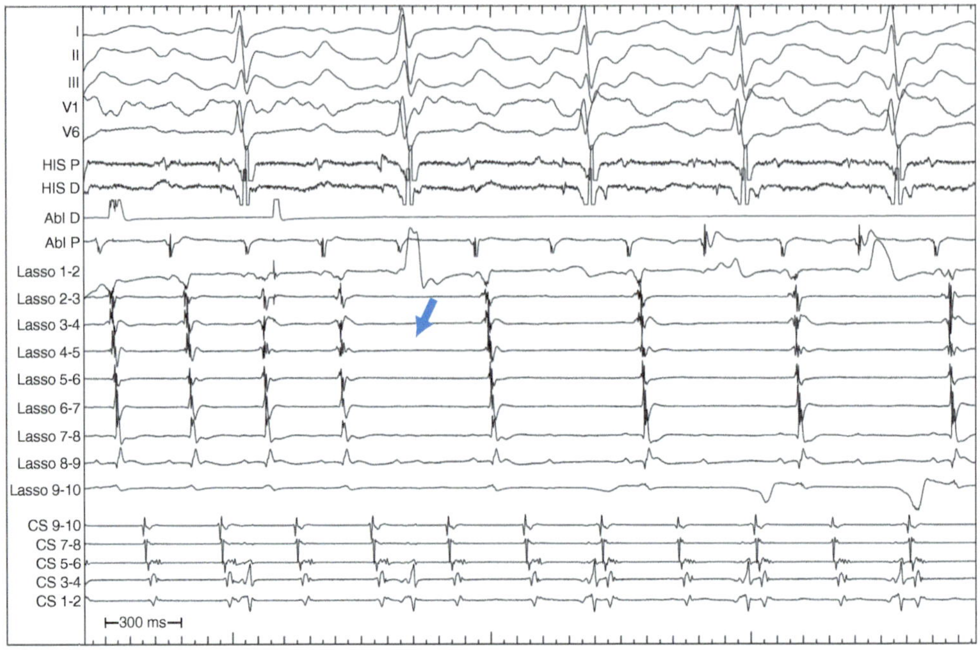

Figure 17-16

In Fig. 17-16, ablation around the right pulmonary veins was continued; in a similar way as previously (PAC; not shown here), the flutter-like arrhythmia began again. Here, PV potentials from the right superior PV go from 1:1 with the arrhythmia to every other cycle *(arrow)*, indicating that this PV is not responsible for the ongoing arrhythmia. PV isolation can be performed during sinus rhythm, atrial pacing, or atrial flutter/fibrillation equally well.

Full Isolation

Right PV Wide Area Circumferential Ablation

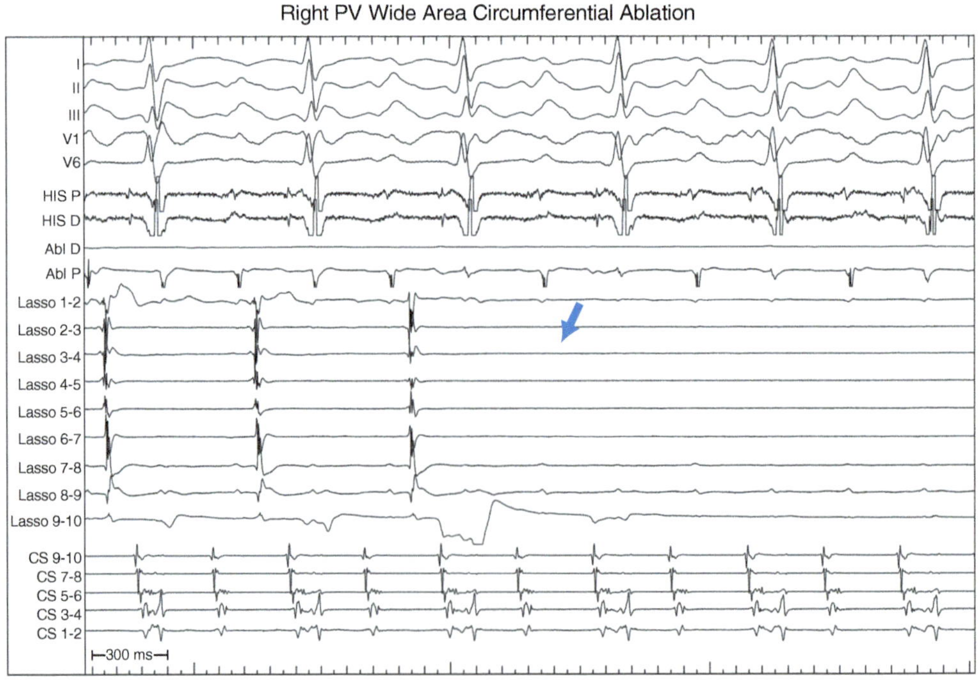

Figure 17-17

Ablation around the right pulmonary veins continues. In Fig. 17-17, PV potentials from the right superior PV are suddenly eliminated *(arrow)*. Obviously, this PV is not responsible for the flutter-like arrhythmia that continues (already known from the prior figure).

Dissociated Potential Seen After Right WACA

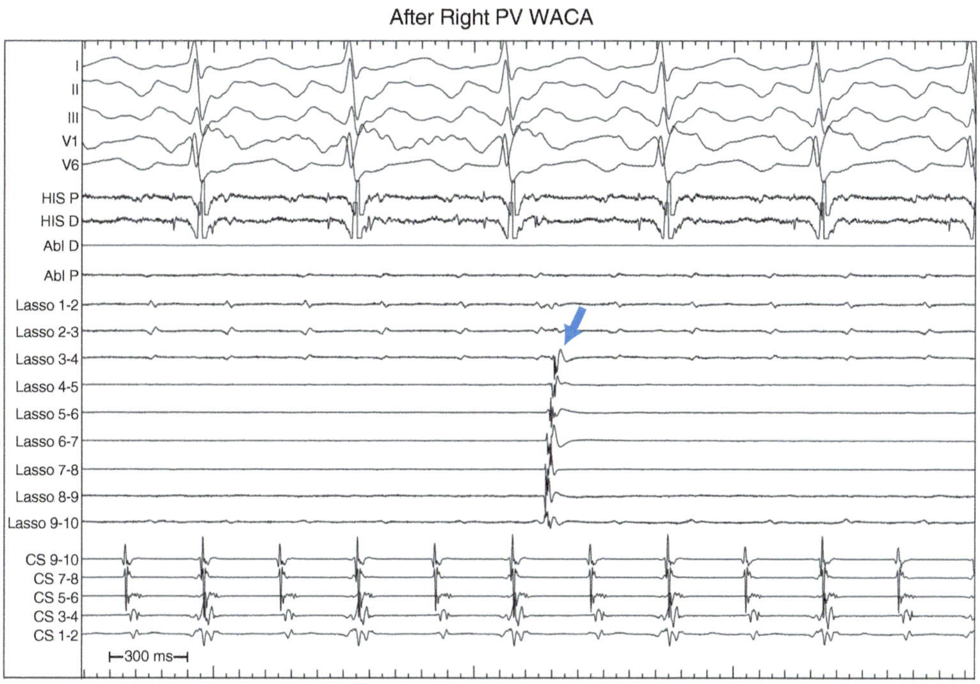

What Is Demonstrated? [Fig. 17-18]

A. Entrance block
B. Exit block
C. Both
D. Neither

Figure 17-18

The flutter-like arrhythmia continues after the right superior PV has been isolated; a single spontaneous discharge (dissociated potential, *arrow* in Fig. 17-18) occurs during a short waiting period to ensure that the PV does not reconnect to the left atrium. This shows entrance block to the PV, but not exit block (which cannot be demonstrated until the rate in the PV is faster than the rate in the atrium).

Exit Block Can't Be Demonstrated When Pacing in Vein After Right WACA During Flutter. What Is Demonstrated? [Fig. 17-19]

A. Entrance block
B. Exit block
C. Both
D. Neither

Figure 17-19

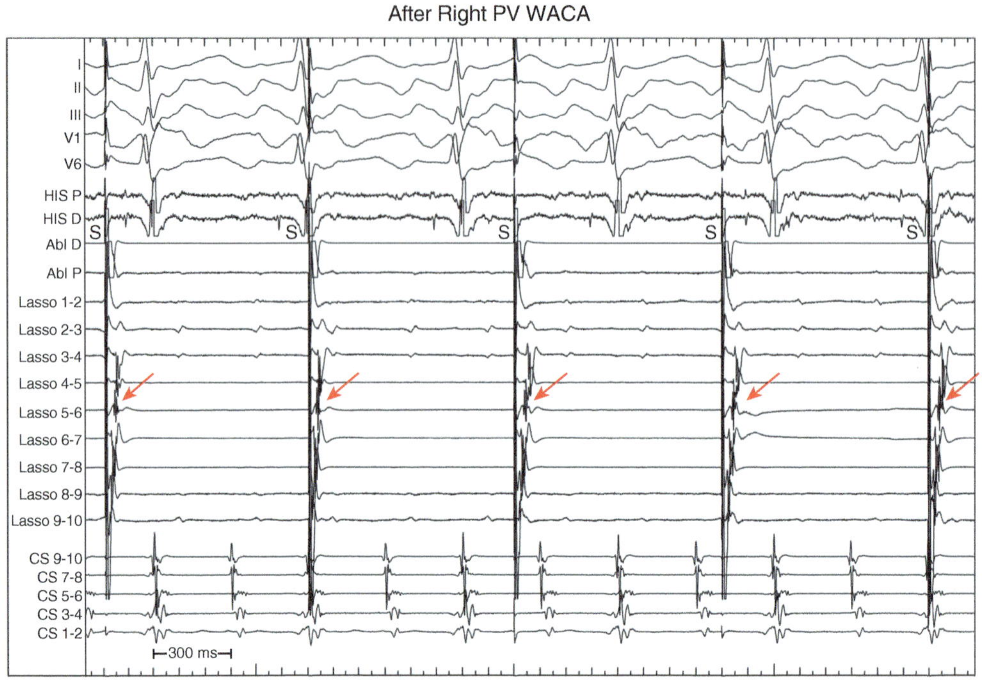

Here, pacing the right *inferior* PV inferentially captures that PV and conducts to the right *superior* PV (where the ring catheter remains; controlled PV potentials are shown by *arrows*) (Fig. 17-19). This again shows entrance block to the PV, because if there were *not* entrance block, the PV potentials would be related to the ongoing flutter-like arrhythmia rather than the stimulus artifacts (as here). This again does not demonstrate *exit* block, which requires dissociation between PV and LA in the presence of a more rapid input from the PV. Although exit block cannot be shown at this time, there is still value in finding a location at which PV capture is possible: after sinus rhythm is restored, the catheter can be maneuvered back to that spot to easily determine whether exit block is present (even without a separate catheter recording from the PV, as here).

Exit Block Testing When Pacing in Vein After Right WACA During Flutter. Which Is Demonstrated? [Fig. 17-20]

A. Entrance block
B. Exit block
C. Both
D. Neither

Figure 17-20

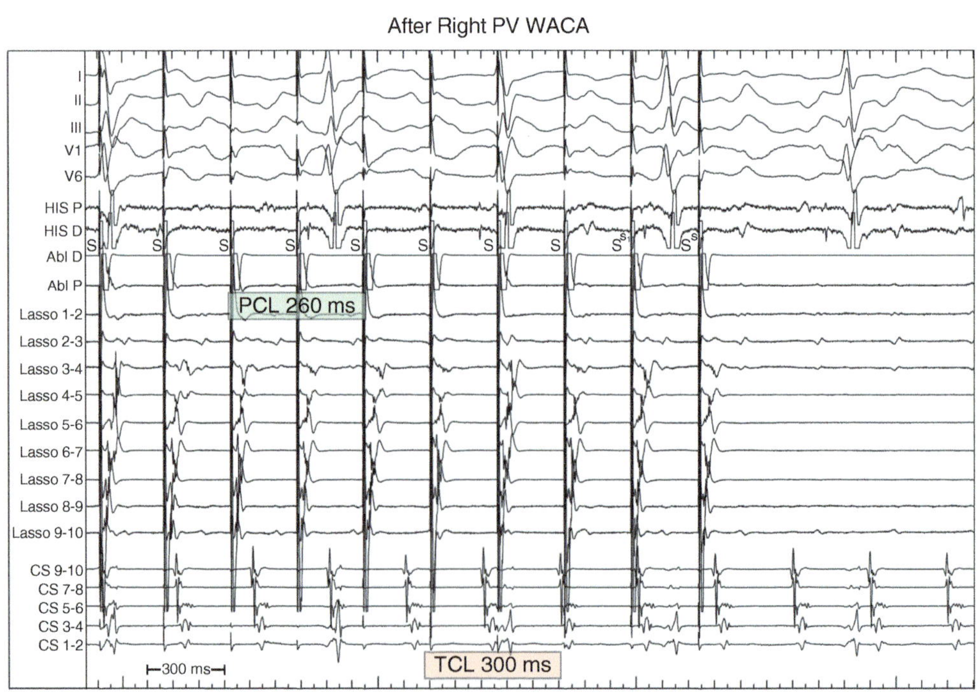

Now, pacing the right inferior PV captures that PV and conducts consistently to the right superior PV at 260 ms, whereas the flutter-like arrhythmia's cycle length is 300 ms and quite regular (Fig. 17-20). Because there is no influence of the pacing on the ongoing arrhythmia, exit block—from both right PVs, because the inferior PV is paced and the superior PV is recorded—has now been reasonably demonstrated.

Pacing During Flutter

From Midcoronary Sinus

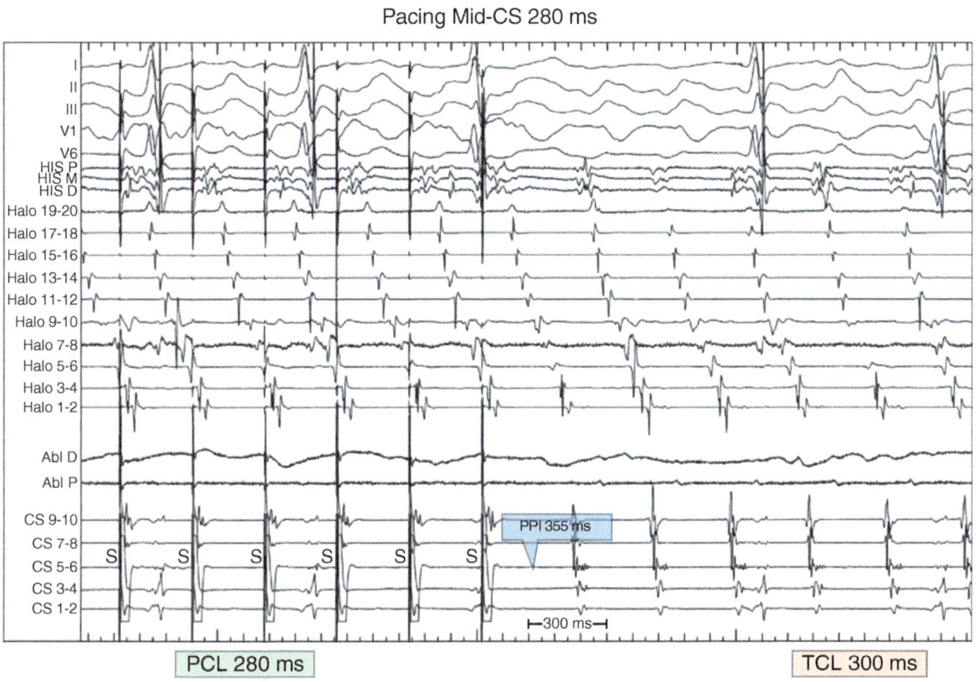

Figure 17-21

Now that all four PVs have been fully isolated with entrance and exit block demonstrated, attention is turned to the flutter-like arrhythmia. In Fig. 17-21, the last several cycles of overdrive pacing from the midcoronary sinus are shown. Because there has been no prior ablation within the right atrium that could alter the expected activation sequence along the tricuspid annulus, the fact that the atrial activation sequence during CS pacing has the configuration shown rather than the expected "chevron" sequence (equivalently early at Halo 1-2 and Halo 19-20, latest at Halo 11-12) is a demonstration of fusion and is diagnostic of macroreentry. Further, the postpacing interval (PPI) at the mid-CS is 355 ms, substantially longer than the tachycardia cycle length (TCL) and suggests that this portion of the CS is not part of the circuit. This is curious, because the prior spontaneous termination event (Fig. 17-15) suggested a left atrial source.

From Proximal Coronary Sinus

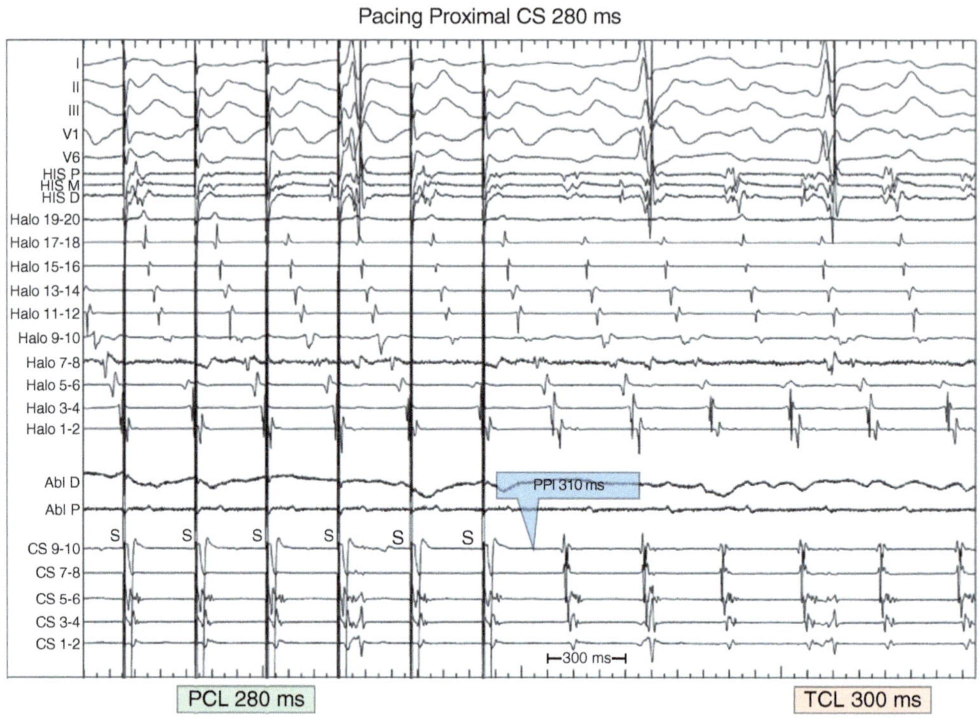

Figure 17-22

In Fig. 17-22, the last several cycles of overdrive pacing from the proximal coronary sinus electrodes (at the ostium) are shown. The atrial activation sequence along the tricuspid annulus is the same as in the prior figure, but the PPI from this site is now 310 ms, nearly the same as the TCL, suggesting that this portion of the CS is very near or part of the circuit.

From Midtricuspid Annulus

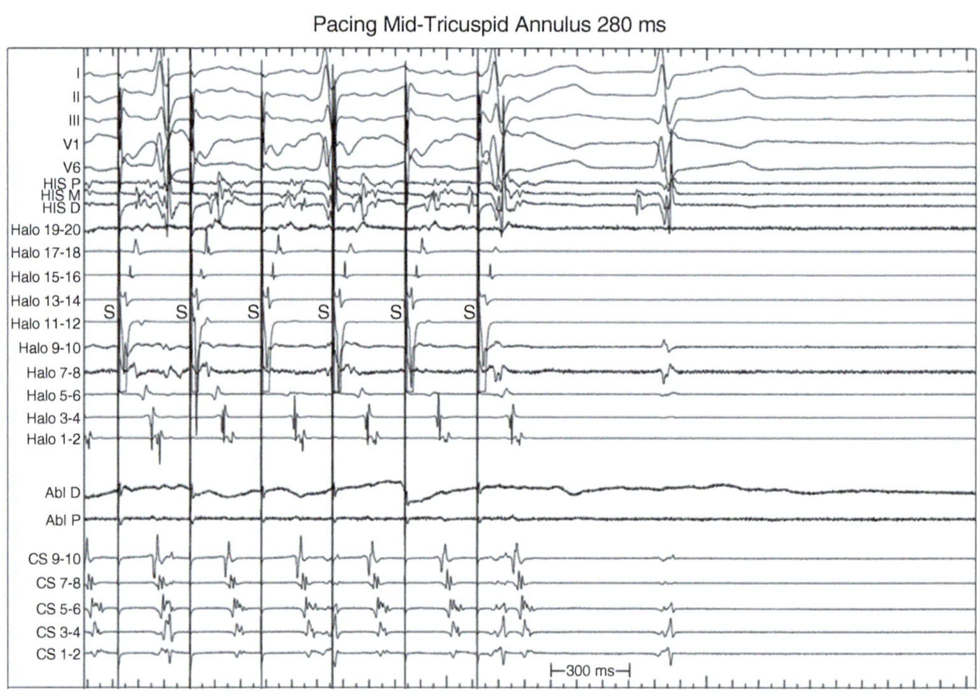

Figure 17-23

In Fig. 17-23, the last several cycles of overdrive pacing from the midtricuspid annulus electrodes are shown. Whereas multiple attempts at overdrive pacing from the coronary sinus (some not shown) did not terminate tachycardia, it was nonetheless terminated by the first attempt at pacing from the tricuspid annulus. When this unexpected result occurs, it is always worth looking back earlier during the episode of stimulation to see if something unusual happened.

Earlier in That Episode of Tricuspid Annulus Pacing

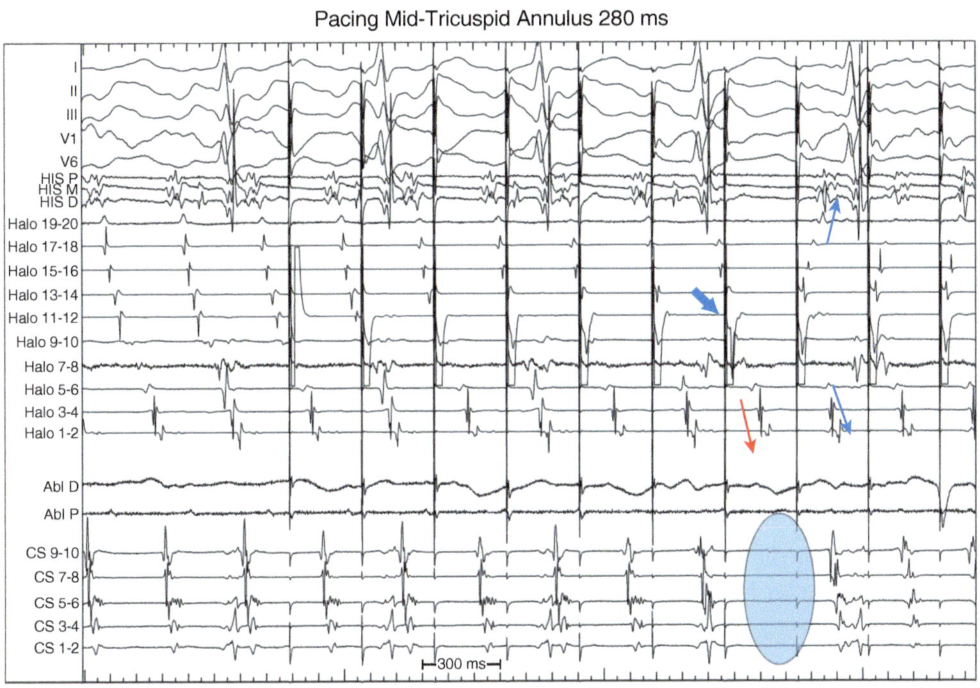

Figure 17-24

In Fig. 17-24, the first several cycles of overdrive pacing from the midtricuspid annulus electrodes are shown. The stimulus indicated by the *large blue arrow* captures the tricuspid annulus tissue and sends the impulse forward *(red arrow)*; however, it does not arrive at the CS *(translucent oval)*. The subsequent stimulus artifact conducts in both directions from the stimulation site *(blue arrows)*, because there is no wavefront from the prior cycle proceeding around the tricuspid annulus. This indicates that tissue close to the proximal CS recordings was essential for perpetuation of the tachycardia (because, in the absence of activation of this site, tachycardia terminates), and that the arrhythmia is most likely right atrial macroreentry (typical, counterclockwise atrial flutter). This is despite the unusual ECG appearance of the flutter waves. Why, then, did a previous figure show this arrhythmia spontaneously terminating in a fashion suggesting a left atrial source (Fig. 17-15)? The answer is in the figure shown here, demonstrating (as noted earlier) that there is a portion of the medial cavotricuspid isthmus where conduction is not robust, and subject to termination when input arrives before full recovery from refractoriness at that site.

Single Extrastimulus from Lateral Tricuspid Annulus

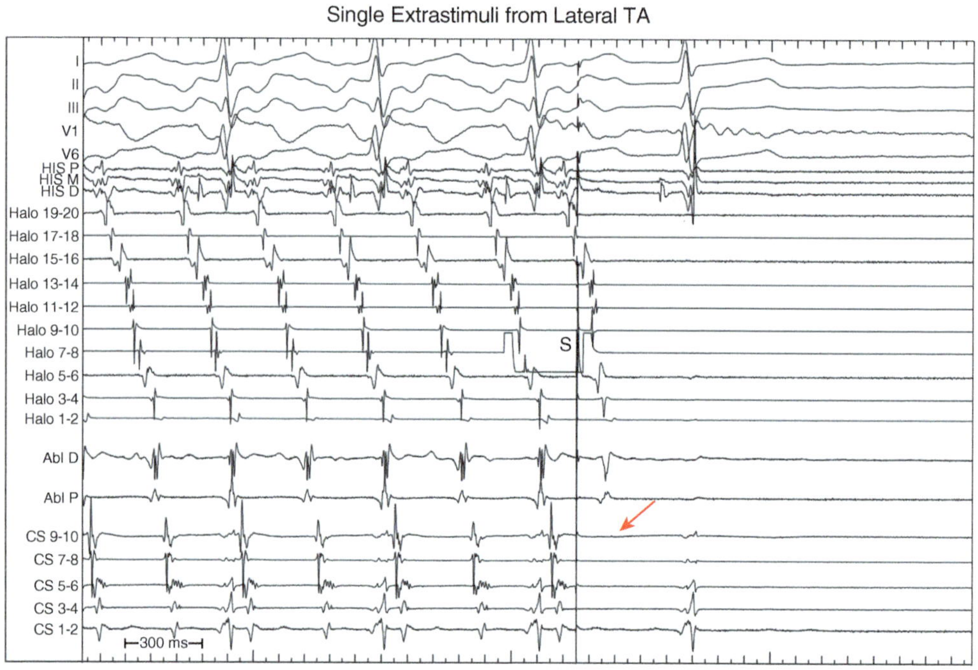

Figure 17-25

To further prove the point, the arrhythmia was reinitiated and a single extrastimulus was given during flutter from another site on the tricuspid annulus (Fig. 17-25); this too propagates distally along the tricuspid annulus toward the CS but fails to reach the CS *(arrow)* because of local refractoriness of that portion of the cavotricuspid isthmus (CTI). This once again shows that the right atrium, not the left, is responsible for this arrhythmia. This phenomenon was reproduced several times after easy reinitiation of flutter. Because of the same phenomenon, overdrive pacing from the CTI (not shown) repeatedly resulted in tachycardia termination rather than entrainment.

Ablation from Cavotricuspid Isthmus

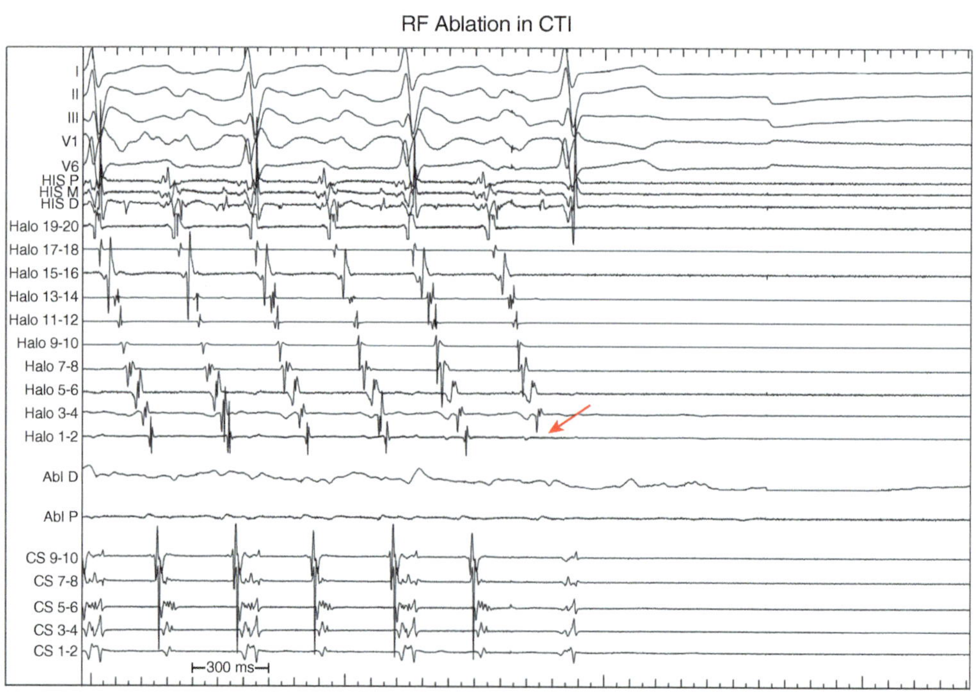

Figure 17-26

Based on the prior findings, ablation in the CTI was begun. This readily terminated flutter, as predicted (Fig. 17-26). Block occurs between electrodes near the tip of the tricuspid annulus catheter (*arrow*, at the medial aspect of the CTI), and proximal CS recordings (at the ostium). This is where spontaneous termination had occurred previously.

Completion of Cavotricuspid Isthmus Ablation

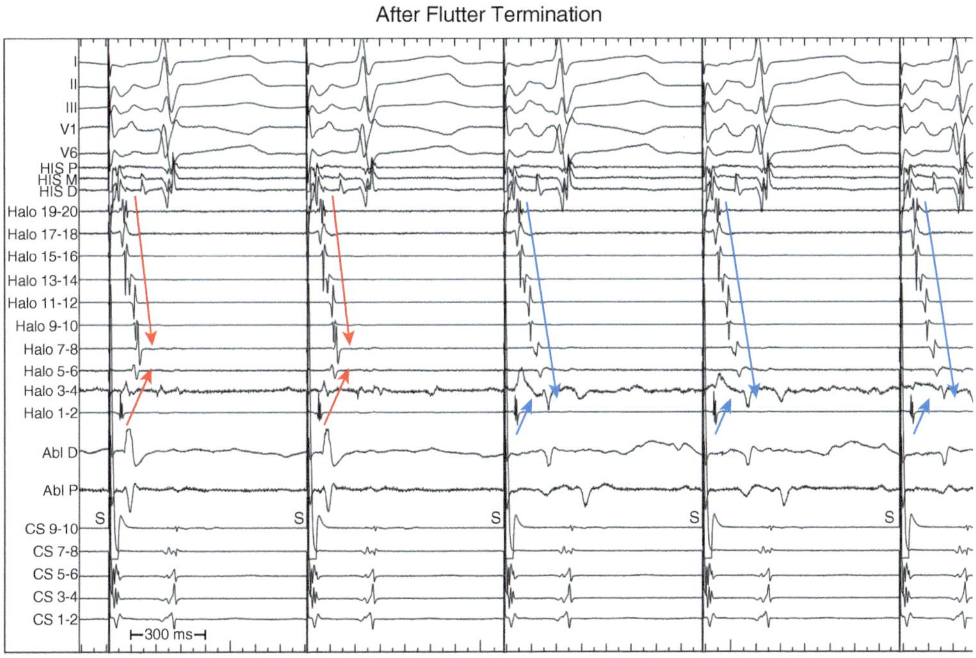

Figure 17-27

As is so often the case, termination of flutter is not equivalent to having bidirectional CTI block. In Fig. 17-27, immediately after termination of flutter, CS pacing shows persistence of conduction in the CTI *(red arrows)*. Additional RF energy is delivered, resulting in medial-lateral block, as shown here *(blue arrows)*. Pacing from the lateral TA (not shown) showed block in the lateral-medial direction as well.

Burst Pacing Initiates Atrial Fibrillation

Burst Pacing During Isoproterenol Infusion

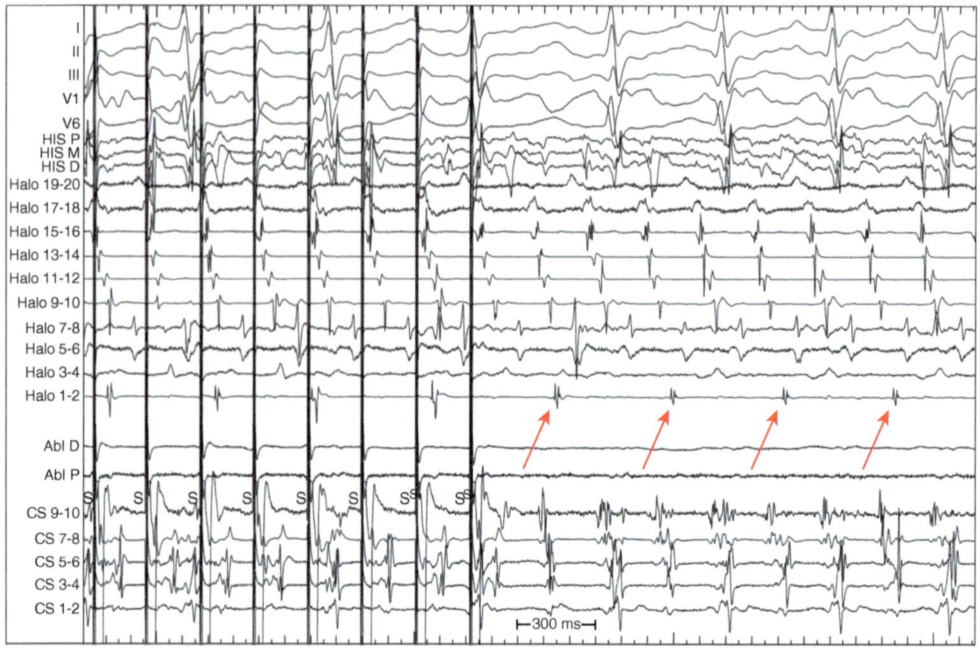

Figure 17-28

Atrial Fibrillation

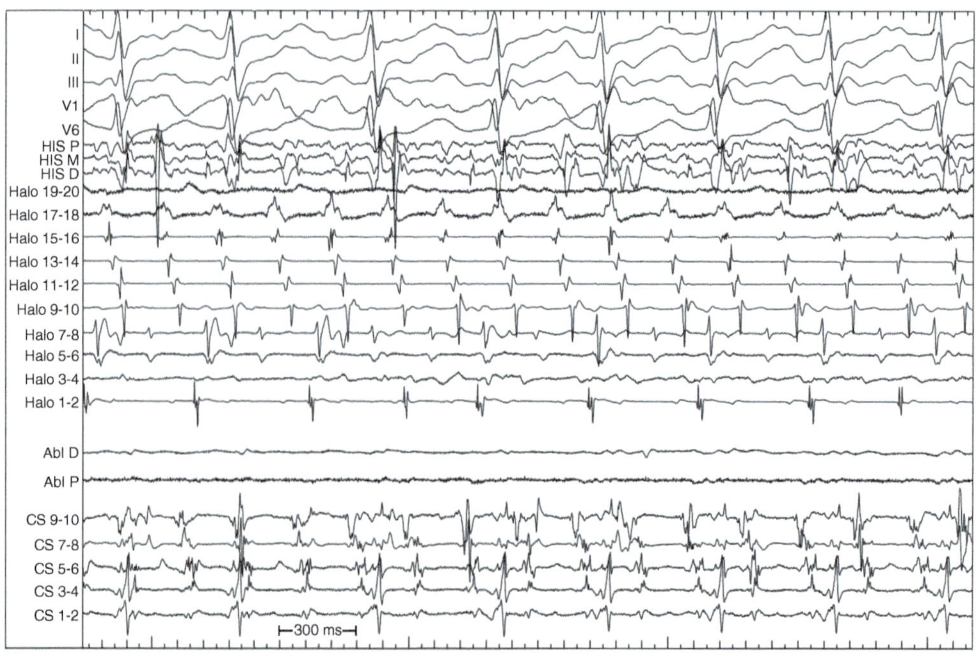

Figure 17-29

Because the patient had a history of only atrial fibrillation by ECG, despite the elimination of atrial flutter, the operators deemed it important to investigate for fibrillation. No arrhythmia was initiated with stimulation in the baseline state, but after isoproterenol infusion at 5 mcg/min, burst pacing initiated the arrhythmia shown in Fig. 17-28. Of note, electrodes at the medial tricuspid annulus (Halo 1-2) are not activated with every atrial cycle *(red arrows)*. At first glance it appears organized, but quickly degenerated to fibrillation (shown in Fig. 17-29), as shown especially in the CS and His recordings.

Standard Intracardiac Recordings and Basket Catheter Recordings in AF

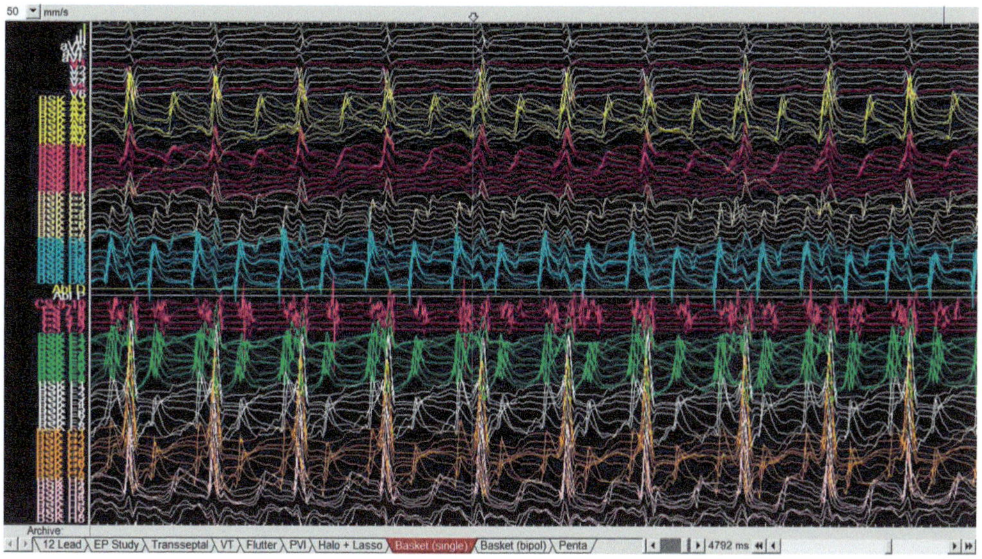

Figure 17-30

Based on the greater degree of disorganization in the CS recordings than those on the tricuspid annulus (right atrium), a 64-pole basket catheter was deployed in the left atrium and recordings were made during fibrillation (Fig. 17-30). Note that, while the CS recordings (*maroon*, at center) are still quite disorganized, the unipolar recordings from the basket catheter appear to be much more uniform from cycle to cycle. One minute of these recordings was acquired and analyzed by a proprietary mapping system looking for rotors or focal sources of atrial fibrillation.

Fluoroscopy of Catheters Including Basket in Left Atrium

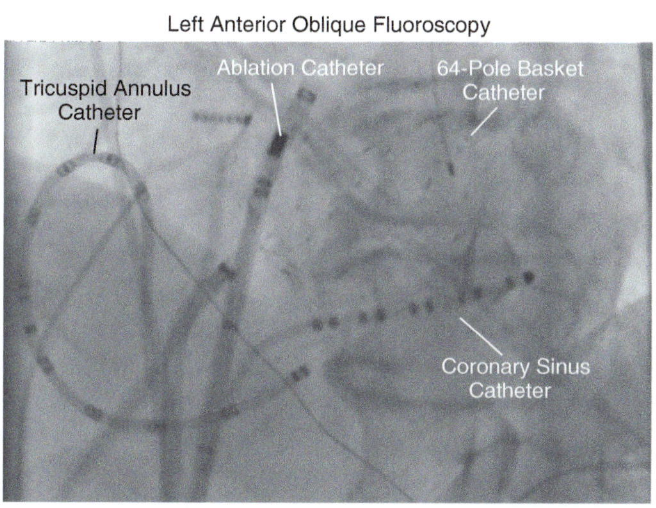

Figure 17-31

Fig. 17-31 shows a fluoroscopic view of catheter locations, including the 64-pole basket catheter in the left atrium; the ablation catheter is still inside a sheath, the tip of which is also in the left atrium. Note the location of the tip of the tricuspid annular catheter in relation to the coronary sinus proximal electrodes (positions the same as during flutter ablation).

Rotor Movie/Still

Figure 17-32

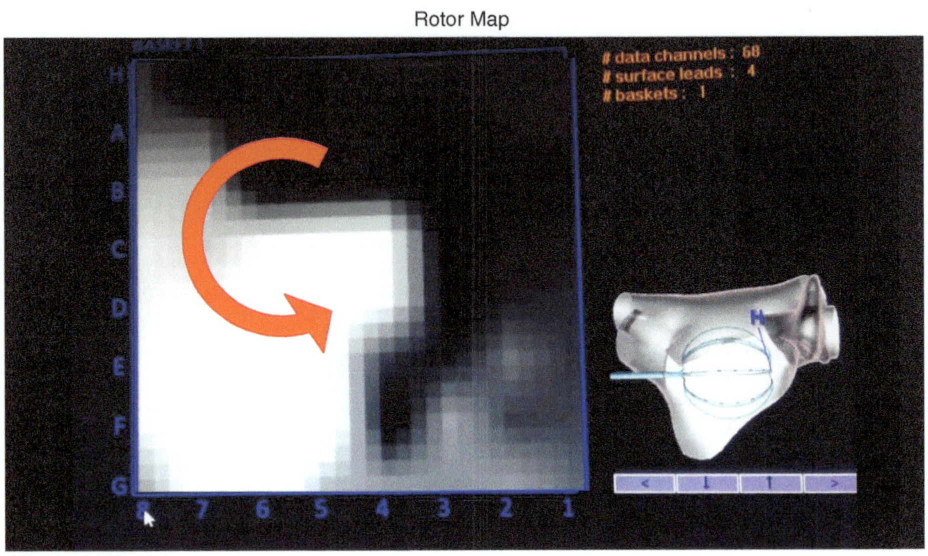

In this 4-second movie (Video 17-1 and Fig. 17-32), a counterclockwise left atrial rotor is seen with a center of rotation at about B-6 on the axial coordinates. This area, corresponding to the inferomedial free wall/floor of the left atrium, was targeted for ablation.

Ablation at Rotor "Core" Terminates AF

Figure 17-33

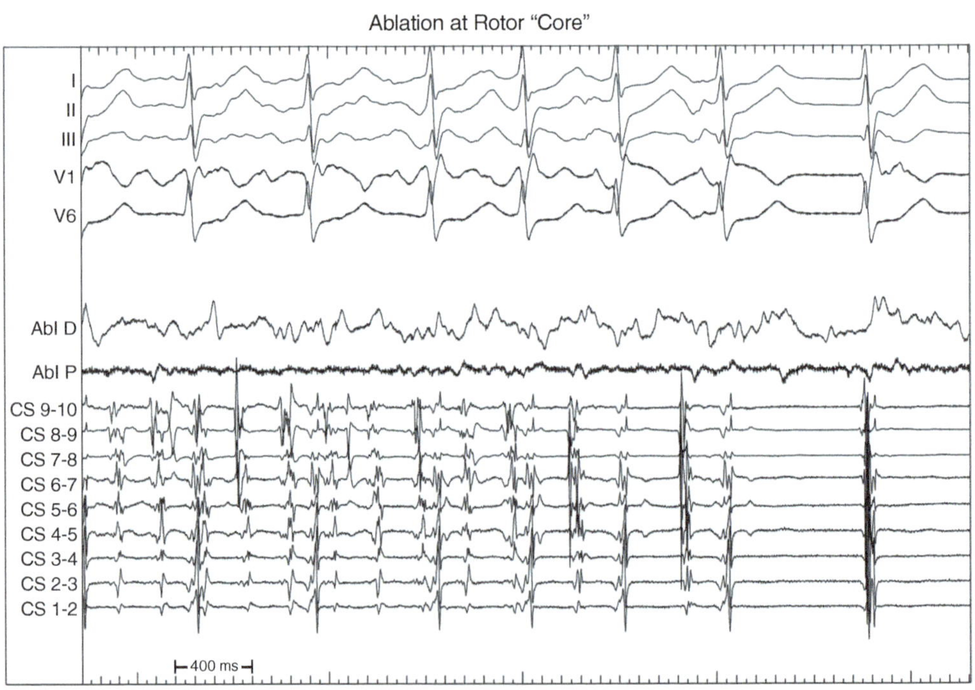

RF ablation near the center of rotation of the previously shown rotor (located on the inferomedial left atrial free wall) resulted in termination of the arrhythmia to junctional rhythm (Fig. 17-33). Fibrillation was reinitiated (with some difficulty) during continued isoproterenol infusion; a second left atrial rotor (located on the inferior portion of the septal aspect of the left atrium) was identified, and during RF ablation at the center of rotation of this rotor, fibrillation terminated to sinus rhythm (not shown). Thereafter, despite higher dose isoproterenol infusion, no arrhythmias could be initiated; the pacing protocol consisted of single- and double-atrial extrastimuli as well as burst pacing for >30 repeated attempts at cycle length 190 ms (shortest cycle length with 1:1 capture at high output).

Adenosine Administration

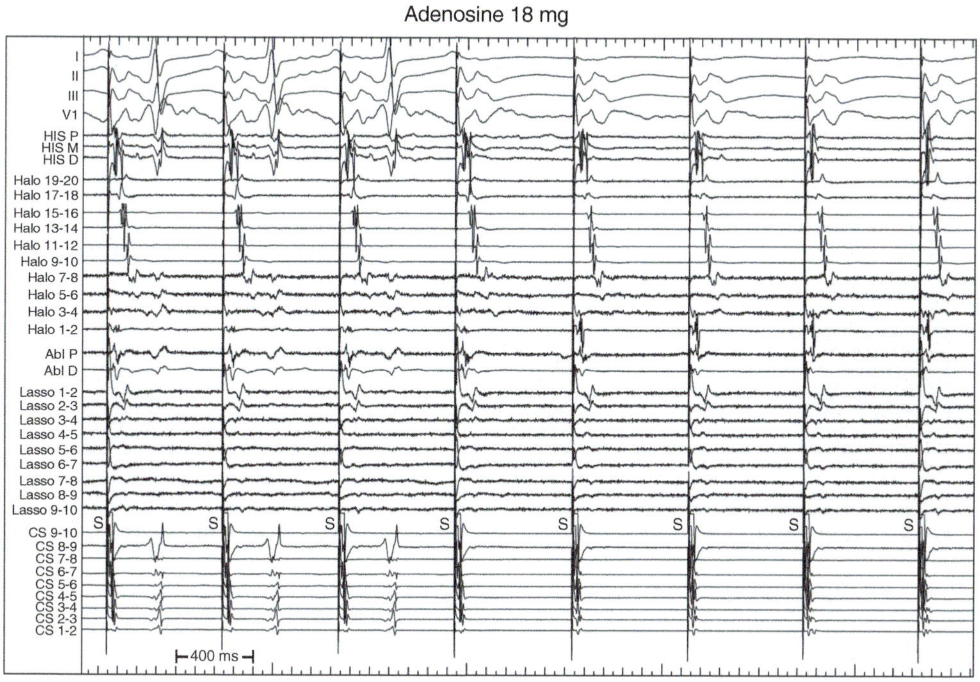

Figure 17-34

After completion of stimulation and checking for bidirectional block in the CTI as well as four PVs in the resting state before and after discontinuation of isoproterenol, adenosine (18 mg) was administered by intravenous bolus while recording from tricuspid annulus as well as right superior PV ("Lasso") and left superior PV (Abl) (Fig. 17-34). Adenosine-mediated hyperpolarization of atrial cells can transiently restore dormant conduction and show that additional ablation is needed. Here, at the time of atrioventricular block *(center)*, pacing from the proximal CS shows persistence of medial-lateral CTI block; there are no PV potentials recorded from either left or right superior PVs.

Adenosine 18 mg

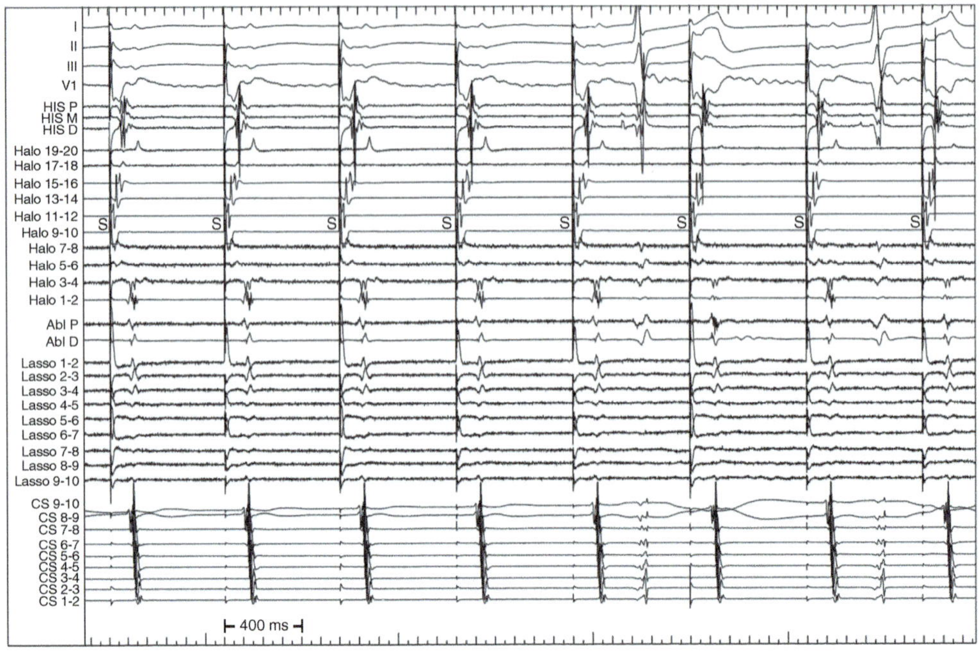

Figure 17-35

Seconds later, the site of simulation is changed to the lateral aspect of the CTI, showing persistence of block in the lateral-medial direction (Fig. 17-35). Again, no PV potentials are recorded from either left or right superior PVs. Not shown is attempted stimulation from the left superior PV, at a site in which capture had been demonstrated previously, without conduction to left atrium. The patient has had no recurrent atrial arrhythmias in long-term follow-up.

Electroanatomic Mapping Showing Ablation Regions

Electroanatomic Mapping

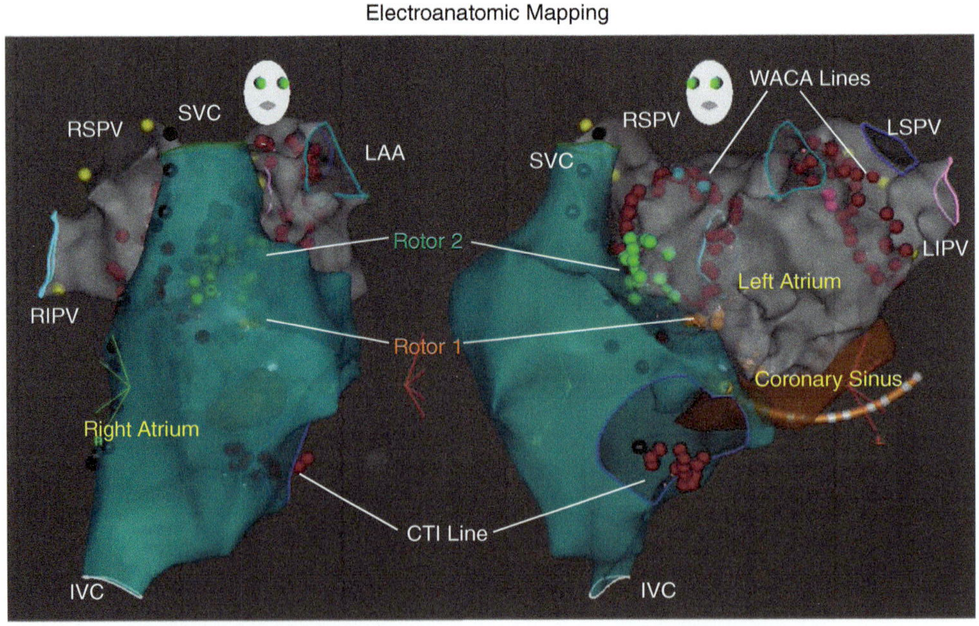

Right Anterior Oblique Left Anterior Oblique

Figure 17-36

In this electroanatomic mapping diagram in Fig. 17-36, the right atrium is *green*, left atrium *gray*, and coronary sinus *brown*. Wide-area circumferential ablation (WACA) lines encircling the PVs are shown as well as sites of rotor mapping (#1 *[orange dots]*, inferomedial left atrial free wall; #2 *[green dots]*, inferior portion of the septal aspect of the left atrium). It is clear that both of these rotor locations are well outside the standard WACA lines and were "missed" by PV isolation. *CTI,* cavotricuspid isthmus; *IVC,* inferior vena cava; *LAA,* left atrial appendage orifice; *LIPV,* left inferior PV; *LSPV,* left superior PV; *RIPV,* right inferior PV; *RSPV,* right superior PV; *SVC,* superior vena cava.

Electroanatomic Mapping

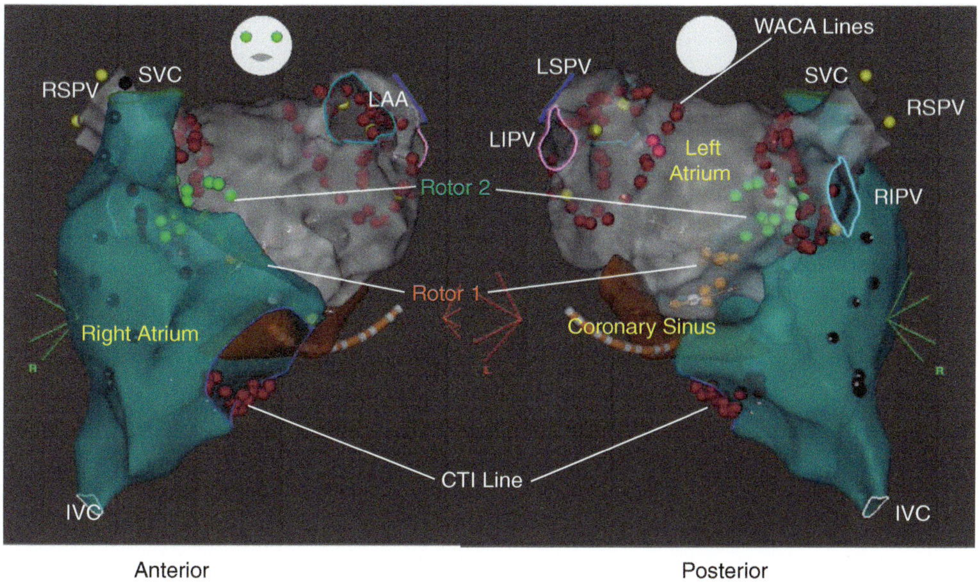

Figure 17-37

The same maps as in the prior figure are displayed in Fig. 17-37 in different orientations. *CTI,* cavotricuspid isthmus; *IVC,* inferior vena cava; *LAA,* left atrial appendage orifice; *LIPV,* left inferior PV; *LSPV,* left superior PV; *RIPV,* right inferior PV; *RSPV,* right superior PV; *SVC,* superior vena cava.

Summary

- Atrial fibrillation can be transformed to atrial flutter by sodium-channel–blocking agents such as amiodarone (which also slows the flutter cycle length)
- Spontaneous termination of atrial flutter is rare but can occur at the narrowest part of the circuit (CTI)
- Careful use of overdrive pacing during tachycardia—analyzing events both at the end and at the beginning of pacing—can be very useful diagnostically
- In patients with predominant atrial fibrillation clinically who are in flutter at the time of the procedure, fibrillation should usually still be treated
- Rotors that maintain fibrillation may reside near typical ablation lines for PV isolation, or outside these zones

Idiopathic Focal Right Ventricular Outflow Tract Ectopy 18

Case Presentation

The patient was a 39-year-old woman referred for management of palpitations for the last 2 years. Episodes began after birth of the eighth child and often worsened when she was upset. Ambulatory recorder showed premature ventricular complexes (PVCs) comprising about 25% of all complexes. Baseline ECG showed sinus rhythm with PVCs having a left bundle branch block (LBBB) and right-inferior axis with a precordial R-wave transition at V3 and smooth R-wave contours in inferior leads. Metoprolol was ineffective at controlling her symptoms (palpitations and fatigue), which were increasingly bothersome. Physical examination finding was normal aside from skipped beats. Echocardiogram showed mild global hypokinesis (ejection fraction 45%). She underwent an EP study elsewhere; the right ventricular outflow tract (RVOT) was thoroughly mapped, and multiple sites were ablated without altering the PVC frequency. She was referred for a repeat EP study and ablation.

Baseline ECGs and Intracardiac Recordings

Where Is the Likely Origin? [Fig. 18-1]

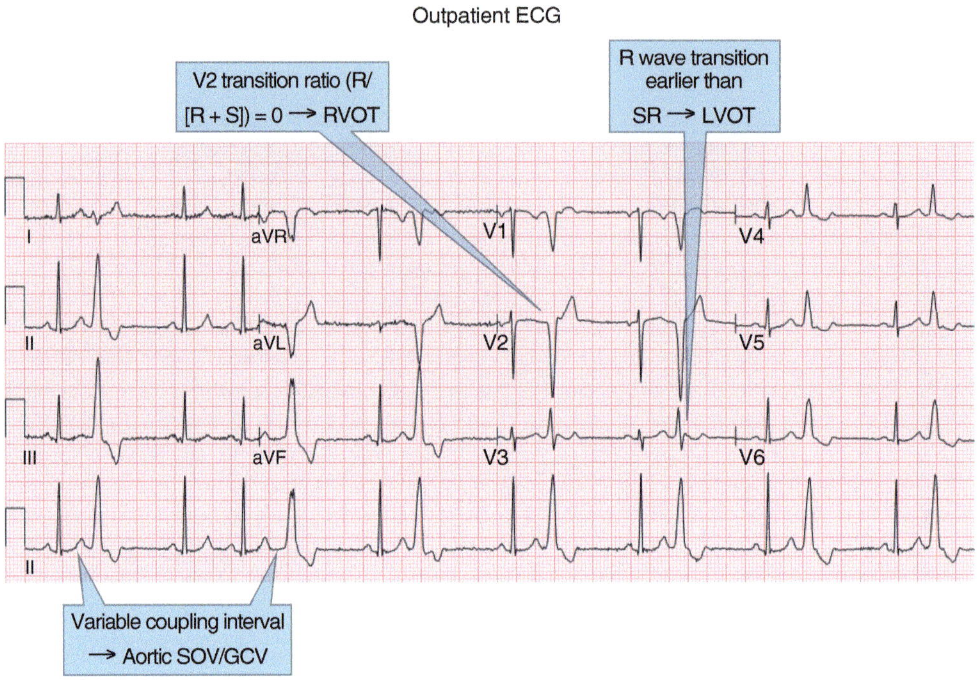

Figure 18-1

A 12-lead ECG of the patient's sinus rhythm with ventricular ectopy is shown in Fig. 18-1. As indicated, several morphologic criteria of the PVCs yield disparate indicators of its origin. For instance, in lead V2, the ratio $R/(R + S)$ of 0 suggests RVOT origin, whereas R-wave transition occurring earlier in the PVC than in sinus rhythm (V3 vs V4) suggests left ventricular outflow origin; finally, the variable coupling interval from the prior sinus complex to the PVC in the rhythm strip suggests aortic sinus of Valsalva (SOV) or great cardiac vein (GCV) origin.

Is This the Same as What We Saw Earlier? [Fig. 18-2]

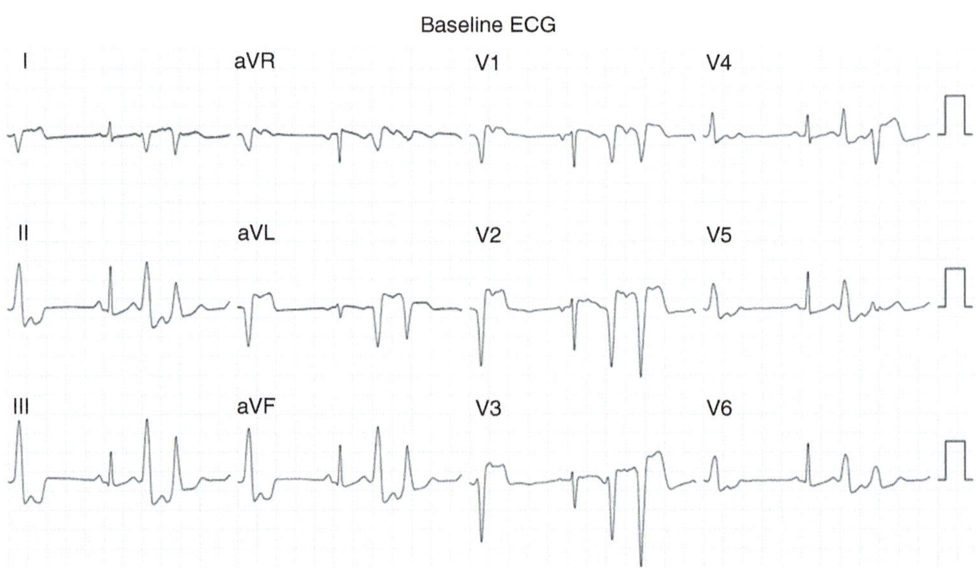

Figure 18-2

With the patient in the electrophysiology laboratory, PVC coupling intervals appear to be more constant (Fig. 18-2); the V2 ratio still suggests RVOT origin but the precordial transition occurs in V4, the same as in sinus. In many cases, precordial leads positioning in the electrophysiology laboratory is slightly different from that in the clinic because of defibrillation patches and electrode patches for the electroanatomic mapping system, if used.

In general, the ECG leads are the last of these to be applied to the chest, and are placed as close to standard locations as possible, but working around patches that are already in place for other purposes. Thus ECGs taken at this setting may not be identical to those obtained in other settings.

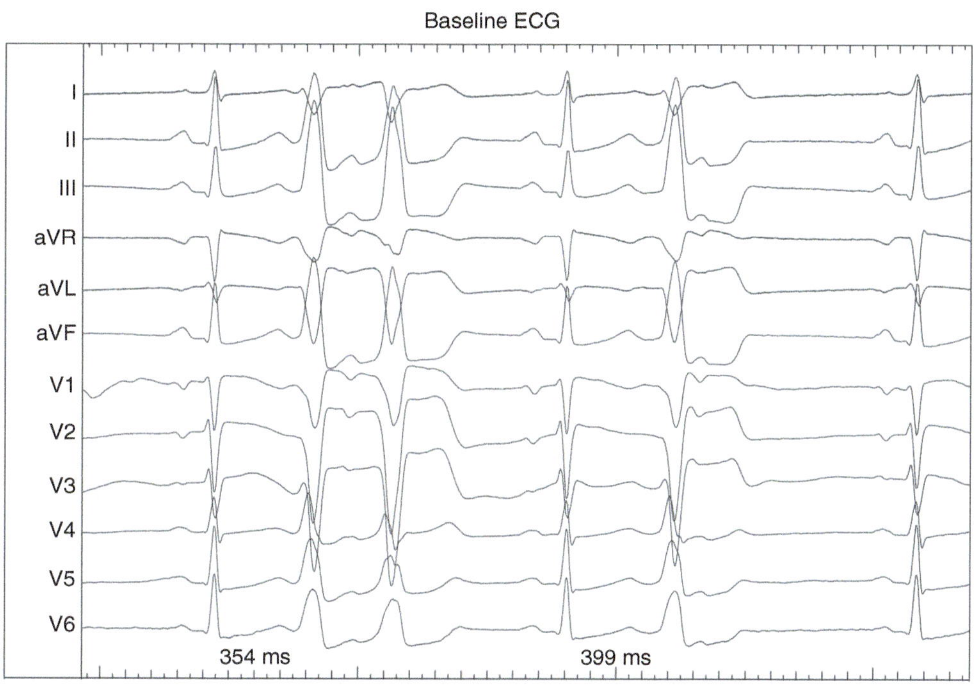

Figure 18-3

A few minutes later in the procedure, PVC coupling intervals in Fig. 18-3 are less constant. It is important to acquire several examples of spontaneously occurring PVCs, as well as noting their coupling intervals, before placement of any endocardial catheters that could cause catheter-induced ectopy and introduce confusion as to morphology and timing of PVCs. Does this indicate anything about target site location?

Figure 18-4

Baseline Intracardiac Recordings

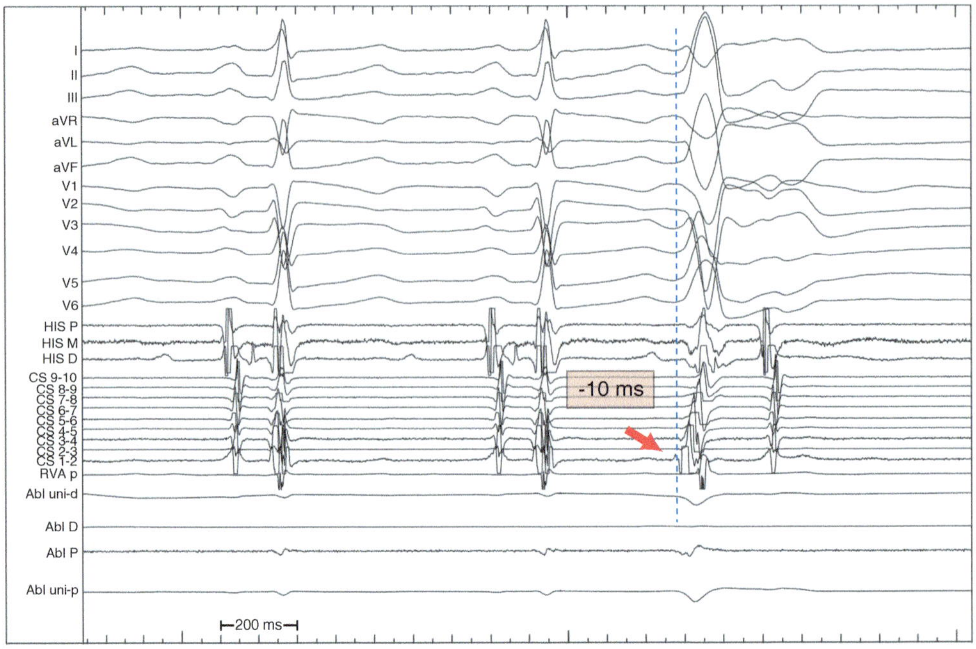

In Fig. 18-4, the coronary sinus (CS) catheter tip has been positioned at the top of the mitral annulus (as distally as possible); the onset of the QRS complex is denoted by a *dashed line.* A far-field component of the distal CS ventricular recording precedes the QRS onset by 10 ms. This suggests that the actual focus is nearby, but probably not exactly at this location (timing at the actual source should be 20 to 40 ms before PVC's QRS onset).

Mapping Different Sites

Does This Mean Anything? [Fig. 18-5]

Figure 18-5

Mapping RVOT

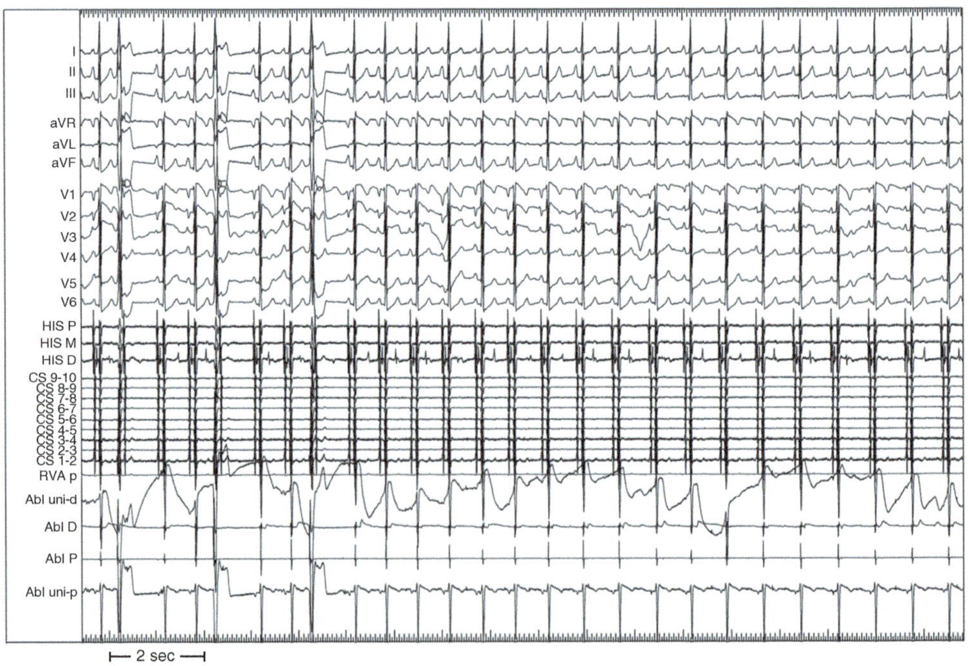

Manipulation of the mapping catheter in the right ventricular outflow tract, where mapping was started, resulted in sudden cessation of ventricular ectopy whereas it previously had occurred every 4 or 5 complexes (seen at left in Fig. 18-5). This probably means that the catheter has "bumped" into the tissue at the source, rendering it transiently depolarized and unable to discharge again until recovery has occurred. If this is a correct interpretation, it is reasonable evidence that the origin is nearby—endocardial RVOT, and not in the great cardiac vein, left ventricle, epicardial surface, or sinus of Valsalva.

Is This a Good Ablation Site?

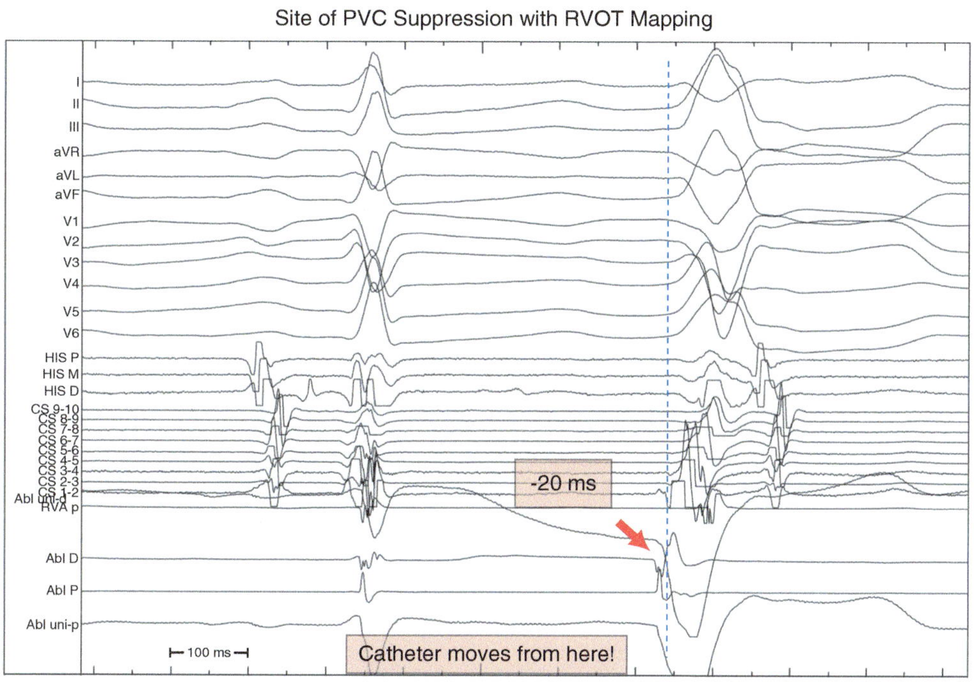

Figure 18-6

Recordings displayed in Fig. 18-6 were made just before inadvertant catheter dislodgement from the site, after which ectopy transiently ceased. Catheter-mediated trauma that eliminates pathway conduction or focal firing suggests proximity to an important site for the arrhythmia. Often, however, trauma has occurred during somewhat vigorous catheter movement (not just gentle "bumping"), so the effect may not be very localizing, and (more important) the catheter tip has often moved on from where the contact actually affected the rhythm—such that the location where it is first observed after the event may not be where the effect occurred. However, the electrogram at this site just before catheter movement had a timing 20 ms before QRS onset and suggests it was, in fact, close to the origin.

Is This a Good Site?

Figure 18-7

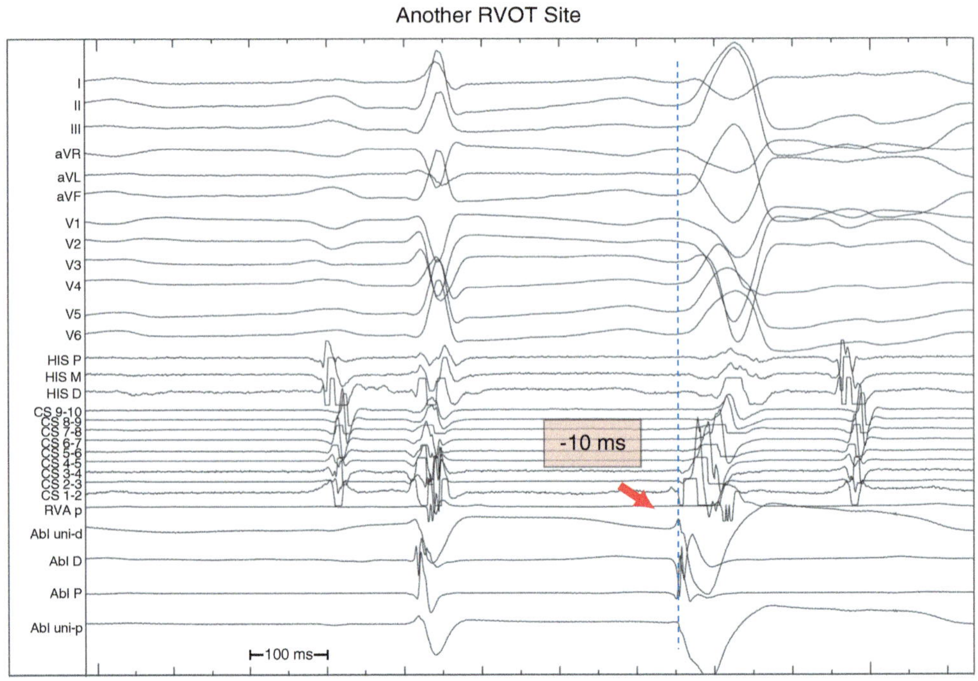

Mapping was continued after resumption of PVCs (Fig. 18-7). This is not such a good site; the distal unipolar recording has an R wave, and the proximal bipolar recording is almost as early as the distal, neither of which are as good as the prior site.

Algorithm Says 94% Match. Ablate Here?

Figure 18-8

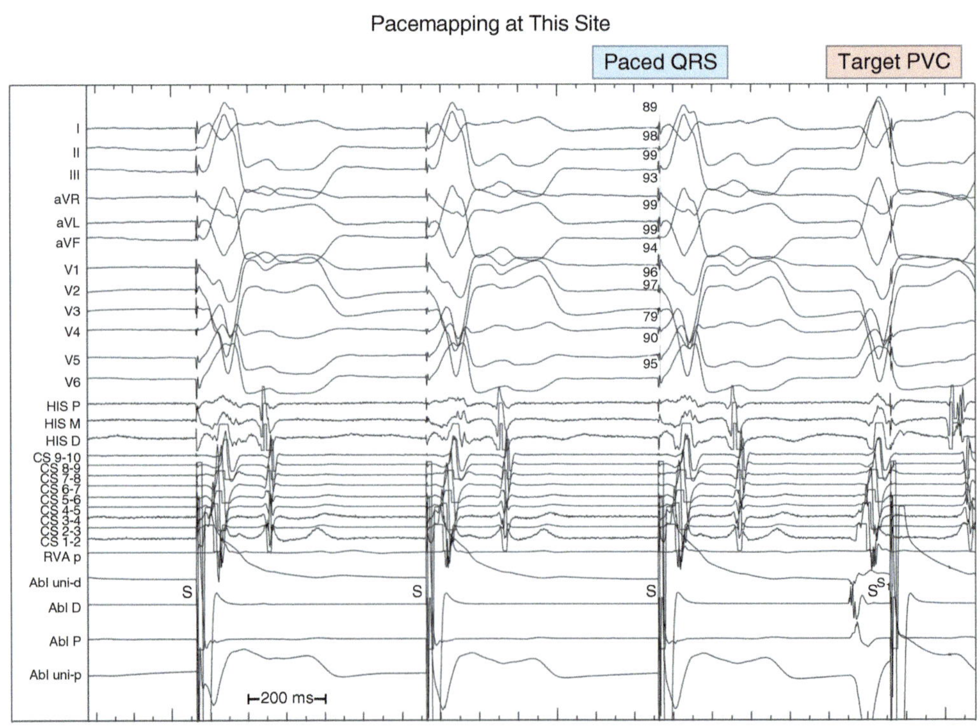

Pacing at this site (Fig. 18-8) yields a reasonable, but far from perfect, match. Ablation was not attempted here. Numbers to the left of each QRS complex on the 3rd paced cycle indicate percentage of morphology match (aggregate, 94%), using an algorithm in the recording system.

Algorithm Says 92% Match. Ablate Here?

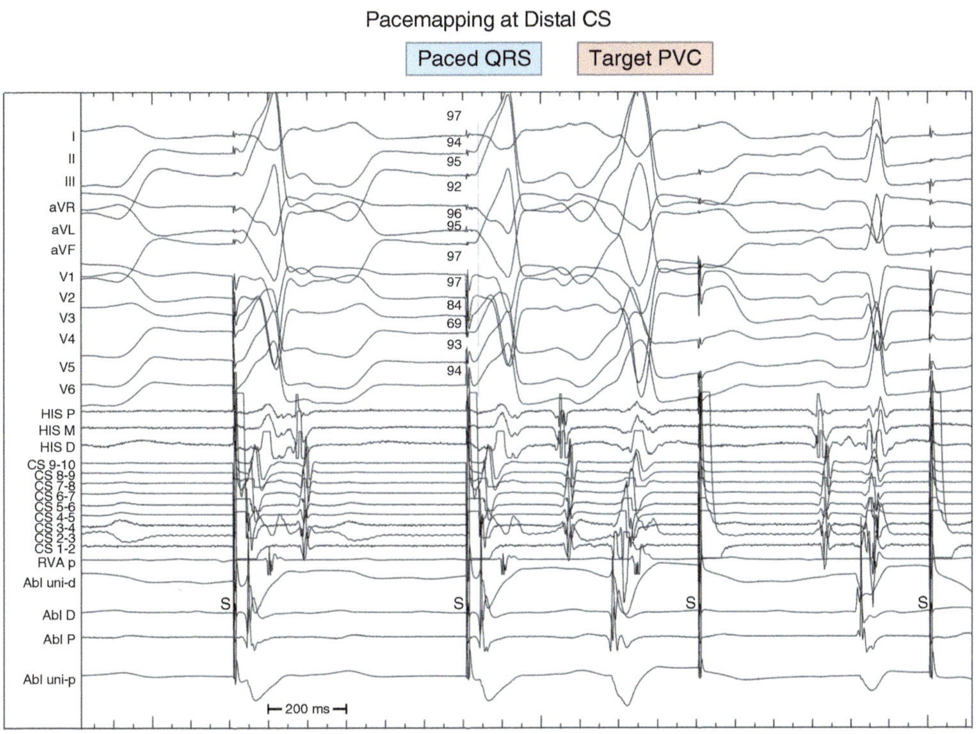

Figure 18-9

Pacing from the distal CS electrode pair yields a reasonable, but inexact, match with the PVC (Fig. 18-9). Ablation was not attempted here.

Is This a Good Site?

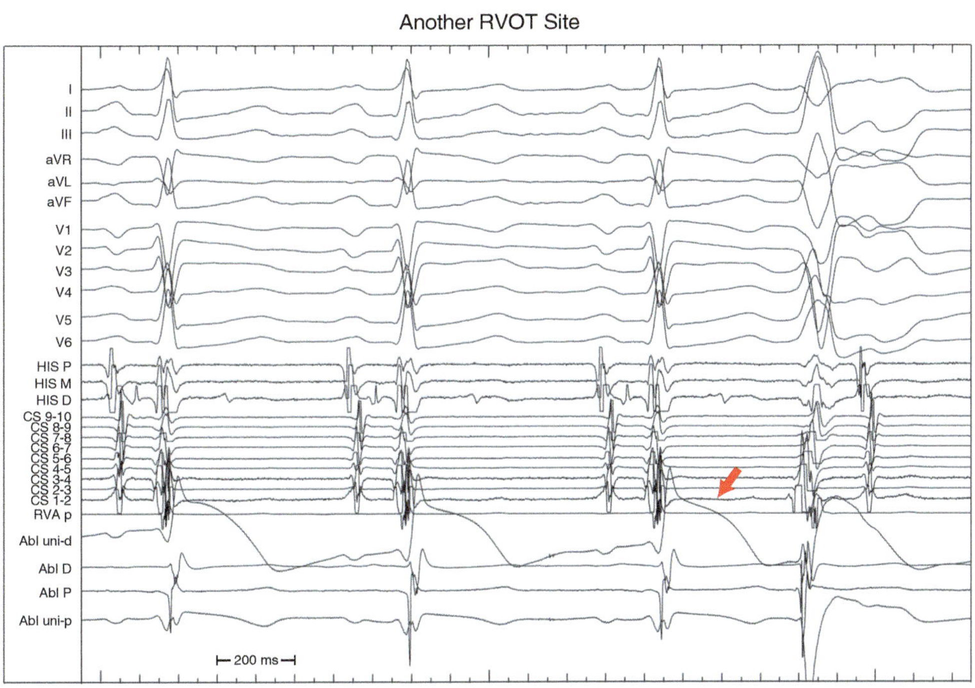

Figure 18-10

Mapping is continued back in the RV outflow tract. ST elevation on the unipolar recording (Fig. 18-10, *red arrow*) indicates too-good contact, threatening perforation. The catheter tip should be withdrawn somewhat from this point.

Is This a Good Site?

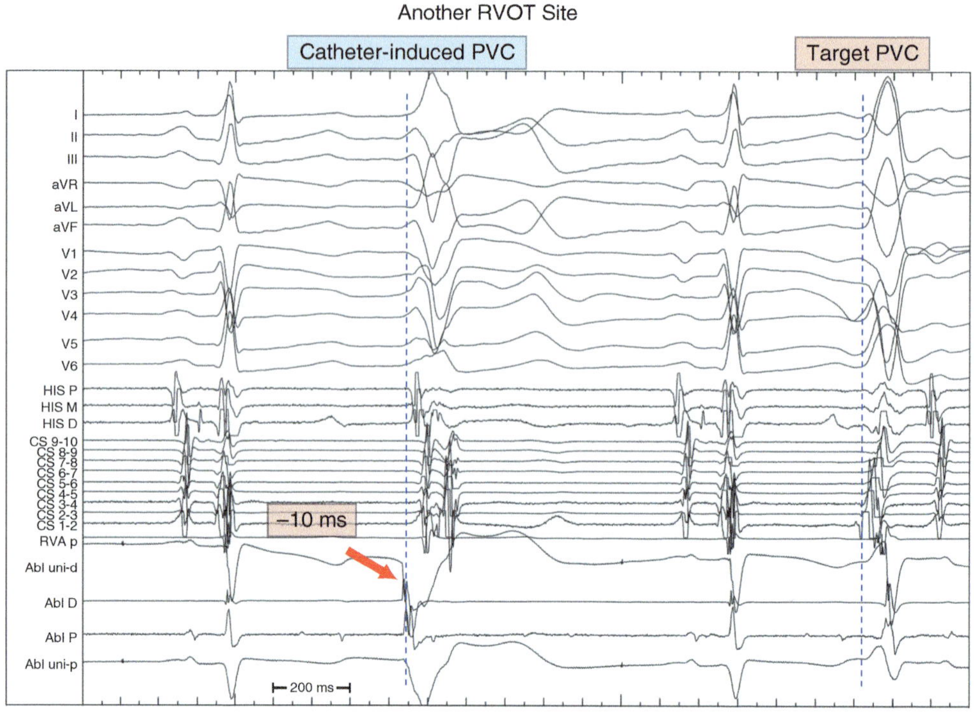

Figure 18-11

Mapping continues; in Fig. 18-11, a reasonably good site is shown; the unipolar recording has no R wave, and it is reasonably early. However, this is a catheter-induced PVC. The beginning of the QRS is difficult to see because of partial obscuration by the P wave. This site is not early during the real PVC (at right).

Is This a Good Site?

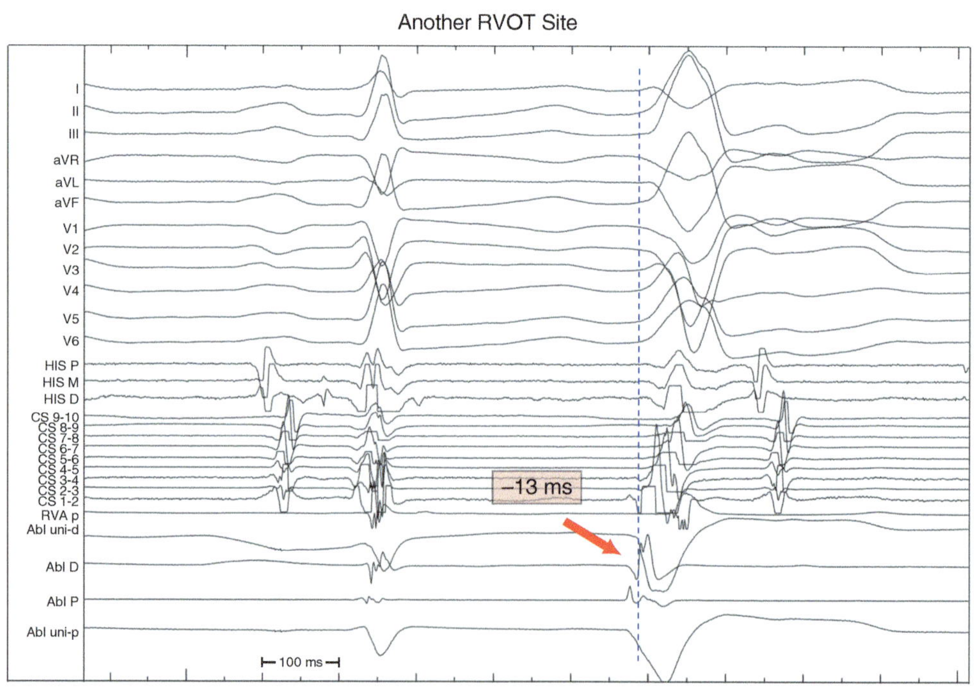

Figure 18-12

Additional mapping in the RV outflow tract shows another reasonably good site in Fig. 18-12; the unipolar has no R wave, and it is reasonably early. However, the proximal bipolar is almost as early as the distal, and distal unipolar and bipolar do not "agree." This was very near the "bump" site and directly across from the CS tip electrode.

Pacemapping to Corroborate Activation Mapping Data

Algorithm Says 94% Match. Ablate Here?

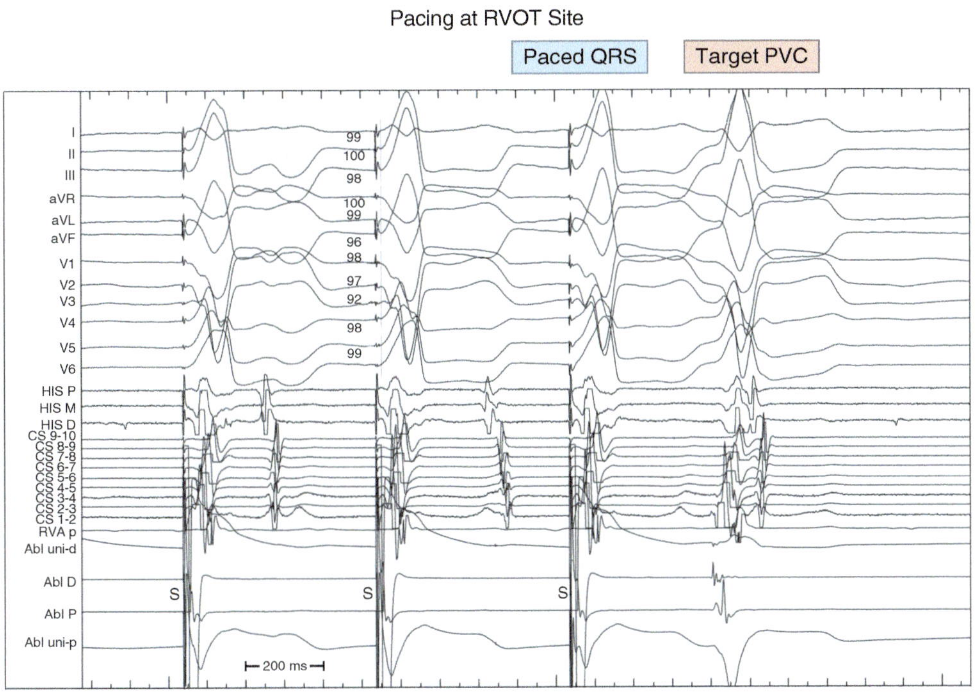

Figure 18-13

In Fig. 18-13, pacing at the site shown in Fig. 18-12 yields the best match yet, which visually/qualitatively seemed better than the 94% match calculated by machine reading. Ablation was attempted here.

First Ablation Attempted

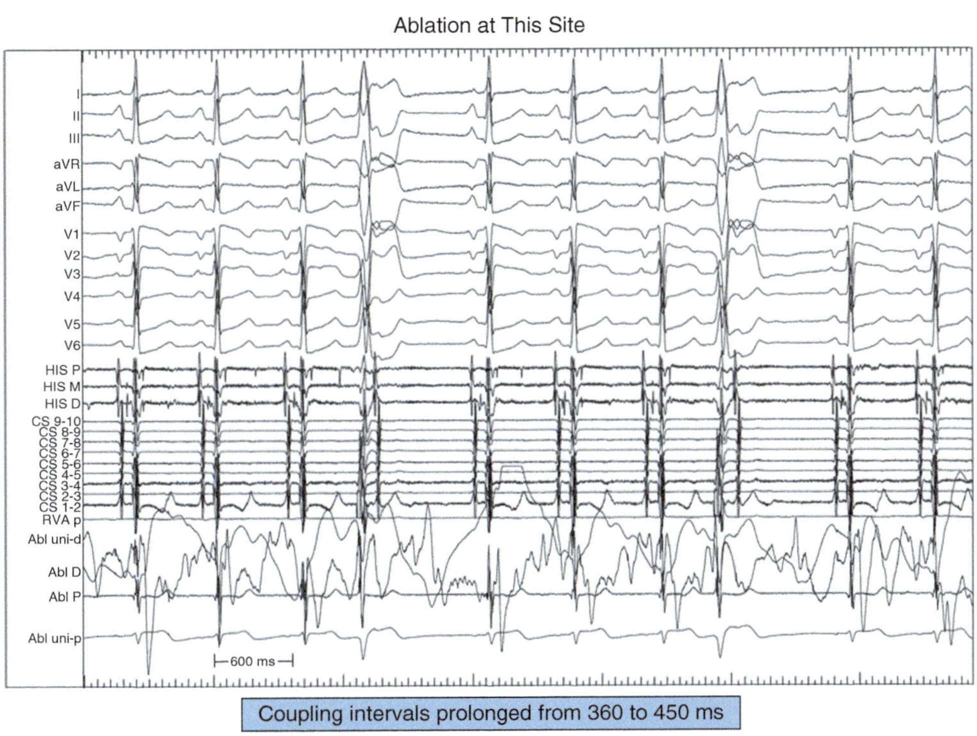

Figure 18-14

As a result of ablation, the coupling intervals of the PVCs from prior complexes increased substantially (Fig. 18-14); nevertheless, PVCs persisted. This probably indicates that the ablation site was near enough to the focus to have an effect on it, but not eliminate it.

Status Update

- RVOT has been thoroughly explored; no better sites were found
- Distal coronary sinus (CS)/great cardiac vein (GCV) has early potential, but we cannot advance the catheter further and cannot get the ablation catheter close to the same site in GCV
- What next?
  - Pericardial access and epicardial mapping?
  - Aortic sinus of Valsalva/left ventricular mapping?
  - Try harder to get the ablation catheter out the CS/GCV?

Mapping Other Sites

Is This a Good Site? [Fig. 18-15]

Figure 18-15

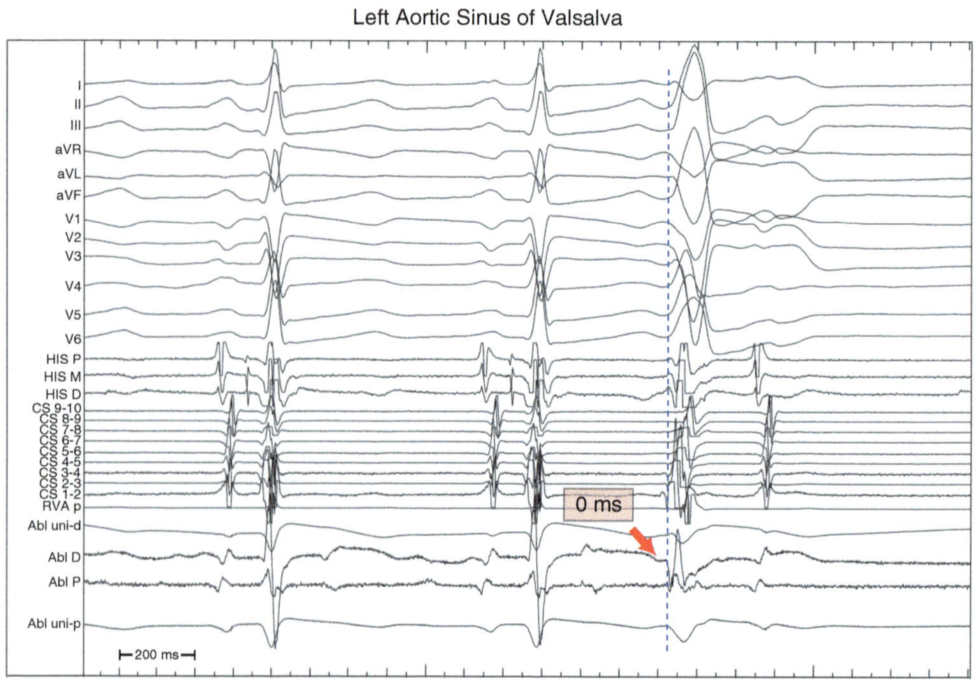

Mapping in the left aortic sinus of Valsalva (SOV) shows a site with poor features (Fig. 18-15); timing is not good at all. Because LV myocardium is some distance away, the unipolar signal is less helpful in the left SOV than when in contact with ventricular myocardium.

Algorithm Says 85% Match. Ablate Here?

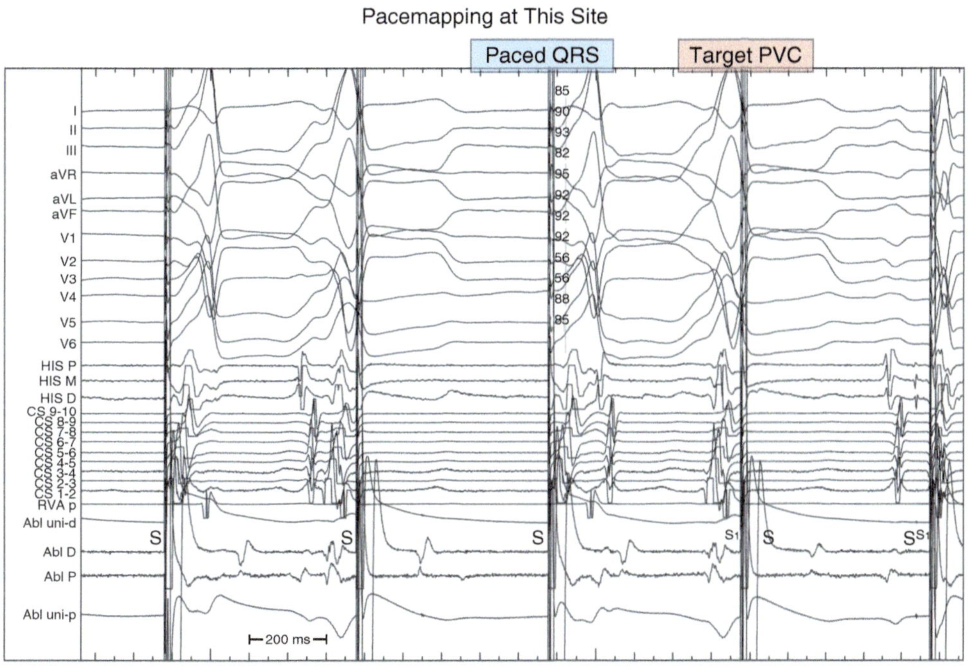

Figure 18-16

Pacing at the site shown in Fig. 18-16 (left aortic SOV) yields the poorest match yet; however, some PVCs can be ablated from this site with poor electrogram and pacemap features. Ablation was attempted here after left coronary arteriography showed >6 mm from this site to the left main ostium. PVCs continued unaffected by a 30-second application of ablation energy.

Is This a Good Site?

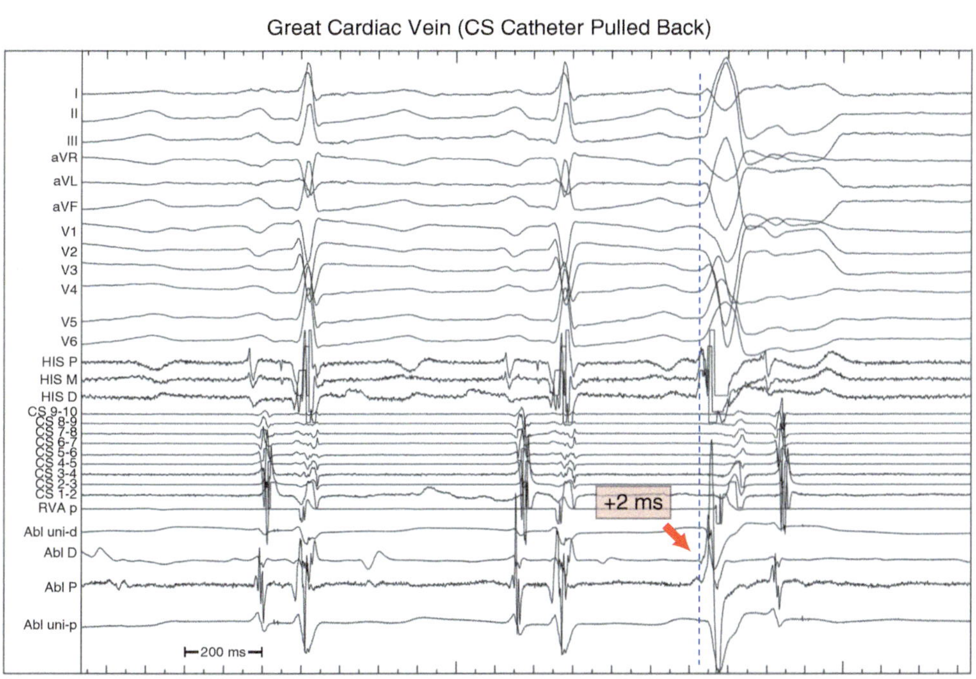

Figure 18-17

Next, the ablation catheter was inserted into the CS and advanced to the great cardiac vein (required partial withdrawal of the CS catheter to fit). Mapping here (Fig. 18-17) showed a poor site; the catheter tip could not be advanced further. The proximal recording has a far-field signal suggesting that something nearby is early (very gained up).

Algorithm Says 79% Match. Ablate Here?

Figure 18-18

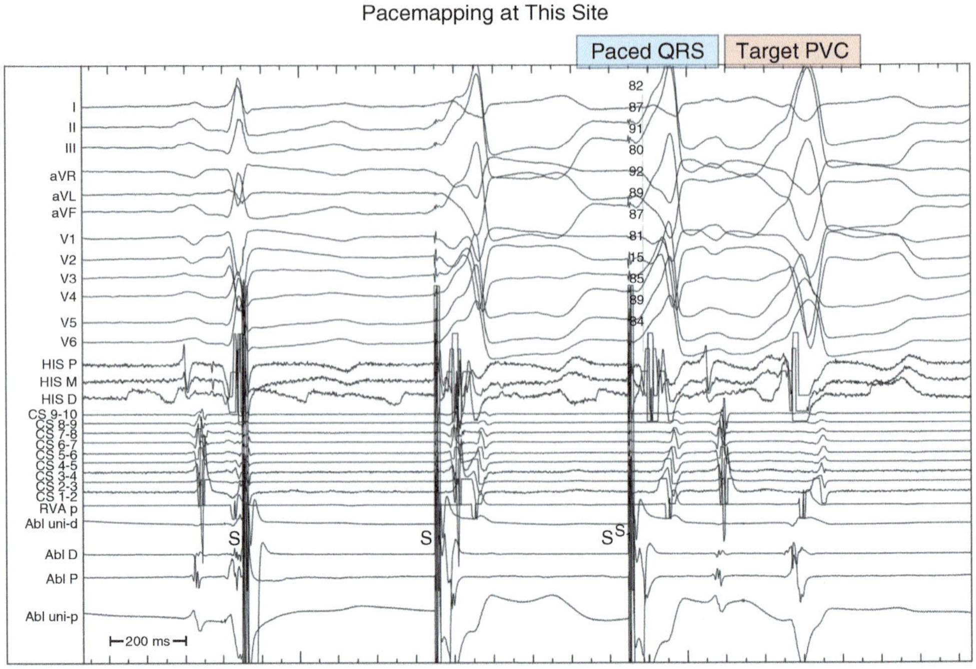

Pacing at this site (Fig. 18-18) in the distal CS yields the poorest match of all (aggregate match 79%); there is no point in attempting ablation in this small vessel with such poor mapping features.

Status Update

- RVOT has been thoroughly explored; no better sites were found
- Aortic sinuses of Valsalva showed poor sites
- Distal CS/GCV was even less promising
- What next?
  - Pericardial access and epicardial mapping?
  - Go back to RVOT where best sites were, and where “bump” mapping was observed?

Repeat Right Ventricular Mapping and Ablation

Is This a Good Site?

RVOT Again

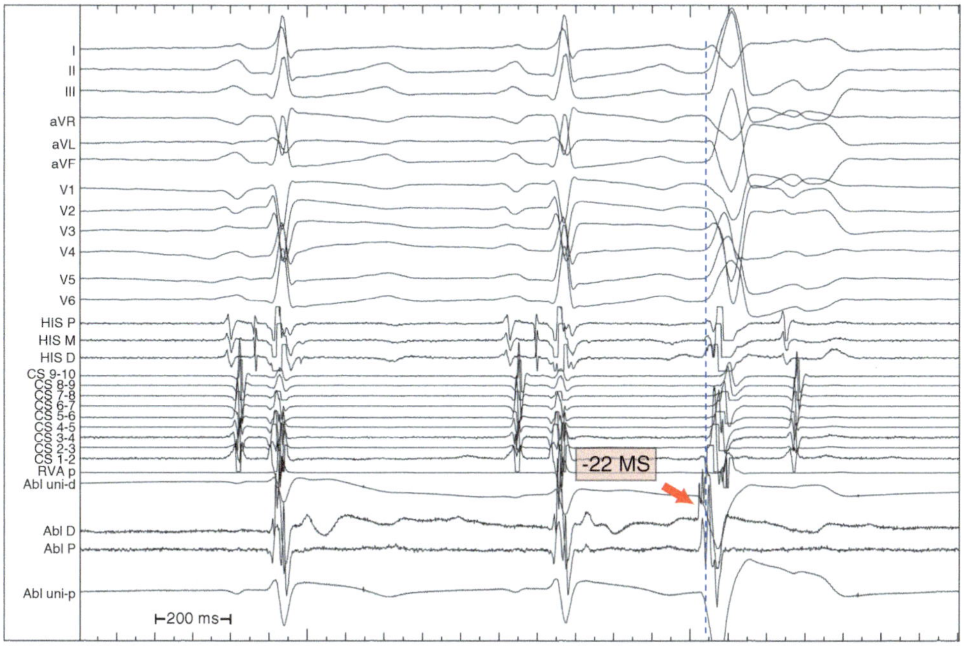

Figure 18-19

Back in the right ventricular outflow tract again, a very good site is encountered in Fig. 18-19; all good target site features are fulfilled.

Algorithm Says 97% Match. Ablate Here?

Pacemapping at This Site

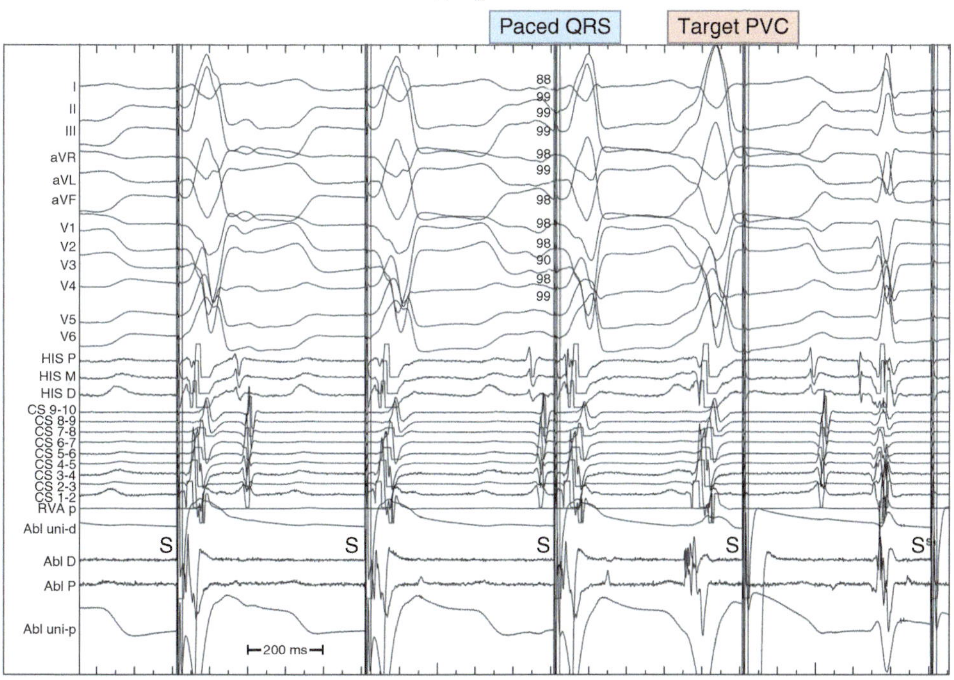

Figure 18-20

Pacing at this site (Fig. 18-20) yields a very good pace-match (aggregate, 97%) with the spontaneously occurring PVC. The pacing output is only 2 mA; the lower the output, the more specific this finding is.

Figure 18-21

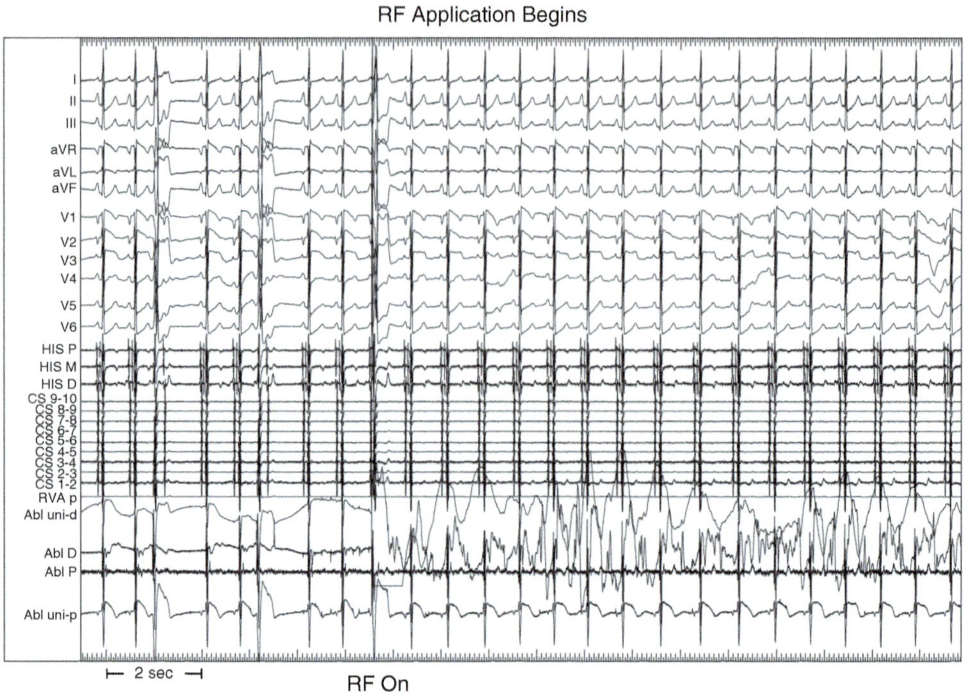

Immediately upon beginning radiofrequency (RF) energy delivery at this site in the RVOT, PVCs ceased and did not recur for the remainder of the procedure (Fig. 18-21).

Figure 18-22

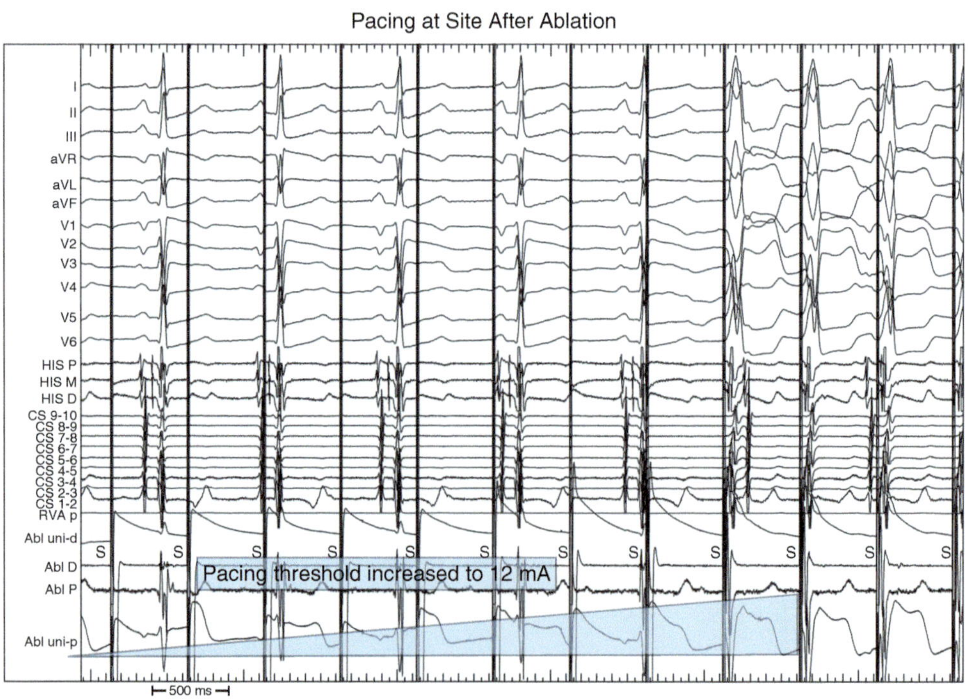

After RF application that eliminated ventricular ectopy, pacing at that site has a markedly elevated capture threshold (Fig. 18-22), indicative of substantial damage to the area. In addition, especially evident on the last two complexes on the right, ST elevation in the unipolar recording is seen, corroborating damage.

Images of Catheters and Maps

Anatomy

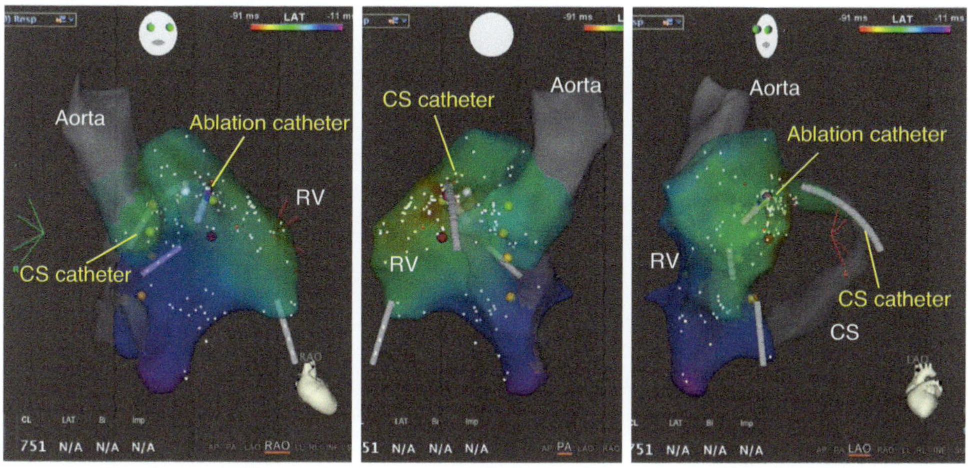

Right Anterior Oblique | Posterior | Left Anterior Oblique

Figure 18-23

Fig. 18-23 displays electroanatomic mapping views of activation timing obtained during PVCs. Different chambers mapped are shown with labels (aorta [root], RV = right ventricle, CS = coronary sinus). In the left anterior oblique view, it is easy to see how the distal CS recordings could have early activation and yet the arrhythmia originates in the leftward aspect of the right ventricular outflow tract, with the two catheters (CS and ablation) nearly touching.

Fluoroscopic Anatomy

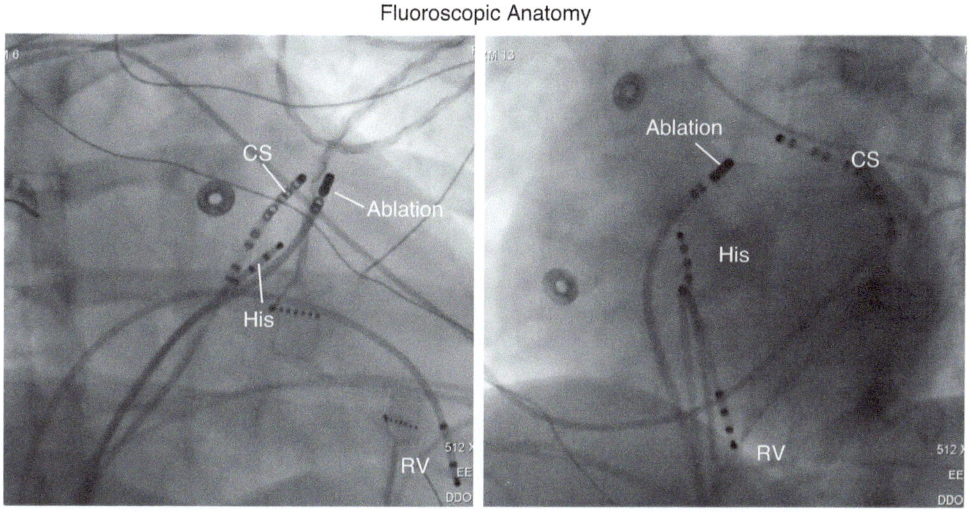

Right Anterior Oblique | Left Anterior Oblique

Figure 18-24

Right and left anterior oblique fluoroscopic views of catheter positions, noting especially successful ablation site in the right ventricular outflow tract, are shown in Fig. 18-24.

Final ECG

Figure 18-25

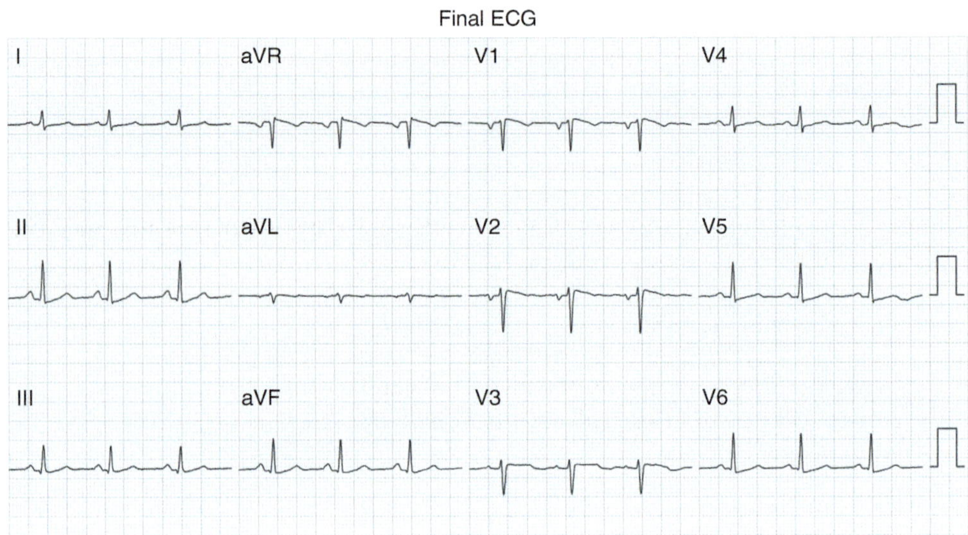

The final sinus rhythm ECG (Fig. 18-25) shows no ventricular ectopy. The patient was discharged the next morning, having had no palpitations or ectopy overnight, or on follow-up as an outpatient.

Mapping Sites Compared

Figure 18-26

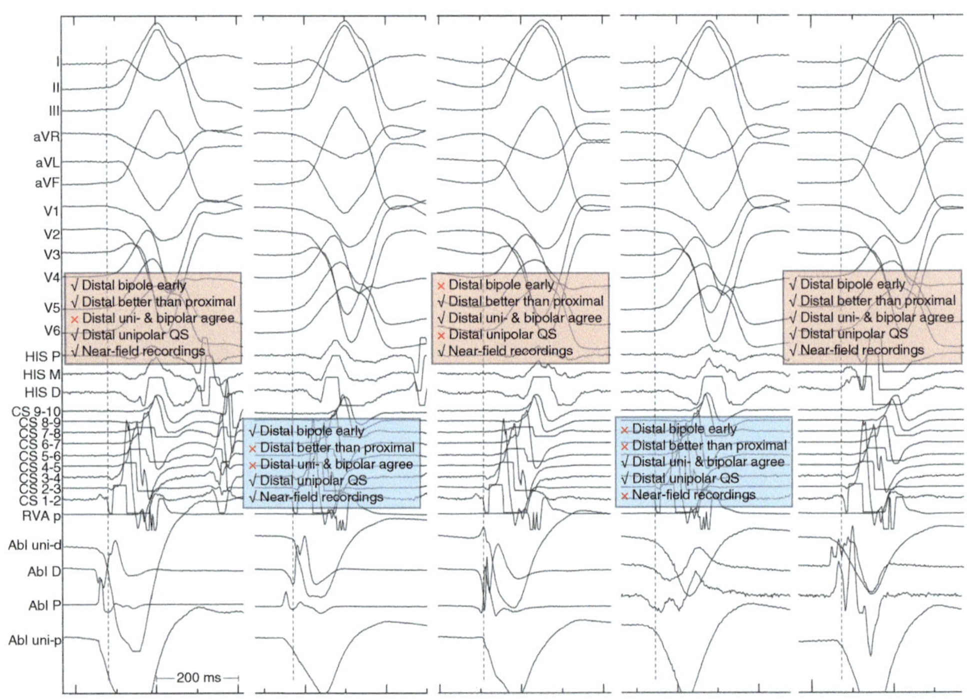

Fig. 18-26 provides a summary of electrogram features at different mapping sites, noting good and bad features.

Summary

- LBBB-inferior axis PVCs and VT may arise from:
  - RVOT/pulmonary artery
  - Right aortic sinus of Valsalva
  - LV or RV endocardium
  - LV or RV epicardium
  - Left aortic sinus of Valsalva/great cardiac vein (rare)
- Preprocedure ECG is an indicator of probability of location, but is not entirely specific
- After disappointing mapping and ablation in other areas, it is worth revisiting areas that had reasonable target features earlier
- Electrogram features of successful ablation sites:
  - Pre-QRS timing 15 to 40 ms
  - Unipolar "QS" configuration
  - "Agreement" between unipolar and bipolar recordings
  - Near-field characteristics (high amplitude, high frequency)
  - Consistent appearance from beat to beat (contact)

19 Coronary Sinus Ventricular Ectopy

Case Presentation

A 65-year-old man experienced symptomatic premature ventricular complexes (PVCs) for years. He initially sought evaluation 5 years ago because of palpitations: he was found to have an irregular pulse and a soft systolic murmur; ECG showed frequent PVCs; stress test was equivocal for ischemia and had no effect on PVCs; coronary arteriography showed normal epicardial arteries. After all this, he preferred no treatment. However, he developed increasing fatigue in the last few months. Ambulatory ECG showed very frequent PVCs and nonsustained ventricular tachycardia (~57% of complexes were ventricular in origin). Echocardiogram showed ejection fraction of 28% and moderate to severe valvular aortic stenosis. He was referred for consideration of transcutaneous aortic valve replacement (TAVR) and electrophysiologic evaluation and possible ablation.

Baseline ECGs

Figure 19-1

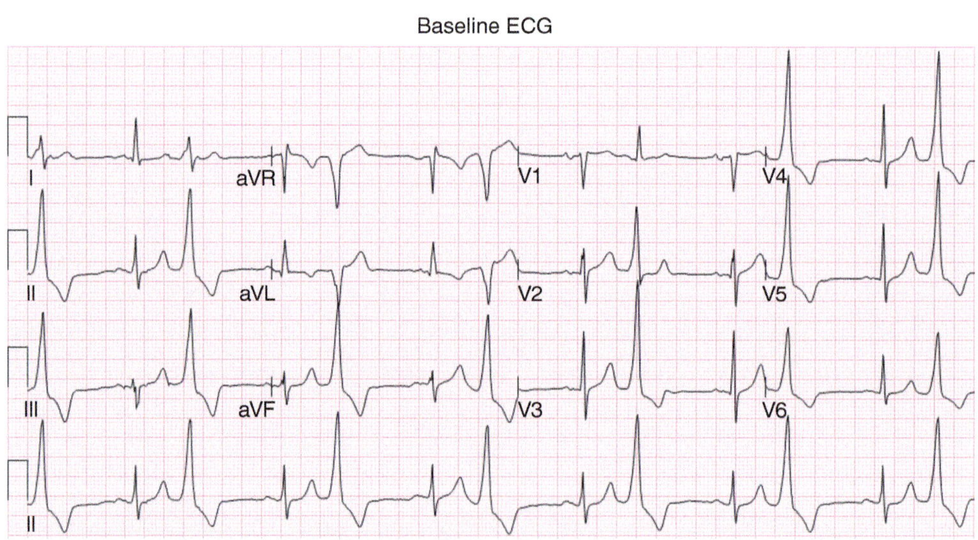

In Fig. 19-1, bigeminal ventricular ectopy is present with fixed coupling to the prior normal QRS.

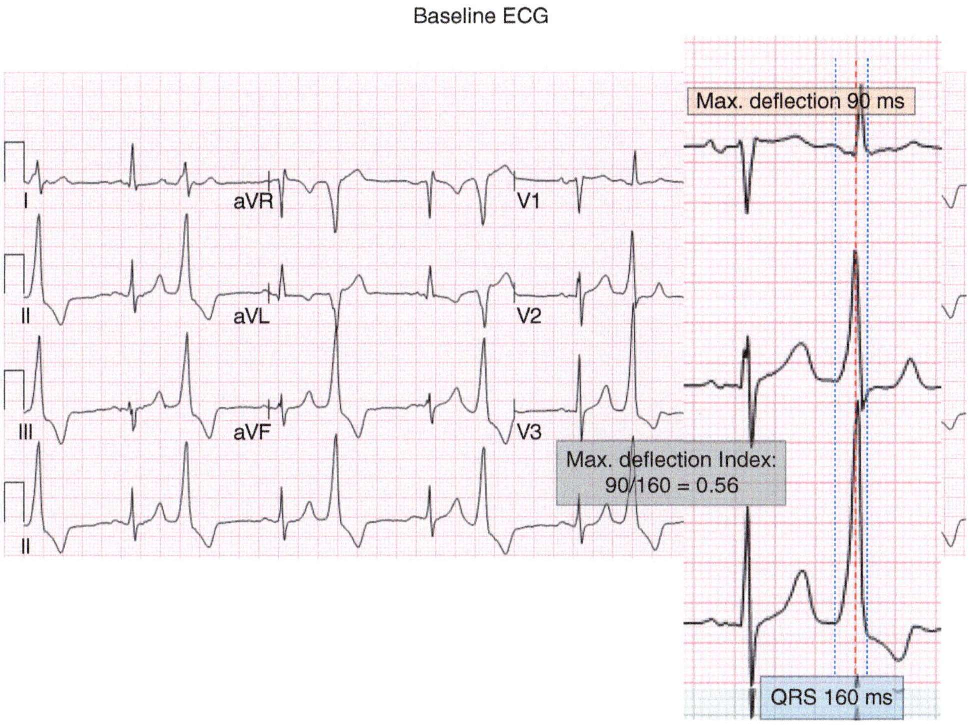

Figure 19-2

The QRS configuration in Fig. 19-2 suggests a possible epicardial source of ventricular ectopy because of the maximum deflection index (0.56). Another potential source, the left aortic sinus of Valsalva, might well become difficult to access (or be completely inaccessible) if he underwent TAVR or surgical valve replacement. Thus EP evaluation and potential ablation before an aortic procedure were reasonable.

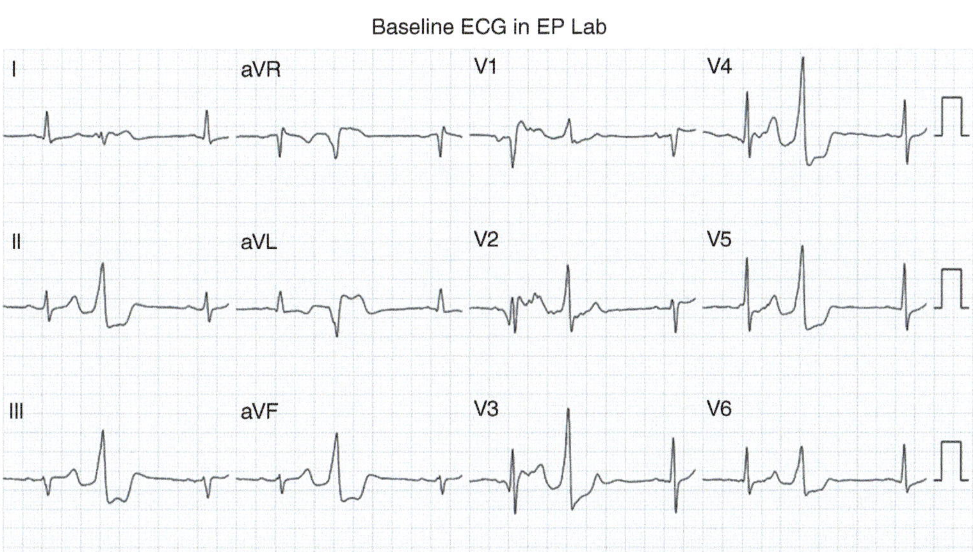

Figure 19-3

PVCs have a slightly different configuration in lead 1 of Fig. 19-3 compared with the office ECG, likely because of lead placement variation. This is a significant limitation of matching ECG morphologies (ventricular tachycardia [VT], Wolff-Parkinson-White syndrome [WPW] of spontaneously recorded episodes with those recorded in the EP laboratory; the ECG leads are typically the last things to go on the patient's chest when they are being prepared for the procedure (defibrillation pads and mapping system surface patches claim their territory first, with whatever skin is left over available for precordial ECG lead placement). It is well-known that differences in limb lead position can influence frontal plane ECG lead appearance.

Figure 19-4

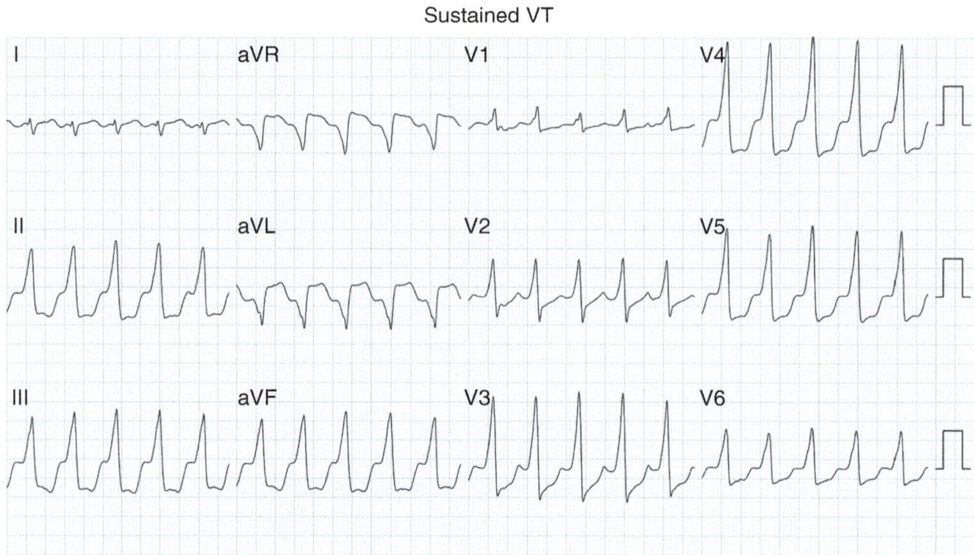

Sustained VT developed while operators were getting vascular access (no catheters in the heart at this time). See Fig. 19-4. This was hemodynamically tolerated and came and went during the procedure (went back to sinus with bigeminy, then VT intermittently).

Mapping Various Sites

Figure 19-5

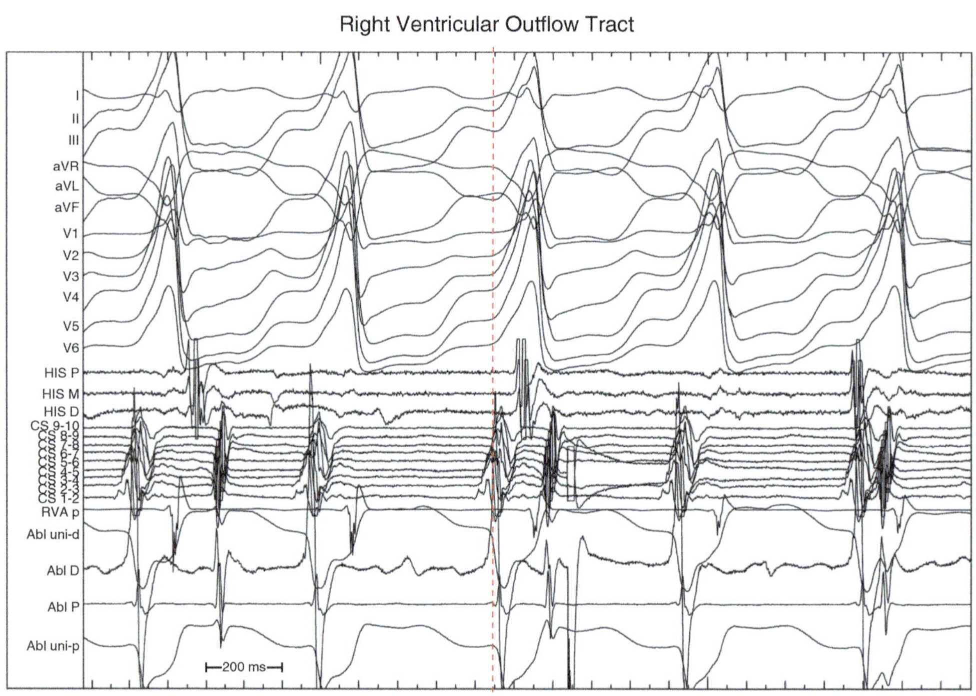

A coronary sinus (CS) catheter, positioned as distally as possible, can often show early activation times and provide clues as to whether the origin is likely to be remote from the recording site (endocardial or aortic sinus of Valsalva, indicated by late activation in the CS), nearby on the epicardial surface (presystolic but far-field appearing), or associated with the coronary venous system (presystolic and near-field). In Fig. 19-5, the distal CS recording occurs well before the QRS onset *(dotted line)* and is relatively sharp, suggesting a nearby source (epicardial, coronary venous, or possibly aortic sinus of Valsalva depending on how close this is to the recording site). Mapping usually starts in the right ventricular outflow tract because, though an unlikely source in this case, it is nonetheless easy to reach. The ablation recording is just at the QRS onset so no ablation was performed.

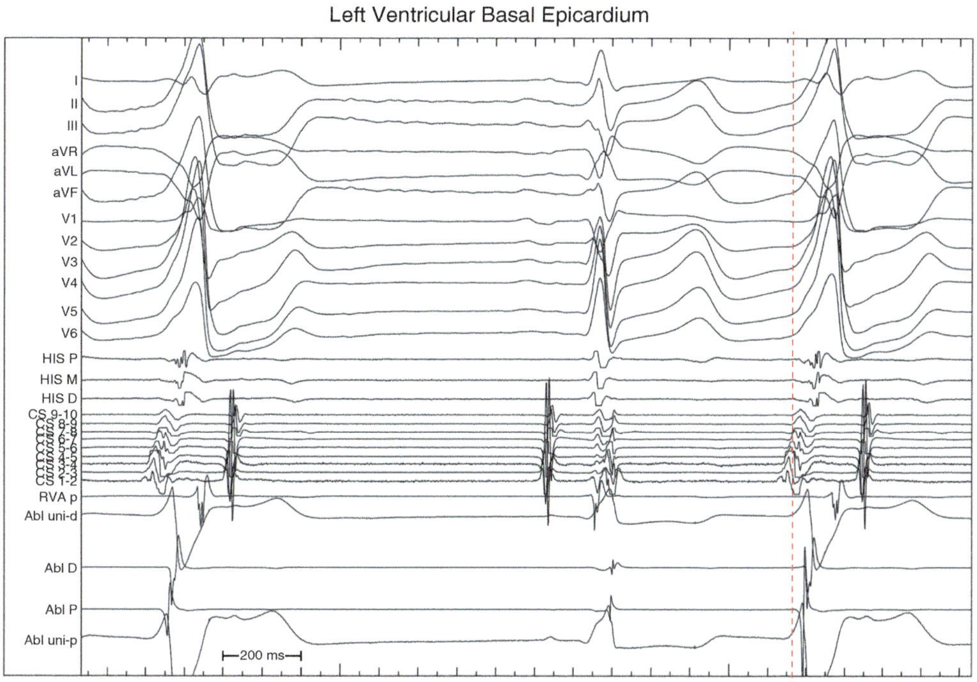

Figure 19-6

Because no attractive ablation sites were found in the right ventricular outflow tract and ECG and electrogram features suggested a possible epicardial source, pericardial access was obtained. In Fig. 19-6, mapping the epicardial surface near the distal CS recording site shows a late activation time, not suitable for ablation. Pacing here (not shown) yielded a poor match with PVCs.

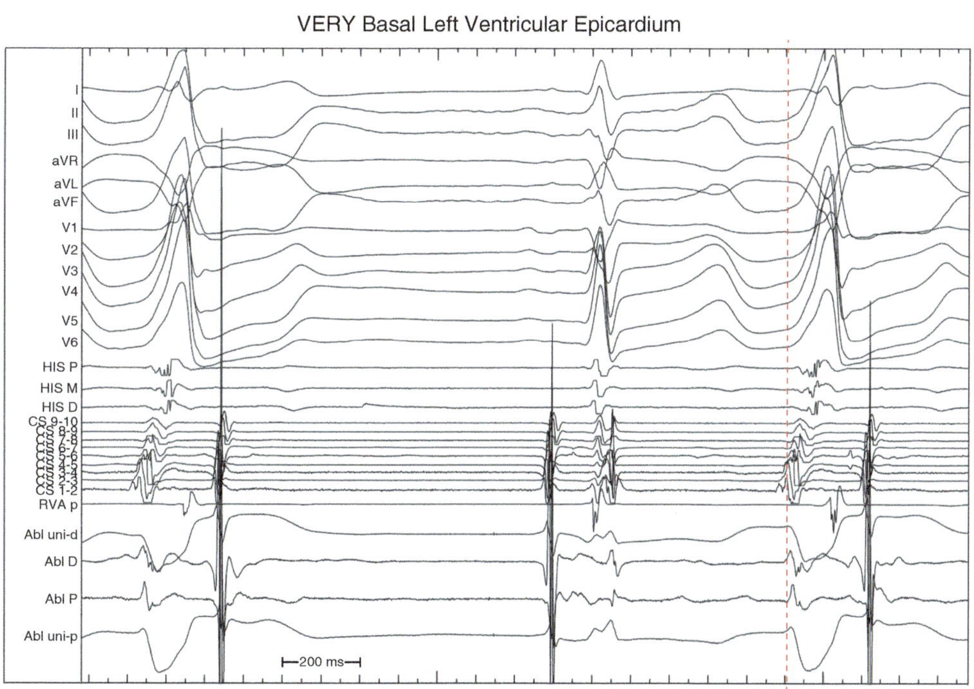

Figure 19-7

A site on the left ventricular epicardial surface even more basal than the prior site (Fig. 19-7, indicated by the large atrial signal) has an electrogram with very minimal presystolic activation with a "QS" in the unipolar recording; the distal bipolar recording precedes the proximal bipolar recording. These features would ordinarily suggest a reasonable ablation site, but earlier recordings remain in the distal CS. Thus this is not an attractive ablation site. Full exploration of areas around this site (that had the best recordings) failed to show any sites more suitable for ablation.

Figure 19-8

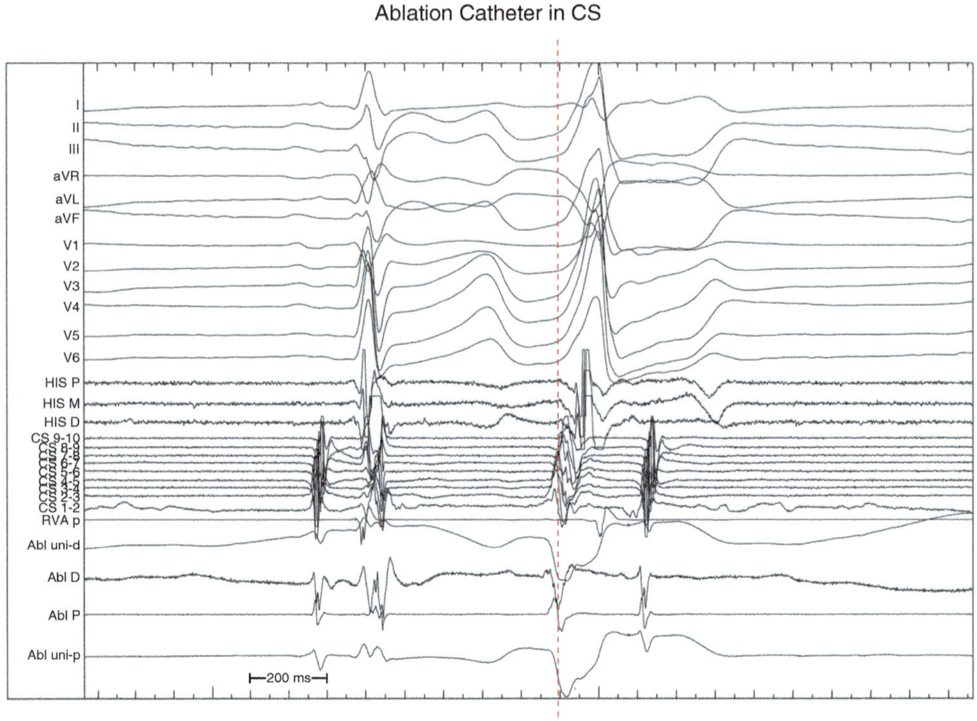

The ablation catheter was removed from the pericardial sheath (and replaced with the dilator and guidewire), and mapping of the aortic root and sinuses of Valsalva was performed. No sites with either presystolic activation or reasonable pace-matches were observed (Fig. 19-8). The catheter was then removed from the arterial system and positioned in the CS alongside the CS catheter. Now, the distal bipolar recording has a timing equivalent to the distal CS recording.

Figure 19-9

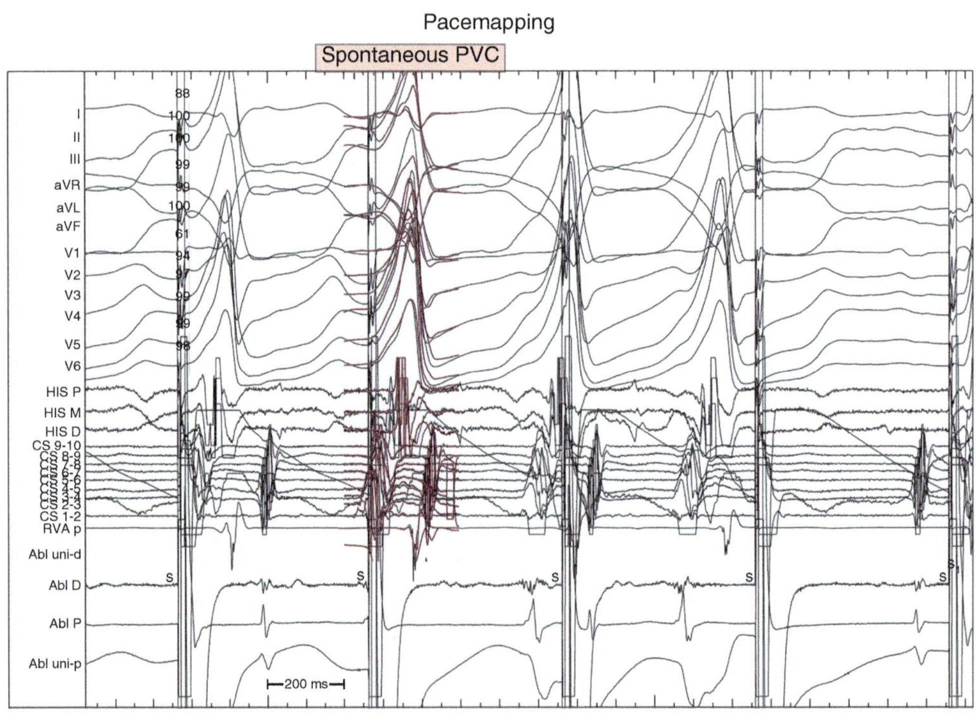

Pacing from the ablation catheter at this site yields at 98% electronic pace-match with the spontaneous PVC (Fig. 19-9, superimposed in *red*). This corroborates the early activation in the distal ablation electrode within the distal CS.

Imaging (Fluoroscopy, Electroanatomic Mapping)

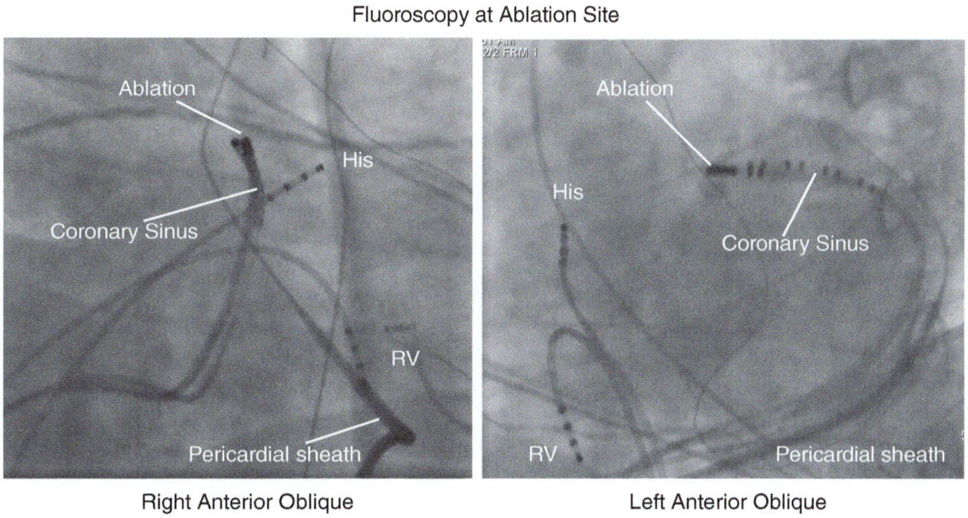

Figure 19-10

Catheter positions during ablation are displayed in Fig. 19-10; note that the ablation catheter tip is slightly distal to the CS catheter (which was pulled back somewhat to allow further advancement of the ablation catheter in the CS). Injection of a diluted solution of radiographic contrast through the irrigation ports of the ablation electrode showed that it was at the junction of the anterior interventricular vein and great cardiac vein. Coronary arteriography showed that the distance to the diagonal artery (closest branch) was about 0.8 cm.

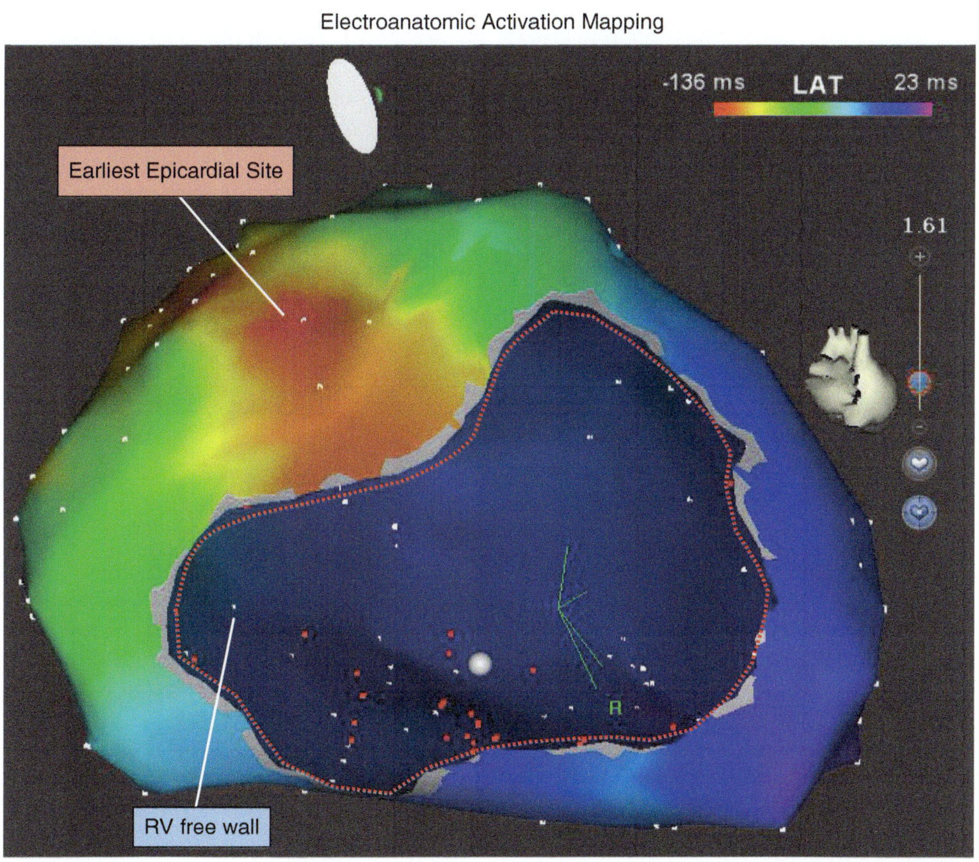

Figure 19-11

Fig. 19-11 provides an activation map of the PVCs on the epicardial surface. The earliest site *(red)* is surrounded by progressively later sites, typical of a focal process. This was at the junction of the great cardiac vein (distal CS) and anterior interventricular vein. Attempts at ablation here would likely have no effect on the ectopy, because of epicardial fat that is always relatively thick in this area.

Figure 19-12

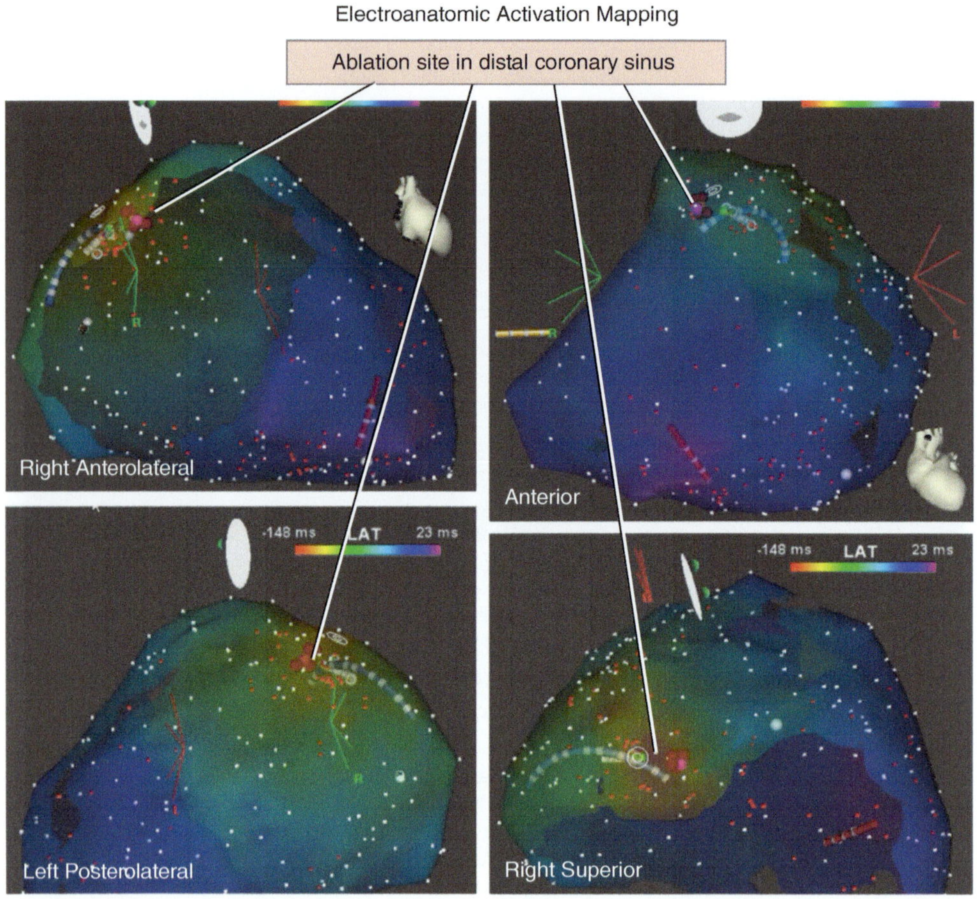

Electroanatomic activation mapping from coronary venous system and epicardium combined is shown in Fig. 19-12. The epicardial map shown previously has been made slightly transparent to allow visualization of the coronary venous mapping sites. *Red dots* indicate ablation sites in the distal portion of the CS, whereas the *purple dot* indicates the site at which ablation eliminated PVCs. It is evident that this site is fundamentally identical to the epicardial site of earliest activation during the PVC.

Ablation

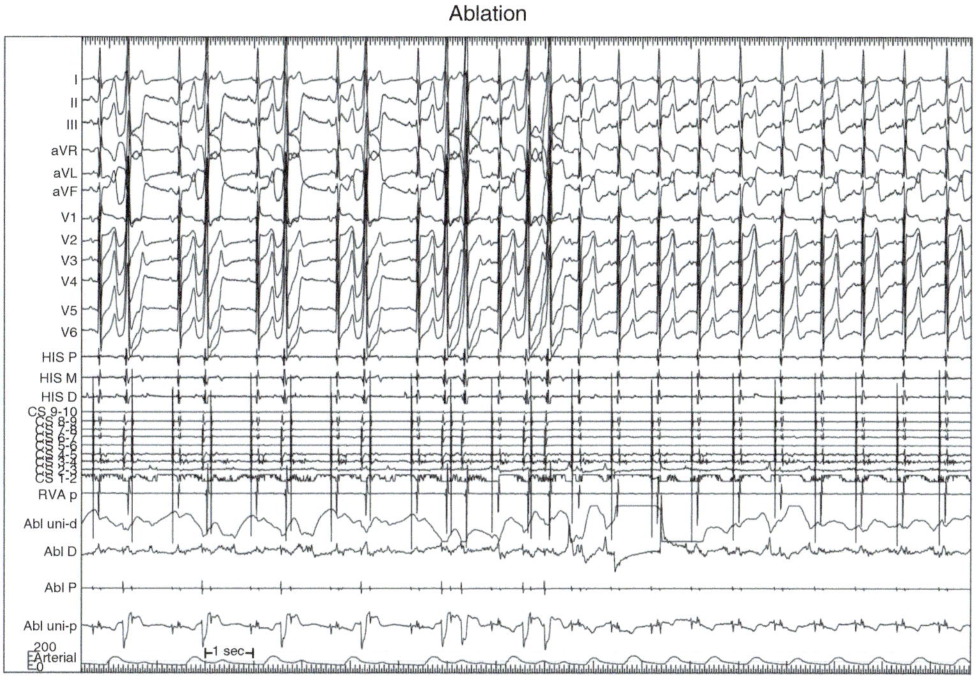

Figure 19-13

Ablation at this site (Fig. 19-13) in the distal CS (15 W) eliminates ventricular ectopy shortly after starting energy delivery. The amount of power delivered in this area should be as little as is needed to achieve the desired effect, because coronary arteries are nearby (left anterior descending, circumflex, or even left main artery). Because the distal CS (actually, great cardiac vein/anterior interventricular vein) is a relatively small vessel, with a relatively small amount of blood to cool an ablation electrode, ablating with a standard (nonirrigated) ablation electrode may not be successful because of rapid heating of the electrode with relatively little power delivery. Using an irrigated electrode overcomes this limitation, allowing greater power delivery without electrode overheating. This does not prevent tissue overheating and steam pops, however. After this RF application, no further ventricular ectopy was observed either spontaneously or after isoproterenol provocation. If this effort had been unsuccessful, ablation in the left aortic sinus of Valsalva would have been attempted.

Hemodynamic Study

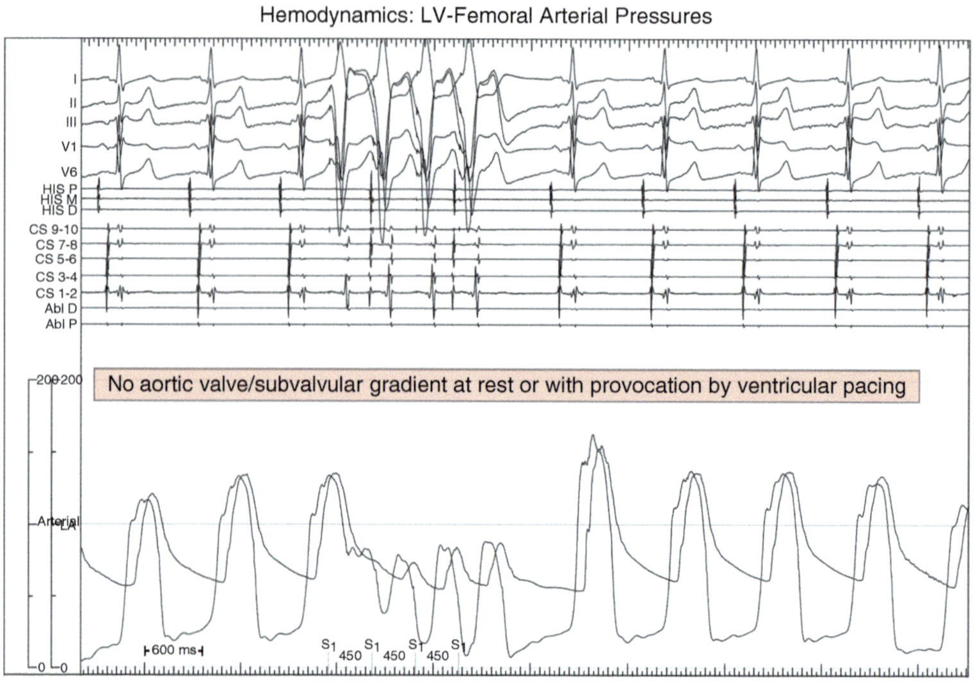

Figure 19-14

A short hemodynamic study after the ablation procedure showed no valvular or subvalvular left ventricular outflow gradient. A burst of ventricular pacing is used to try to provoke a gradient (Fig. 19-14).

Final ECG

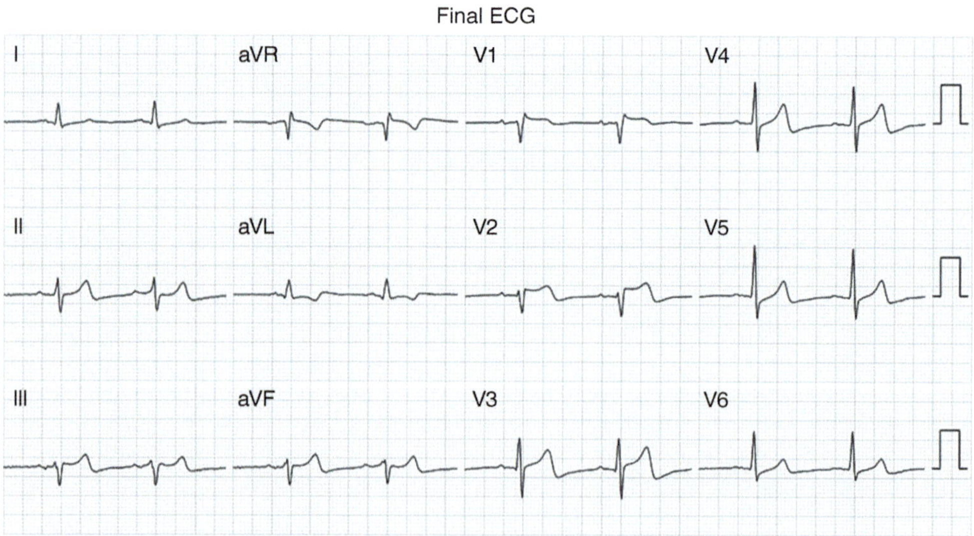

Figure 19-15

The ECG (Fig. 19-15) has entirely normalized, with no residual ectopy. The patient was monitored overnight to ensure no complications related to either pericardial access or ablation in the region of the coronary arteries. Repeat echocardiogram about 10 weeks after the procedure showed ejection fraction 52% and minimal aortic valve gradient.

Summary

- PVCs and ventricular tachycardia that have a configuration that suggests an epicardial source may arise from the actual epicardial surface, or the coronary venous system or aortic sinuses of Valsalva
- Ablation within the coronary venous system is feasible, sometimes necessary, and generally safe, but the veins restrict catheter movement to their lumens; epicardial mapping offers greater versatility, but a layer of epicardial fat interposed between the epicardial surface and catheter in the pericardial space may limit ablation efficacy
- The appearance of abnormal hemodynamics may be related to frequent ventricular ectopy (or other causes of irregular ventricular filling, such as atrial fibrillation)

20 Papillary Muscle Ventricular Ectopy

Case Presentation

A 63-year-old man without prior cardiac history was referred for evaluation of frequent premature ventricular complexes (PVCs). His initial complaint was dizziness and fatigue; finding an irregular pulse led to obtaining an ECG that showed frequent monomorphic PVCs. An ambulatory monitor showed monomorphic PVCs comprising 18% of all complexes. Echocardiogram showed mildly decreased left ventricular ejection fraction (43%). He was referred for electrophysiology study and possible catheter ablation.

Baseline Recordings

Figure 20-1

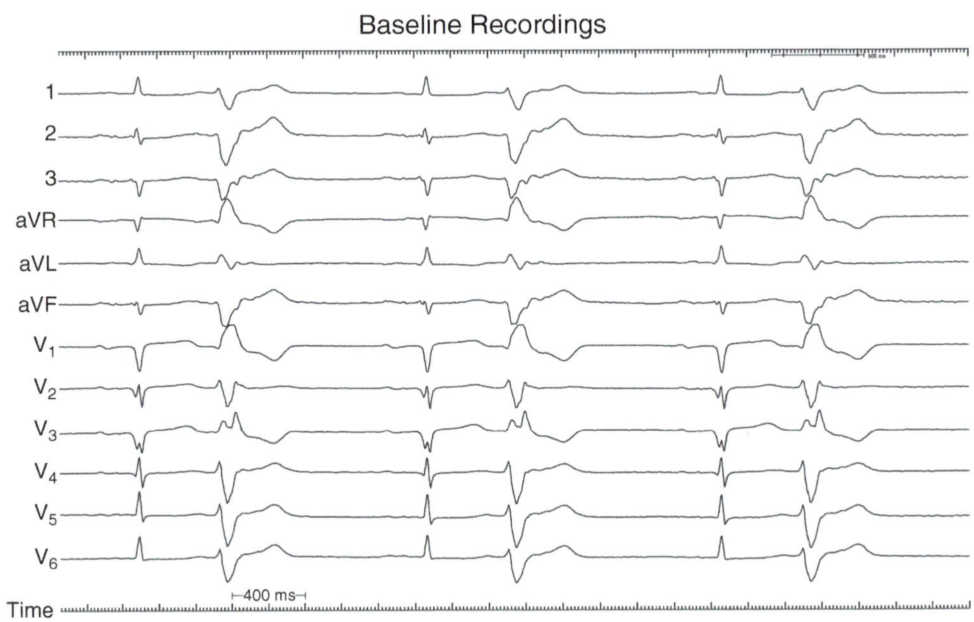

Baseline recordings made at the time of EP study (Fig. 20-1) show bigeminal PVCs with a right bundle branch block, rightward superior axis morphology. In a structurally normal heart such as his, the morphology overall suggests an inferolateral, somewhat apical left ventricular (LV) origin (negative in leads 1, 2, and 3 and relatively early R-wave regression in precordial leads). There is a tiny Q wave in lead V1; sometimes this points to a papillary muscle as the origin of the PVC. It is important to make recordings of the spontaneous PVCs before inserting catheters into the heart so that the true target is known, because catheters can themselves cause ectopic complexes that can confuse mapping.

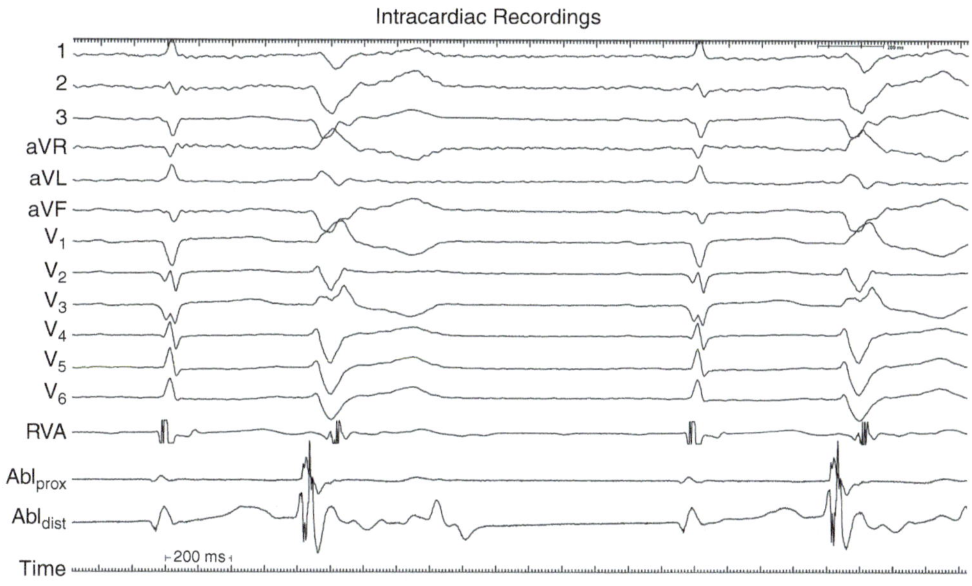

Figure 20-2

Intracardiac recordings from right ventricle and a catheter in the left ventricle (Abl) are shown in Fig. 20-2 during sinus rhythm with ventricular bigeminy.

Mapping

Figure 20-3

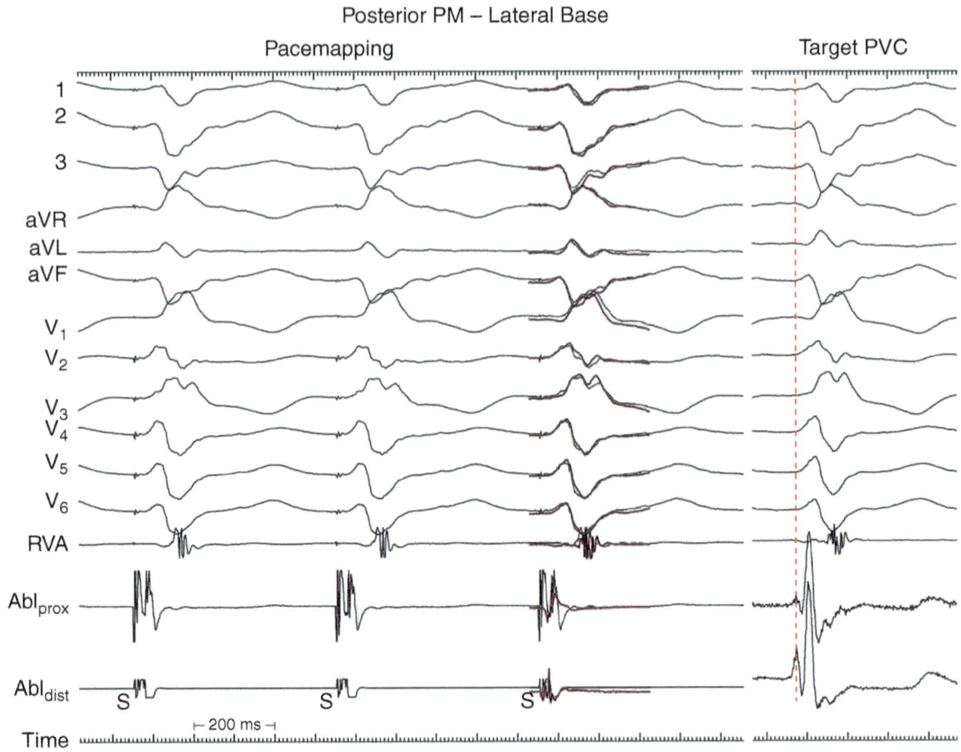

The process of mapping in this case consisted of activation mapping (manipulating the ablation catheter to various locations in the heart seeking earliest presystolic activation) corroborated by pacemapping (pacing at candidate sites to see how closely the resulting QRS complex corresponds to the native PVC). For either purpose, it is important to have adequate gain of surface ECG leads to be able to determine (1) the true QRS onset, because this will serve as a point of reference for determining whether a mapping site is early or late, and (2) being able to compare subtle differences in paced versus target PVC complexes. In Fig. 20-3, the activation time at a site on the lateral base of the posterior papillary muscle is shown at right; a *dashed line* indicates the onset of the QRS complex. Pacing at this site for three complexes is also shown. A single beat of the target PVC is superimposed on the last paced complex. The activation time at this site is about −15 ms, with distal electrode earlier than proximal, but the paced morphology is not a very good match. Mapping will continue.

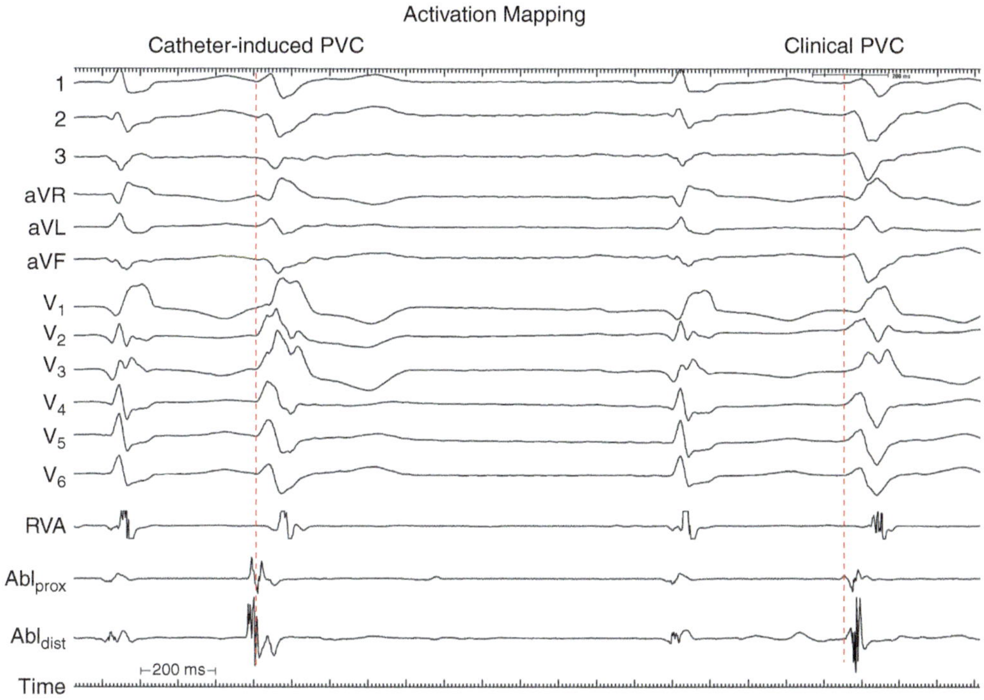

Figure 20-4

At another site, the PVC on the left has an activation time about −33 ms, with the distal electrode earlier than proximal (Fig. 20-4). This looks like a great ablation site, but careful inspection shows that the PVC morphology is different from the target PVC at right (where the activation time is not good at all). The PVC on the left is thus catheter-induced ectopy and illustrates one of the hazards of mapping in such cases. Catheter–tissue contact is important for both mapping and ablation, but can cause PVCs that look like good ablation targets, but are not.

It is no surprise that the activation time is so early, because the catheter tip (where this distal recording is made) caused the ectopy. Of note, catheter-induced right bundle branch block (RBBB) is now present during sinus complexes.

Figure 20-5

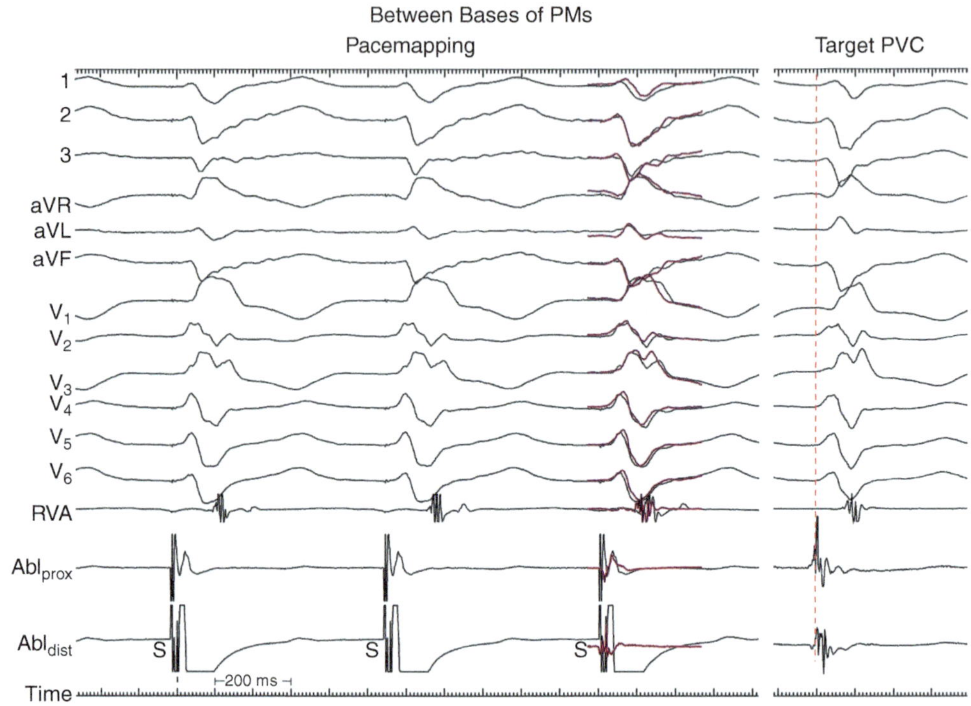

At a site between the bases of the anterior and posterior papillary muscles (Fig. 20-5), the activation time is about −15 ms; however, the proximal and distal electrodes have similar timing, and for ablation, the distal should be earlier. Pacing at this site again shows a good, but not exact, match with the target PVC. Mapping will continue.

Figure 20-6

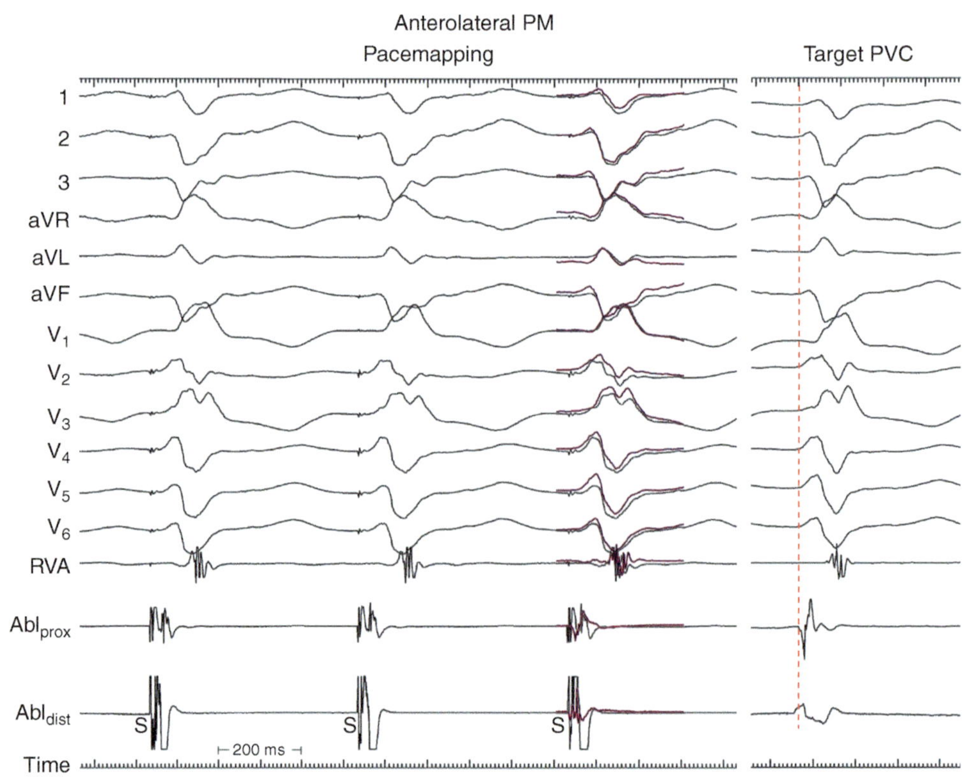

A site on the anterolateral papillary muscle (Fig. 20-6) has an activation time at the distal electrode of about −15 ms, but the proximal electrode is even earlier; pacing was performed at the site (even though it would not serve as a good ablation site because of the timing of activation), and again was not a very good match with the target PVC.

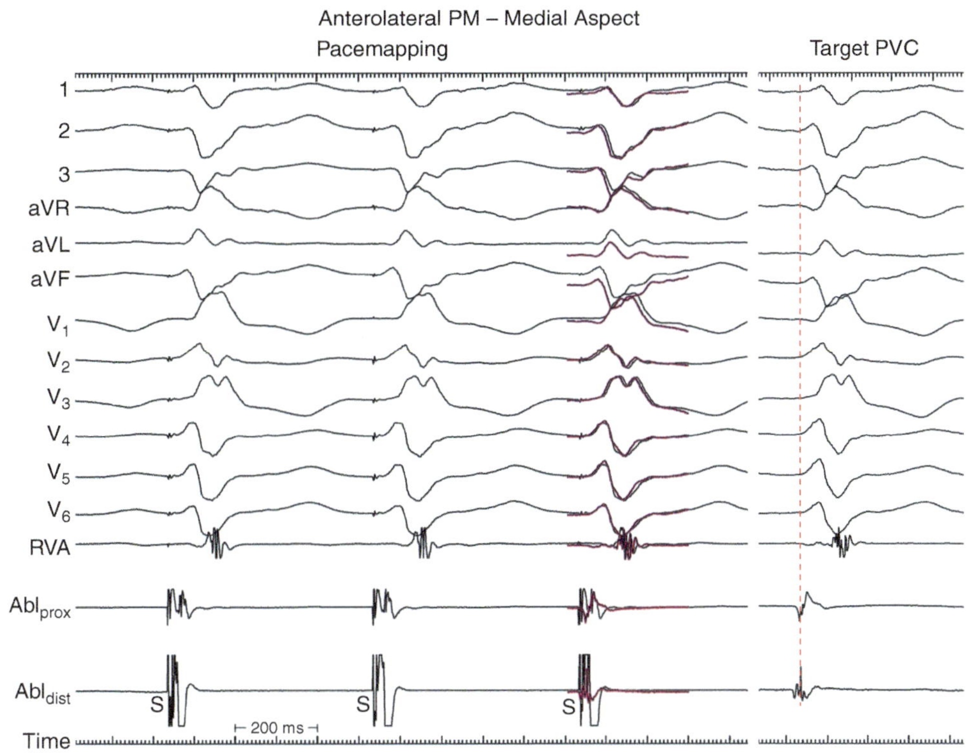

Figure 20-7

In Fig. 20-7, a site on the medial aspect of the anterolateral papillary muscle shows an activation time about −25 ms; this is the earliest that has been found thus far. The location is away from where the Purkinje network should be and the electrogram does not suggest Purkinje tissue (typically a very sharp potential preceding and often separated from a larger ventricular signal by 5 to 10 ms). Thus this seems to be myocardial in origin. Pacing at this site exactly replicates the target PVC. This should hopefully serve as a good ablation site.

Figure 20-8

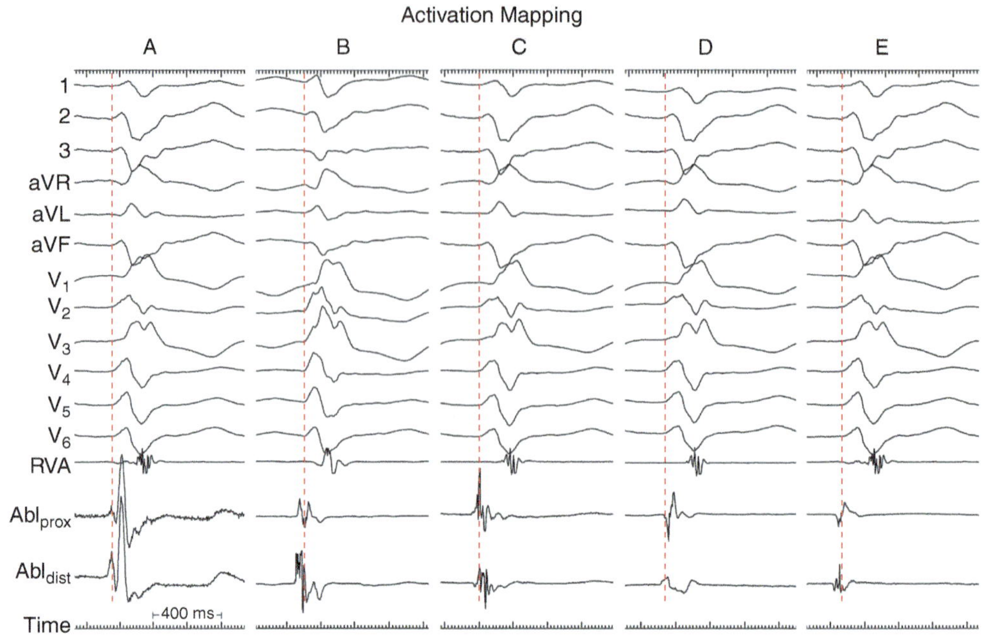

Fig. 20-8 is a compilation of activation times from five different LV sites. At site A, the distal electrogram is somewhat early relative to the QRS onset (−15 ms) and precedes the proximal electrogram, but its timing is not particularly early. At site B, the activation time looks great at −33 ms, but the QRS complex is different from the target PVC (our catheter-induced PVC from earlier). Site C has a relatively early electrogram timing (−15 ms), but the proximal electrode is earlier (−20 ms). At site D, the timing of the distal electrogram is about −20 ms, but its shape is rounded rather than sharp, indicating relatively poor contact. None of these candidate sites are suitable for attempting ablation. At site E, a sharp electrogram precedes the QRS complex by about 25 ms and is earlier than the proximal electrode. This is the site at which the perfect pace match was obtained.

Ablation

Figure 20-9

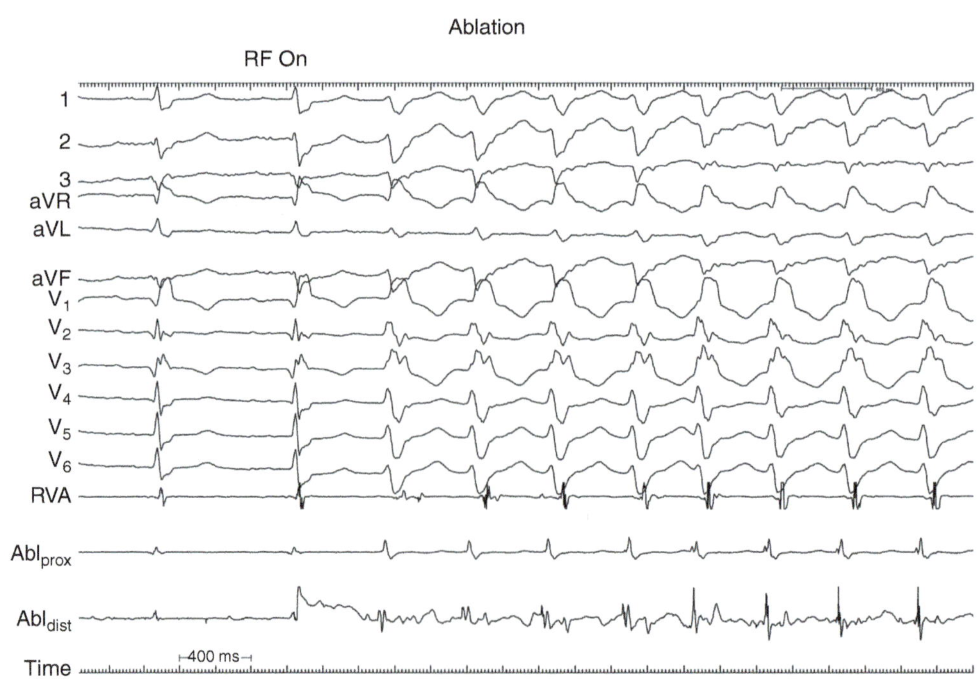

In Fig. 20-9, radiofrequency (RF) ablation is begun at the site shown in Fig. 20-7. The first thing to notice is that the first two complexes at left are sinus complexes with RBBB; the previously bigeminal PVCs have been transiently suppressed by catheter pressure at the site. Almost as soon as RF energy is turned on, a flurry of ventricular tachycardia (VT) with the same morphology as the target PVCs occurs. This is a common finding with focal arrhythmias, so much so that if one does not see RF-induced ectopy during the first few seconds of ablation in such cases, it is worth considering stopping energy delivery and mapping elsewhere or getting better contact on the site.

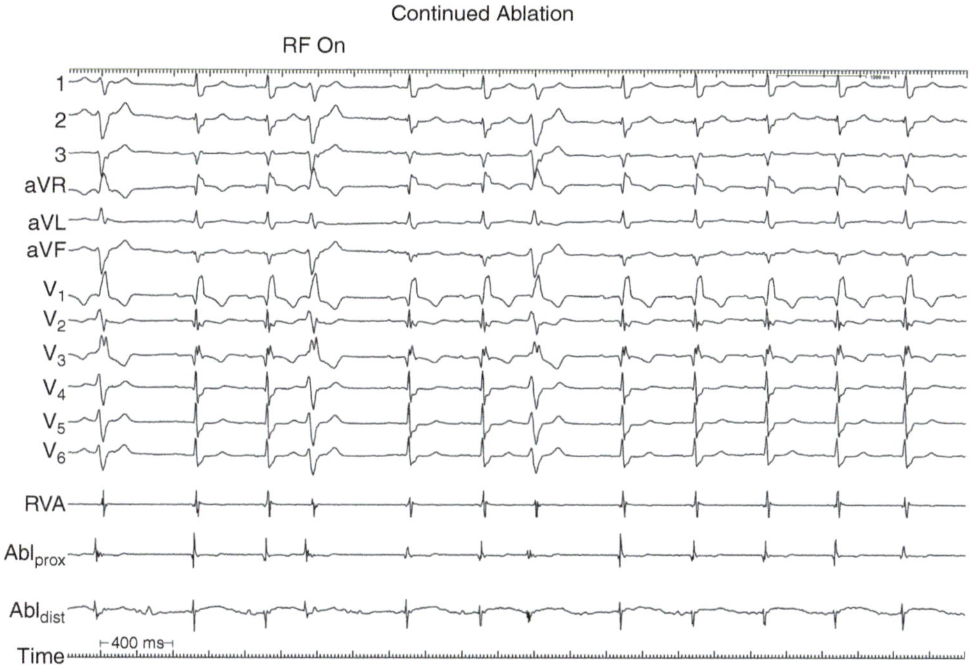

Figure 20-10

After stopping RF delivery at the site, rare PVCs persisted. Here (Fig. 20-10), PVCs have become trigeminal. Additional RF energy is delivered that results in sudden cessation of ectopy. Several more RF applications were delivered in the same general area, because foci of ectopy are sometimes deep and/or diffuse. Despite extensive ablation, papillary muscle dysfunction with mitral regurgitation is rare.

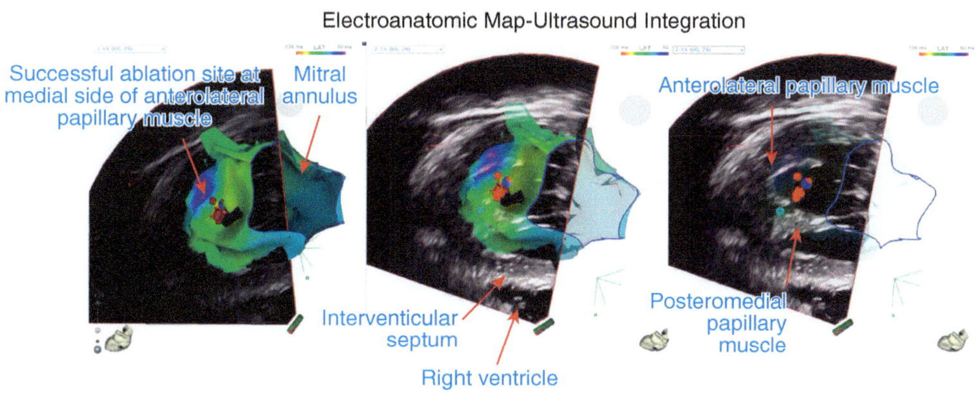

Figure 20-11

Intracardiac echocardiography is often useful for delineation of structures, such as papillary muscles, and stabilization of catheters especially in cases such as this. Stability of catheter contact on papillary muscles is notoriously difficult to achieve. Here (Fig. 20-11), integration of electroanatomic mapping and intracardiac echocardiography shows where ablation was performed (*red dots*, medial aspect of anterolateral papillary muscle).

Summary

- PVCs and VT arising from a papillary muscle are relatively rare and must be distinguished from fascicular ectopy as well as verapamil-sensitive VT
- PVCs more commonly originate from the posterior than anterior papillary muscle, but can arise in a right ventricular papillary muscle as well
- Intracardiac echocardiography may help in localizing the anatomic site of origin of the PVC/VT and aid in stabilization of the ablation catheter, but is not mandatory
- Ectopic foci from papillary muscles may be difficult to ablate because of catheter stability and depth of penetration needed

21 Focal Fascicular Ventricular Tachycardia

Case Presentation

The patient was a 37-year-old man with palpitations for many years and had occasional lightheaded episodes. ECG showed right bundle branch block (RBBB) and rightward inferior axis QRS. The rhythm was incessant (present 100% of the time) and atrioventricular (AV) dissociation was evident. Echocardiogram revealed low-normal left ventricle (LV) systolic function (ejection fraction [EF] 40%). He had undergone three catheter ablation attempts in the past, without noteworthy benefit. He was referred for repeat electrophysiology (EP) study and possible ablation, but he expressed skepticism about whether it was worth it to proceed in light of prior failures.

Baseline ECG and Intracardiac Recordings

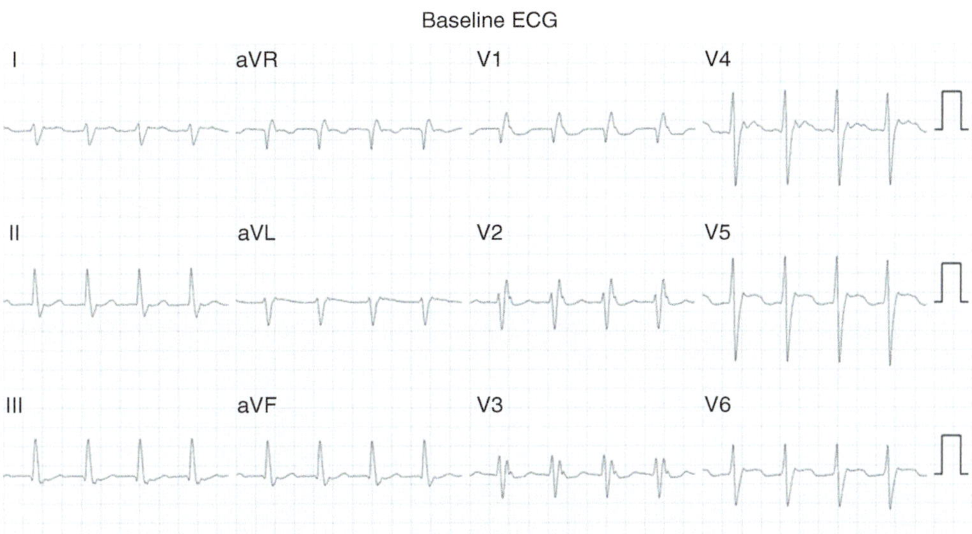

What Is the Rhythm?

- Ventricular tachycardia (VT)?
- Supraventricular tachycardia (SVT) with aberration?
- Fascicular? [Fig. 21-1]

Figure 21-1

The ECG in Fig. 21-1 shows a wide-complex tachycardia with RBBB-rightward inferior axis. P waves are not clearly seen. Using standard morphologic criteria, most suggest that this is a supraventricular (SVT) QRS complex rather than ventricular in origin (QRS duration, axis, precordial QRS onset to S nadir <100 ms, time to peak in lead 2 <50 ms, sharp Q in aVR). However, an arrhythmia from the infranodal conduction system (junctional with aberration, or fascicular) could look like this and meet the same criteria (suggesting SVT with aberration).

What Does This Say About the Nature of the Arrhythmia? How Can the Mechanism Be Assessed?

Figure 21-2

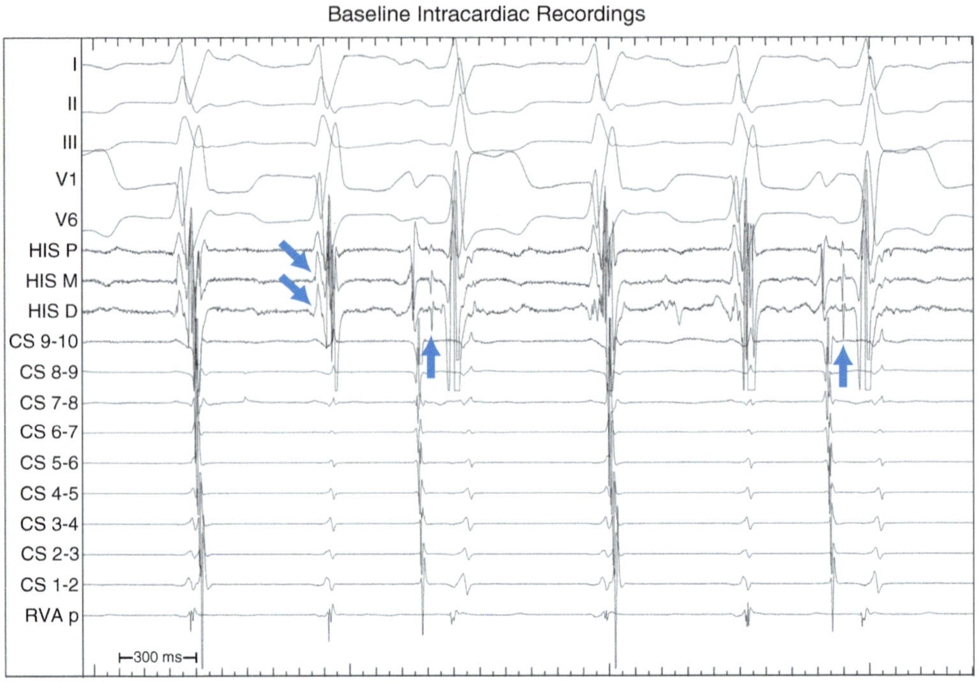

Baseline intracardiac recordings (Fig. 21-2) show AV dissociation during the wide-complex tachycardia; the third and sixth QRS complexes are different from the others, being either fusion complexes or complete capture complexes as a result of fortuitous timing of a P wave at such a time that anterograde conduction over the normal conduction system is possible. Both of these QRS complexes have His potentials (inscribed anterogradely; *slanted arrows*) before the QRS complex, identifying them as fusion/capture complexes. The His potential during tachycardia complexes is not as easily seen; *vertical blue arrows* point to possible retrograde His potentials. This also shows that the baseline rhythm is fascicular in origin rather than junctional with RBBB/left posterior fascicular block; in the latter case, conducted complexes should also show RBBB/right axis.

Effects of Right Ventricular Overdrive Pacing

Figure 21-3

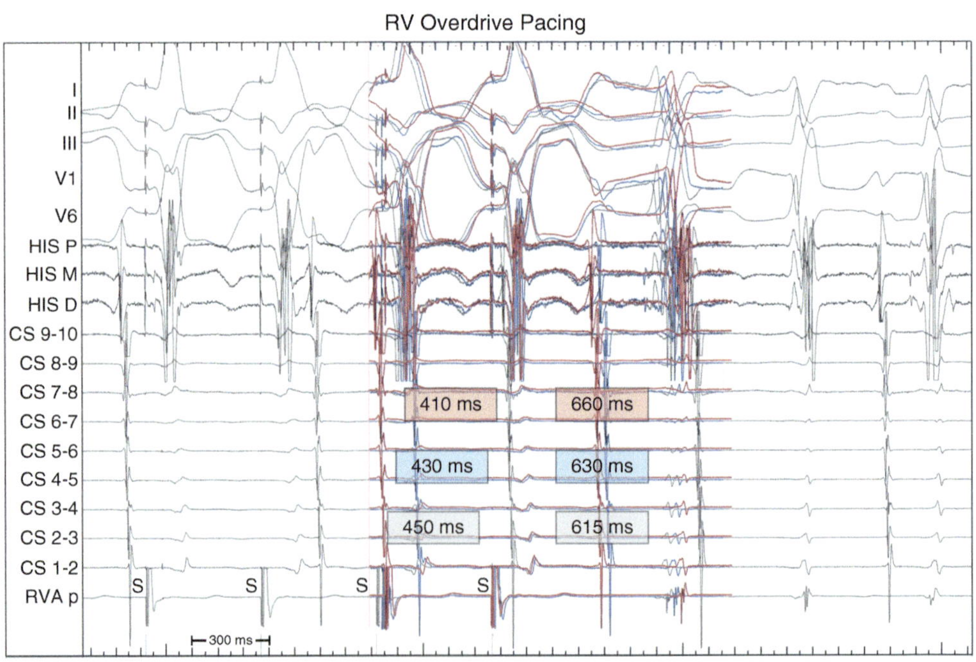

To determine whether the tachycardia mechanism was macroreentry or a focus (most likely automatic), overdrive pacing was performed at progressively more rapid rates and the timing of the first return VT cycle measured. In Fig. 21-3, for pacing at cycle length (CL) 450 ms, the first VT complex returns after 615 ms; for pacing at 430 ms (in *blue*), the VT returns at 630 ms; and for pacing at 410 ms (in *red*), the VT returns at 660 ms. This response shows overdrive suppression, a characteristic of automatic foci. In reentrant rhythms, the return cycle is typically relatively constant over a wide range of overdrive paced CLs, whereas in tachycardias due to classical triggered activity related to delayed afterdepolarizations, the first complex of the resumed arrhythmia returns progressively sooner following more rapid paced rates.

Different Mapping Sites ("Purkinje Potential")

Is There a Good Ablation Site Shown? [Fig. 21-4]

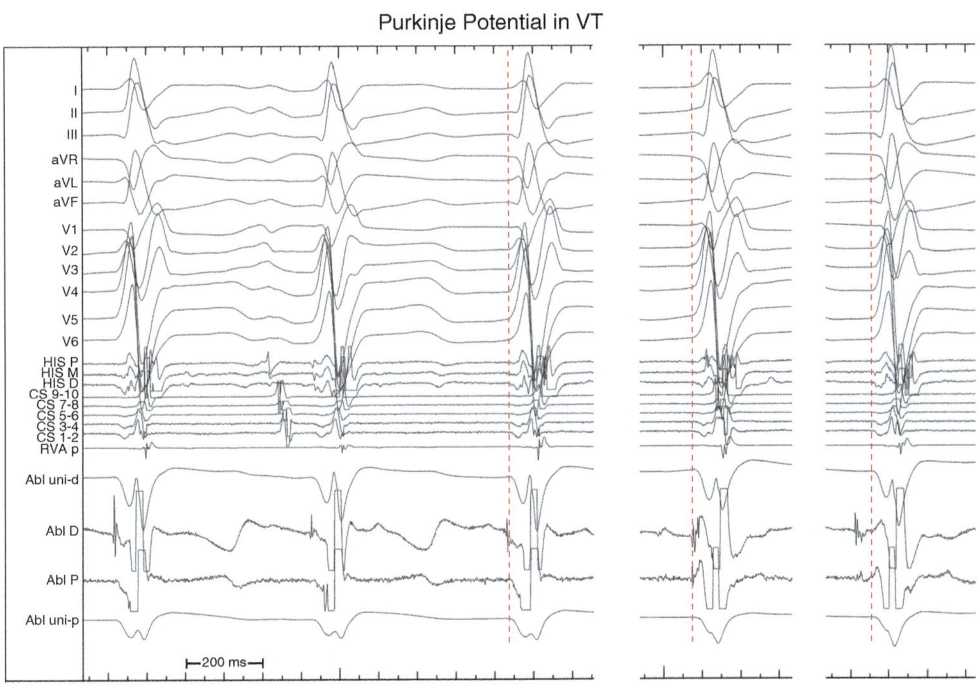

Figure 21-4

Based on the foregoing tests, a diagnosis of a focal, automatic fascicular tachycardia has been made and its origin will be sought. In Fig. 21-4, multiple sites are mapped during the arrhythmia, seeking the earliest Purkinje recording; this should be 15 to 40 ms before QRS onset *(dashed red line).* Ablation at a site other than that of earliest activation (the focus) will have no effect on the focus but may alter its exit (QRS morphology); see below (Fig. 21-12). Thus it is important to take the time to carefully map and determine the earliest site, from which all other recordings emanate. While each panel shows a Purkinje spike in Abl D recordings, only in the far right panel is it significantly prior to the QRS onset; this was the very earliest site found of about 90 sites sampled during tachycardia.

Catheter Manipulation Terminates VT

Figure 21-5

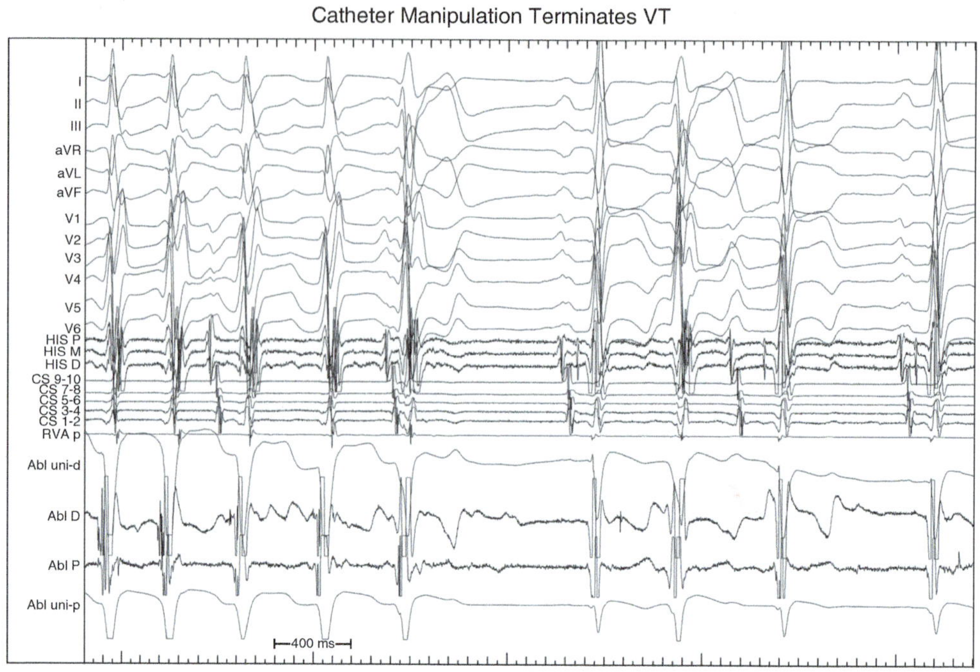

The focus is often very superficial on the endocardial surface and thus susceptible to catheter-induced trauma, resulting in arrhythmia termination (as shown in Fig. 21-5) and subsequent quiescence for prolonged periods. In many (but not all) cases, the focus recovers within minutes and mapping can continue. Careful mapping (minute catheter movements) allows logging of the site on an electroanatomic mapping system at the moment of catheter-related arrhythmia termination so that it can still be targeted for ablation even if the arrhythmia remains quiescent. This so-called "bump-mapping" implies a very small discrete target that is superficial (ie, not in deeper layers) and furthermore has been encountered by the catheter (it was "bumped").

Pacemapping Anteroseptal Wall, Superimposed on Baseline VT ECG

Figure 21-6

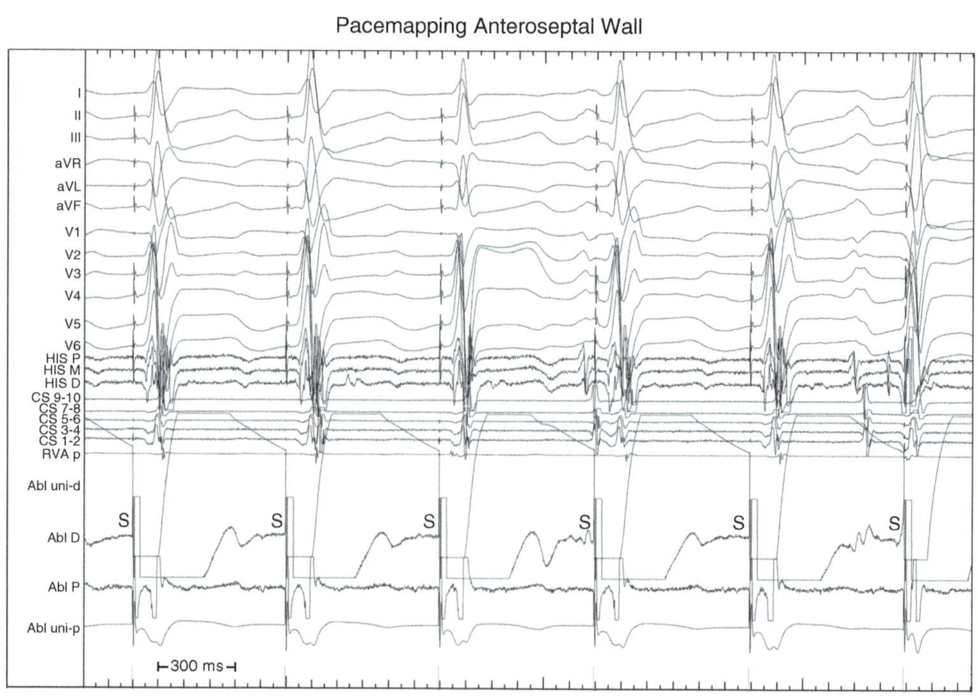

Pacemapping can corroborate activation mapping data; in Fig. 21-6, pacing at a site with an early Purkinje potential during VT perfectly replicates the arrhythmia on 12-lead ECG with an electrocardiographically quiet, discrete interval from stimulus-QRS that correlates with the interval from the Purkinje potential to QRS onset during VT.

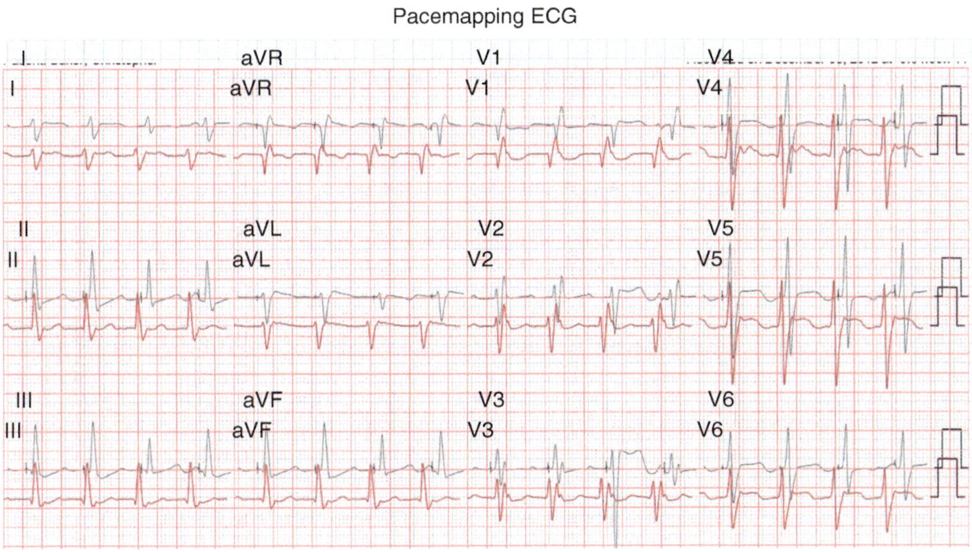

Figure 21-7

Superimposition of the VT ECG atop the pacemapping ECG (in red, aligning the first complex in each panel) shows a perfect match with VT (Fig. 21-7).

RF Energy Delivery

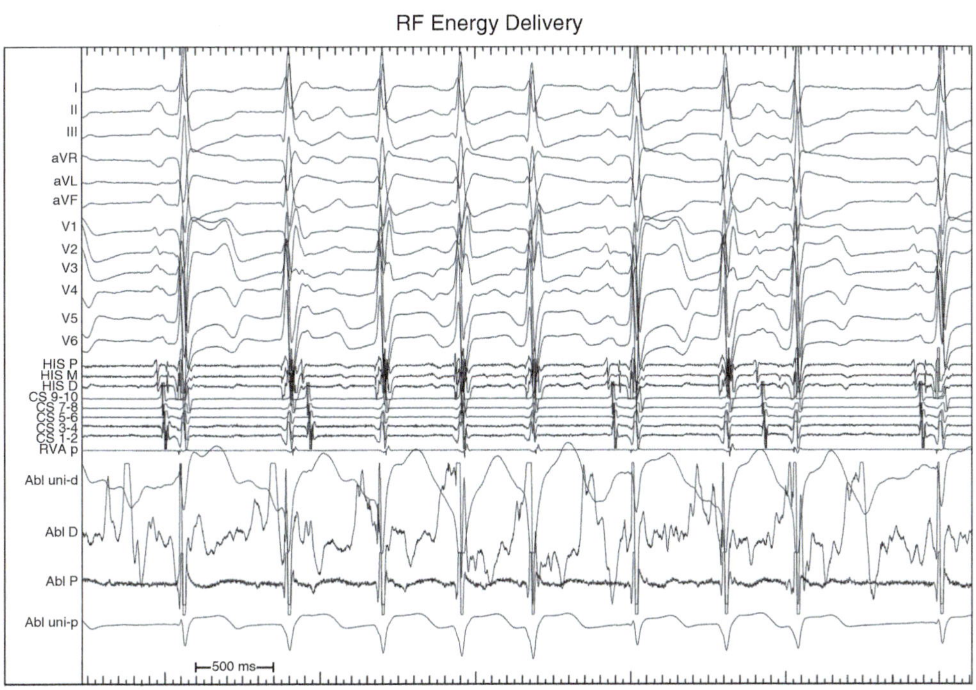

Figure 21-8

During RF delivery at the site of earliest Purkinje activation during VT, a flurry of activity with the same QRS complex occurs followed by termination to sinus rhythm (Fig. 21-8). This effect is characteristic of focal emanation (in contrast, reentrant VTs typically slow before termination).

Final ECG and Intracardiac Recordings

Final ECG

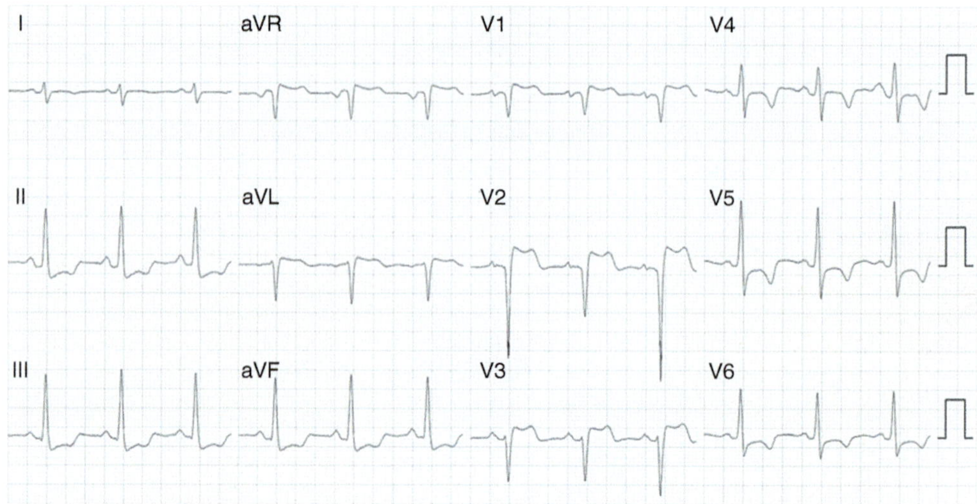

Figure 21-9

The final ECG (Fig. 21-9) shows sinus rhythm without bundle branch block or axis deviation; ST-T wave abnormalities are an artifact of the recording system.

Final Intracardiac Recordings

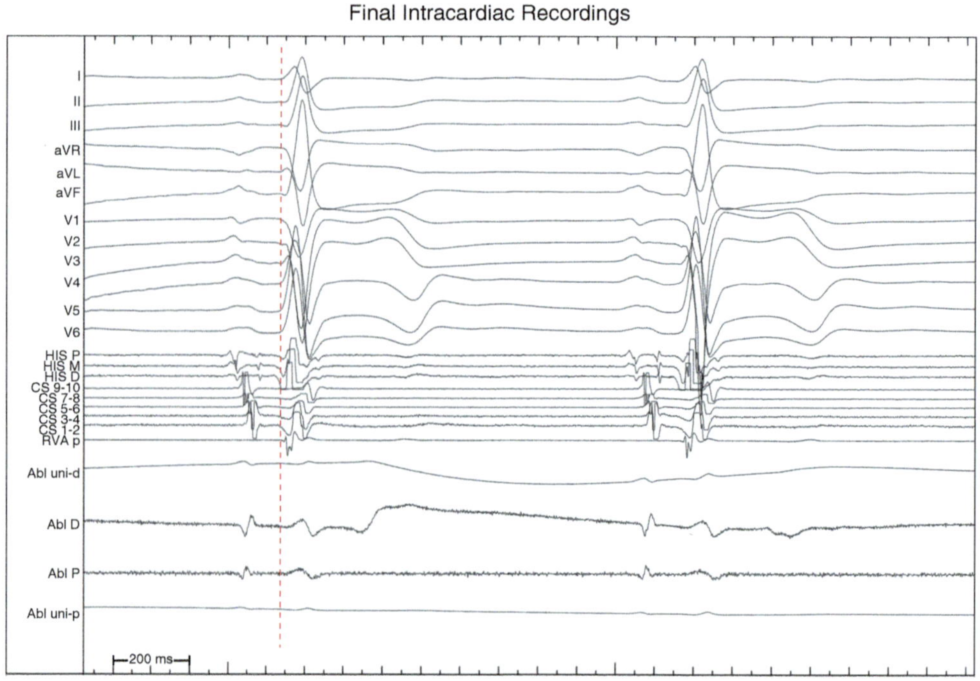

Figure 21-10

The final intracardiac recordings (Fig. 21-10) show sinus rhythm without bundle branch block or axis deviation.

Electroanatomic Maps

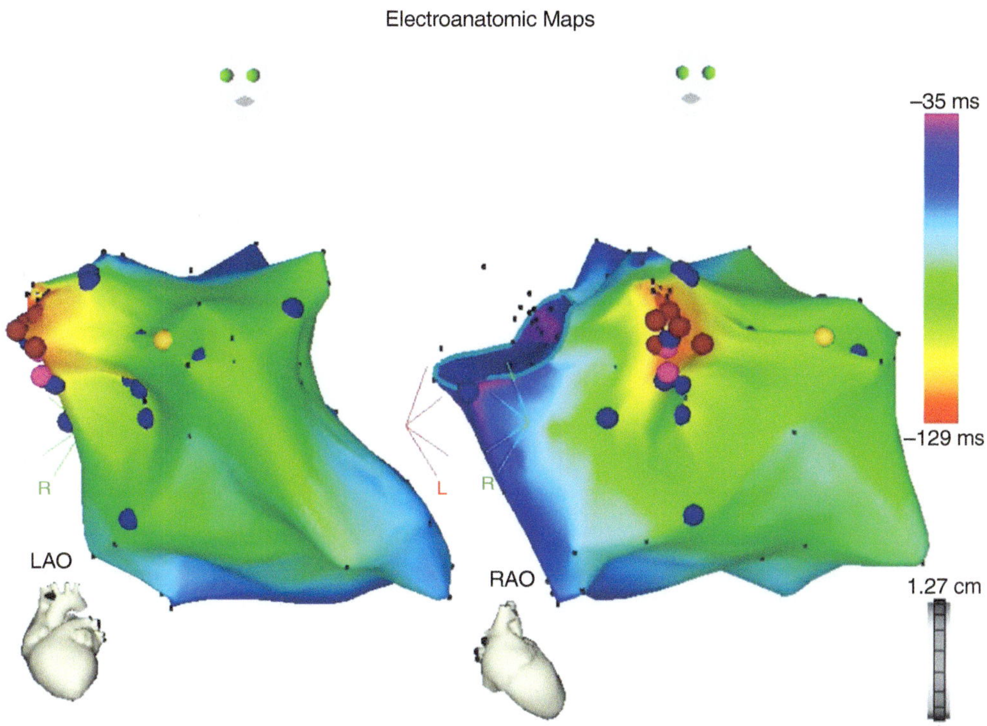

Figure 21-11

Fig. 21-11 displays the right and left anterior oblique views of the left ventricular activation during VT. The *purple dots* signify where perfect pace-matches were obtained as well as ablation sites where tachycardia terminated; *red dots* are consolidation ablation sites; *blue dots* denote where other Purkinje potentials were identified. The activation map shows earliest recordings during VT at the upper basal septal/anterior wall junction, with all other activations proceeding centrifugally from this region (consistent with a focal process).

Points on Mapping Fascicular VTs

Figure 21-12

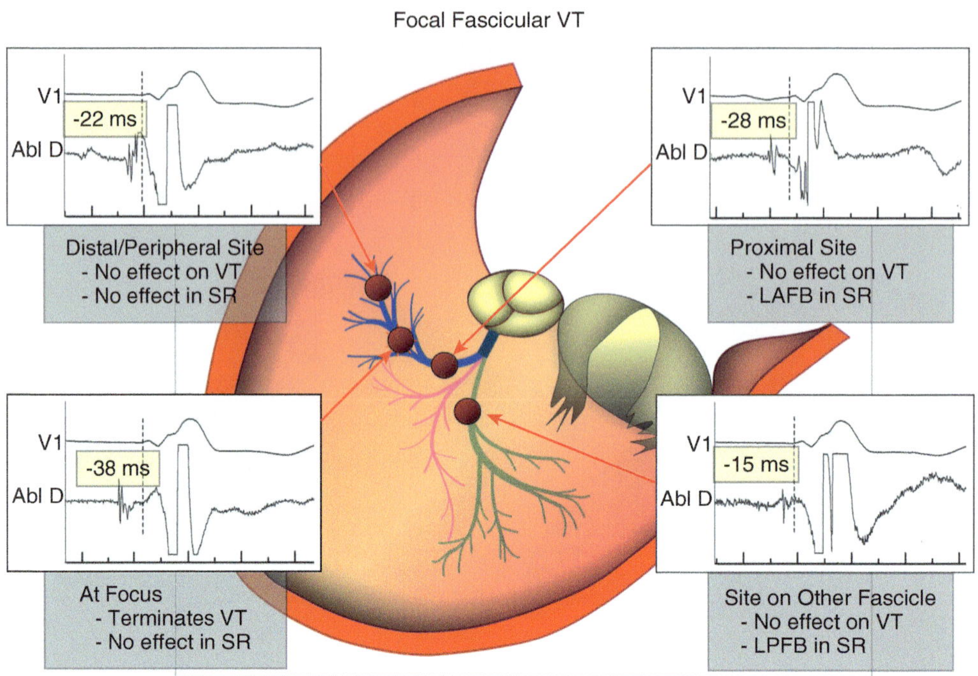

Fig. 21-12 shows the importance of ablation at the best site and implications of ablation at incorrect sites. SR, sinus rhythm; LAFB, left anterior fascicular block; LPFB, left posterior fascicular block.

Follow-up

- No further arrhythmias overnight, discharged the following morning
- Seen in follow-up 3 months later:
  - Sinus rhythm, no ectopy
  - Energy significantly improved
  - Very glad now that he had the procedure

Summary

- Fascicular tachycardias can be reentrant or focal (as in this case); overdrive pacing can differentiate these two causes
- It is important to determine whether the arrhythmia is junctional with bundle branch block/fascicular block or fascicular rhythm
- "Bump-mapping" can be useful but has limitations
- Correct targeting of the focus is critical for eliminating it and not causing unwanted "collateral damage" to other areas

22 Reentrant Fascicular Ventricular Tachycardia

Case Presentation

The patient is a 30-year-old man with four episodes of severe palpitations. In the first episode, the patient had palpitations and near-syncope while playing basketball. He was taken to the local ER, and his blood pressure was 110/80 mm Hg and wide complex tachycardia was 200/min. He was given adenosine, metoprolol, and diltiazem, but there was no effect. Arrhythmia was ultimately slowed and terminated. He was hospitalized and underwent an electrophysiology (EP) study; no arrhythmia was initiated. He was diagnosed with probable atrial tachycardia and treated with metoprolol, and subsequently discharged. Subsequent episodes were with and without exertion and stopped spontaneously after 15 to 40 min. He was found to have normal exercise capacity, and findings of physical examination and echocardiogram were normal; baseline ECG was normal too. The EP study found no inducible arrhythmias, and he was referred for a repeat EP study and possible ablation.

Baseline ECGs

What Is the Rhythm? [Fig. 22-1]

- VT?
- SVT with aberration?
- Fascicular?

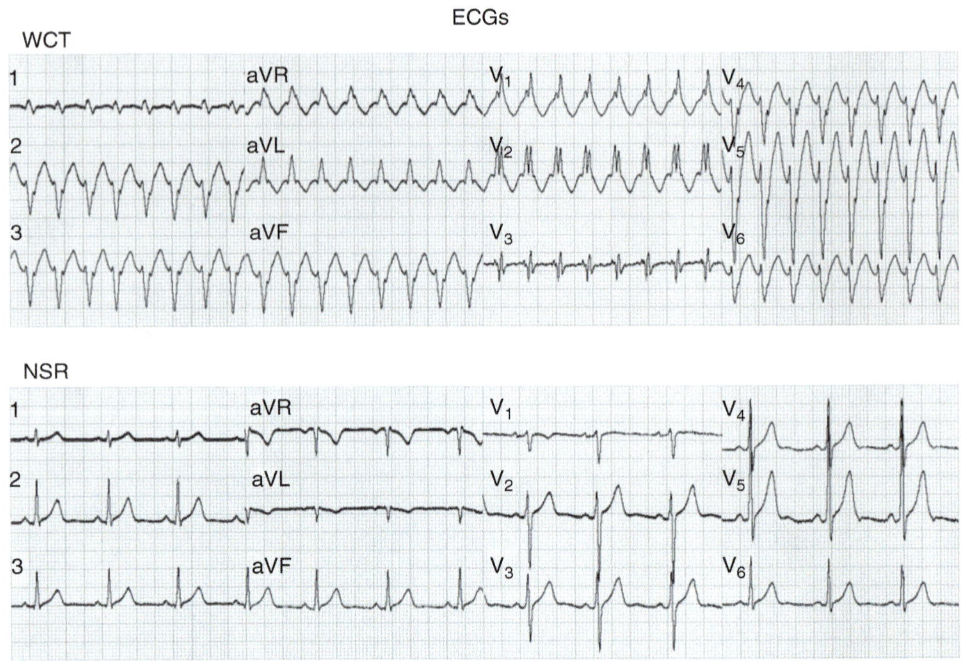

Figure 22-1

As shown in Fig. 22-1, the QRS during the wide complex tachycardia (WCT) is about 130 ms in duration and has RBBB pattern that in V1 and V6 is more consistent with ventricular tachycardia (VT; the rR′ in V1, R/S ratio <1 in V6), but the R-wave peak time in lead 2 (<50 ms), rS interval in a precordial lead <100 ms (Brugada criterion), qR pattern in aVR, and ventricular activation velocity index in V2 and V3 (>1) favor supraventricular tachycardia (SVT). P waves are not clearly evident (thus one cannot determine dissociation of atrial activity). There are no pathologic Q waves during the WCT or sinus rhythm to suggest old infarction. There is no preexcitation or any other abnormality of the QRS or repolarization to suggest a cardiomyopathy. Thus the WCT is either an atypical form of aberration during SVT or it is VT in the absence of structural heart disease. It is notable that no arrhythmias could be initiated at the prior EP study, but some VT in normal hearts as well as some focal atrial tachycardias may be difficult to initiate.

Baseline Atrial Pacing and Arrhythmia Induction

What's Going on Here? [Fig. 22-2]

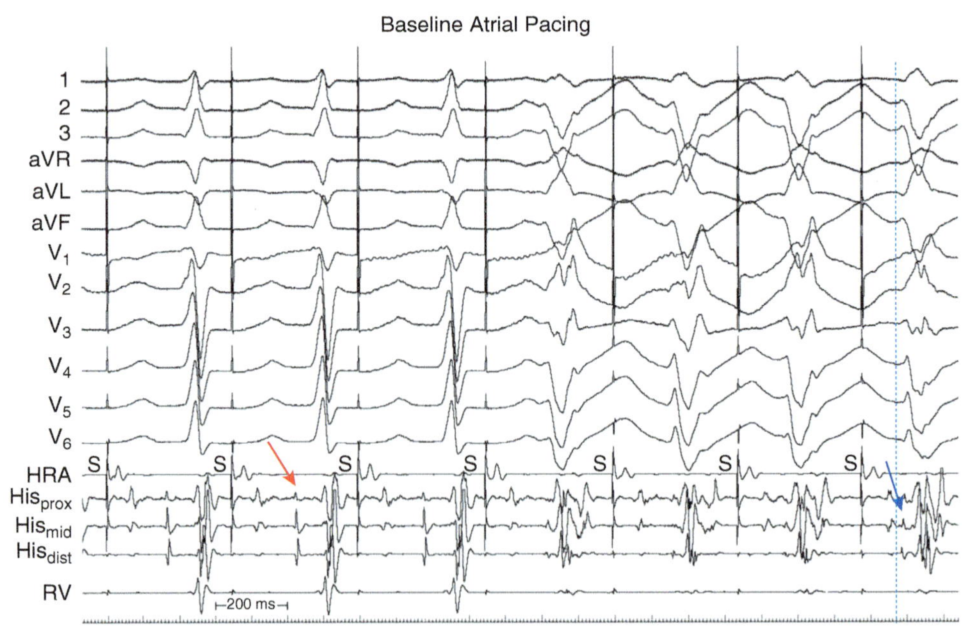

Figure 22-2

During atrial pacing (S) at the beginning of the study (to determine AV Wenckebach cycle length), the WCT occurs (Fig. 22-2). Note the His potential *(red arrow)* with a normal HV interval (45 ms) during atrial pacing on the left half, and the much shorter HV interval during WCT on the right half (in fact, a negative HV interval—the His *[blue arrow]* is after the QRS onset *[dashed line]*). Three situations exist during which the His potential consistently occurs after the QRS onset: 1) ventricular preexcitation, 2) ventricular pacing, and 3) ventricular ectopy/tachycardia. Because this would be an unusual pattern of preexcitation and is definitely not ventricular pacing, VT is favored as the diagnosis. Although many electrophysiologists do not routinely use His recording catheters during EP studies, the simple recording of a consistent His potential can have great diagnostic benefits.

Baseline Arrhythmia

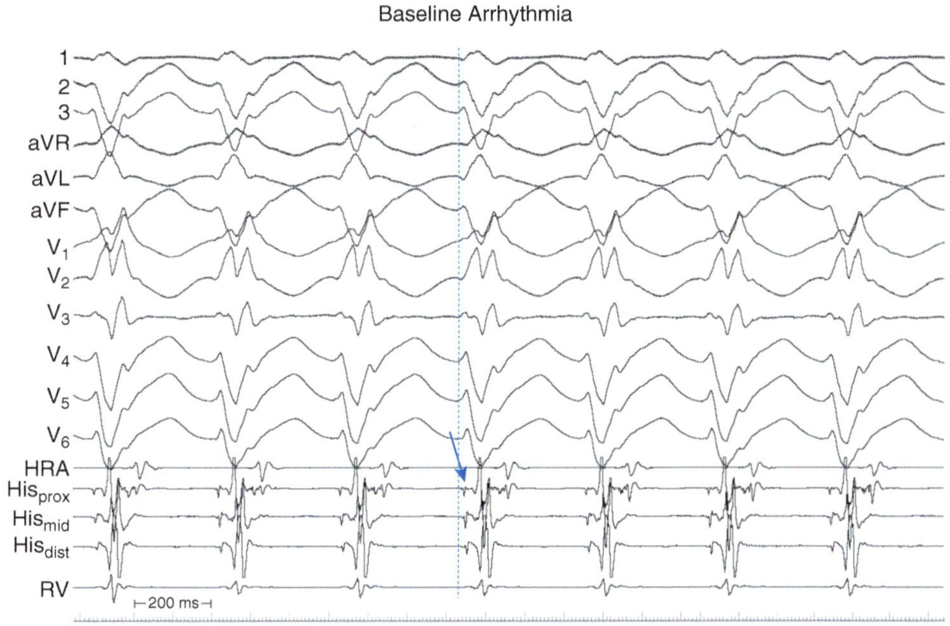

Figure 22-3

After cessation of atrial pacing, VT continues as shown in Fig. 22-3. The *blue arrow* is clearly seen after the QRS onset *(dashed line)*. Note that there is a 1:1 V:A relationship (explaining why dissociation was not evident on the regular ECG). The direction of propagation of the His recordings appears to be proximal to distal; this would be unusual with a retrogradely activated His during VT, but in this case, only the proximal electrodes are actually at the His bundle (with a modest atrial recording in sinus and VT), whereas the middle and distal electrode pairs are probably recording a right bundle potential. The VT spreads from the left ventricle (with RBBB pattern), ascends the left bundle branch, conducts retrogradely through the His bundle, and turns around to activate the right bundle branch anterogradely (whereas the right ventricle may be directly activated across the ventricular septum).

Table of Differential Diagnosis

RBBB WCT in the Absence of Structural Heart Disease:

- Verapamil-sensitive left posterior fascicular (LPF) reentry
- SVT with aberration
- Focal fascicular VT
- Papillary muscle focal VT
- Other myocardial VT

The differential diagnosis of an RBBB WCT includes several possibilities as noted above. Table 22-1 offers some useful distinguishing features. In our case, already determined to be VT, there is a Q wave in lead 1 but not V1, and the rhythm did not terminate with adenosine.

TABLE 22-1 Differential Diagnosis of RBBB WCT

	Verap. Sens. LPF VT	SVT + Aberration	Focal Fascicular VT	Papillary Muscle VT
QRS duration	Rel. narrow	Rel. narrow	Rel. narrow	Wider
Q in lead 1	Yes	Yes	No	No
Q in lead V1	No	No	No	Yes
AV relationship	Variable	1:1	Variable	Variable
Adenosine effect	None	Termination	Termination	None
HV interval	−20 ms	45 ms	−15 ms	−10 ms
Earliest Purkinje	(throughout)	After His	Before His	Before His
Overdrive pacing	Constant return cycle	Variable effects	Overdrive suppress	Overdrive suppress
Pacemapping	Not helpful	Not helpful	Excellent	Excellent

Right Ventricular Pacing in VT

Figure 22-4

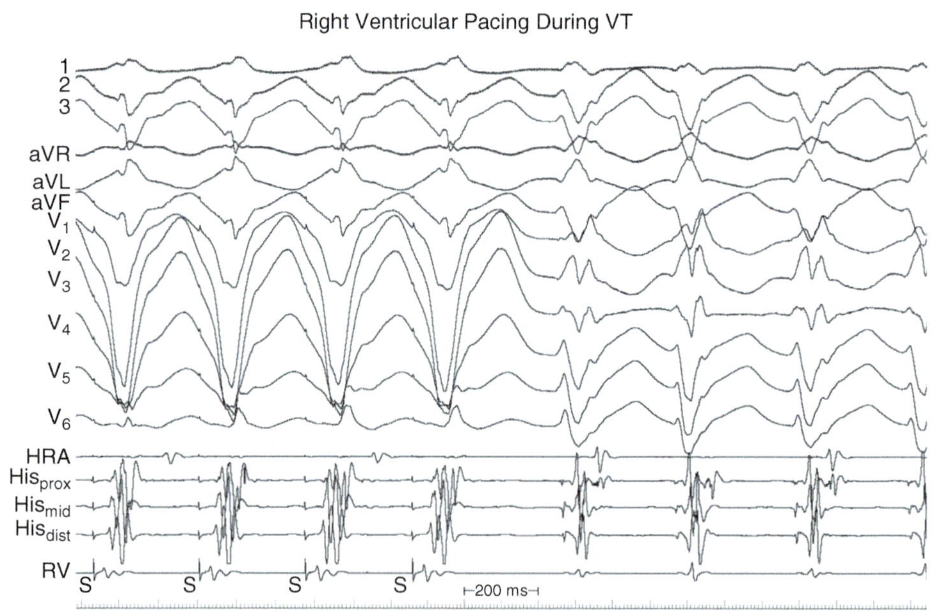

As seen in Fig. 22-4, VT had a stable cycle length of 315 ms; the timing of the first beat of VT after the end of right ventricular overdrive pacing during VT did not vary over a range of cycle lengths (310 ms, shown here, to 280 ms); pacing at 270 ms terminated VT. This would not be expected with a focal process, in which overdrive suppression of an automatic focus occurs (faster overdrive pacing results in longer delay until VT resumes); termination of a focal arrhythmia with overdrive pacing is also unusual. A constant return cycle over a range of overdrive paced cycle lengths and eventual termination of VT with more rapid pacing is entirely consistent with reentry, however.

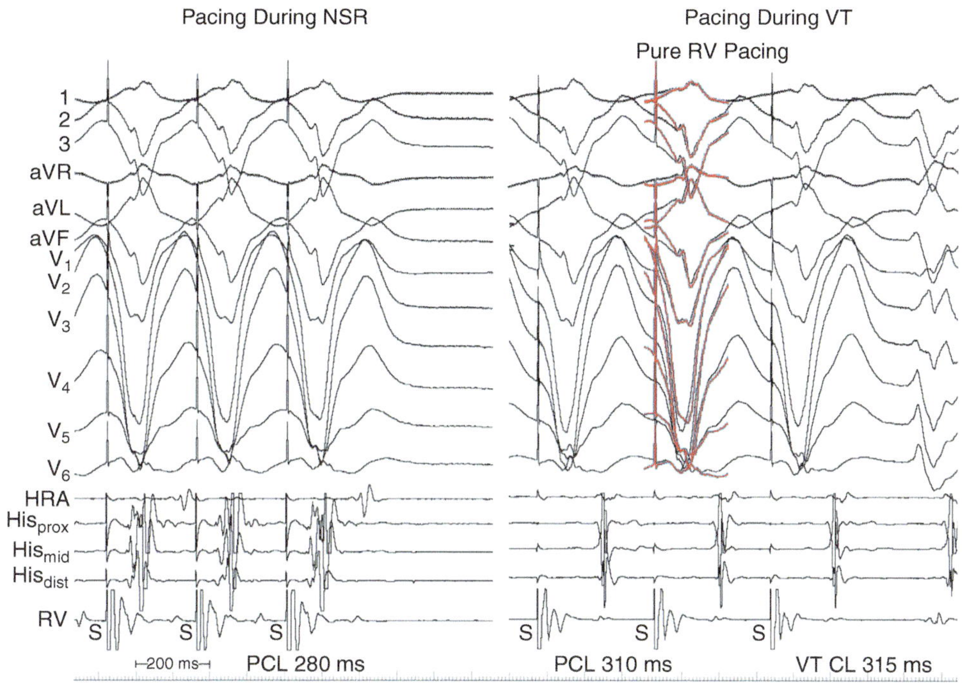

Figure 22-5

Pacing during VT may show fixed fusion (every QRS complex a consistent blend), and if so, is diagnostic of macroreentry. In Fig. 22-5, RV pacing during VT at a rate just slightly faster than VT is shown at *right*, and pure RV pacing (during sinus rhythm) at *left*. A single complex of pure RV pacing superimposed on RV pacing during VT shows little difference; it can be argued that V4 to V6 show some slight differences but these are minimal. Based on this one example, one may be tempted to conclude that because fusion is not evident, the rhythm is not macroreentry. This is an unwise conclusion, because although a single episode of pacing that shows fusion can diagnose macroreentry, it often takes pacing at many cycle lengths and different sites to show fusion. Based on all the information now available, the diagnosis of left posterior fascicular–related reentry ("verapamil-sensitive VT") seems secure at this point. Even though many VTs in the absence of structural heart disease terminate with adenosine injection, this one characteristically does not (although it does respond to verapamil). Before availability of adenosine, many cases of this VT were erroneously diagnosed as SVT because of their occurrence in otherwise healthy people, relatively narrow QRS in tachycardia, and termination with verapamil injection.

Mapping and Cartoons of Circuits

Figure 22-6

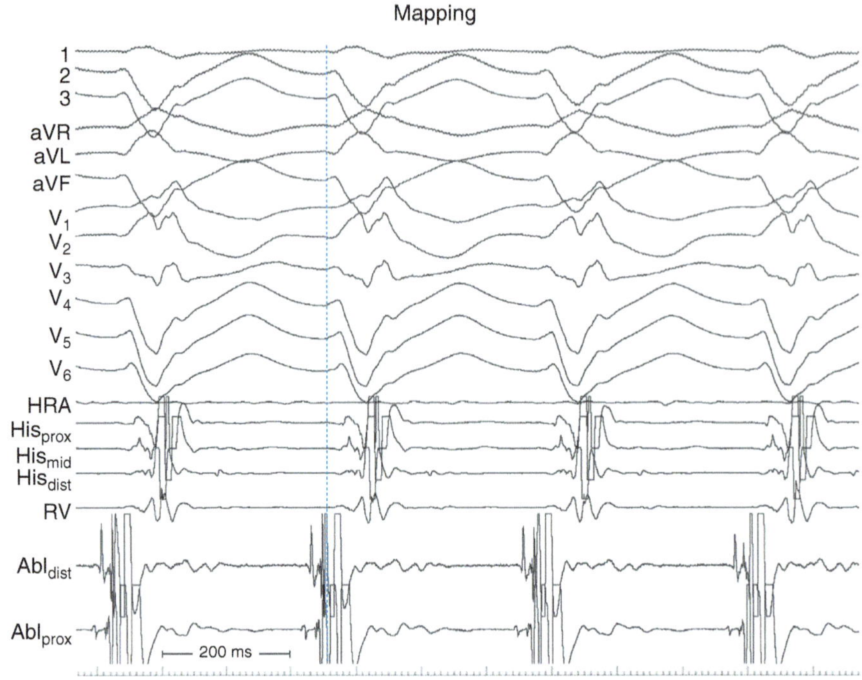

Having established a diagnosis of verapamil-sensitive left posterior fascicular VT, mapping can begin to find an appropriate ablation target. In previous years, finding the most presystolic Purkinje potential (10 to 40 ms, as in Abl_{dist} in the figure) was the goal; more recently, with the understanding that the posterior fascicle is the retrograde limb of tachycardia whereas a diastolic pathway composed of possibly partially depolarized Purkinje cells with calcium channel–dependent activation, or Purkinje cells in a false tendon, the target of ablation has become the lower turnaround site where the anterograde diastolic pathway joins the retrograde posterior fascicle. Recordings from the site in Fig. 22-6 may be >50 ms presystolic and have multiple deflections (as in Abl_{prox}), perhaps signifying activation of the two pathways.

Figure 22-7

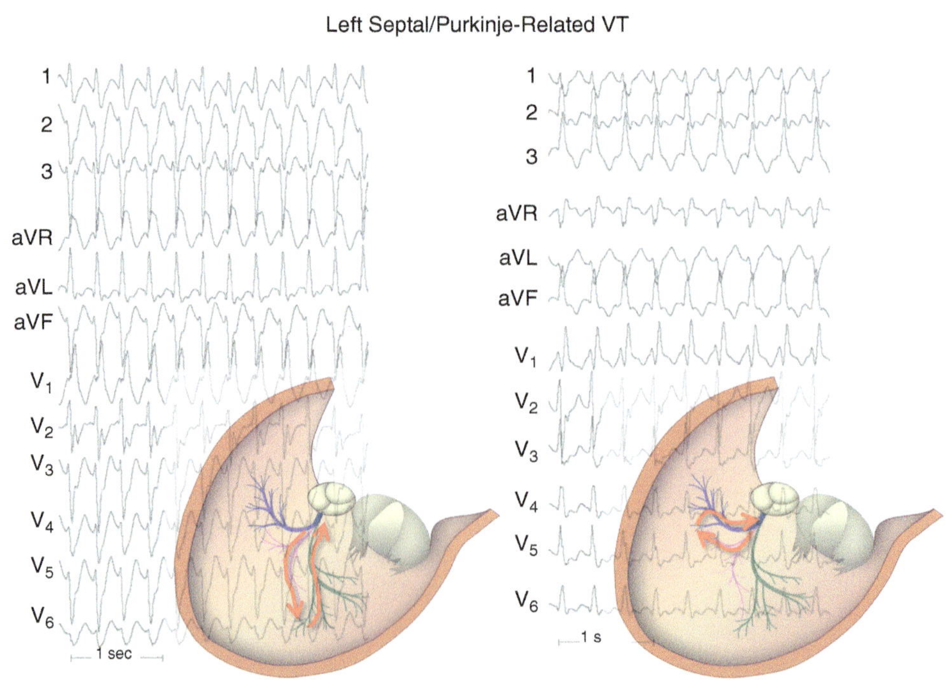

The verapamil-sensitive Purkinje-related VTs displayed in Fig. 22-7 usually involve the posterior fascicle, at left, but can also involve the anterior fascicle, as shown at right.

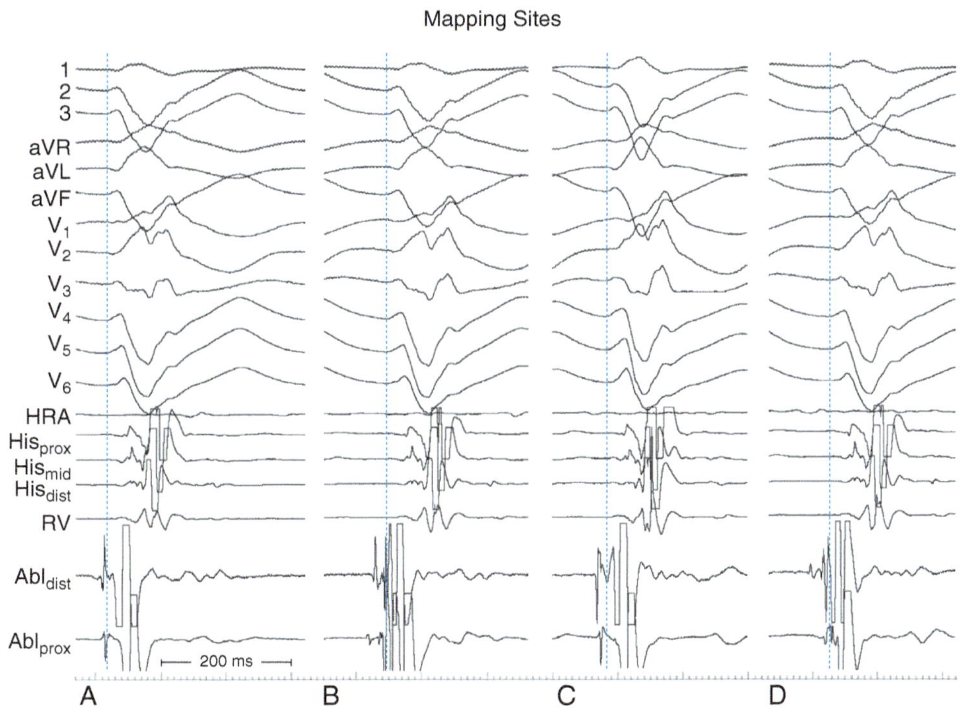

Figure 22-8

Several other mapping sites are shown in Fig. 22-8 (*dashed line* denotes onset of the VT QRS). Though all have presystolic potentials, which is the ideal target site? At site A, the distal electrogram precedes the proximal, but neither is very presystolic. At site B, the distal electrogram is earlier than that in A, but is later than the proximal recording and because ablation can only be done from the distal electrode, this site is not suitable either. At site C, the distal electrogram precedes the proximal, and both are reasonably presystolic, but the deflection is single rather than multiple and suggests posterior fascicle recording only. At site D, the distal electrogram precedes the proximal, is very presystolic, and is very complex (with multiple deflections). This is a very reasonable target site for ablation. Pacemapping during sinus rhythm at this site may or may not replicate the VT (because capture of surrounding myocardium may occur). Thus pacemapping is not a reliable tool for choosing ablation targets in this arrhythmia. Of note, these sites may be very sensitive to even mild catheter trauma, so great care must be taken to move the catheter tip slowly and cautiously; "bump termination" of VT may be followed by noninducibility for the rest of the procedure. Electroanatomic mapping systems that can record a three-dimensional location at which catheter trauma terminates VT can be used to guide ablation even when VT cannot be reinitiated (as long as location of the site was recorded at the actual time of catheter trauma and not seconds later, after the catheter may have moved).

Ablation

Figure 22-9

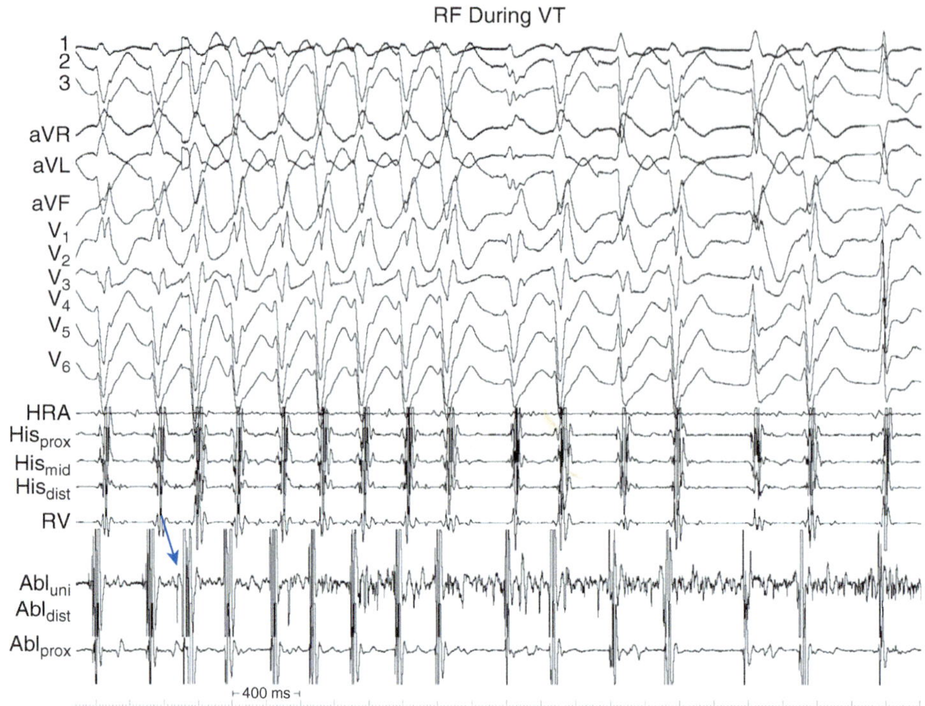

Radiofrequency energy is delivered at the target site during VT *(blue arrow)*. This causes a nearly immediate acceleration of the arrhythmia (more typical for focal automatic or triggered arrhythmias) and then "stuttering" of cycle length before termination (last complex), as seen in Fig. 22-9. VT could not be reinitiated thereafter, with or without isoproterenol infusion; the sinus rhythm ECG at the end of the procedure was unchanged (ie, no axis shift related to ablation near the His-Purkinje system). Ablation may lead to either acceleration or deceleration in this arrhythmia, whereas most reentrant tachycardias slow before termination during ablation.

Other Mapping Strategies

Left Septal/Purkinje-Related VT Ablation Strategies

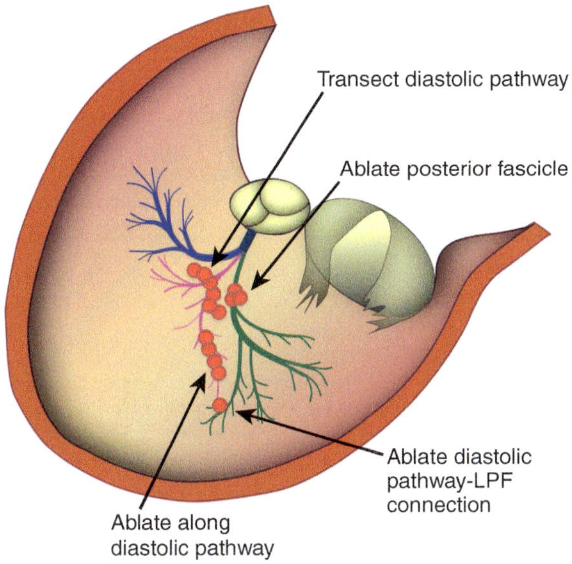

Figure 22-10

In Fig. 22-10, the left ventricle is shown opened along the lateral wall; the anterior fascicle is *blue*, the posterior fascicle is *green*, and the diastolic pathway during VT is shown in *purple*. Ablation strategies in this disorder include ablation at the site of connection of the left posterior fascicle and diastolic pathway (usually on the inferior left ventricular septum, as in our case); ablation along the diastolic pathway indicated by very delayed (and usually very small) potentials during sinus rhythm until these are eliminated; or linear ablation in the basal septum to try to transect the diastolic pathway. The latter may be the only option in cases in which VT cannot be initiated despite a reasonably clear diagnosis from the ECG during a prior spontaneous episode, or when catheter trauma during mapping precludes subsequent VT induction and thus mapping. Ablation of the posterior fascicle is not advised because this is a rather widely distributed structure and its elimination may require very extensive ablation (unwise in a normal heart).

Final Recordings

Figure 22-11

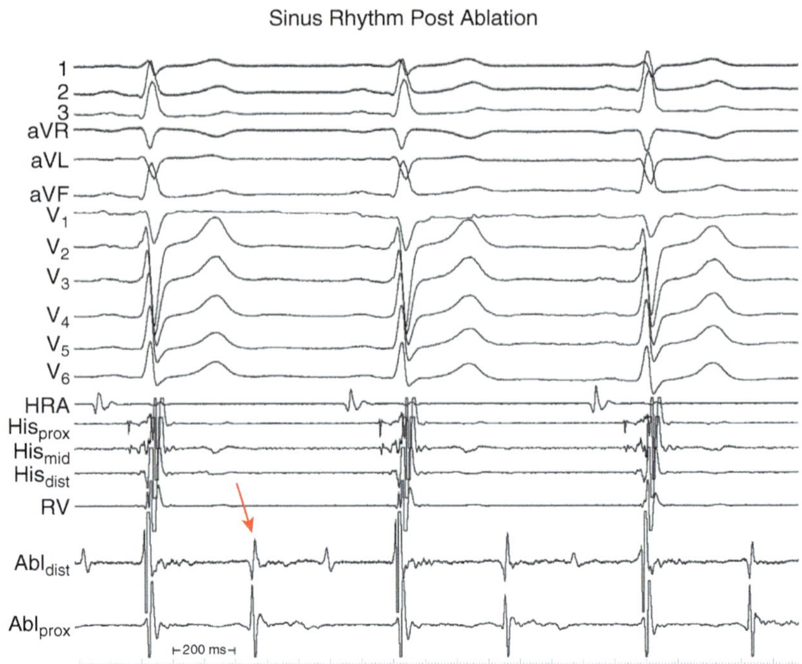

The large deflection indicated by the *red arrow* in Fig. 22-11 may be because of repolarization or recording artifact, or it may be a recording from the diastolic pathway used anterogradely during VT in these cases. Ablation at sites where these potentials are recording, eliminating them, is an effective ablation strategy when VT cannot be induced. Most often, if they can be recorded at all, they are much smaller than those shown here and may show multiple deflections.

Summary

- VT in the absence of structural heart disease often resembles, and is mistaken for, SVT on the ECG
- RBBB VT in the absence of SHD may be
  - Focal fascicular
  - Focal myocardial (including papillary muscle)
  - Verapamil-sensitive left posterior fascicular reentry
- In verapamil-sensitive left posterior fascicular VT, the diastolic pathway is very susceptible to catheter trauma
- Available mapping and ablation strategies include the following:
  - Targeting complex late diastolic potentials in VT
  - Targeting diastolic potentials in sinus rhythm
  - Transecting the presumed location of the diastolic pathway

Focal Cause of Ventricular Fibrillation

23

Case Presentation

The patient was a 45-year-old woman presented with cardiac arrest from polymorphic ventricular tachycardia (VT). Her history included ascending aortic disease with repair of aortic root and mechanical aortic valve replacement two months previously. She recovered well, but suffered unheralded cardiac arrest while shopping. She was hospitalized on cooling protocol, and she recovered well. The ejection fraction was 45%. Unfortunately she suffered recurrent polymorphic ventricular tachycardia/fibrillation. She was treated with amiodarone, beta blockade, and beta agonists, but there was no effect (i.e., she continued to have recurrent episodes of polymorphic VT). She was referred for electrophysiology (EP) study and possible ablation. What is the strategy?

Clinical Rhythm Strips

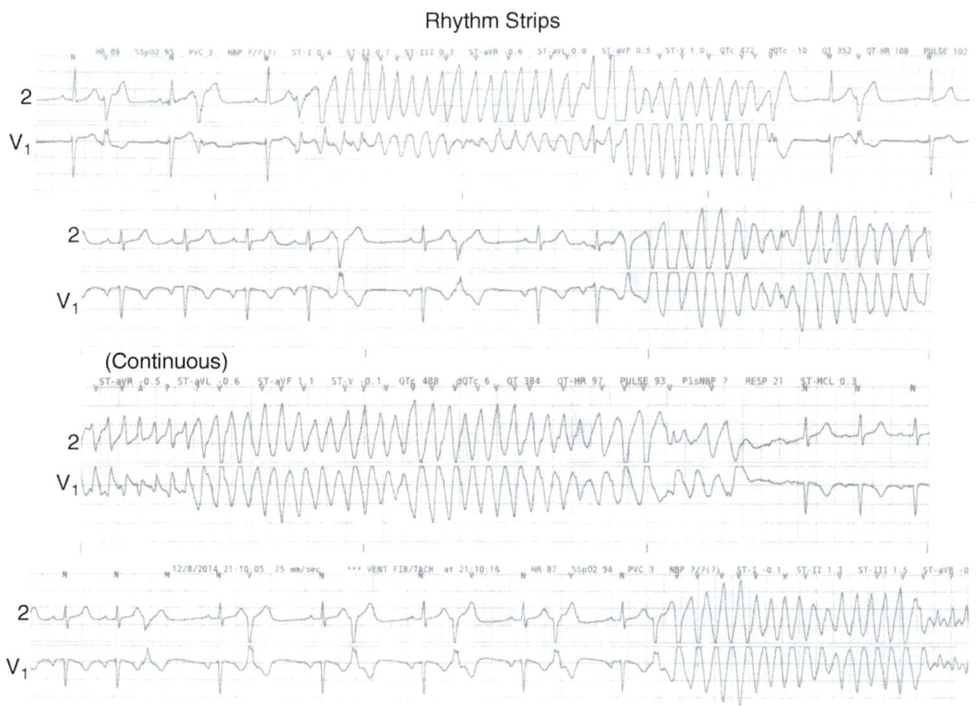

Figure 23-1

Repeated episodes of polymorphic VT (PMVT) are initiated by relatively narrow QRS premature ventricular complexes (PVCs) (Fig. 23-1).

Baseline ECG and Intracardiac Recordings

Figure 23-2

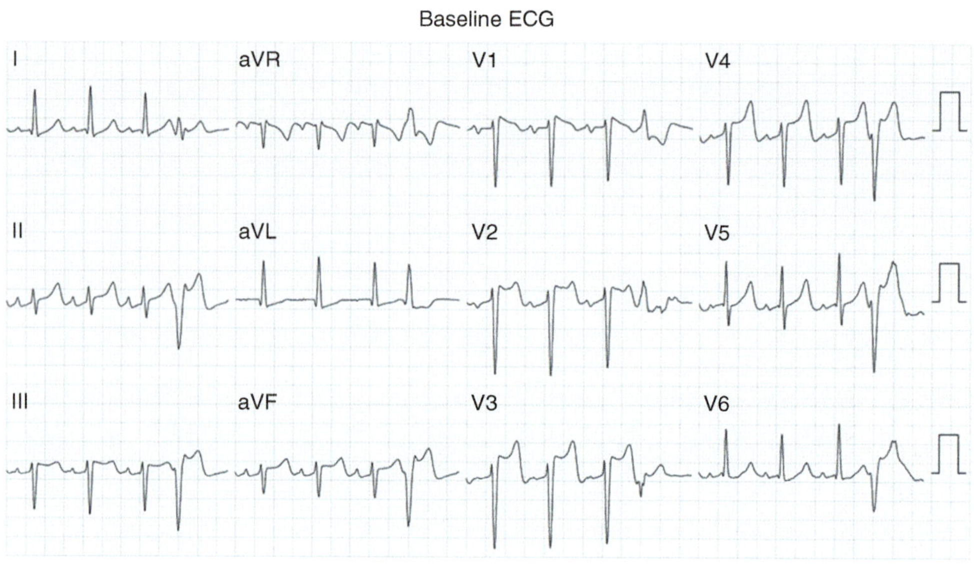

ECG (Fig. 23-2) is otherwise normal (apparent ST elevation in right precordial leads is an artifact of the recording system). The PVC morphology is clearer, having RBBB, leftward superior morphology, and the QRS complex is relatively narrow. Although not clearly fascicular, it is consistent with an origin in or near the Purkinje network.

Figure 23-3

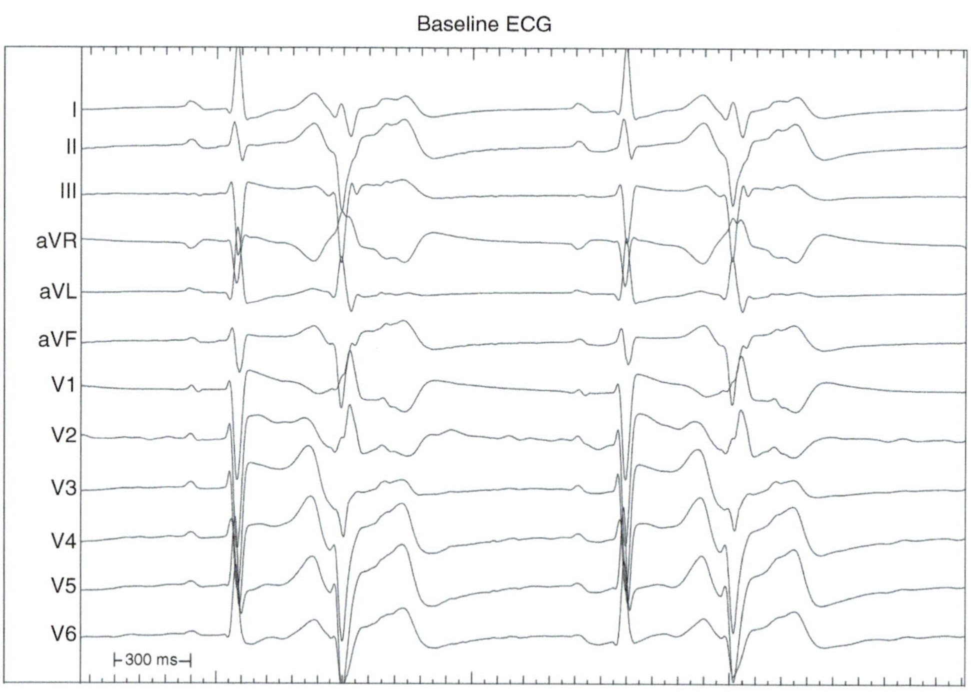

Fig. 23-3 is the typical PVC morphology that led to repeated episodes of PMVT.

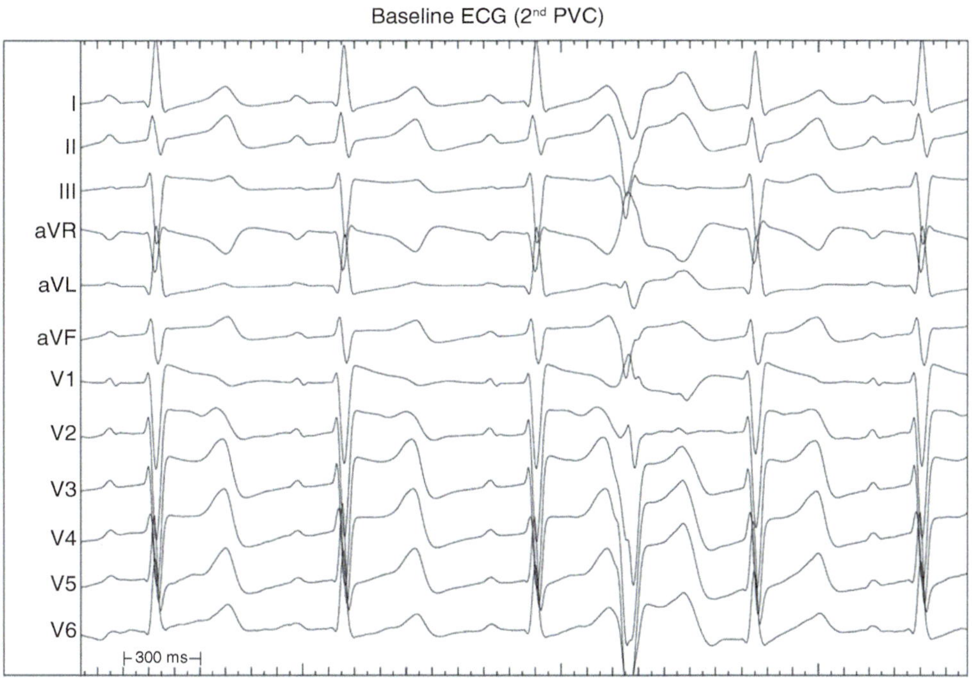

Figure 23-4

Fig. 23-4 is a second PVC morphology that occasionally preceded PMVT episodes (distinct from the main PVC, this has a rightward axis).

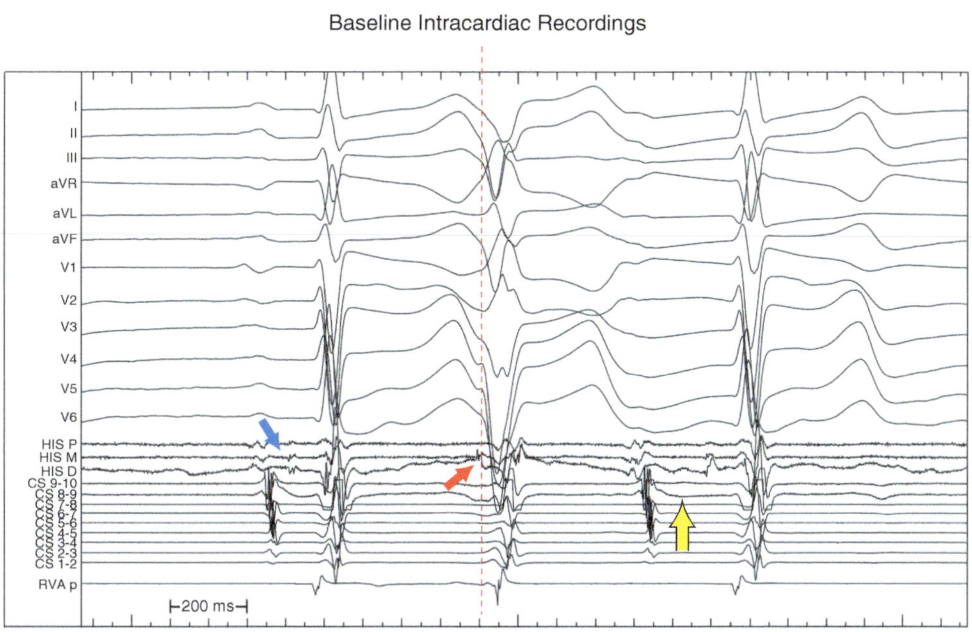

Figure 23-5

Once catheters are in place, an early indicator that the target PVC *(center)* is part of the Purkinje network is the finding that a His potential (Fig. 23-5, *red arrow*) precedes the PVC QRS onset *(dashed line)*. The *blue arrow* shows the same potential in sinus rhythm. The *yellow arrow* shows a longer AH interval on the following sinus complex, indicating retrograde penetration into, but not through, the AV node (concealed conduction).

Polymorphic VT Episodes

Figure 23-6

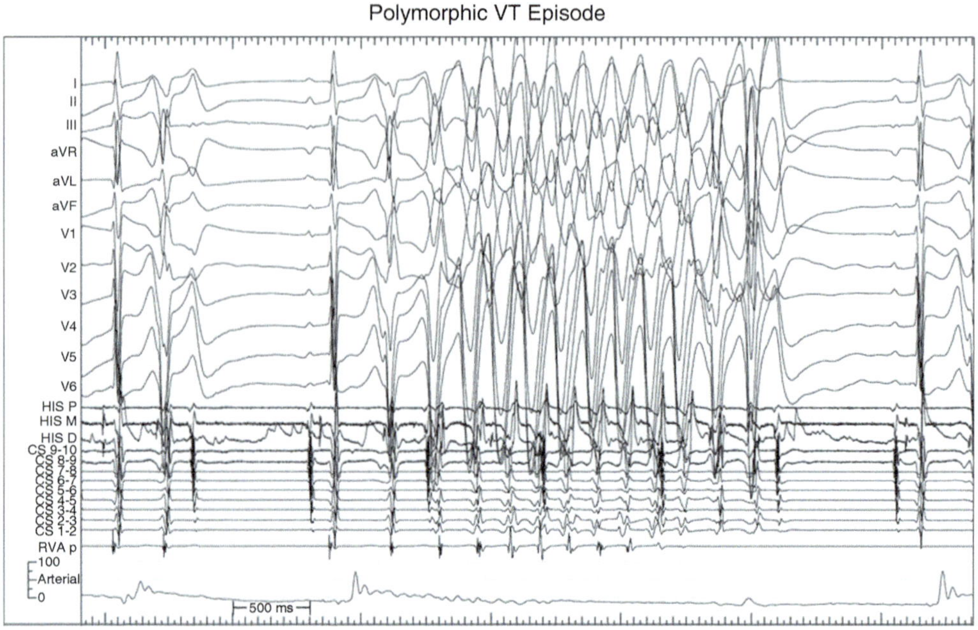

While setting up for transseptal catheterization to access the left ventricle, PVCs initiated several episodes of PMVT (Fig. 23-6). Note that this particular episode was initiated by a relatively narrow QRS PVC with a rightward axis (not the same as the original PVC). Note also that blood pressure *(bottom tracing)* practically disappears for the entirety of the PMVT episode (about 3 seconds).

Figure 23-7

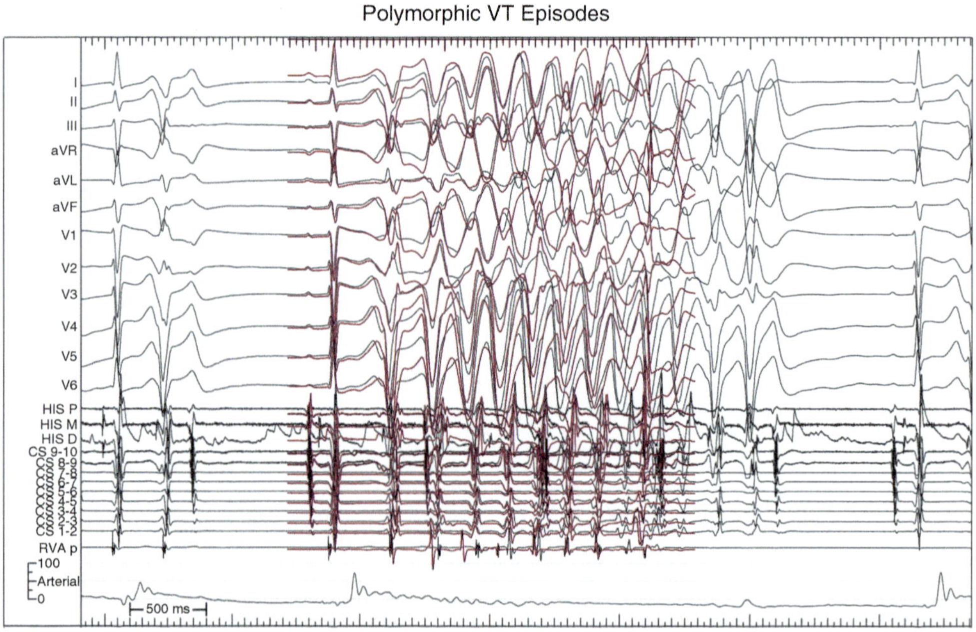

Two episodes of PMVT are shown in Fig. 23-7 with one superimposed on another; this illustrates that the first several cycles of episodes, although polymorphic, may be nearly identical. This suggests a consistent pattern of activation for these cycles until it becomes more disorganized.

Polymorphic VT Episode

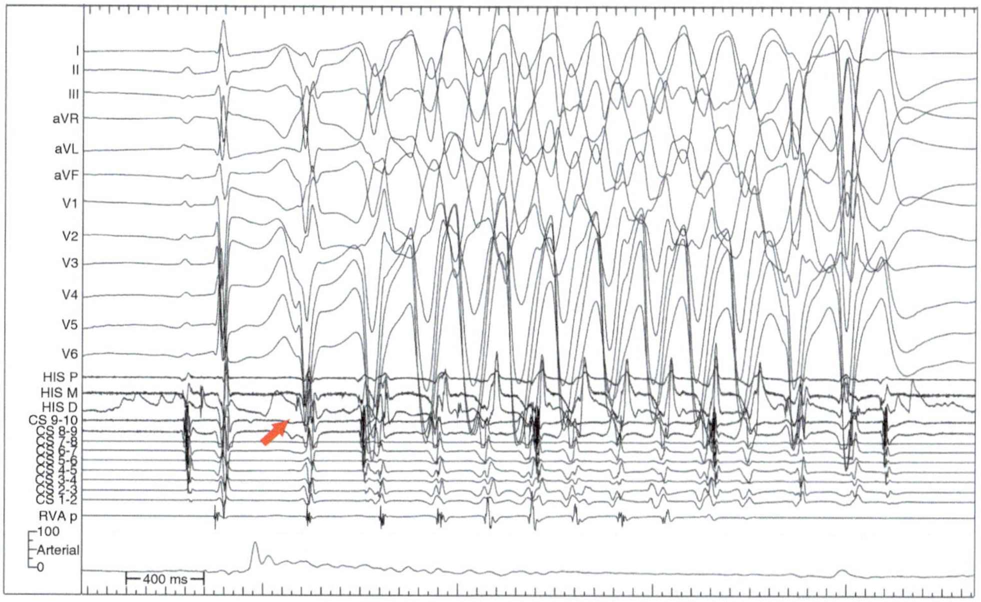

Figure 23-8

Fig. 23-8 is the same episode enlarged, to show the initiating PVC (right axis deviation) and the His potential at its QRS onset *(red arrow)*. This His timing can occur only when the origin is within the His-Purkinje system.

Polymorphic VT Episode Onset

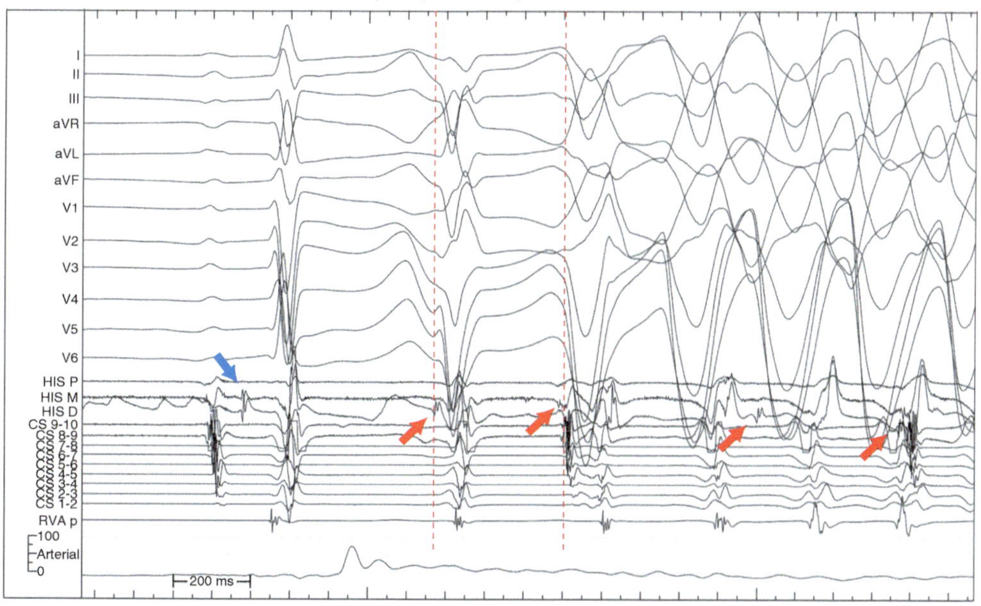

Figure 23-9

Fig. 23-9 shows the same episode enlarged further, to show the initiating PVC (right axis deviation) and the His potential (first *red arrow*) at its QRS onset *(dashed line)*. This sequence repeats, with a nearly identical QRS configuration, on the second complex. His potentials are seen with some, but not all, subsequent complexes. His potential in sinus rhythm is shown with a *blue arrow*.

Mapping Ventricular Ectopy

Is This a Good Ablation Site?

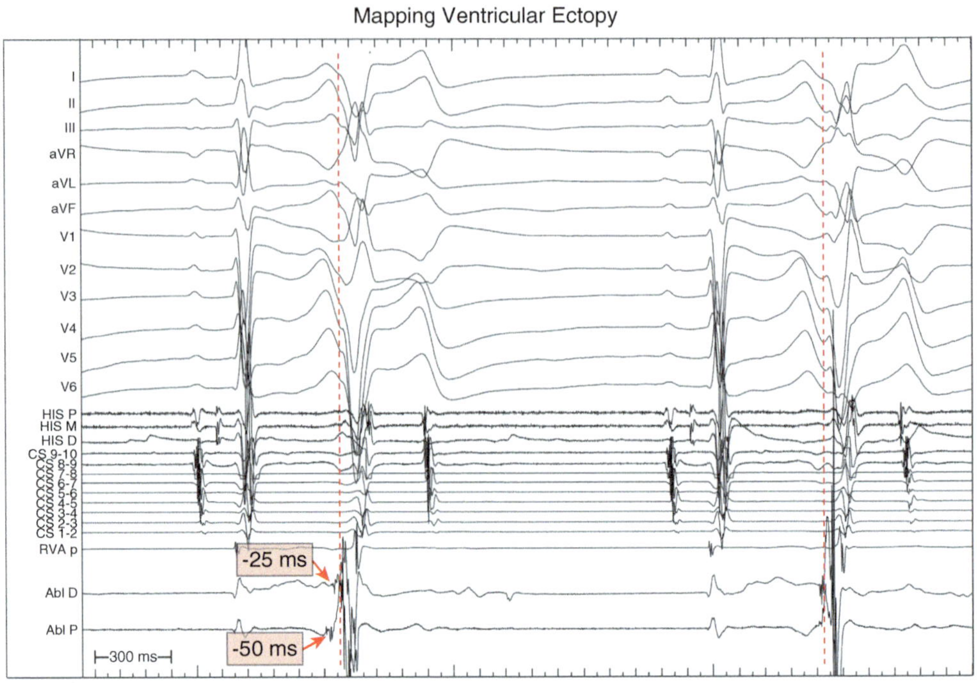

Figure 23-10

In Fig. 23-10, the ablation catheter has been introduced into the left ventricle via transseptal access (mechanical aortic valve). The PVC is of the rightward axis variety (which has caused PMVT episodes); the His potential is not well-seen with the PVC complex in this instance but an origin in or near the Purkinje network is suspected based on the sharp potentials on the ablation recordings. Whereas the distal mapping electrode has a potential 25 ms before QRS onset, which should be adequate for an ablation target, the proximal electrode has an even earlier potential. A Purkinje origin would be more strongly supported if such a potential were present in sinus rhythm (but it is not evident).

Where's the His? [Fig. 23-11] Is This a Good Ablation Site?

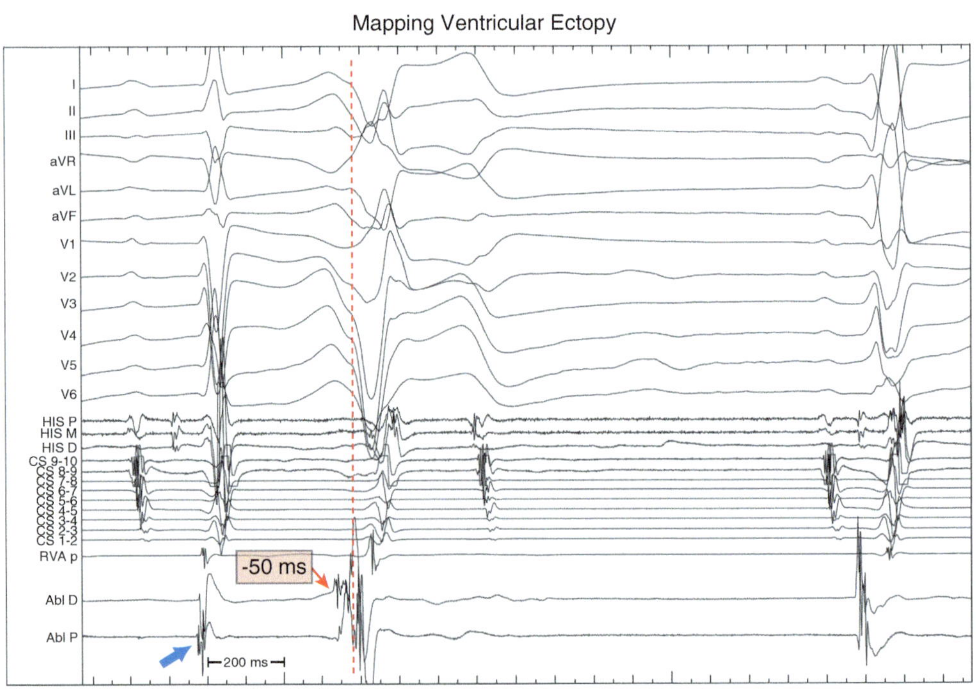

Figure 23-11

Fig. 23-11 shows another mapping site, this time with the distal electrode having a potential 50 ms before PVC onset. The His is again not clearly present during this PVC; the proximal electrode shows a potential consistent with Purkinje origin in sinus rhythm *(blue arrow)*. Attempts at pacemapping at these sites to confirm the same morphology as the PVCs produced inconsistent capture (not shown).

Site of RF and RF Delivery

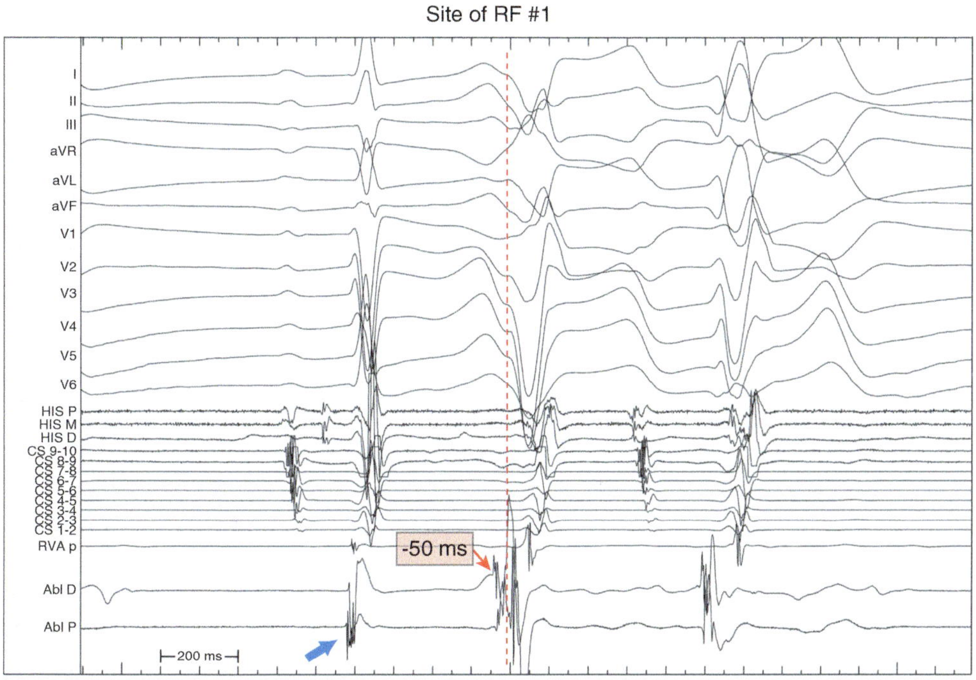

Figure 23-12

Fig. 23-12 displays the same mapping site, this time with the distal electrode having a potential 50 ms before PVC onset. The His is again not clearly present during this PVC; the proximal electrode shows a potential consistent with Purkinje origin in sinus rhythm *(blue arrow)*.

Figure 23-13

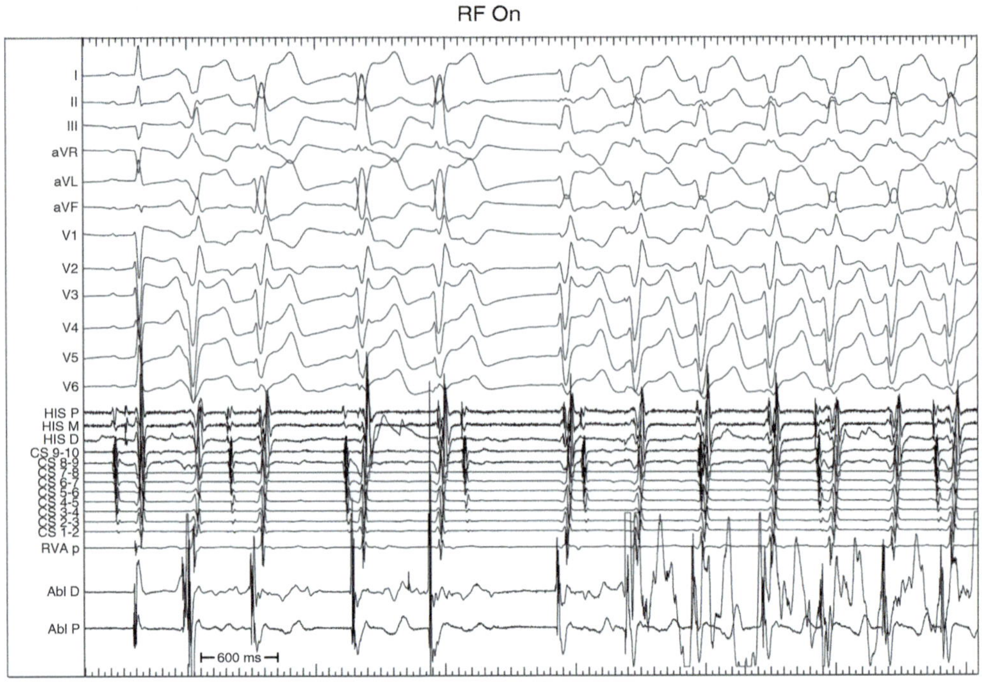

With onset of RF energy delivery *(right of center)*, a run of ventricular tachycardia occurs in Fig. 23-13, suggesting heating of tissue with the property of automaticity. This continued for another 25 seconds, then became nonsustained for 3 to 5 complexes, and then ceased.

Figure 23-14

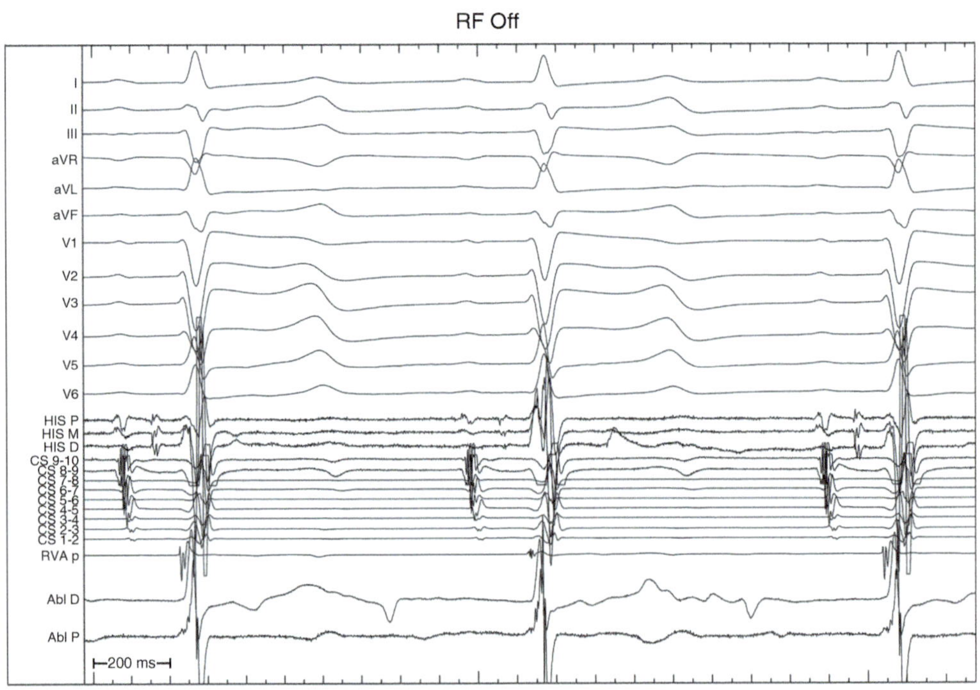

Purkinje potentials are no longer evident at the ablation site (Fig. 23-14). Note also the presence of left anterior fascicular block (not present until ablation). This was transient.

Additional Findings

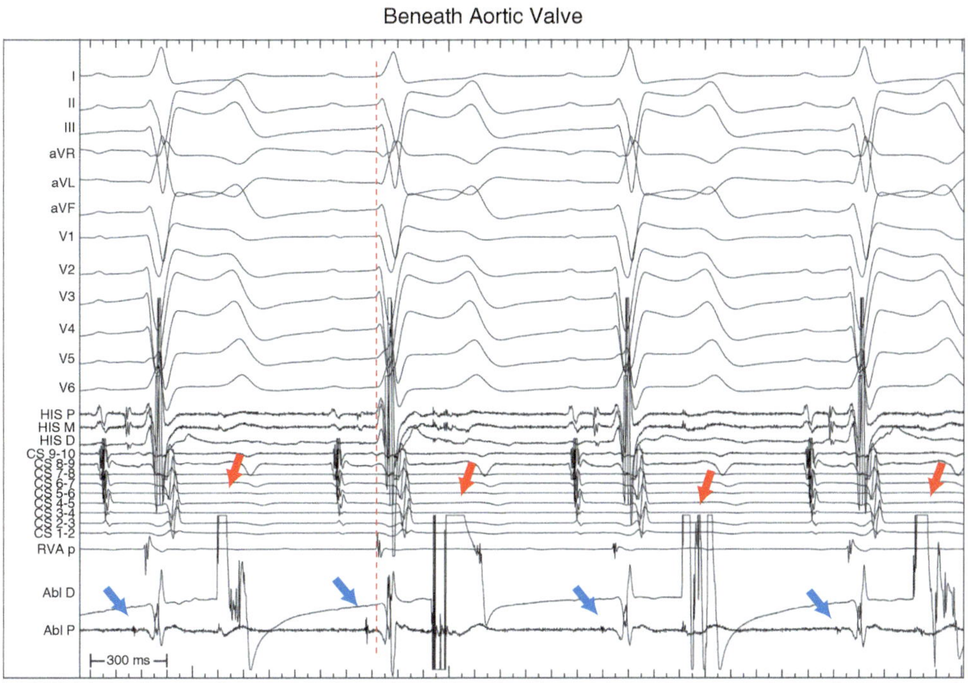

Figure 23-15

In Fig. 23-15, *blue arrows* are Purkinje potentials well before the QRS and without any discernible atrial activity—and recorded beneath the aortic valve. The location and timing are such that these are left bundle branch potentials. Mechanical injury to these can result in transient (or rarely, permanent) LBBB.

Red arrows denote electrical artifact generated by contact of the ablation electrode with the prosthetic valve struts. The signal is unphysiologically large, sharp, multicomponent, and not completely repetitive. It does not occur randomly, but periodically with cardiac motion.

Figure 23-16

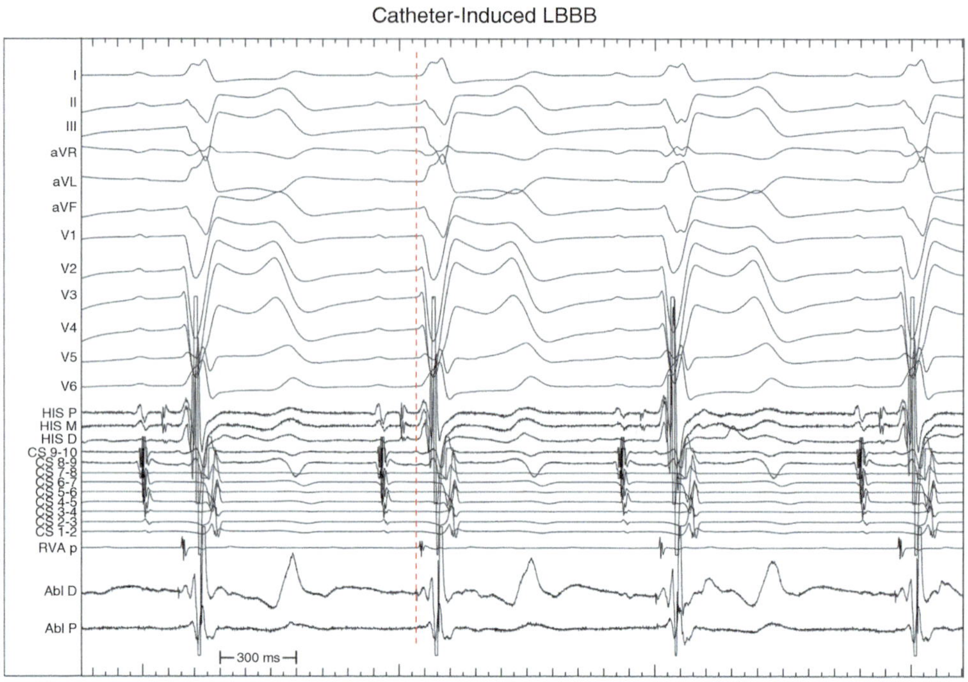

In Fig. 23-16, with development of catheter-induced LBBB, the LB potential is no longer before the QRS onset *(dashed line)* but coincident with or even slightly after it. This may not be actual *block,* but possibly significant *delay.*

The patient had no further arrhythmias over a 5-day in-hospital follow-up; LBBB resolved; an ICD was implanted before discharge.

Electroanatomic Mapping

Figure 23-17

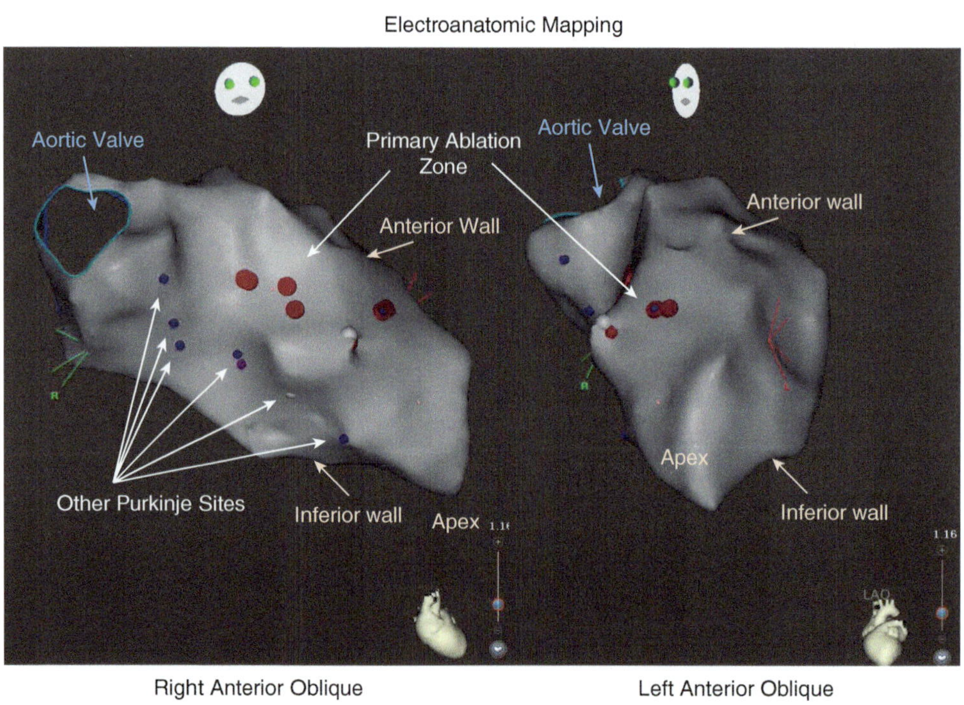

Fig. 23-17 displays an electroanatomic map during sinus rhythm showing sites with purple tags denoting Purkinje potentials as well as red tags denoting ablation sites where PVCs with the morphologies implicated in PMVT initiation were mapped, having Purkinje potentials preceding QRS complexes.

Summary

- Patients with recurrent polymorphic VT/VF should be investigated for severe ischemia, drug/electrolyte derangements, and progressive heart failure as well as the possibility that a focal source of fibrillation is responsible
- Focal-origin PMVT/VF has several features:
  - Episodes start with relatively closely coupled PVCs
  - Initiating PVCs generally have a consistent morphology
  - The first few cycles of PMVT are often identical
  - QRS complexes of initiating PVCs are relatively narrow
- Patients with suspected focal-origin PMVT/VF should have continuous telemetry with multiple leads (ideally full 12 leads) to determine whether initiations are stereotypic as well as defining morphology for potential ablation targets
- Ablation can be life-saving in such patients

24 Ventricular Tachycardia After Remote Infarction

Case Presentation

The patient was a 58-year-old man referred for catheter ablation of incessant ventricular tachycardia (VT). He had a history of inferior wall myocardial infarction (MI) and bypass surgery 5 years earlier. A ventricular fibrillation arrest occurred ~3 months after bypass surgery; he received a secondary prevention implantable cardioverter-defibrillator (ICD). At a routine office visit, his heart rate was 120/min, without symptoms; he was sent to the emergency room, where a tentative diagnosis of supraventricular tachycardia (SVT) was made (no response to adenosine). He was sent home, still in the arrhythmia, knowing that he had a scheduled visit with his electrophysiologist (EP) in several days. During the EP outpatient visit, VT was diagnosed and pace-terminated, and he was scheduled for elective ablation. Episodes recurred, and he was admitted to hospital for ablation more urgently.

Baseline ECG

Figure 24-1

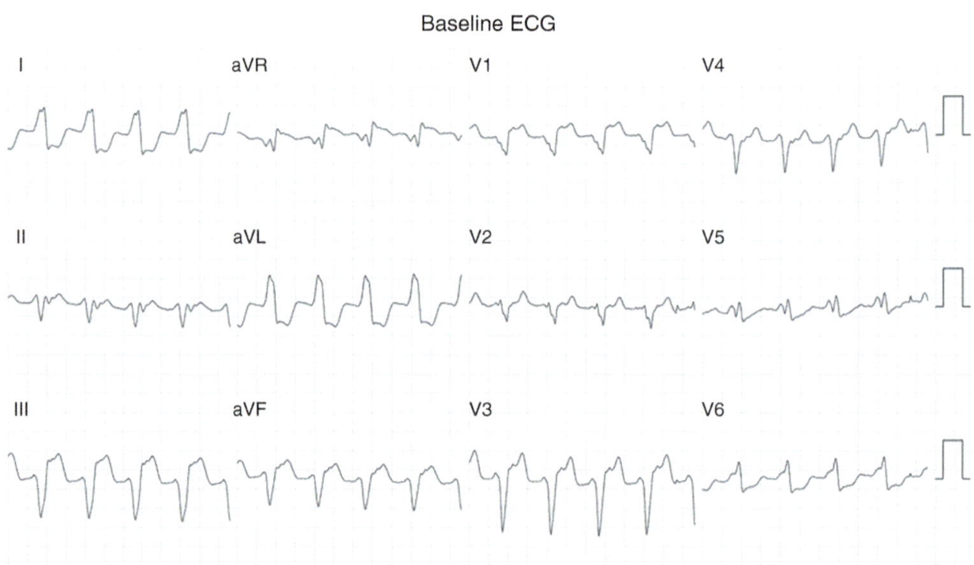

In Fig. 24-1, this appears to be ventricular tachycardia with 1:1 retrograde conduction (*arrows* show P waves). Consistent with his history of inferior infarction, this appears to have a source (focus or exit from circuit) on the inferobasal septal wall, according to published algorithms.

Atrial Pacing Initiates VT

Coronary Sinus Atrial Pacing

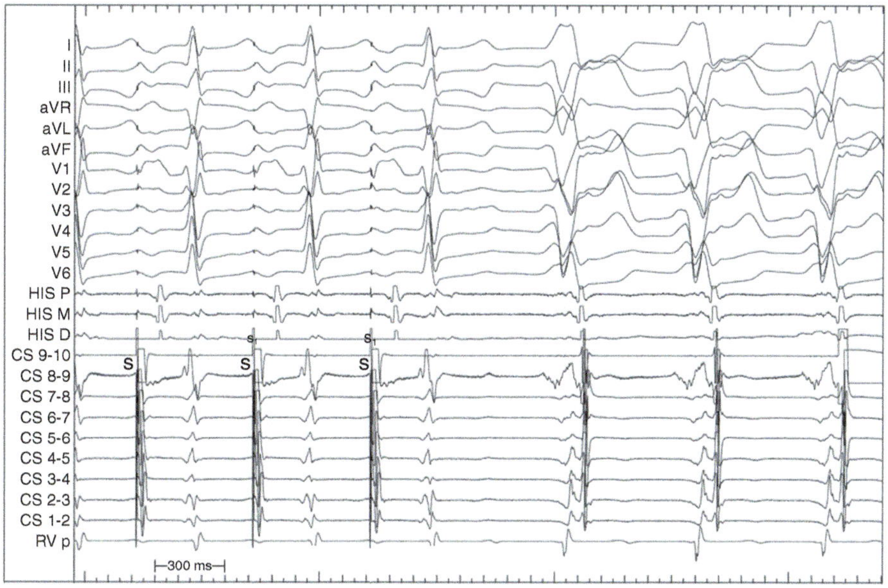

Figure 24-2

VT was accidentally terminated during catheter insertion and manipulation; in Fig. 24-2, during baseline atrial pacing, it is reinitiated. This unanticipated finding is quite unusual with VT at all, but when it occurs, most often a triggered (focal) mechanism is responsible for the VT.

Right Ventricular Overdrive Pacing

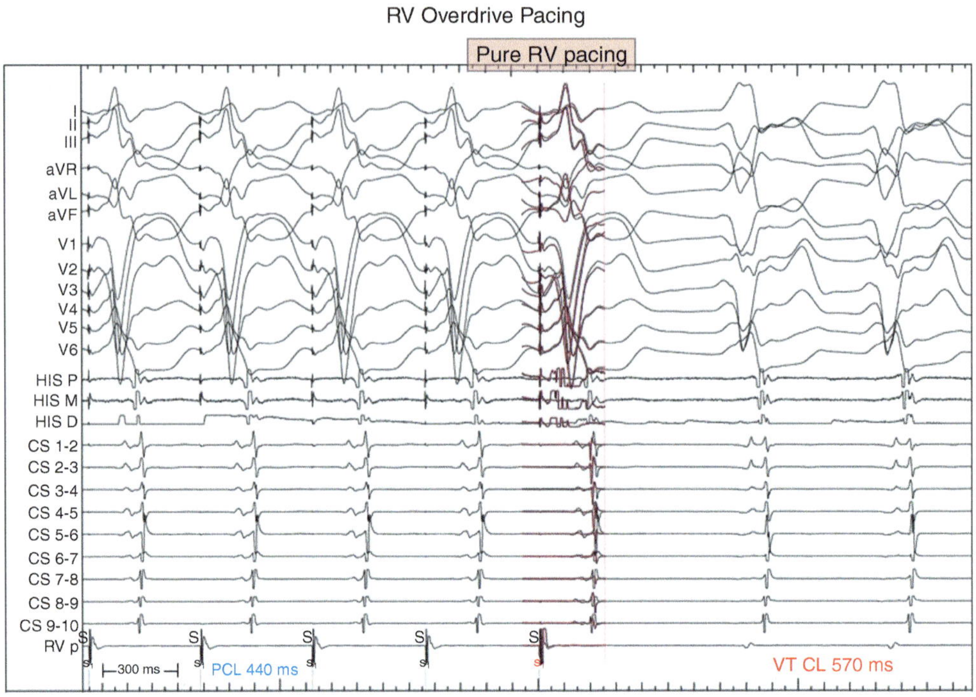

Figure 24-3

Incessant VT may be either focal or reentrant in origin. Because there was a question as to the VT mechanism (focal vs macroreentry) based on how it was initiated with atrial pacing, overdrive ventricular pacing was performed to investigate further. In Fig. 24-3, overdrive pacing at 440 ms is performed from the right ventricular (RV) outflow region, to maximize differences between VT and paced wavefronts. A single complex of pure RV pacing from later in the procedure is superimposed in *red*. This looks very similar to the paced complex during VT with only some minor differences. Because there is no clear fusion, macroreentry cannot be diagnosed; however, the absence of clear fusion on one example of pacing does not allow us to conclude that the VT has a focal origin. As such, this provides no definitive diagnostic information. (PCL, paced cycle length; VT CL, VT cycle length.)

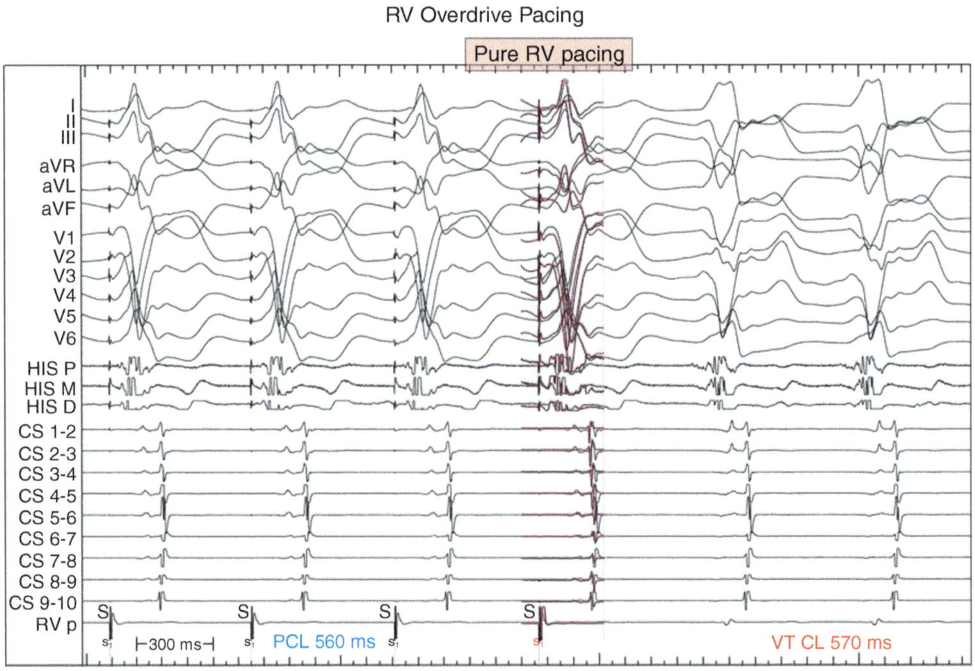

Figure 24-4

In Fig. 24-4, overdrive pacing is performed at a slower rate (560 ms) than before to further amplify differences between VT and paced wavefronts. Again, a single complex of pure RV pacing from later in the procedure is superimposed in *red*. This shows more differences between pure pacing and pacing during VT than were seen in Fig. 24-3: just as the more rapidly one paces during VT, the more all complexes will resemble pure pacing, it is also true that the *slower* one paces during VT (closer to VT cycle length), the contribution of the paced wavefront to the QRS will be less and fusion will be easier to discern. In this example, only minor differences are seen between pure pacing and pacing during VT (lead 1, V1-V2).

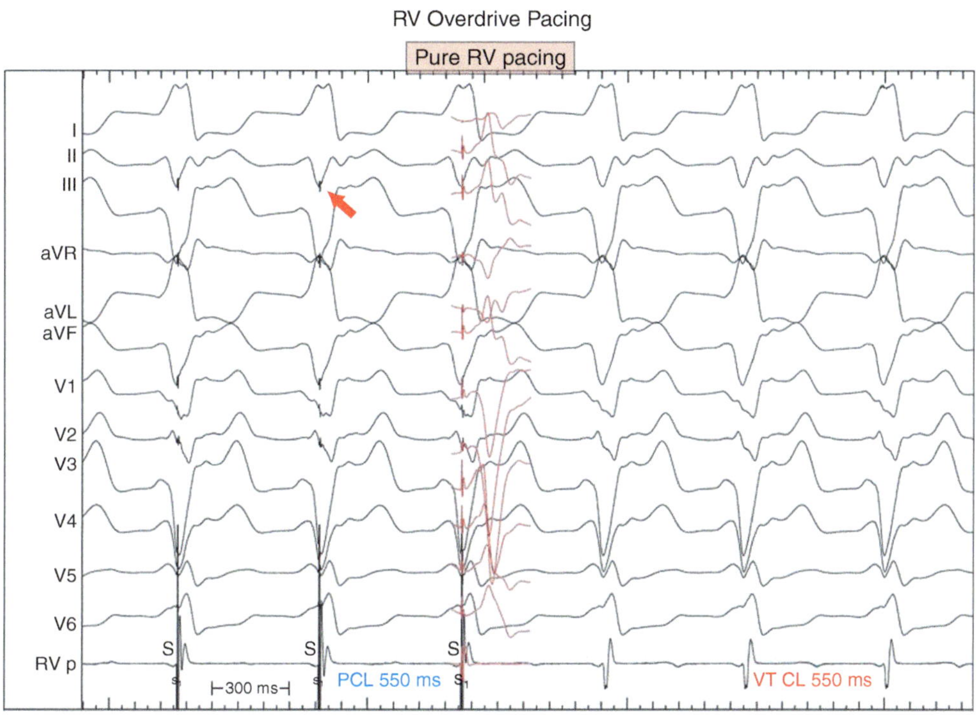

Figure 24-5

Fig. 24-5 shows RV overdrive pacing during VT a few minutes later; again, a single complex of pure RV pacing is superimposed for comparison. Now, it appears that there is a clear difference between pure pacing and pacing during tachycardia—indicating fusion—and thus implicating macroreentry. Note also that the stimulus artifact *(arrow)* occurs after the onset of a paced complex, another hallmark of macroreentry. Why is this so clear now when it was not before, pacing at the same site and rate? Careful inspection of the figure shows that one of the primary requirements for making an assessment has not been met: the VT has accelerated slightly such that its CL and the paced CL are the same. In fact, the RV electrogram starts before the stimulus—so none of it is actually captured (thus explaining why the "paced" QRS complexes are so similar to those of VT). This shows the importance of ensuring that capture is occurring when pacing during VT.

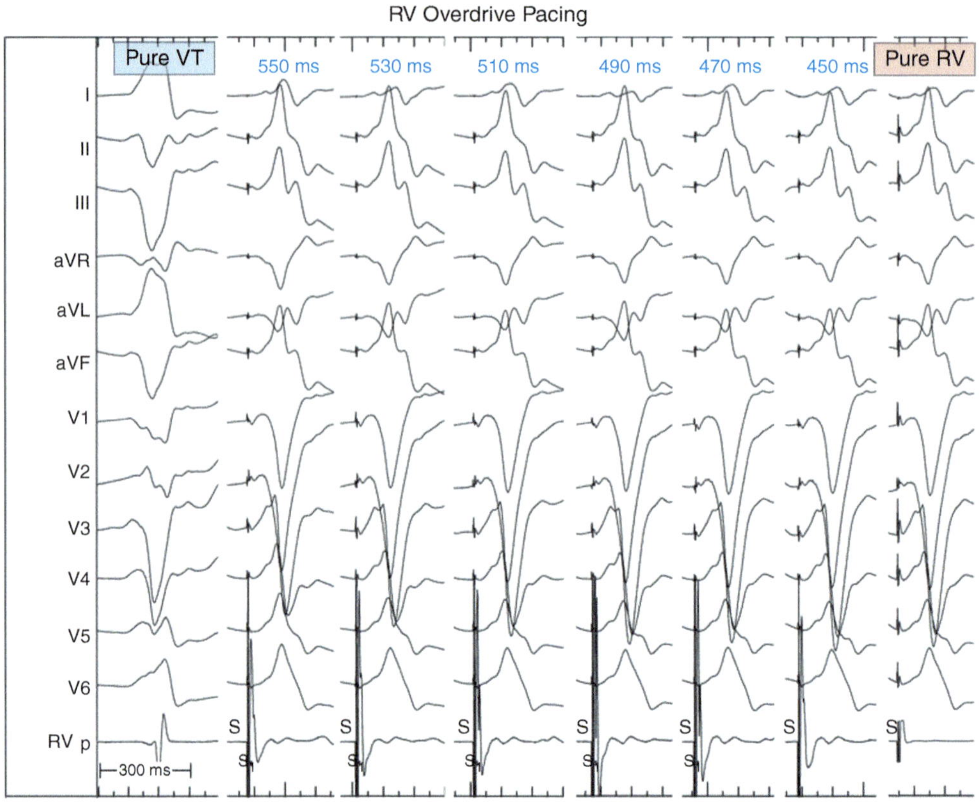

Figure 24-6

Fig. 24-6 shows a single complex of RV overdrive pacing at several different cycle lengths as indicated. Only minimal changes ("progressive fusion") are evident between pure tachycardia and pure pacing as the paced CL changes, mainly in lead 1. This is suggestive of macroreentry but not nearly as strong evidence as it could be.

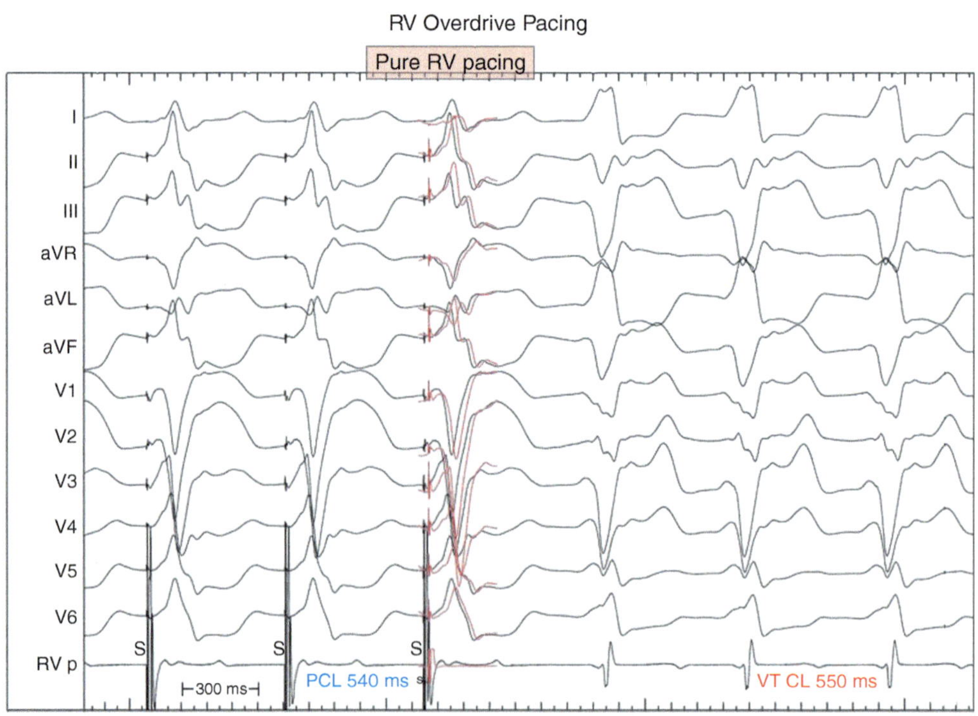

Figure 24-7

In Fig. 24-7, we have another attempt at overdrive pacing at 540 ms (when the VT CL is still 550 ms) that now shows clear differences between pacing during VT and pure RV pacing (again, a single complex of pure RV pacing is superimposed). This is clearly evident in lead 1 (also present in leads 3, aVR, aVL) and now makes a strong case for macroreentry.

Left Ventricular Mapping and Pacing

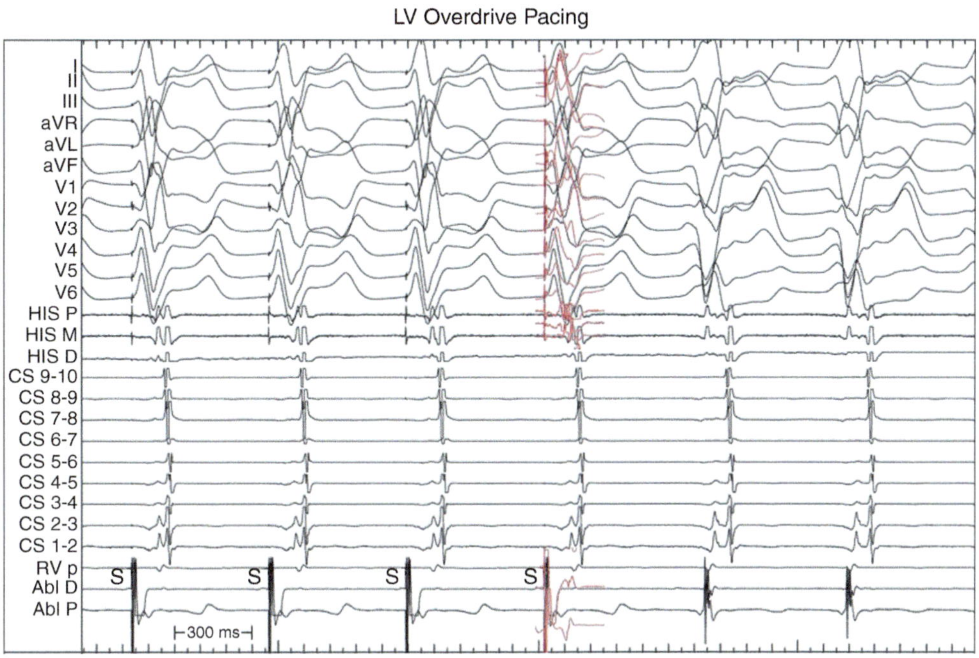

Figure 24-8

Another means of demonstrating fusion, and thus proving macroreentry, is to pace from different sites to accentuate differences between pure pacing and pacing during tachycardia. In Fig. 24-8, a site in the high lateral left ventricle is paced during VT, with a single complex of pacing from this site during sinus rhythm (superimposed in *red*) a few minutes later. Differences between the pure paced complex and those during VT are more marked than were evident with right ventricular pacing. Based on demonstration of fusion with different pacing strategies, macroreentry seems to be a secure diagnosis.

LV Mapping/Overdrive Pacing

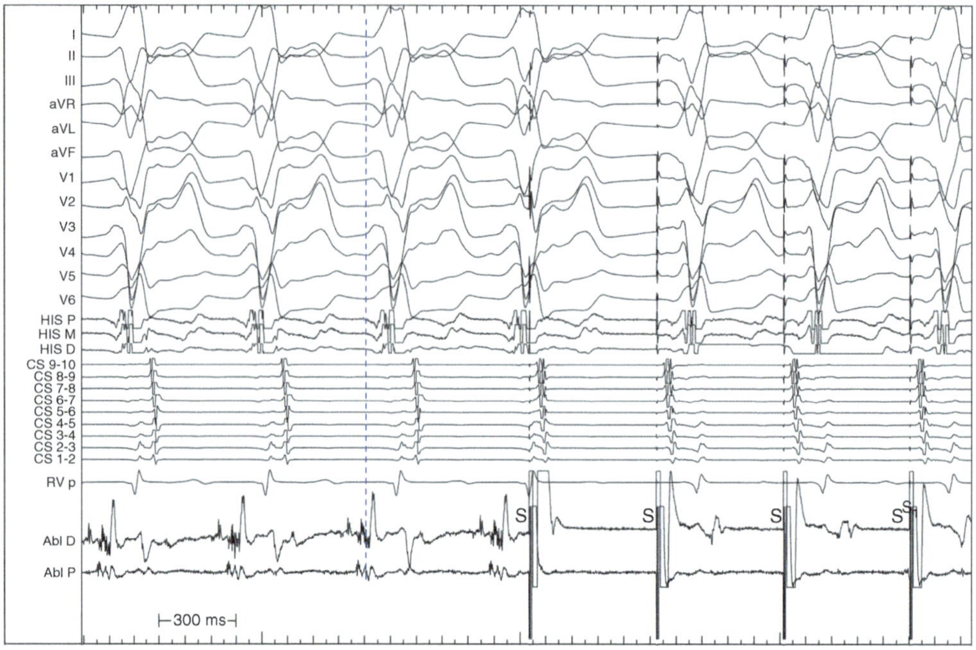

Figure 24-9

Having established a diagnosis of macroreentry, we can now search for a middiastolic electrogram as a reasonable ablation target site. In Fig. 24-9, a site in midlate diastole (*dashed line* denotes QRS onset) with marked fragmentation is shown. When attempting overdrive pacing at this site to determine whether it is a participant in tachycardia, the first stimulus results in termination of tachycardia without propagating to the rest of the heart *(arrow)*. If this is a reproducible phenomenon (ie, not spontaneous termination), it signifies that the site of stimulation is integral to the tachycardia circuit. After this stimulus terminates VT, further stimulation results in capture with a QRS configuration similar to VT, though not identical. Note also that the atrial recordings in the CS are accelerated to the paced CL and occur almost immediately after the stimulus artifact, indicating that there is direct atrial capture with stimulation (thus the catheter is very close to the mitral annulus).

Re-Initiation from LV

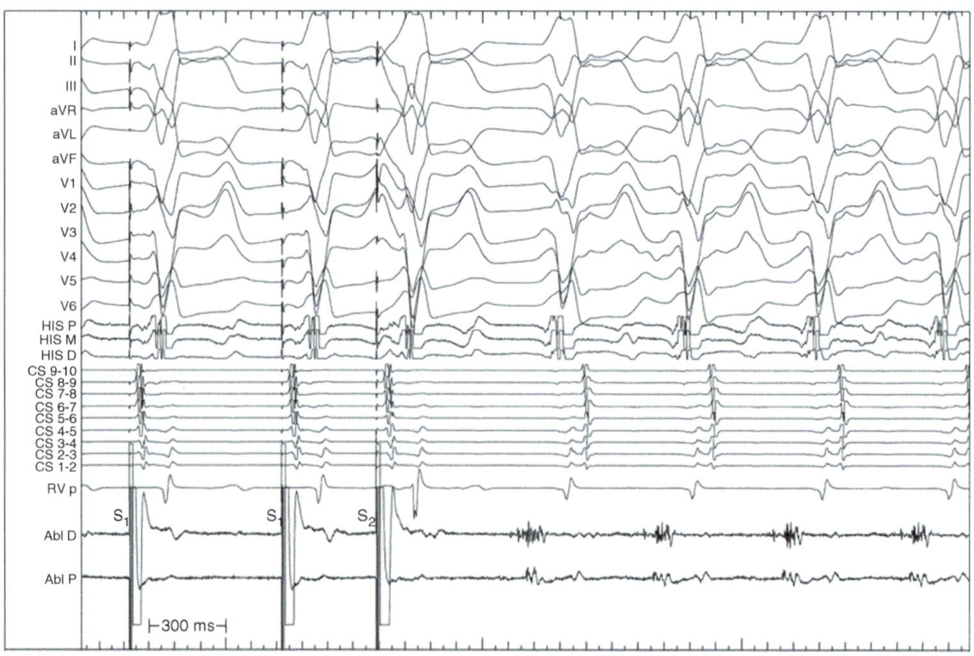

Figure 24-10

In Fig. 24-10, pacing from the same site readily reinitiated the same VT. Of note, the paced QRS complex is similar, but not identical, to that during VT. Part of the difference may be because of atrial capture during stimulation resulting in P-wave distortion of the QRS onset; capture of ventricular tissue outside the diastolic corridor could also contribute to differences between paced and VT QRS complexes.

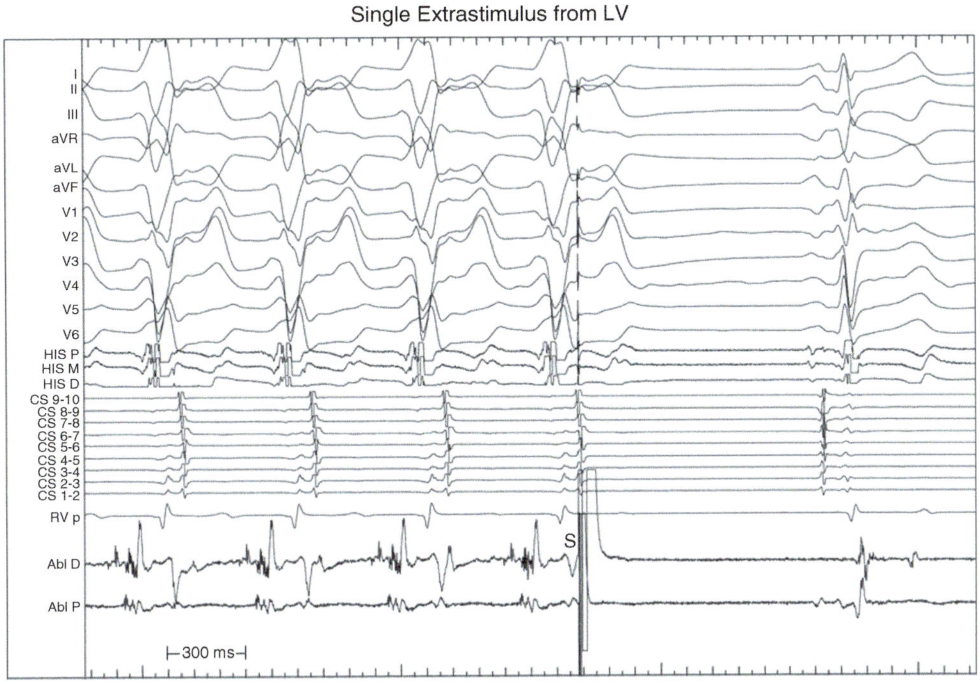

Figure 24-11

After VT was reinitiated, a single extrastimulus was delivered from the same location as in the prior figure; VT again abruptly terminates without propagation (Fig. 24-11). This sequence was repeated twice more, with the same results. This denotes that the site of stimulation is definitely within a critical isthmus of the VT circuit.

Figure 24-12

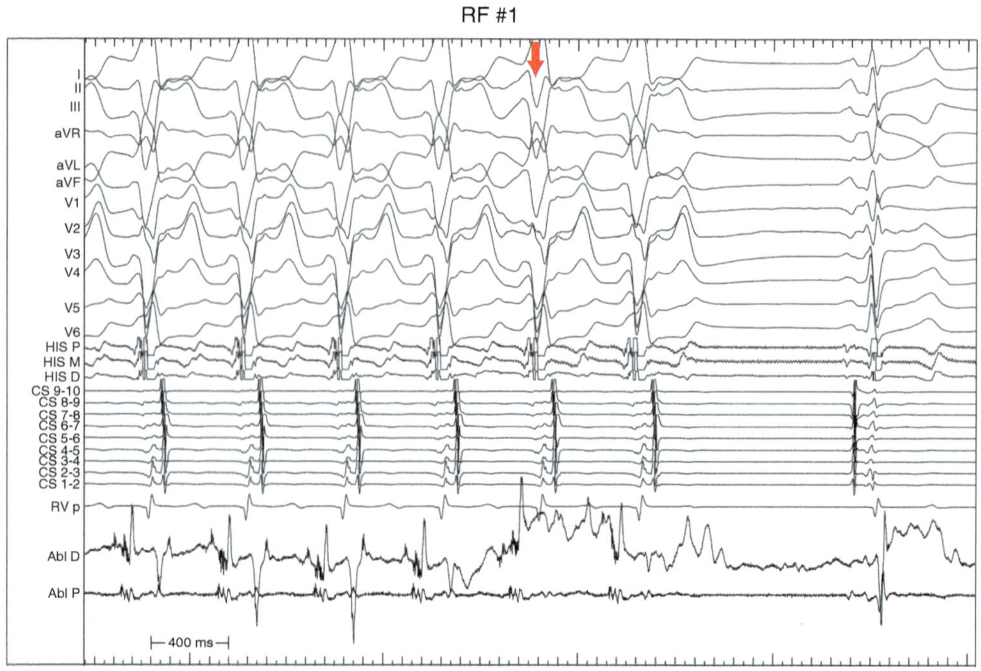

Based on the prior information that identified this site as being a critical part of the VT circuit, radiofrequency (RF) energy was delivered (*arrow*; Fig. 24-12). This resulted in termination of VT after <1 second.

Figure 24-13

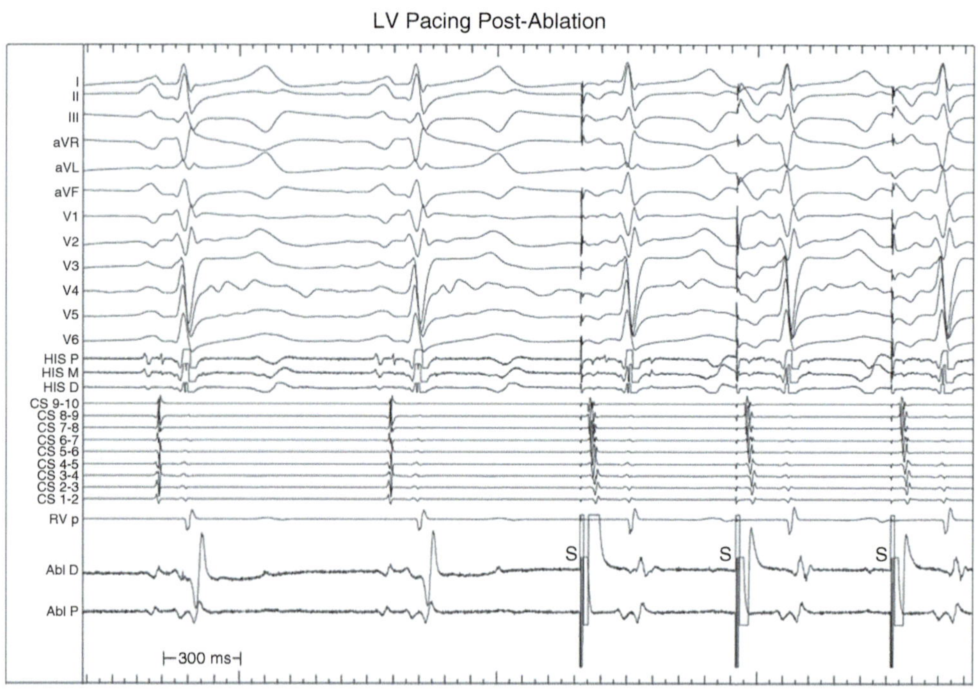

As had been seen earlier, pacing from this site in the left ventricle can also capture the atrium—but here (Fig. 24-13), after ablation, only atrium is captured. This is despite there being a larger ventricular electrogram at the site in sinus rhythm. Before ablation, it was possible to capture ventricular muscle in this area, but ablation has damaged enough remaining muscle that local ventricular capture is not possible. Subsequently, a full stimulation protocol from the right ventricular site as well as a different left ventricular site (at which capture was feasible) resulted in no inducible VT. The patient has had no VT on follow-up.

Electroanatomic Mapping

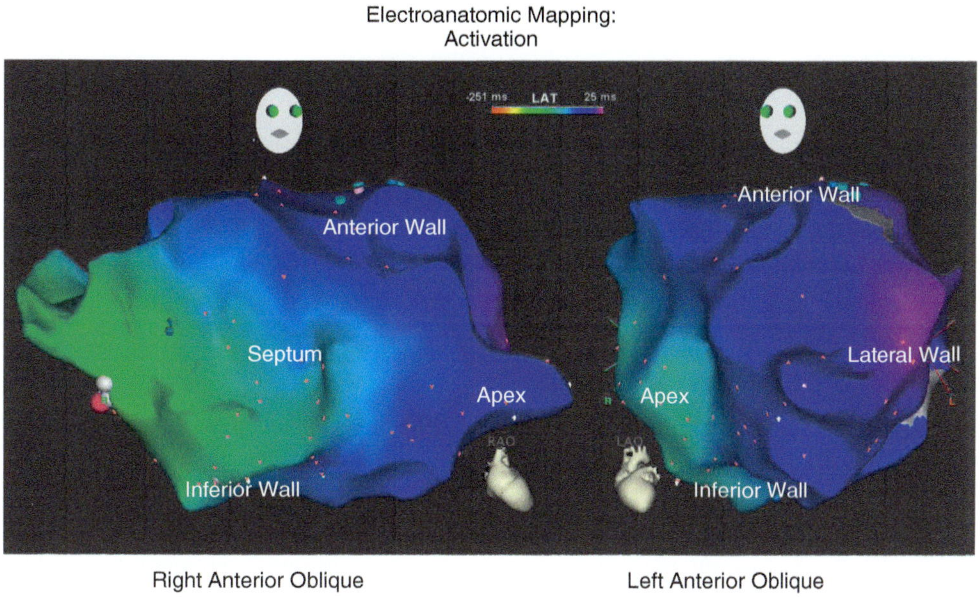

Figure 24-14

Fig. 24-14 (electroanatomic activation mapping) shows relatively late activation from standard right and left anterior oblique views because the pathology is on the inferobasal free wall.

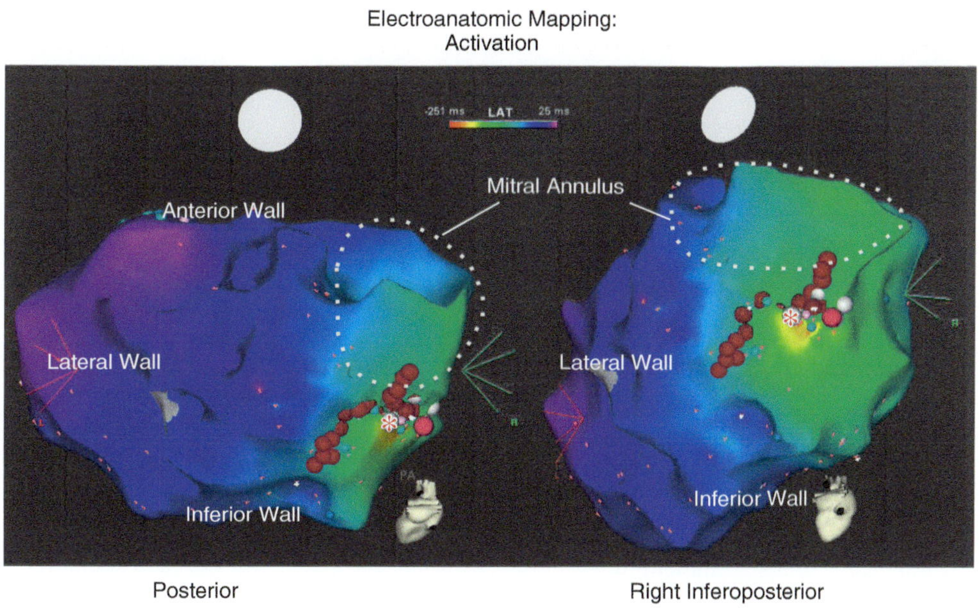

Figure 24-15

In Fig. 24-15, activation mapping viewed posteriorly shows the site of stimulation at which VT was terminated with a nonpropagated stimulus and where RF energy terminated it, rendering it noninducible thereafter *(asterisk)*. The *pink dot* denotes a site of pacemapping that yielded an excellent match with VT. *Red dots* denote sites at which RF energy was applied to connect the mitral annulus *(dashed line)* to more normal myocardium on the inferior wall (better seen on voltage map in Fig. 24-17).

Electroanatomic Mapping: Voltage

Figure 24-16

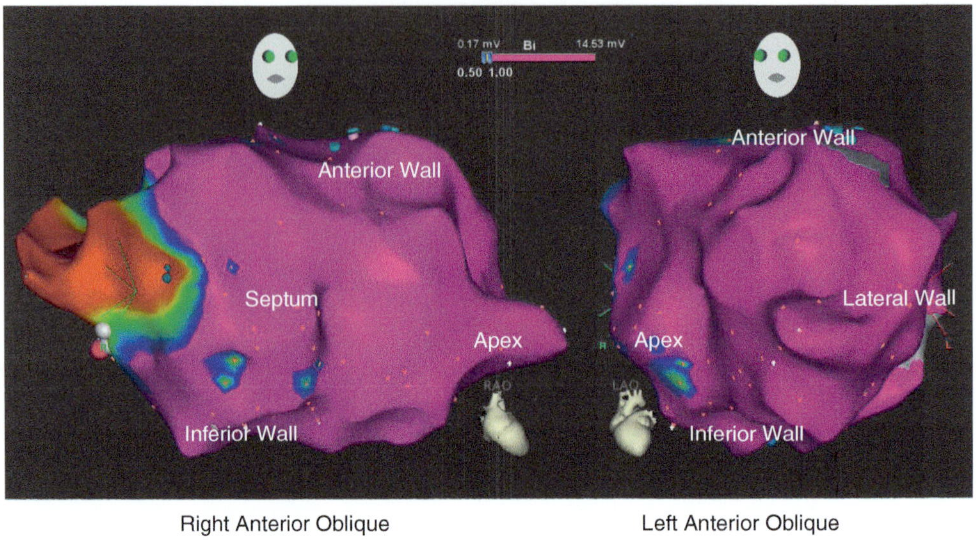

In Fig. 24-16, electroanatomic voltage mapping shows some abnormalities at the basal left ventricle *(red)* in standard right and left anterior oblique.

Electroanatomic Mapping: Voltage

Figure 24-17

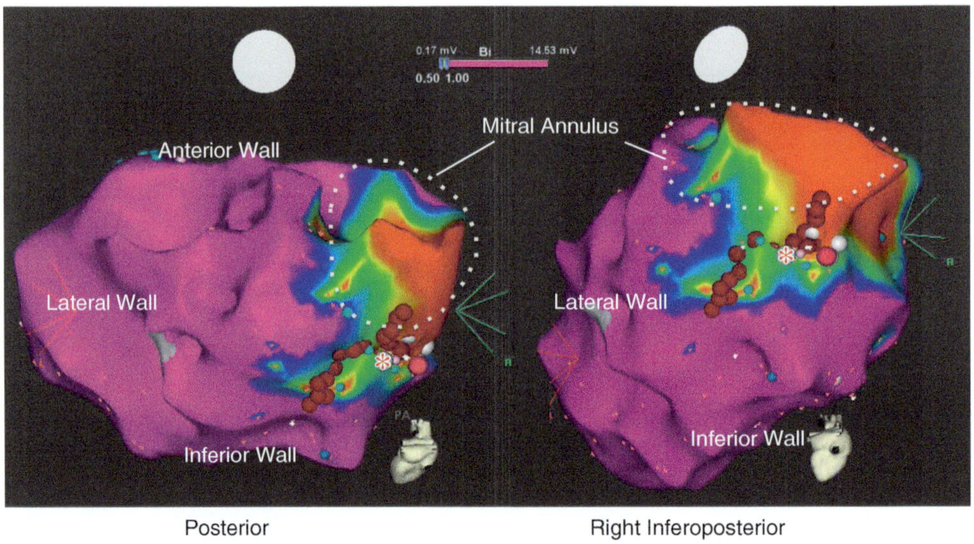

In Fig. 24-17, voltage mapping viewed posteriorly again shows the site of stimulation at which VT was terminated with a nonpropagated stimulus and RF energy delivery *(asterisk). Red dots* again denote sites at which RF energy was applied to connect the mitral annulus *(dashed line)* to more normal myocardium *(purple)* on the inferior wall.

Finally ECG

Interestingly, the final ECG during sinus rhythm (Fig. 24-18) shows no evidence of prior infarction—unusual in cases in which enough damage has occurred to result in relatively slow VT.

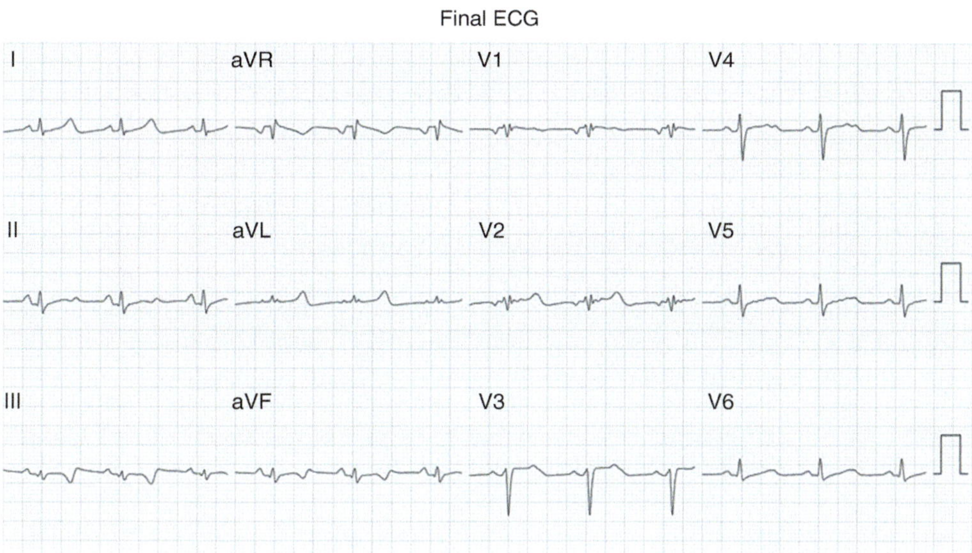

Figure 24-18

Summary

- It is important to determine the mechanism of VT before mapping and ablation in all cases, but especially:
  - In cases of incessant VT (which can be either focal or reentrant)
  - When there are unexpected findings (initiation of VT with atrial pacing or catecholamines)
- Overdrive pacing to determine presence or absence of fusion (and thus macroreentry) may yield data that are equivocal or require careful inspection to make correct conclusions
- Unanticipated diagnostic findings (nonpropagated stimulus terminating arrhythmia) may occur and should not be overlooked, because they have important implications regarding mapping and ablation

25 Focal Ventricular Tachycardia in the Postinfarction Patient

Case Presentation

A 56-year-old man with a history of myocardial infarction (MI) coronary artery bypass surgery had an implantable cardioverter-defibrillator (ICD) placed because of cardiac arrest several months after surgery. He began having episodes of palpitations and was found to have recurrent episodes of slow ventricular tachycardia. Medical therapy (beta blocker, a short course of amiodarone) failed to control episodes. Exercise stress testing 2 months earlier showed no evidence of residual ischemia. Left ventricular function was mildly depressed (ejection fraction 40%) with inferior wall motion abnormality; there was no ventricular thrombus. He was referred for electrophysiologic (EP) study catheter ablation.

Baseline Recordings

Figure 25-1

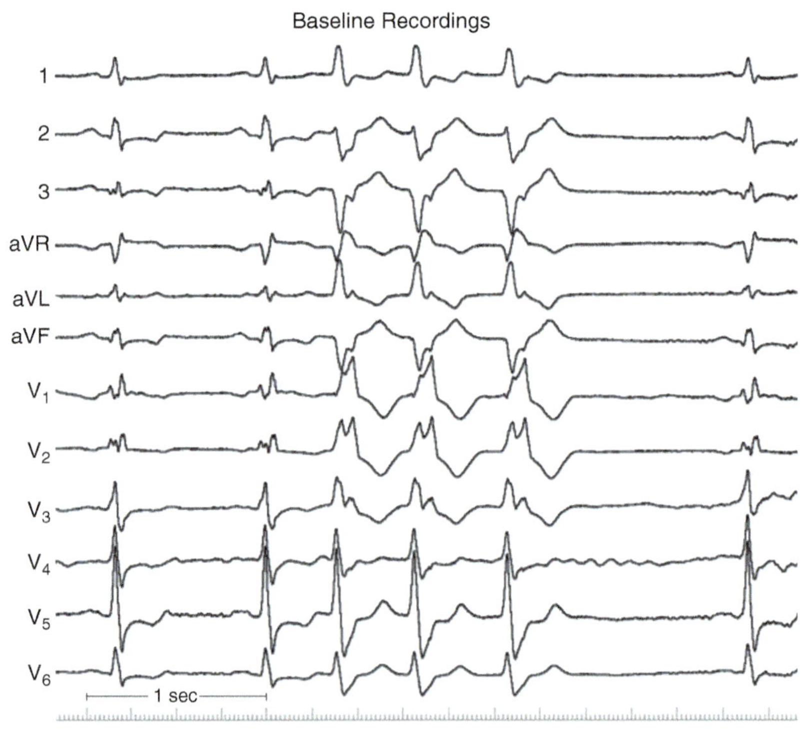

A recording of an episode of his typical VT morphology (right bundle branch block [RBBB], left superior axis, Fig. 25-1) was made before the EP procedure. VT starts spontaneously, with the initiating complex identical to all others, and the rhythm is slightly irregular before terminating. Although most VT in patients with prior MI is caused by reentry in the region of scar, the behavior of this VT is unusual for reentry, in which the initiating complex is often different from the rest of the VT complexes, and episodes tend to be sustained and quite regular. The features of this patient's VT raise the question whether this could be a focal (automatic or triggered) process; this occurs in up to 9% of patients with prior MI. Foci are usually at the periphery of the scarred region. Further investigation is needed to sort out the mechanism of this arrhythmia because ablation-site characteristics (late diastolic signal) are very different from those of the usual macroreentry (middiastolic potential). The VT morphology suggests a left ventricular (LV) source; LV thrombus has already been excluded by echocardiogram (important information before placing a catheter in the LV).

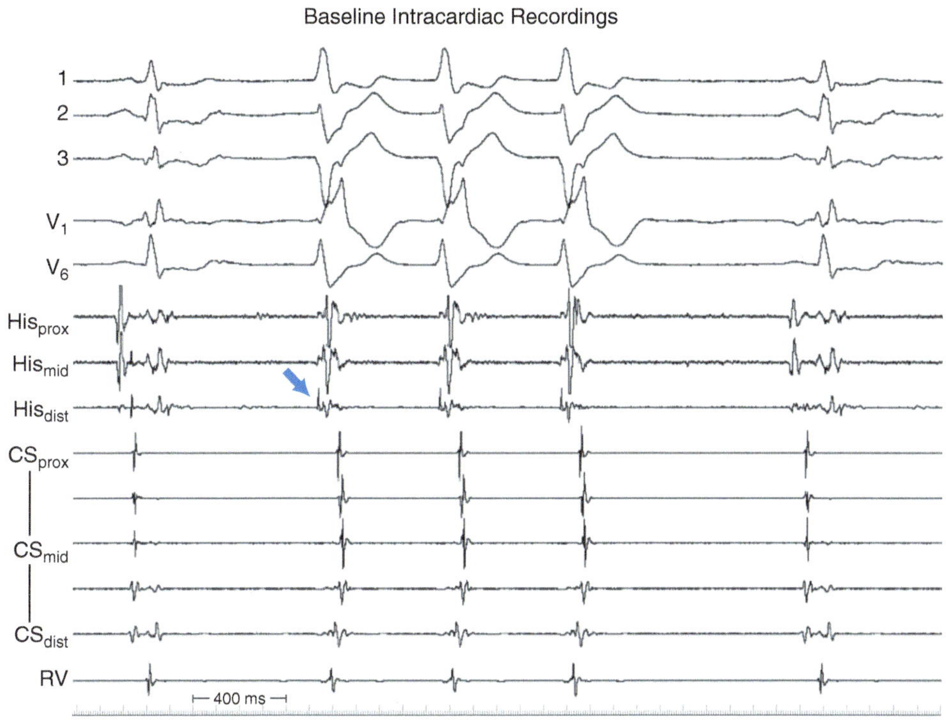

Figure 25-2

At the time of EP study, catheters were placed to be able to record and pace from atrium, His bundle region, and ventricle (Fig. 25-2). An episode of nonsustained VT is seen with corresponding intracardiac recordings. Retrograde conduction is present during VT, which (as seen before) starts spontaneously with the first complex identical to other VT complexes. The *arrow* points to a signal consistent with a His potential (also seen during the sinus rhythm complex at left). This raises the possibility that a focal fascicular tachycardia or reentry within the His-Purkinje system (HPS) could be operative, and the QRS morphology is reasonable for either of these.

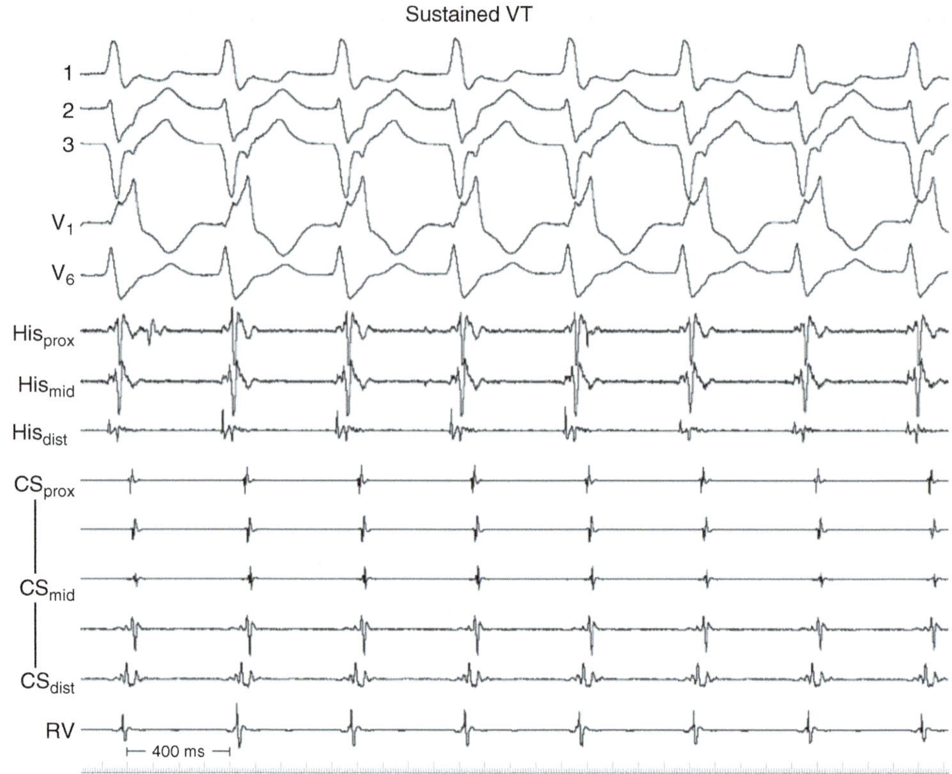

Figure 25-3

With isoproterenol infusion, VT became more sustained and slightly more regular (Fig. 25-3). This is again more consistent with a focal mechanism, but can occur with reentry.

Determining VT Mechanism

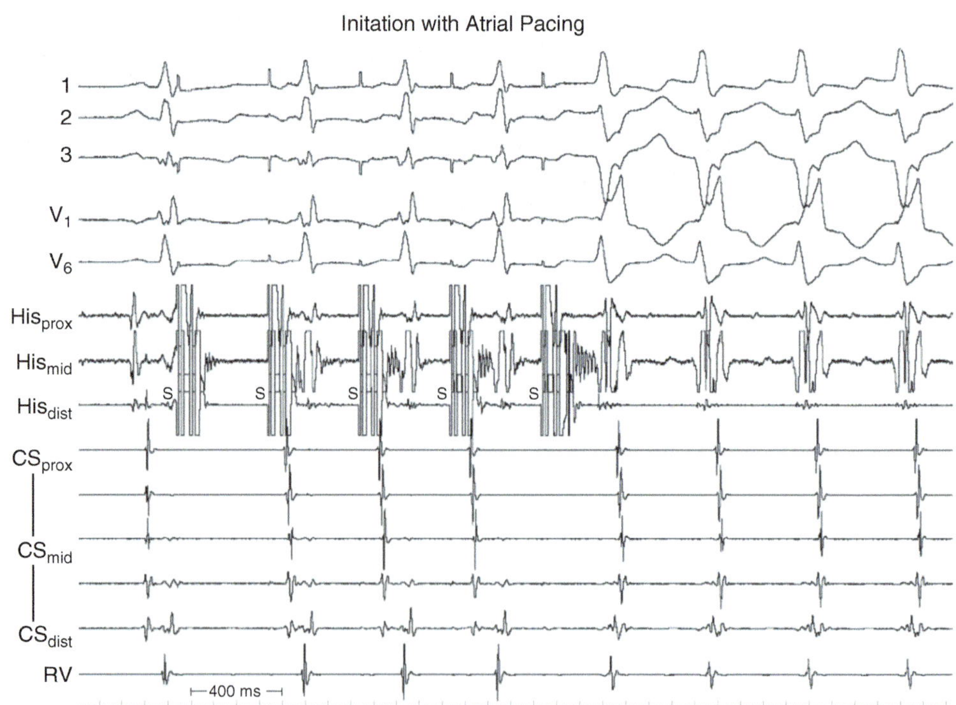

Figure 25-4

VT terminated spontaneously (not shown); in Fig. 25-4, atrial pacing initiates VT again. This was actually an attempt to pace the His bundle region to see if the resulting QRS complex was like that of VT, but instead of His or ventricular capture, only atrial capture occurred and this initiated VT again (of five stimuli [S], only the middle three capture). This finding again favors a focal source of VT, but nothing is certain yet.

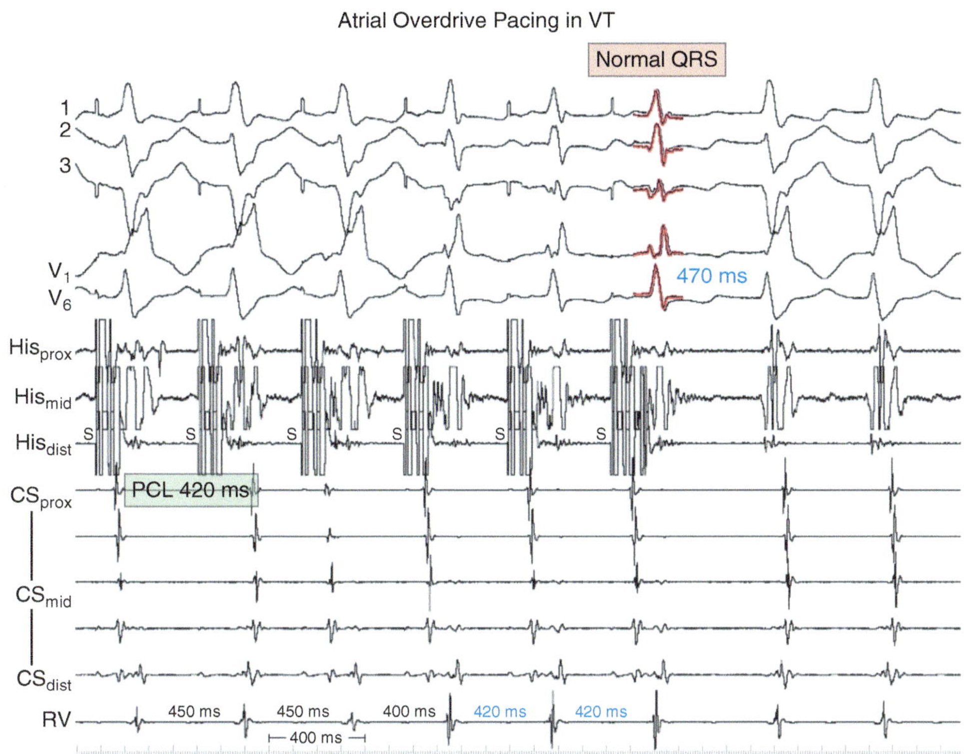

Figure 25-5

Another attempt at pacing from the distal His electrode during VT also results in atrial (not ventricular) capture (Fig. 25-5). Although the last four stimuli capture atrium, the last three affect the QRS complex by having some atrioventricular conduction, and after the last two stimuli, QRS complexes are identical to the sinus complex (superimposed in *red*). This indicates full control of the ventricles (also shown by RR intervals above the RV recording), and should terminate reentry within the HPS; however, the rhythm resumes after the last paced complex. The QRS-QRS interval at the first VT complex is 470 ms, just longer than the tachycardia cycle length (CL). Although HPS reentry is unlikely, a focal mechanism (fascicular or ventricular) is still quite plausible.

Figure 25-6

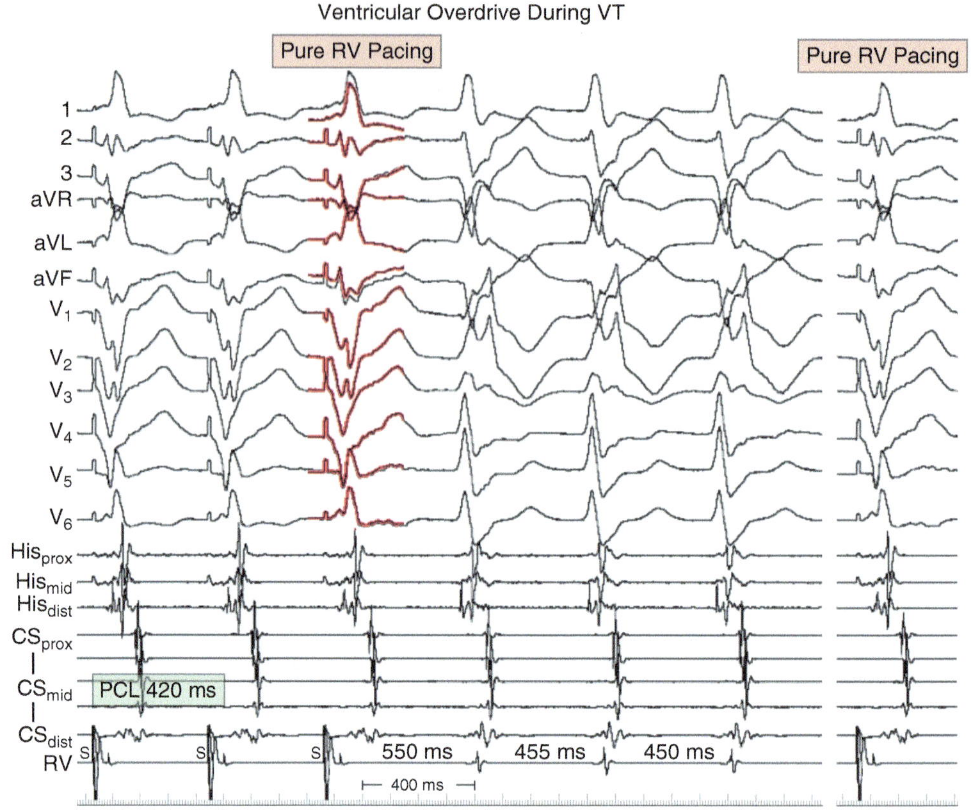

To try to determine VT mechanism more clearly, overdrive ventricular pacing is performed during VT. In Fig. 25-6, pacing from the RV electrode accelerates all complexes to the paced CL and the same VT returns on cessation of pacing. Although many would call this entrainment of VT, it is not possible to say just yet; fusion is necessary to declare that entrainment is present and thus diagnose macroreentry. Here, a single complex of pure ventricular pacing is shown at right, and is superimposed on a complex of pacing during VT; these appear to be identical. However, the absence of fusion on one attempt at overdrive pacing does not thereby diagnose a focal mechanism; one may have to pace at different CLs and different sites without showing fusion to more certainly diagnose a focal process. One additional feature to evaluate is the interval from last paced complex to first subsequent VT complex (the return cycle, here 550 ms); with reentry, this should stay constant no matter what CL or how many complexes of overdrive pacing are performed at the same site, but may show overdrive suppression with a focal mechanism when pacing faster or longer. Finally, the VT CL after resumption is usually the same as baseline with reentry but may be slower for a few cycles if overdrive suppression of a focus has occurred. Here, the VT CL is a little slower than baseline (450 ms). These again suggest a focal process.

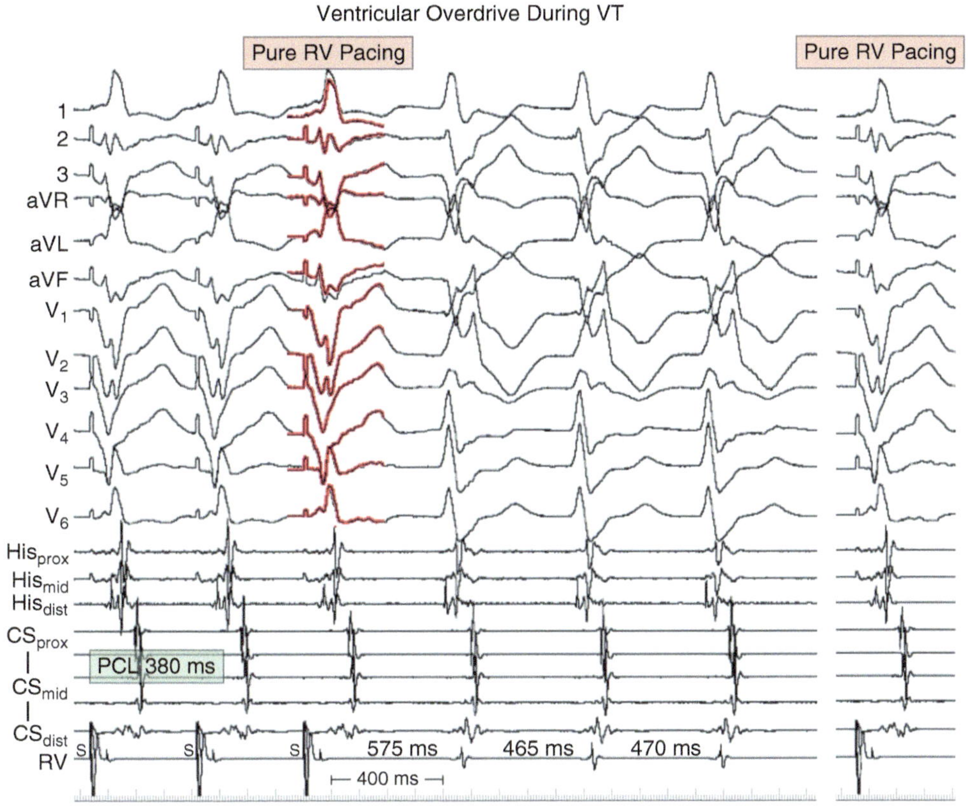

Figure 25-7

In Fig. 25-7, pacing during VT from the same site is performed at a faster CL (380 ms). The return cycle is longer than before (575 ms) and as shown the VT is slower as it resumes. These again suggest a focal process; there is again no fusion on the ECG during pacing, but one would not expect it even if macroreentry were present because if it were not seen at a slower paced CL it will not appear at a faster one. The best chance of showing fusion is to pace well away from where the anticipated exit site (or focus) is, and as close to the VT CL as possible to allow exit from the VT circuit to blend with the paced wavefront.

Figure 25-8

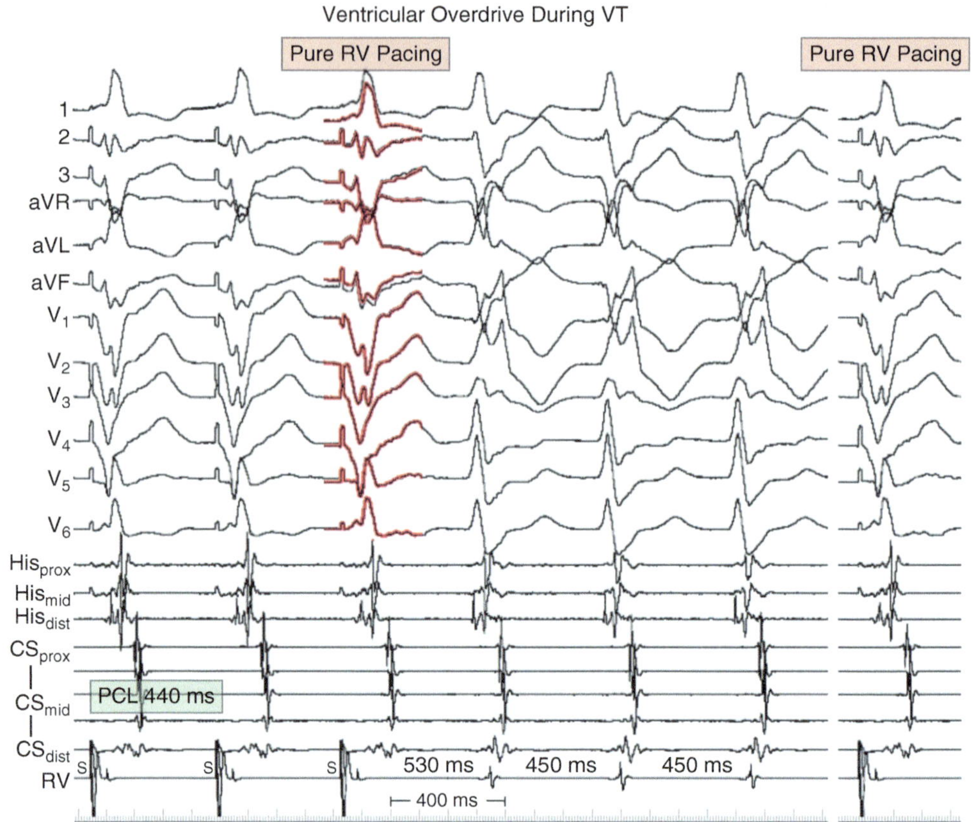

In Fig. 25-8, pacing is performed during VT as slowly as possible and still has capture (440 ms). This again shows no hint of fusion (all complexes look fully paced); the return cycle is shorter and the VT resumes at about the baseline CL. Two other pacing sites were used with the same outcome (not shown). All these data taken together (lack of fusion at multiple CLs and sites of pacing; appearance of overdrive suppression; transient slowing of resumed VT; initiation with atrial pacing) combined with the clinical behavior (irregular bursts of nonsustained VT with the first complex like all others) are very consistent with a focal, automatic process and nothing points to reentry. At this point, we can begin mapping, searching for a site with a late diastolic potential. Scarring around the site may produce some decrease in electrogram amplitude and a longer presystolic interval (50 to 80 ms) than is usually seen in VT in patients without structural heart disease (20 to 40 ms).

Mapping and Ablation

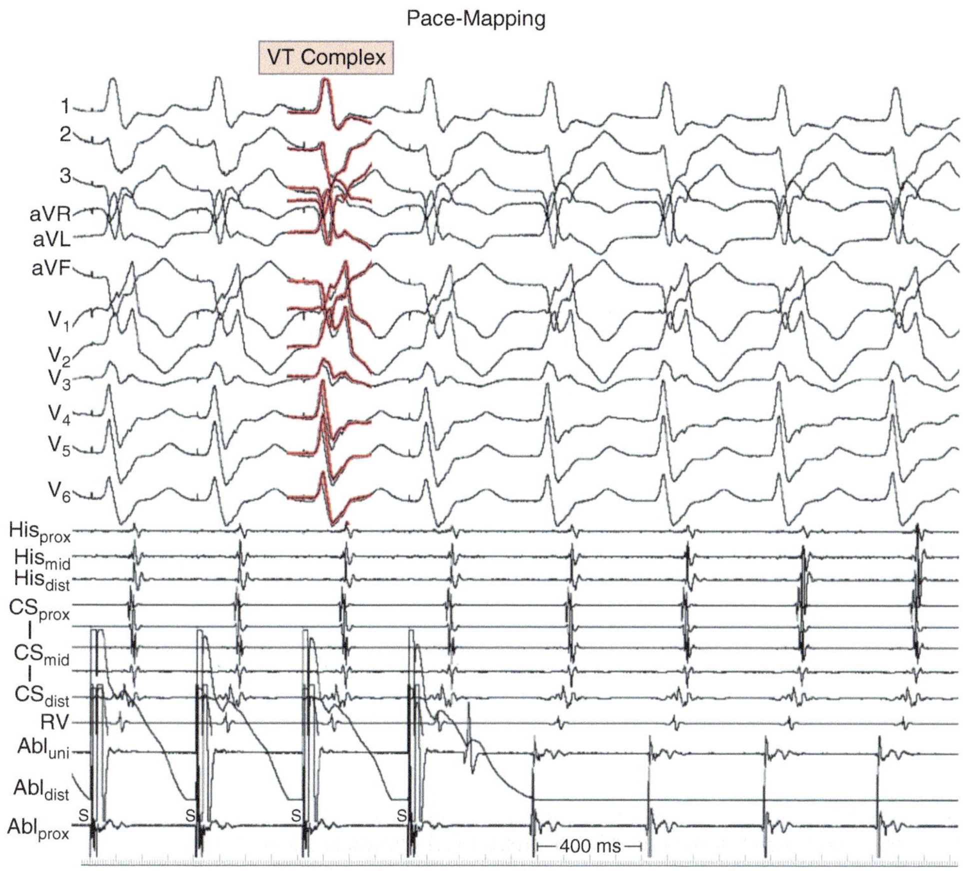

Figure 25-9

In Fig. 25-9, ventricular pacing is performed at a site with a late diastolic electrogram (not shown); a VT complex is shown in *red*, superimposed on a paced complex. Although the overall "match" is quite good, there are some slight differences (leads 2, V2 to V4). If one is pacing from the exact point of emanation from a focal arrhythmia, the resulting paced complex should ideally be identical. Mapping was continued without ablation at this site.

Figure 25-10

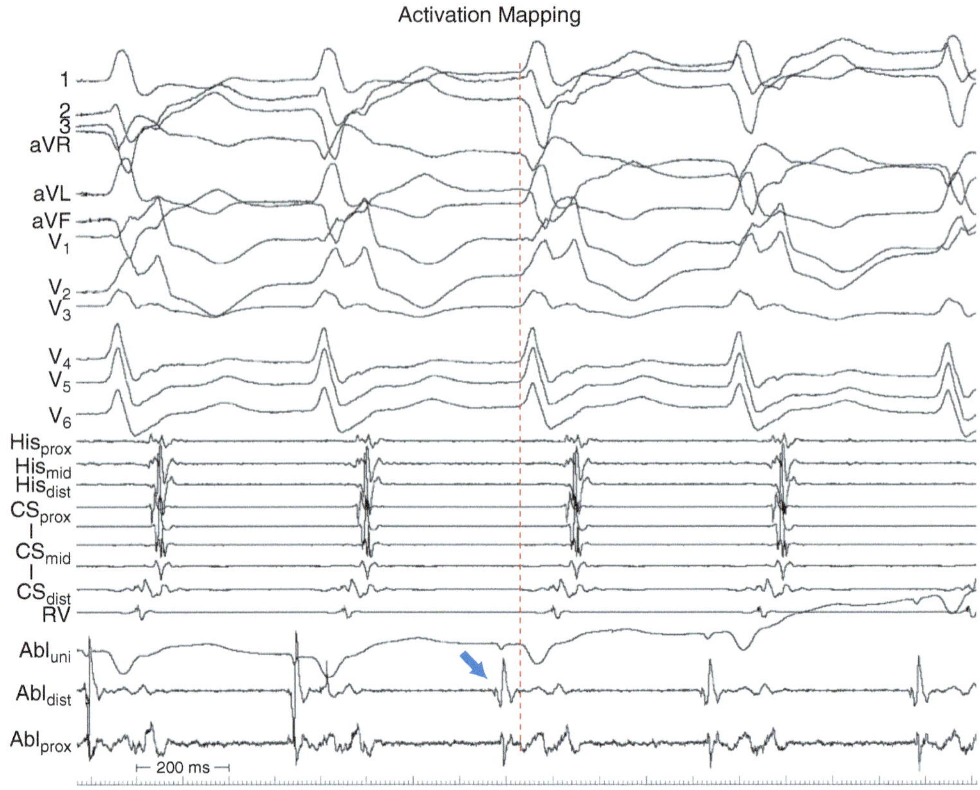

In Fig. 25-10, recordings from a site in the inferior LV are shown; the *dashed line* denotes the onset of the surface QRS complex. The distal ablation recording is complex and has a very small component *(blue arrow)* at its onset that is about 60 ms before QRS onset. It is possible that this small component represents a Purkinje potential (and thus the VT would be a focal fascicular tachycardia); VT was incessant at this point; thus it was impossible to know what the site looked like during sinus rhythm (ie, whether a Purkinje potential was present then). Of note, no such potential was evident after restoration of sinus rhythm with ablation, and the lack of an isoelectric interval between the small potential and the main portion of the local electrogram suggests that this is ordinary myocardium rather than fascicular tissue at the source.

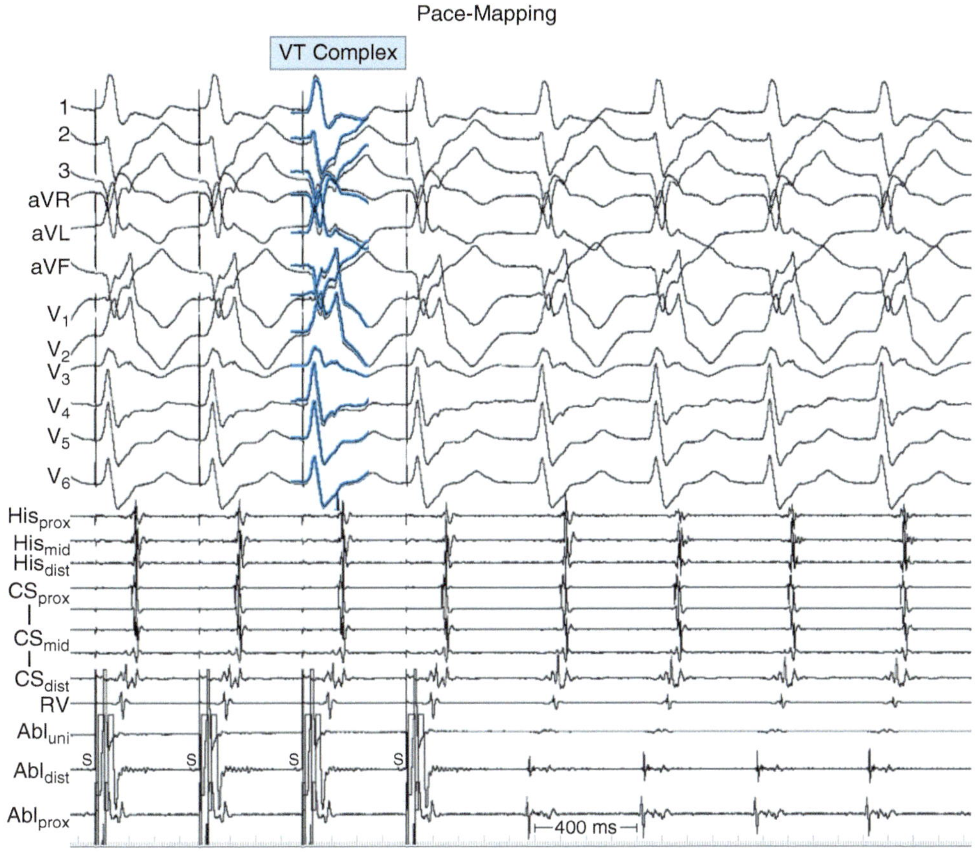

Figure 25-11

In Fig. 25-11, pacemapping is performed from the site shown in Fig. 25-10 to corroborate it as a reasonable site for ablation. As before, a VT complex is superimposed (in *blue*) over a paced complex, showing a perfect "match" with the VT. The stimulus-QRS interval is slightly less than the electrogram-QRS interval during VT, probably signifying the pacing was performed at a slightly excessive output (capturing some tissue beyond the actual focus). Similar to what was observed when pacing at a different site, although VT resumes after stopping pacing, this cannot be considered to be concealed entrainment because to do so, fusion (manifest entrainment) has to be demonstrated at some other time (but could not be in this case because macroreentry is not present).

Figure 25-12

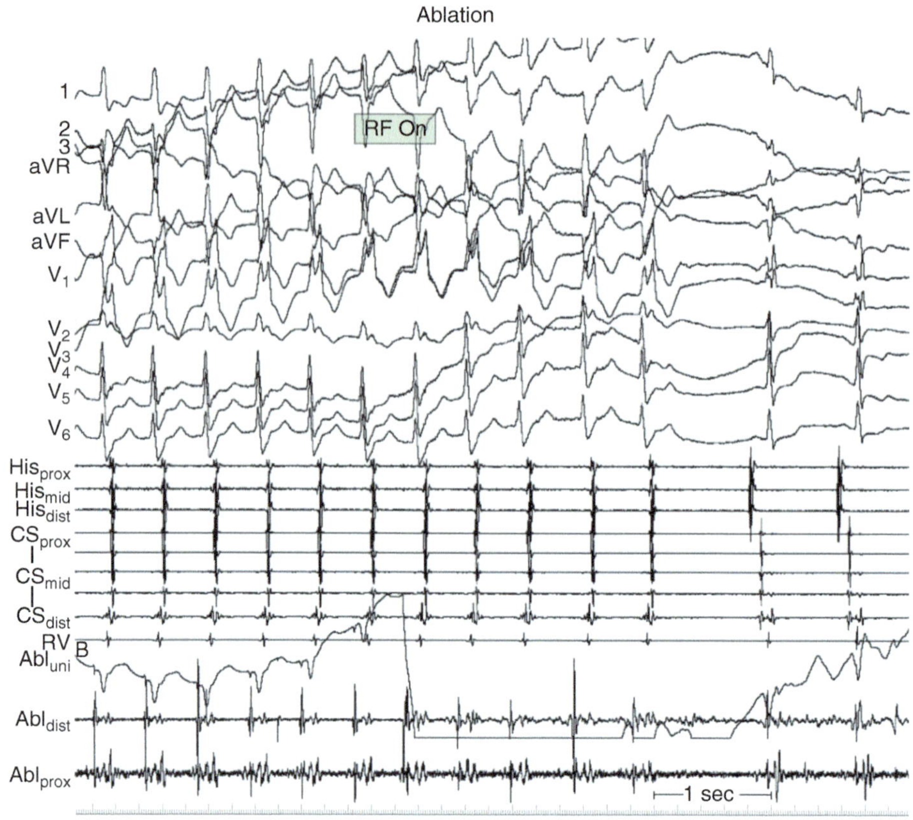

Fig. 25-12 shows the onset of ablation delivered during VT. Less than 3 seconds after the beginning of RF application, VT abruptly ceases after slight acceleration and then slowing. VT could not be initiated thereafter with atrial or ventricular pacing, nor increased isoproterenol infusion.

Figure 25-13

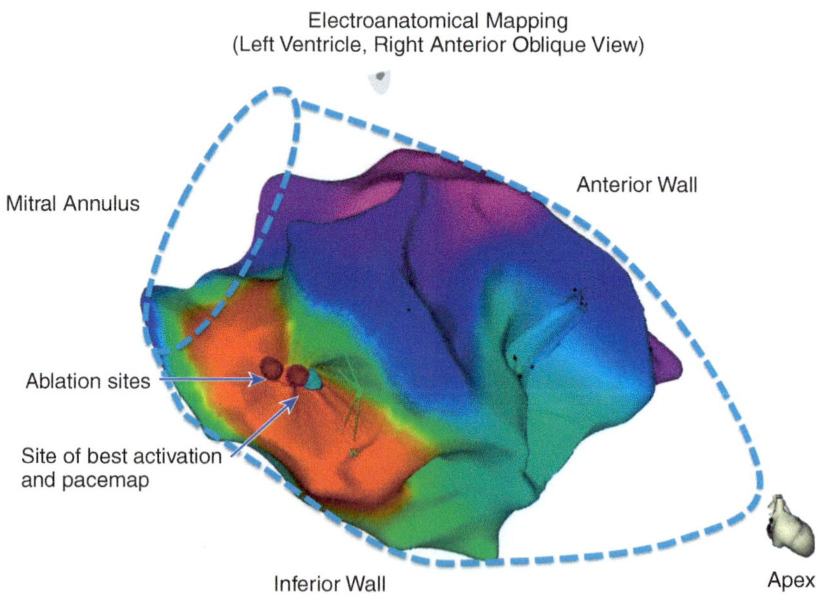

A partial endocardial electroanatomic activation map of the LV made during VT is shown, with an idealized outline of the LV in the left anterior oblique projection (Fig. 25-13). As can be seen, the focus was on the inferior basal portion of the left ventricle.

Summary

- In patients with prior myocardial infarction, a focal mechanism is present in up to 9% of VTs that are induced during electrophysiology study
- Focal VTs often occur in irregular bursts spontaneously or are initiated with atrial pacing, facilitated by catecholamines
- Careful investigation must be performed to ascertain whether a focal process is involved in VT when its behavior is atypical for reentry
- Mechanistic distinction from more typical macroreentrant VT in this population is important because ablation-site characteristics are very different

26 Focal Epicardial Ventricular Tachycardia

Case Presentation

A 38-year-old man was resuscitated from cardiac arrest at home. Ventricular tachycardia (VT) or ventricular fibrillation (VF) was initial rhythm, shocked to sinus, and then "sinus tachycardia with right bundle branch block (RBBB)." His history revealed significant alcohol intake, though none recently. He had been nauseated and bloated for 4 to 6 weeks before the event and had palpitations. Treatment included intravenous (IV) Amiodarone and repeated cardioversions for VT (not "sinus tachycardia with RBBB"); lidocaine was added (with no effect). He was maintained during VT on dopamine and then placed on a cooling protocol. ECG revealed severely dilated left (LV) and right ventricle (RV) with LV ejection fraction 15% to 20%. Catheterization showed a normal left coronary, but could not engage right coronary. VT persisted despite continued amiodarone infusion. Progressive hypotension was refractory to vasopressin, epinephrine and intra-aortic balloon pump.

Baseline VT ECG

The Most Likely Mechanism Is

A. HPS reentry
B. Myocardial reentry
C. Myocardial focus

Figure 26-1

ECG

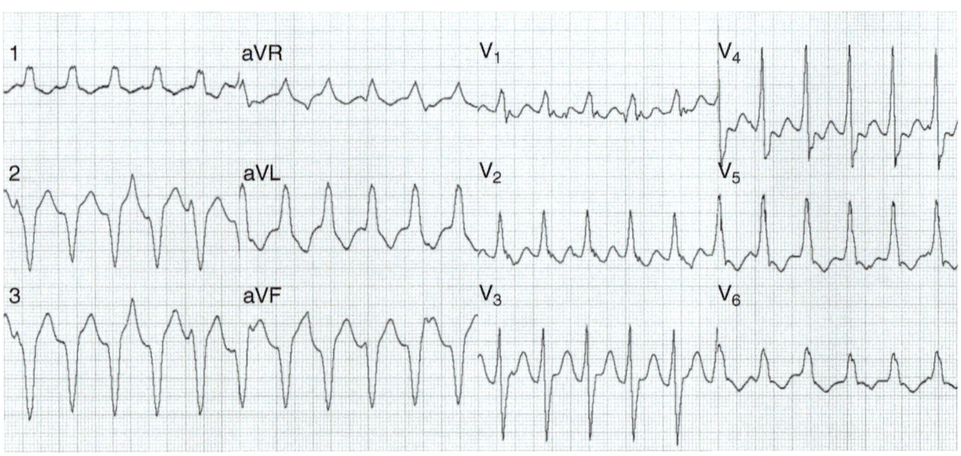

Fig. 26-1 shows a 12-lead ECG of the presenting arrhythmia, diagnosed as VT with AV dissociation (inferior leads) and standard morphologic criteria. The pattern is most consistent with a myocardial source rather than His-Purkinje reentry (which should generally resemble aberrant conduction patterns), but whether this is a focus in the myocardium or exit from a circuit cannot be determined from the ECG.

Overdrive Pacing from RV During VT

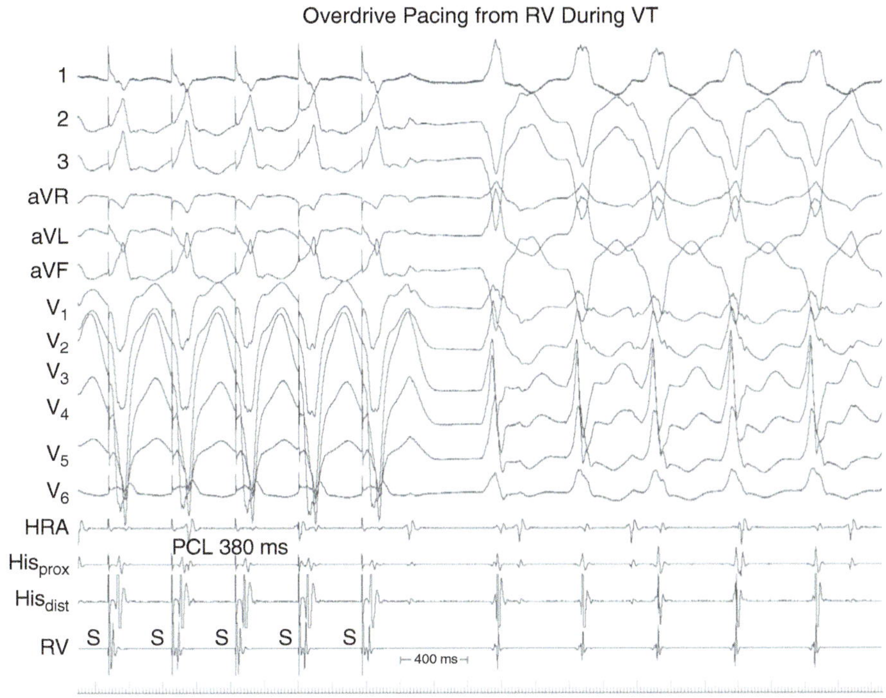

The Most Likely Mechanism Is

A. HPS reentry
B. Myocardial reentry
C. Myocardial focus

Figure 26-2

Once electrode catheters had been positioned, overdrive pacing was performed from the right ventricular catheter. Pacing was initiated during tachycardia, all electrograms were accelerated to the paced cycle length, and upon cessation of pacing, the same tachycardia resumed (Fig. 26-2). Although many would call this an example of entrainment, one essential piece is missing: fusion. It is difficult to demonstrate fusion with a single example of overdrive pacing during a tachycardia, and without demonstrating fusion, it is difficult to make a diagnosis of macroreentry. Making this distinction (macroreentry vs a focal process) is critical, because the characteristics of the ablation site are dictated by which mechanism is involved (late diastolic potential for a focal process, mid-diastolic potential for macroreentry).

What Do You Want to Do Now?

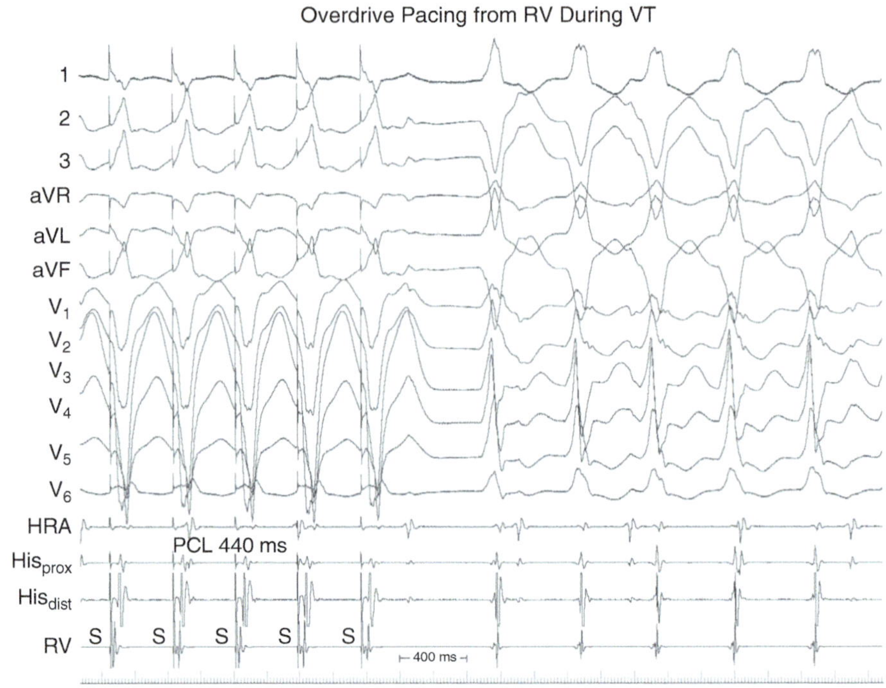

Figure 26-3

One way to ascertain whether fusion is present or not is to pace from the same site at different cycle lengths; the slower the pacing rate (closer to that of tachycardia), the more opportunity there will be to demonstrate fusion, and as the cycle length of pacing changes, the resultant QRS complex (particular blend of pacing vs VT) will change in the presence of macroreentry. In addition, selection of a pacing site can be very helpful: if the pacing site is close to the anticipated exit site of the tachycardia, it will be difficult to demonstrate fusion, whereas if a site is chosen far away from the anticipated exit zone, fusion will be more readily demonstrated. When presented with a RBBB, left superior axis VT, a pacing site was chosen that would produce a LBBB, right inferior axis complex—such that, if fusion were possible, it would certainly be evident when pacing during VT from such a site at a slow cycle length. However, if the VT is because of a focus, there will never be any evidence of fusion, and overdrive pacing from a remote site will always look like pure pacing from that site, no matter what stimulation rate is chosen. In the example shown in Fig. 26-3, pacing is performed at a cycle length (440 ms) just 30 ms shorter than the VT cycle length, yet the complexes during pacing appear to be identical to those when pacing at a more rapid cycle length (380 ms). In addition, the interval from the last paced complex to the first beat of VT that resumes is relatively long compared with the VT cycle length. This would be unusual for macroreentry, but not for an automatic focus that exhibits some degree of overdrive suppression of excitability.

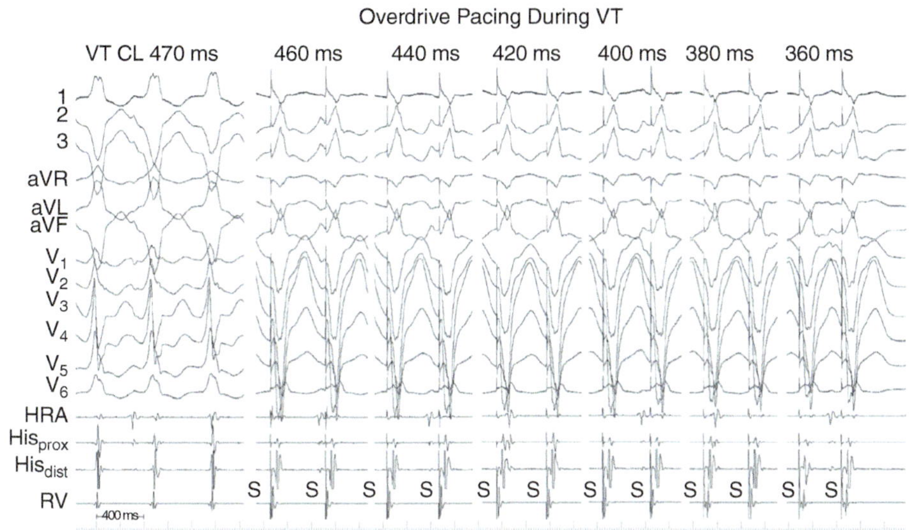

Figure 26-4

In Fig. 26-4, all 12 ECG leads of VT are shown at *left* (470 ms cycle length) as well as 2 complexes of pacing from the right ventricular outflow tract during VT at several different cycle lengths (including 460 ms, just 10 ms faster than the VT). It is evident that, no matter what cycle length of pacing during VT is used, QRS complexes are identical, indicating absence of fusion and strongly suggesting that macroreentry is not present (thus, a focal process). This evidence, taken with the suggestion of overdrive suppression as well as centrifugal pattern of electroanatomic activation mapping (shown later), led to a diagnosis of a focal ventricular tachycardia.

Mapping and Pacemapping

Figure 26-5

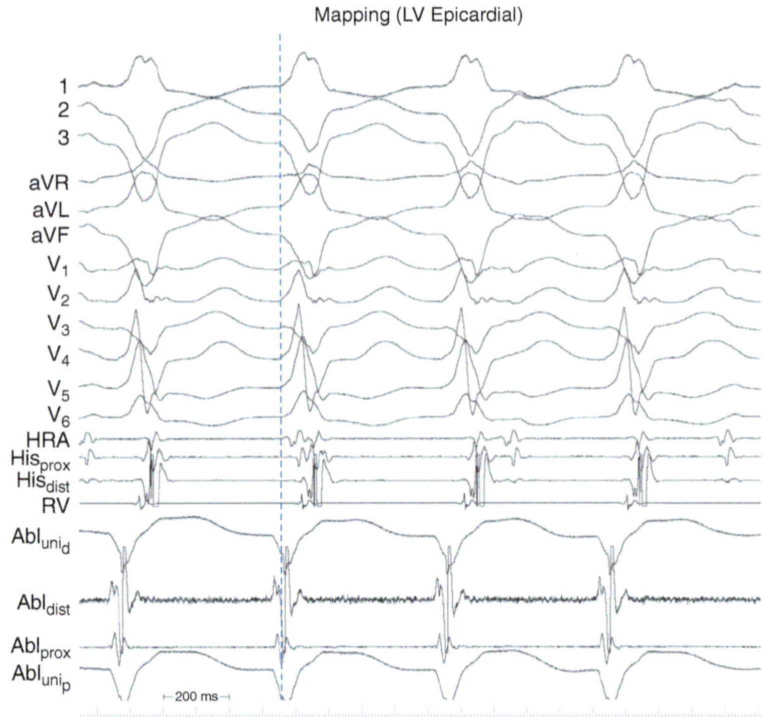

Having established a diagnosis of a focal VT, a site is sought with late diastolic activation (20 to 40 ms before the QRS onset), and a "QS" configuration in the unipolar recording. Thorough and extensive mapping of both right and left ventricular endocardial surfaces did not reveal any sites with timing before the QRS onset. With the "QS" configuration in the inferior ECG leads, in the absence of known infarction, pericardial access was obtained for epicardial mapping. The electrogram shown in Fig. 26-5 is from a site on the inferior left ventricular wall, halfway between apex and base, on the epicardial surface. Its features match those of the ideal target site noted previously; the QRS onset is denoted by a *dashed line*.

Figure 26-6

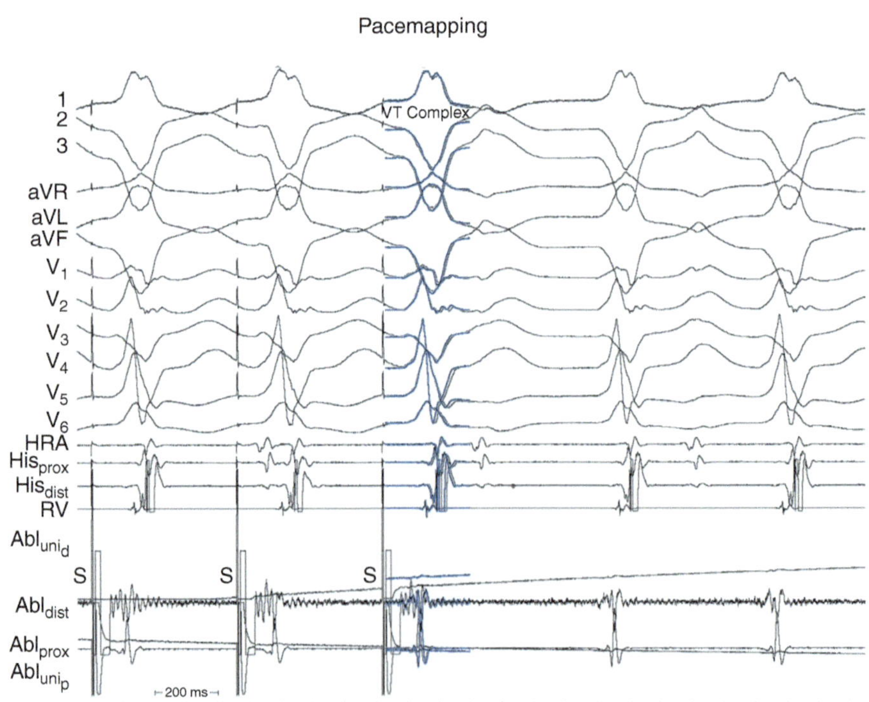

Pacing at this epicardial site (Fig. 26-6) produced a perfect 12-lead ECG (and intracardiac) match with a VT complex (superimposed in *blue*). This corroborates the activation mapping information. Note a relatively short stimulus-QRS interval, also consistent with a focal process.

Ablation and Postablation Pacing at Site

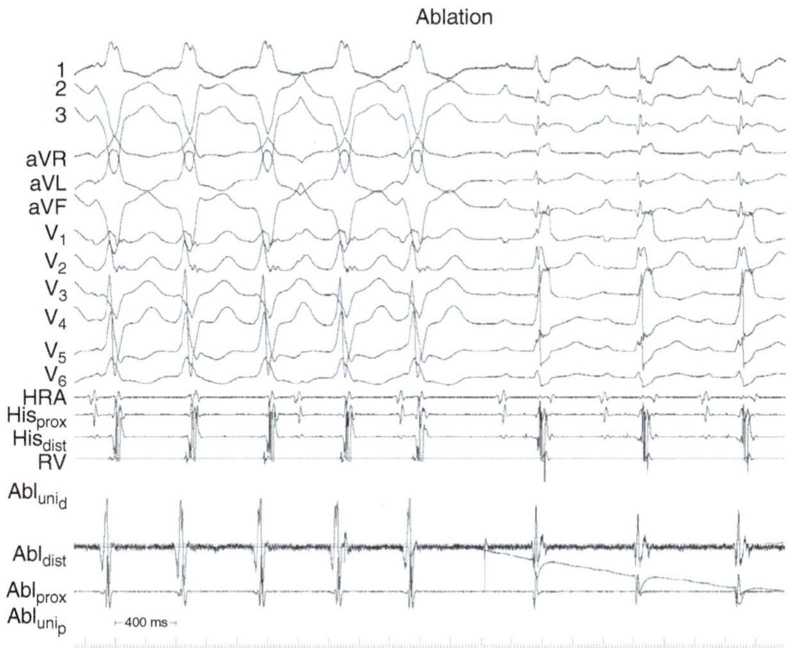

Figure 26-7

During radiofrequency (RF) energy delivery at the site of earliest activation mapping, tachycardia abruptly terminates to sinus rhythm (Fig. 26-7). The arrhythmia did not recur. Several other RF applications were administered in the same area to consolidate the damage.

Figure 26-8

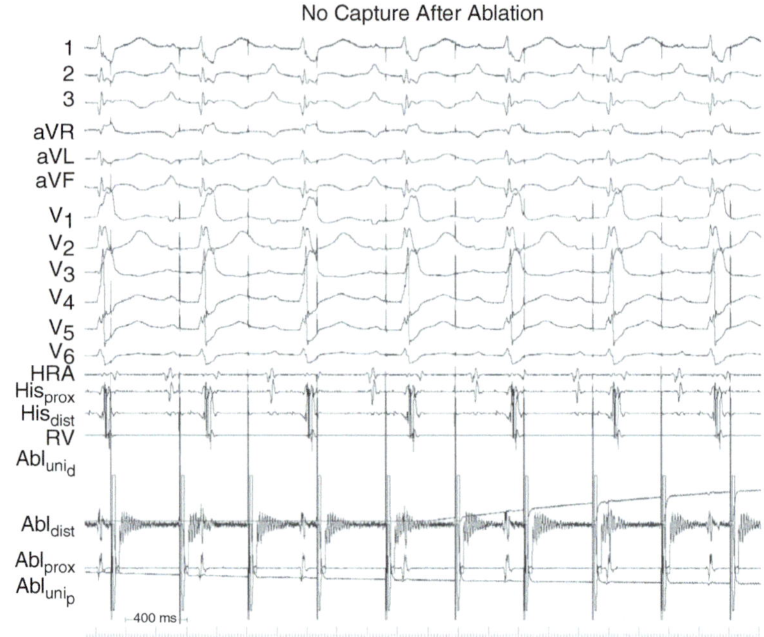

High-output stimulation at the site of ablation shows inability to capture, indicating destruction of excitable tissue in that area (Fig. 26-8). The patient had no further arrhythmias during the course of his hospitalization, during which left ventricular function gradually recovered almost completely (ejection fraction 40% to 45%). He regained full neurologic function and was discharged home.

Before ablation, it is usually important to perform coronary arteriography to avoid injury to a nearby vessel during RF delivery; in this case, because the patient was unlikely to survive unless the VT was controlled, right coronary arteriography was not performed before RF delivery but was done later in the procedure, showing >1 cm from the ablation zone to the posterior descending artery.

Electroanatomic Mapping (Activation and Voltage)

Figure 26-9

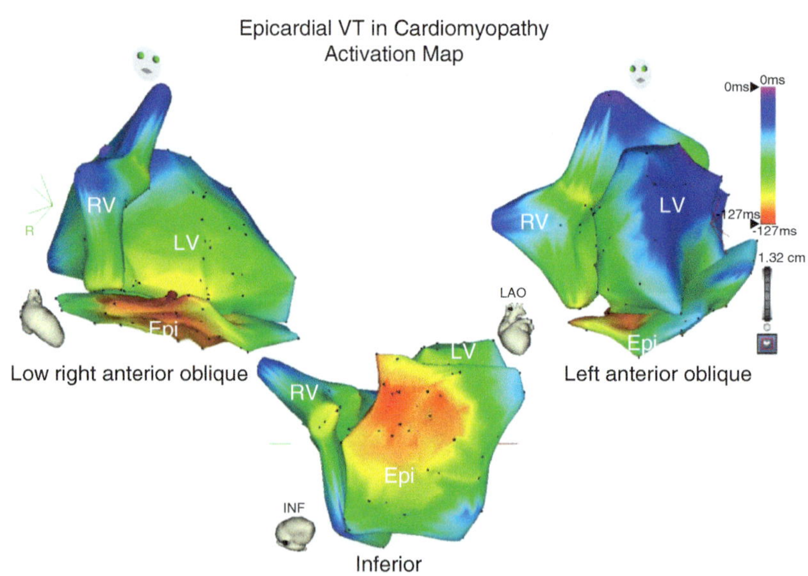

Fig. 26-9 displays electroanatomic activation mapping during ventricular tachycardia of right and left ventricular endocardial surfaces as well as the epicardial surface. *Red coloration* indicates the region of earliest activation, on the inferior wall at the junction of right and left ventricles.

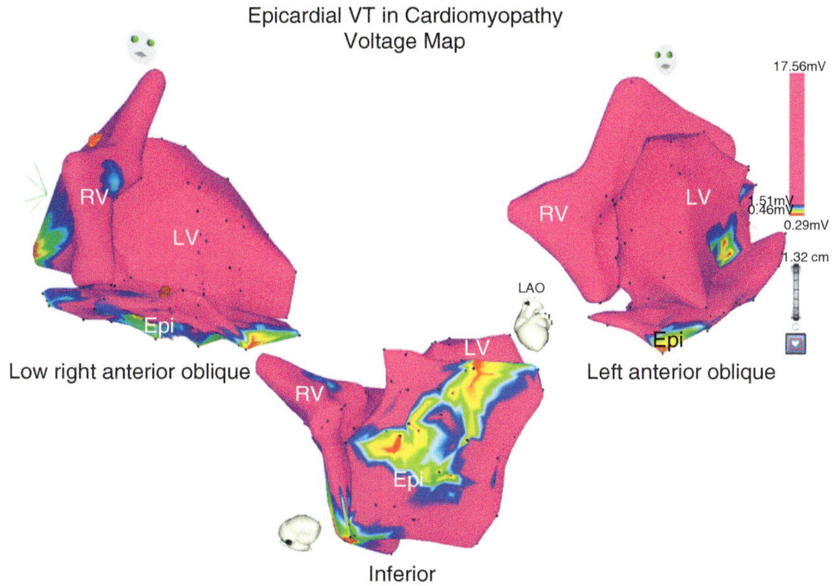

Figure 26-10

Electroanatomic voltage mapping of right and left ventricular endocardium, and epicardial surface of the inferior wall are shown in Fig. 26-10. *Purple color* indicates normal voltage; *red,* very low voltage/scar. The latter was limited to a very small area on the inferior wall of the left ventricle.

Summary

- Patients with nonischemic cardiomyopathy may have different types of VT:
  - Myocardial macroreentry—endocardial versus midwall versus epicardial
  - His-Purkinje reentry (bundle branch reentry [BBR])
  - Focal discharge (myocardial, Purkinje)
- Investigation and mapping attention should be focused:
  - To determine VT mechanism, thus how the ablation target should appear
  - At areas of low voltage/scar (perivalvular)
  - At His-Purkinje system (possibility of BBR)
- Electroanatomic mapping can help:
  - Determining areas of prior damage/scar
  - Delineation of potential channels for ablation
  - Tag sites with abnormal potentials for subsequent targeting
  - Planning and constructing lines of ablation

27 Ventricular Tachycardia in Dilated Cardiomyopathy

Case Presentation

The patient was a 74-year-old man with increasingly frequent implantable cardioverter-defibrillator (ICD) shocks. In 2009, poor left ventricular (LV) function was noted in the setting of prior (small) myocardial infarction (MI). Single-chamber ICD was implanted (primary prevention). In 2012, there was the first appropriate shock for ventricular tachycardia (VT), and amiodarone was initiated. There were more palpitations and shocks. Antitachycardia pacing (ATP) was modified, and there were more episodes and shocks. Mexiletine was added to amiodarone. There were more palpitations and shocks. In 2014, he was referred for electrophysiology (EP) study and possible ablation. Echocardiogram revealed poor LV systolic function (diffuse); there was no LV thrombus. ICD interrogation: repeated episodes of VT, cycle length (CL) 440 ms, not terminated with ATP (requiring shock).

ICD Stored Electrograms from 1 Day Before Ablation

What Else Do You Need to Know Preprocedure? [Fig. 27-1]
What Will Be the Procedural Strategy?

ICD Electrograms 1 Day Before

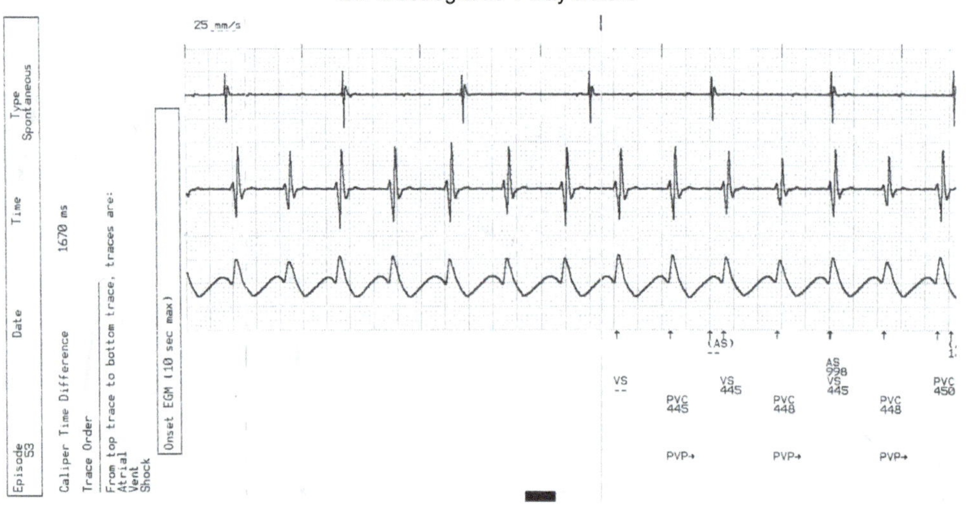

Figure 27-1

What other studies might be useful? Echocardiogram (exclude LV thrombus, demonstrate regional wall motion abnormalities) or magnetic resonance imaging (identification of scar regions), if your institution will do these in patients with ICDs.

ICD electrograms (Fig. 27-1) can be useful to sort out which of possibly several induced arrhythmias at EP study "match" the spontaneously occurring VT.

Which catheters to use? CS can be helpful for anatomic/fluoroscopic landmark as well as showing interesting electrograms in cases of VT arising from the basal region.

Baseline ECG and Intracardiac Recordings

Can You Interpret as far as Infarction? [Fig. 27-2] Anything to See?

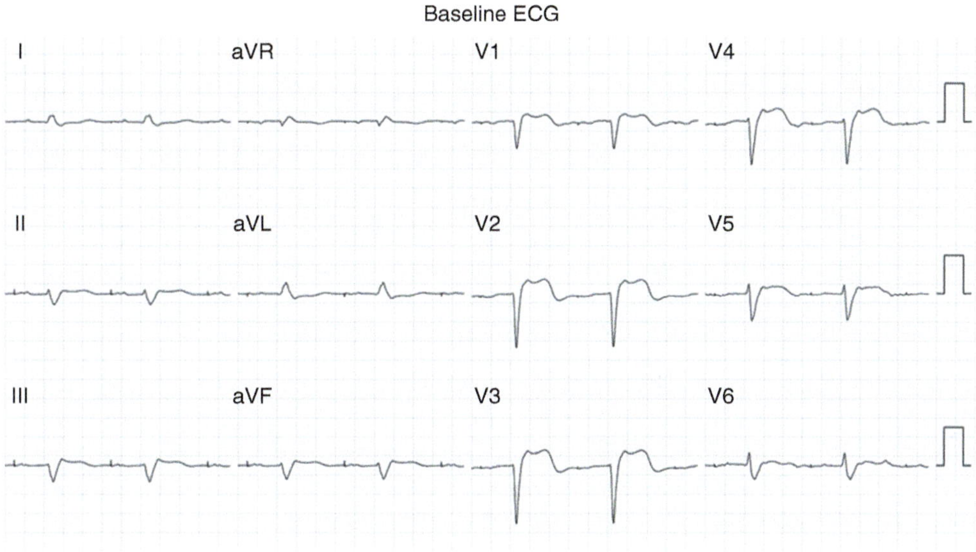

Figure 27-2

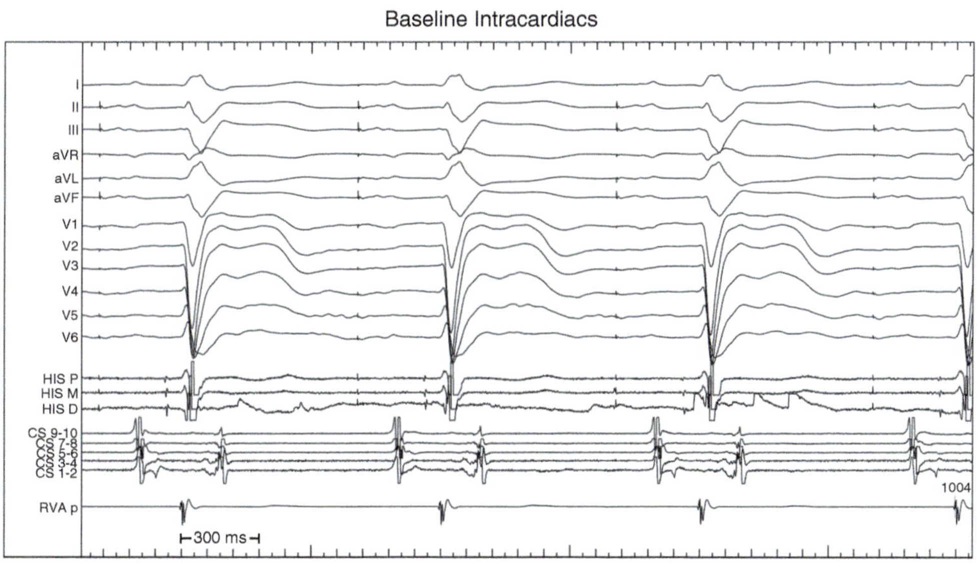

Figure 27-3

ECG during atrial pacing with conduction (Fig. 27-2) shows a wide QRS without clear infarct pattern. Ventricular electrograms (Fig. 27-3) on coronary sinus recordings are very late in the QRS complex—maybe it means something, maybe it doesn't.

Ventricular Pacing Baseline

Is Retrograde Conduction Present? [Fig. 27-4]

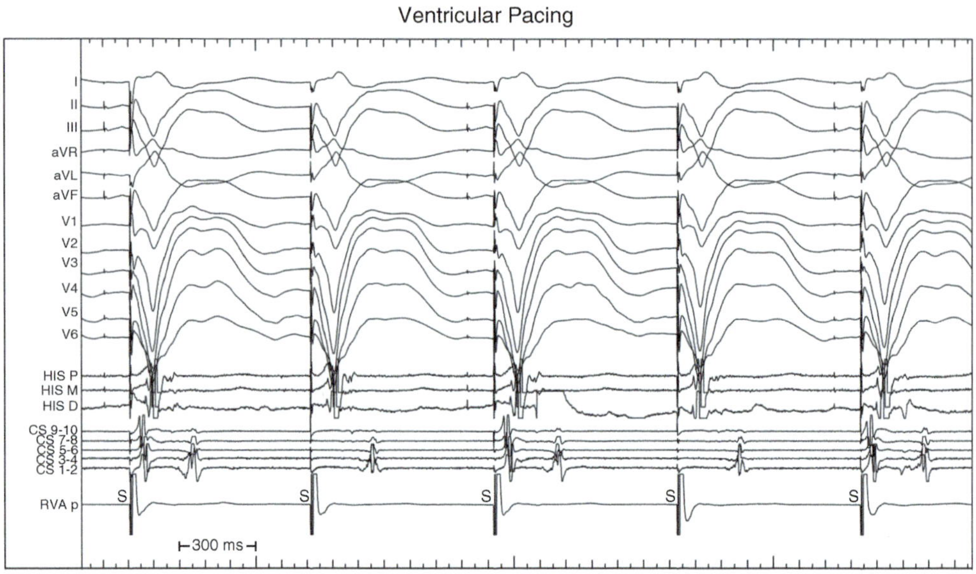

Figure 27-4

Potentials in the coronary sinus recordings that follow each QRS shown in Fig. 27-4 are actually very delayed ventricular signals, not atrial. True atrial signals are driven by atrial pacing from the ICD, and occur immediately after 1st, 3rd, and 5th ventricular stimulus artifact. Thus although retrograde conduction is probably not present, it is difficult to interpret.

VT Initiation and Attempt to Terminate

Is This the VT We're Looking For? [Fig. 27-5]

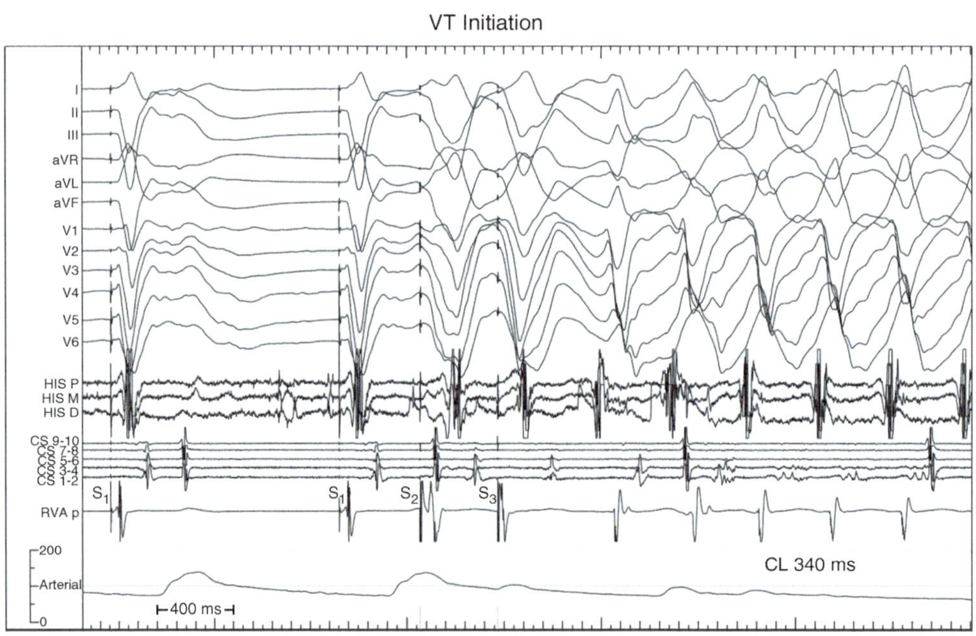

Figure 27-5

VT was initiated with double extrastimuli. The spontaneous tachycardia cycle length was 430 ms; it would be difficult for this one (340 ms) to be the same VT (Fig. 27-5).

Antitachycardia Pacing – No Good

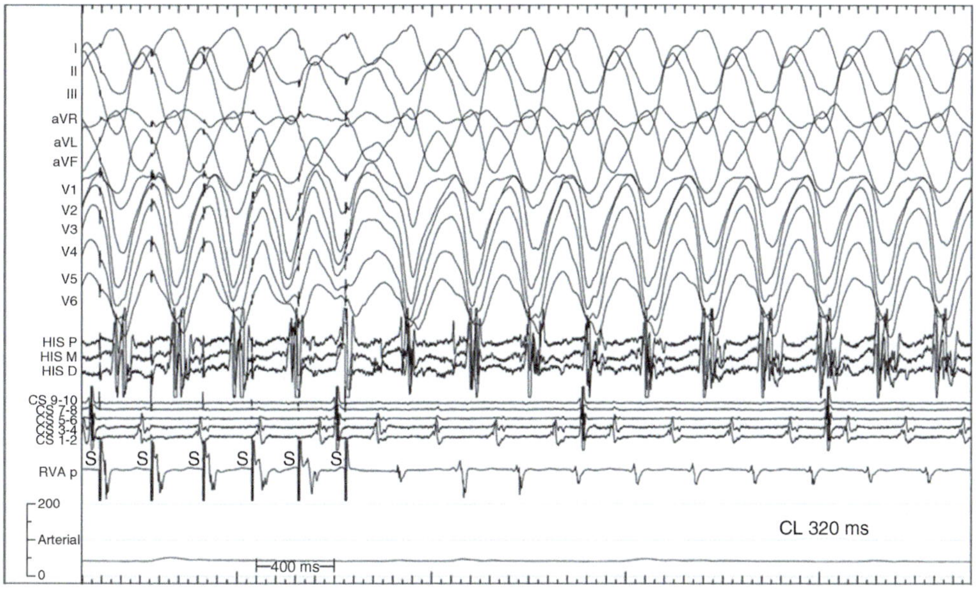

Figure 27-6

Overdrive pacing fails to terminate the rapid VT. At least this phenomenon (Fig. 27-6) is consistent with his clinical behavior—acceleration with antitachycardia pacing.

Why No QRS?

Shock Advised!

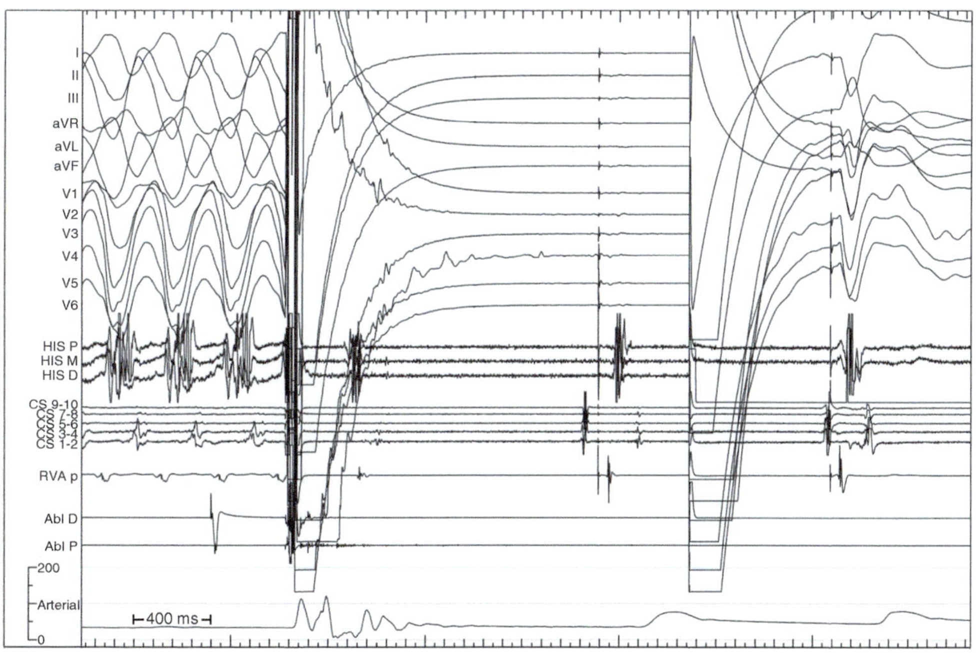

Figure 27-7

In Fig. 27-7, shock terminates rapid VT, but a stimulus from the device after the shock does not seem to capture the ventricle (no QRS complex). There really is one (note ventricular electrogram in RVA signal) and there is a systolic wave in the blood pressure recording, but surface ECG amplifiers have not reset.

VT Reinitiation

Is This the VT We're Looking For?

Figure 27-8

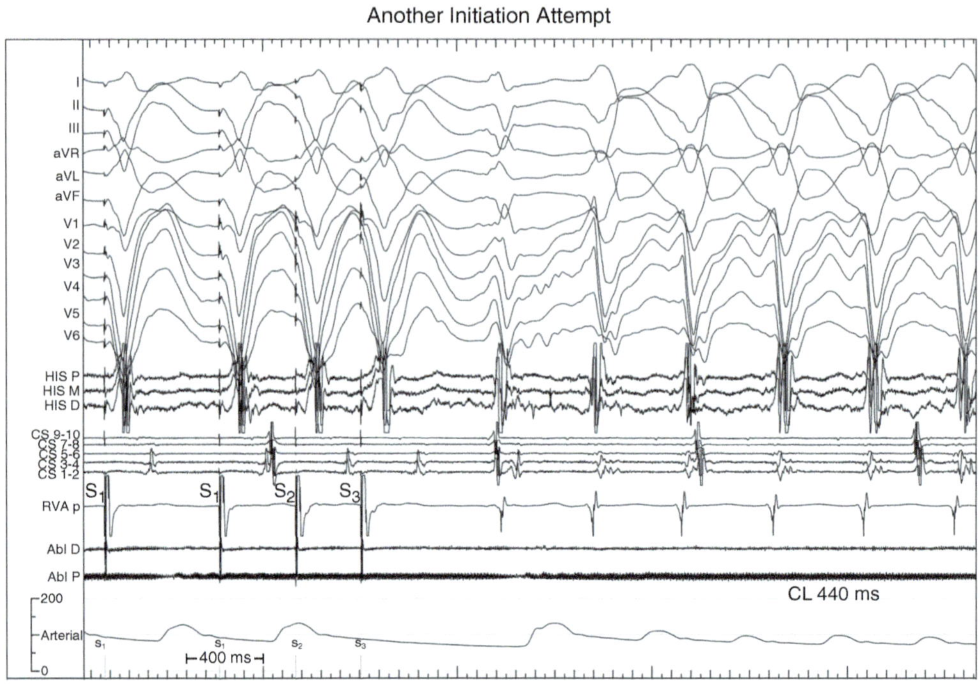

Another attempt is made to initiate VT. The VT shown in Fig. 27-8 has a cycle length very similar to the one that occurred spontaneously and is very likely the VT we are seeking.

Comparison of ICD Electrograms from This Episode and Prior Episode

Figure 27-9

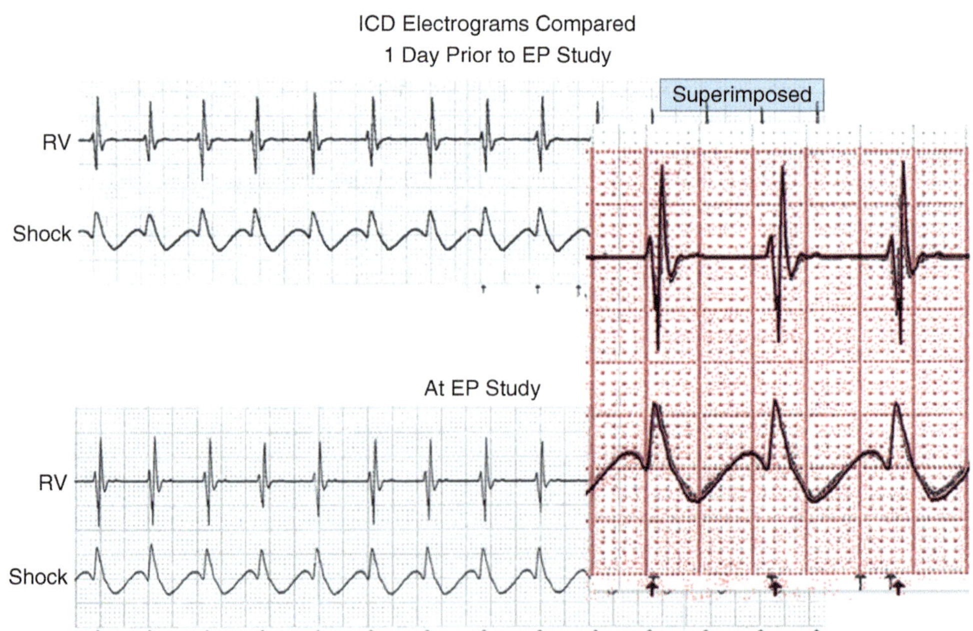

In Fig. 27-9, real-time electrograms from EP study (at bottom) are compared with those from the stored episode (at top); they are identical. Thus the induced VT corresponding to these electrograms is the same as the spontaneously occurring VT.

ECG of Target VT

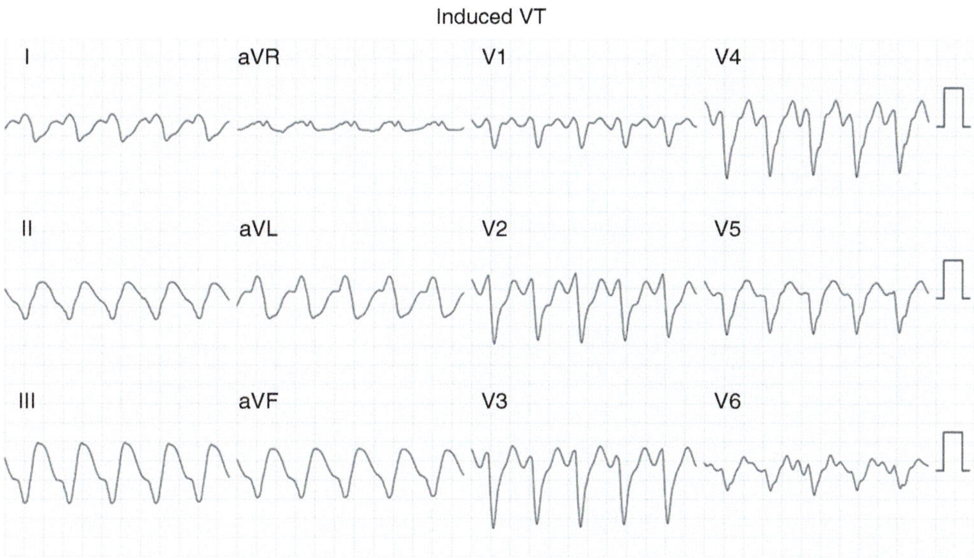

Figure 27-10

In Fig. 27-10, a 12-lead ECG of the induced VT has a left bundle branch block, leftward superior axis. It has findings that suggest a relationship to an inferior scar, though other features (poor R-wave progression) might suggest an apical exit site.

Comparison and Critique of Different Mapping Sites During VT

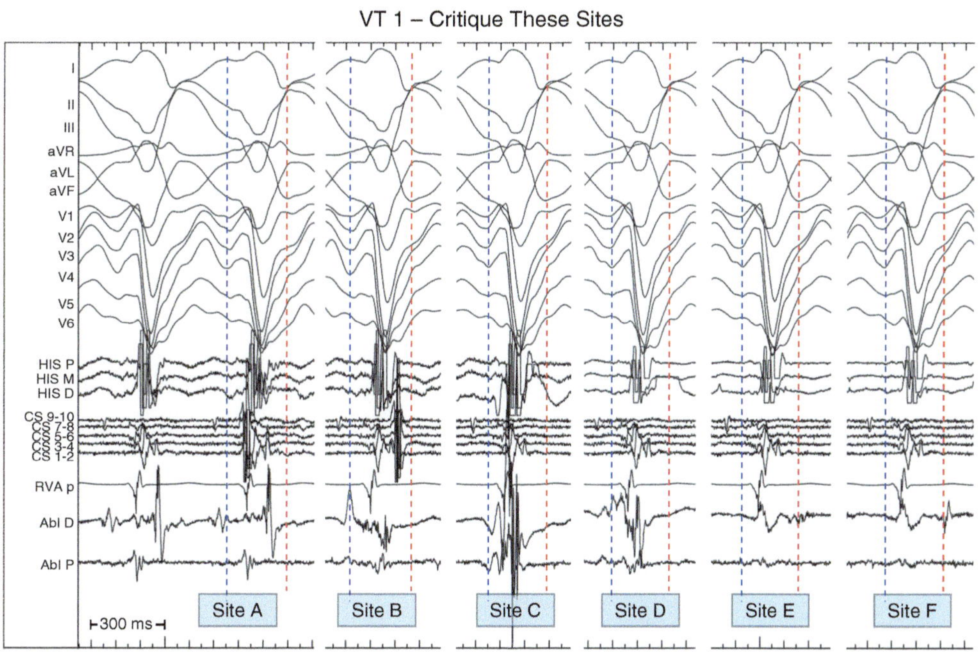

Figure 27-11

Fig. 27-11 displays several mapping sites (*dashed blue line* denotes onset of the QRS complex; *dashed red line,* the end):

A—late diastolic recording looks a little far-field; near-field component occurs during QRS complex
B—fragmented signal during QRS complex, but other portion is barely presystolic
C—high-amplitude, intra-QRS signal, of no interest
D—fragmented signal, with far-field late diastolic component
E—fragmented signal in early diastole—more interesting
F—discrete potential in early diastole—more interesting

Critique This Site . . .

VT 1

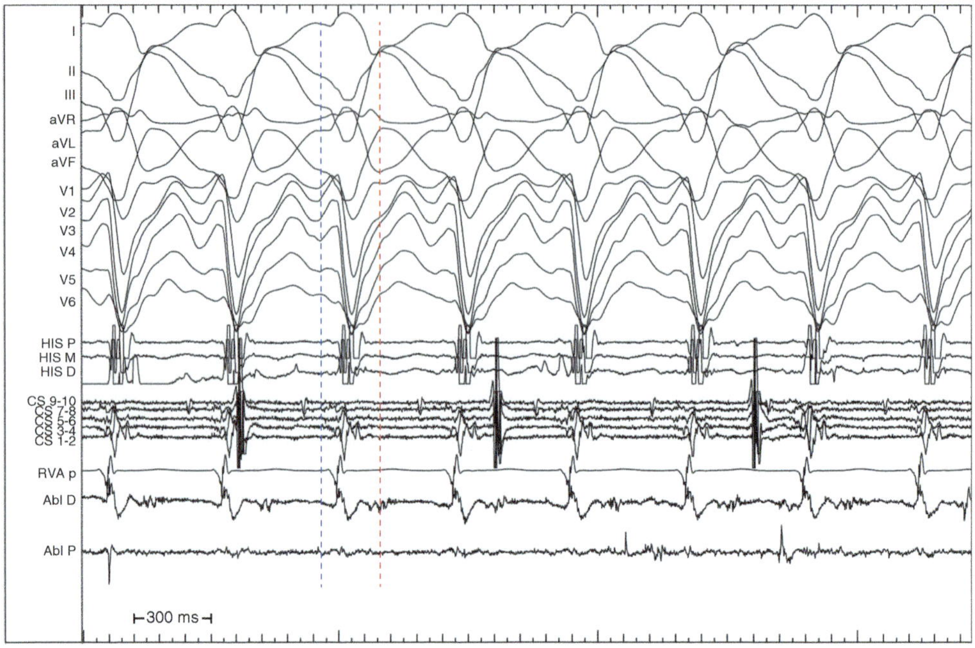

Figure 27-12

The site in Fig. 27-12 is only mildly interesting; though it has a systolic component (inside QRS complex), there is a fragmented portion extending into early diastole.

Critique This Site . . .

VT 1-2 Seconds Later, Adjacent Site

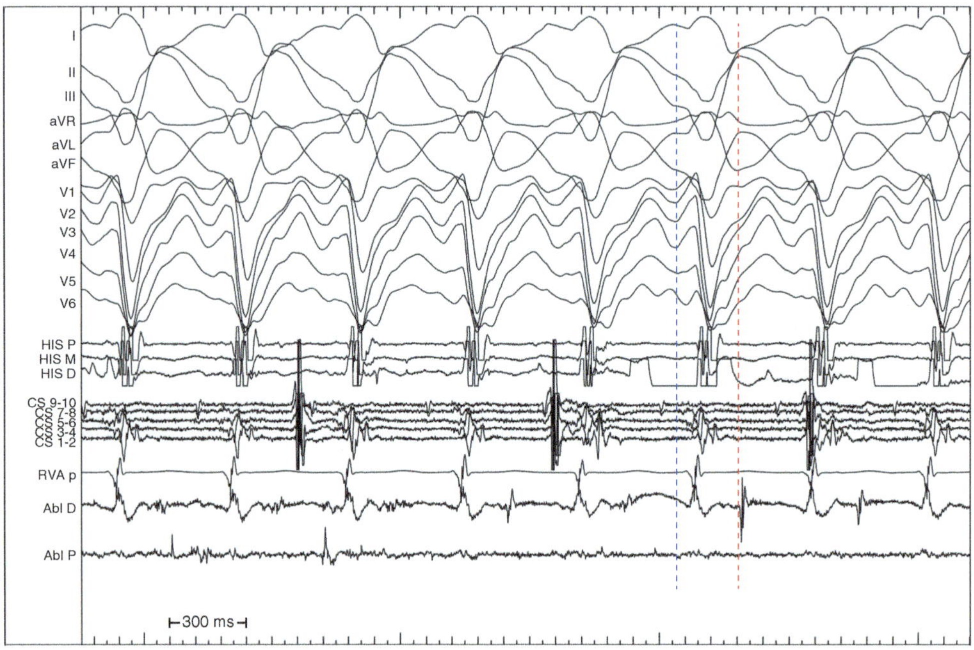

Figure 27-13

Recordings from just a few millimeters away have an interesting early diastolic component (Fig. 27-13), showing that potentially important sites may be extremely close to sites that are not very interesting (Fig. 27-12). This underscores the importance of detailed mapping.

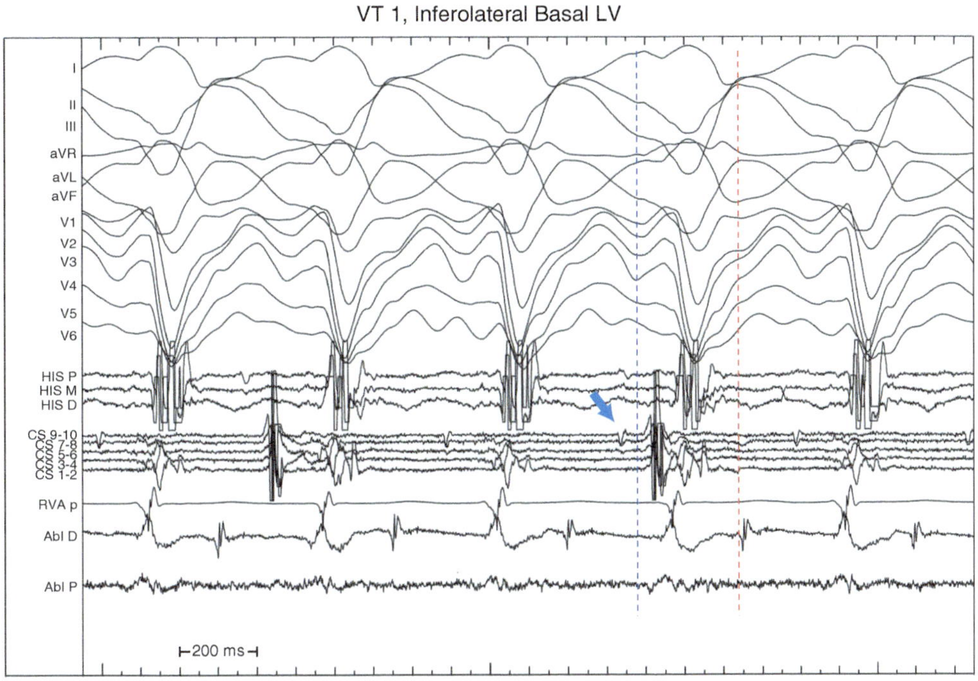

Figure 27-14

All the time we have been mapping, coronary sinus recordings have shown mid-late diastolic potentials (blue arrow) when adequately gained (Fig. 27-14).

What's Going on Here? [Fig. 27-15]

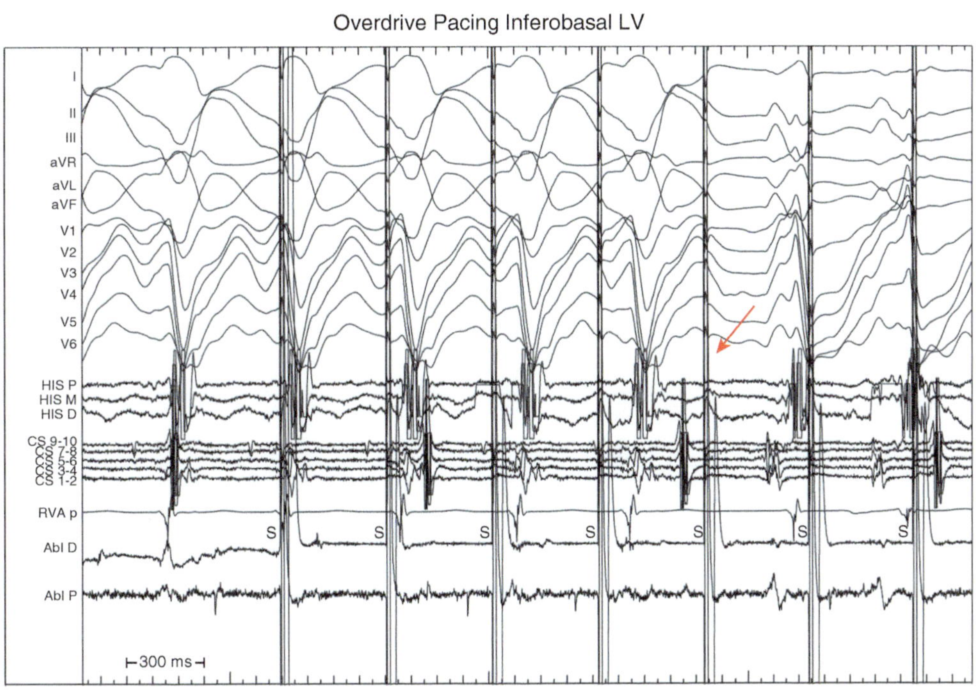

Figure 27-15

An attempt at overdrive pacing during VT results in termination of VT without apparent propagation *(arrow)*; actually, the impulse captures and propagates in the opposite direction as shown by the longer stimulus-QRS and complete change in polarity of the resulting QRS complex (Fig. 27-15). If this is a reproducible phenomenon, it has significant implications regarding the site (within the protected isthmus essential for VT continuation).

Critique This Site . . . 0.15 mV [Fig. 27-16]

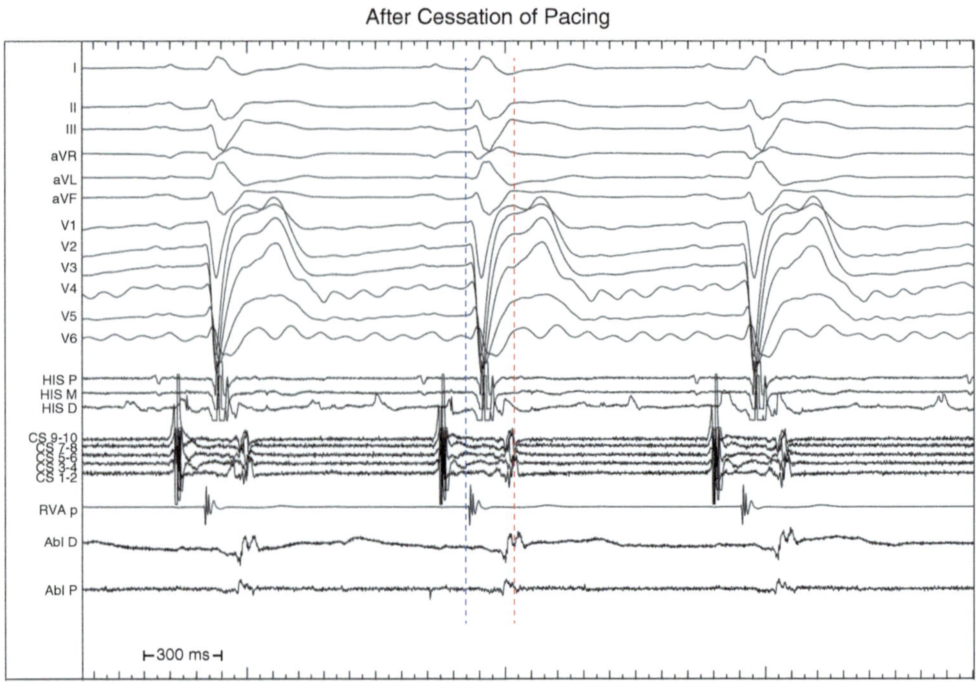

Figure 27-16

The site at which VT terminated with a nonpropagated stimulus is shown in Fig. 27-16 during sinus rhythm—not a very impressive site. This illustrates one of the problems with sinus rhythm/substrate mapping (poor sensitivity).

Comment on Capture at This Site . . . [Fig. 27-17]

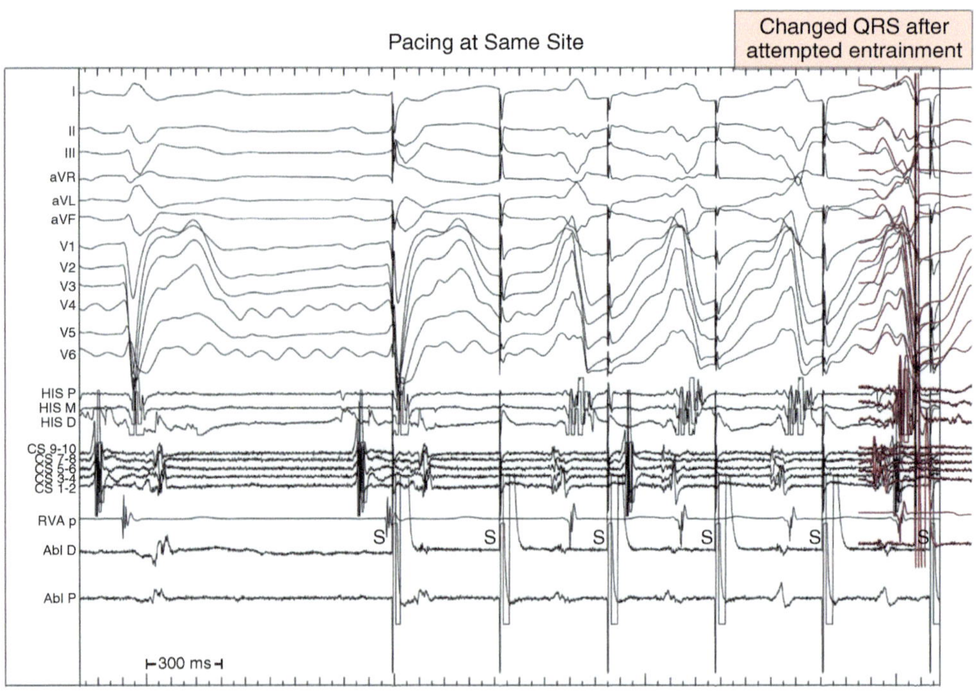

Figure 27-17

Stimulation at this same site (Fig. 27-17) results in a QRS complex very similar to that obtained during overdrive pacing during VT. The interpretation is that it is electrically a shorter distance to propagate in this direction (which would be toward the entrance of the circuit) than toward the exit (that would result in the same morphology as the first VT).

Pacing Induces VT-2

Comment on Capture at This Site . . . [Fig. 27-18]

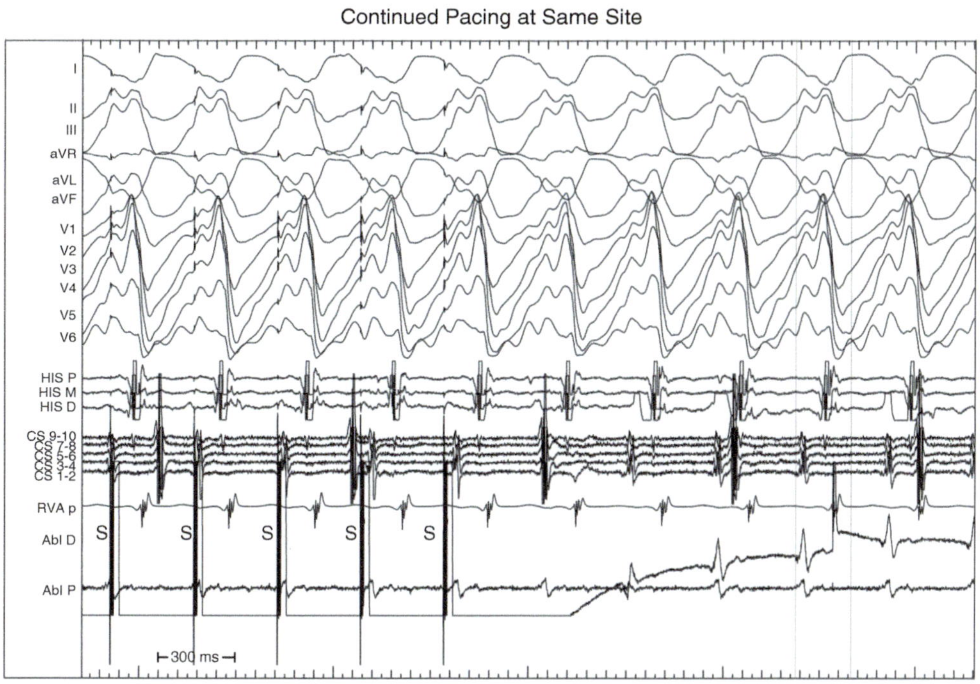

Figure 27-18

As pacing continues in Fig. 27-18, it is clear that another VT has been initiated (note lack of correlation between stimulus artifacts and QRS complexes on the left of the figure).

ECG of VT-2

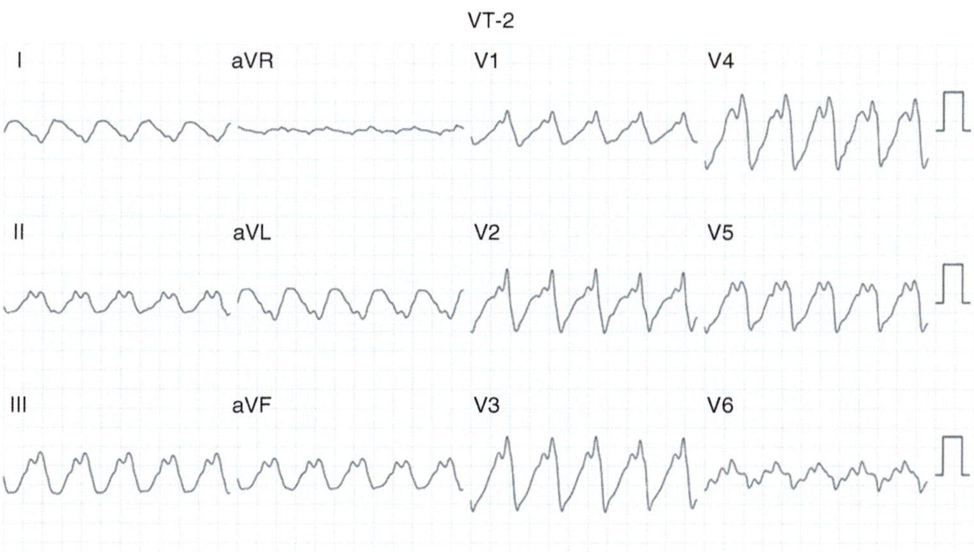

Figure 27-19

Fig. 27-19 shows a 12-lead ECG of the second induced VT.

VT-2, Pacing, and Sinus Rhythm at One Site

Critique This Site . . . and Where Is It? [Fig. 27-20]

Figure 27-20

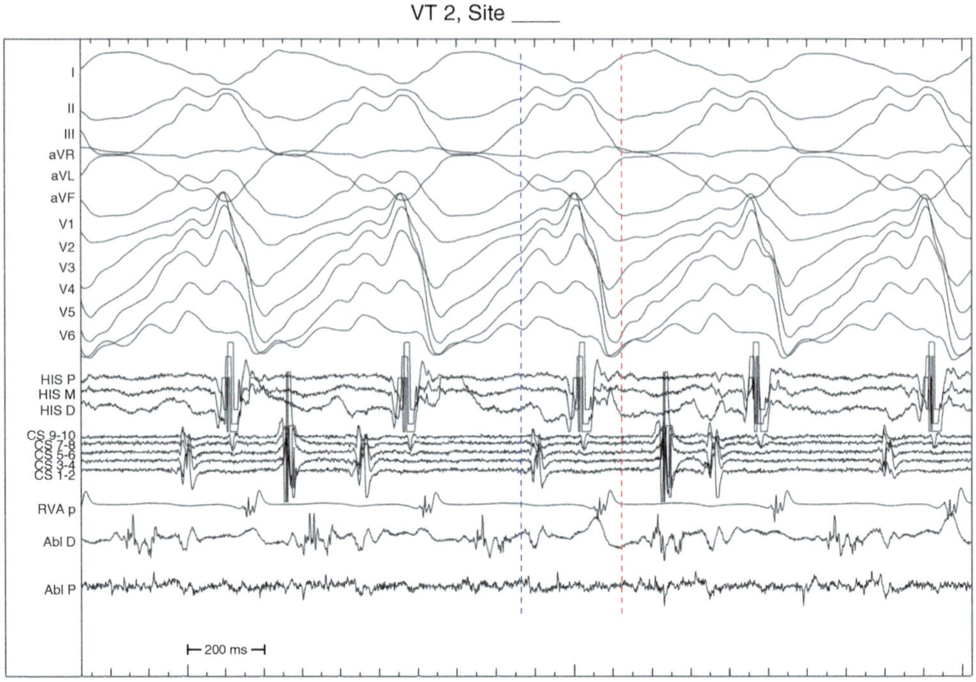

Fig. 27-20 shows a mid-diastolic potential, from the basal lateral LV.

Figure 27-21

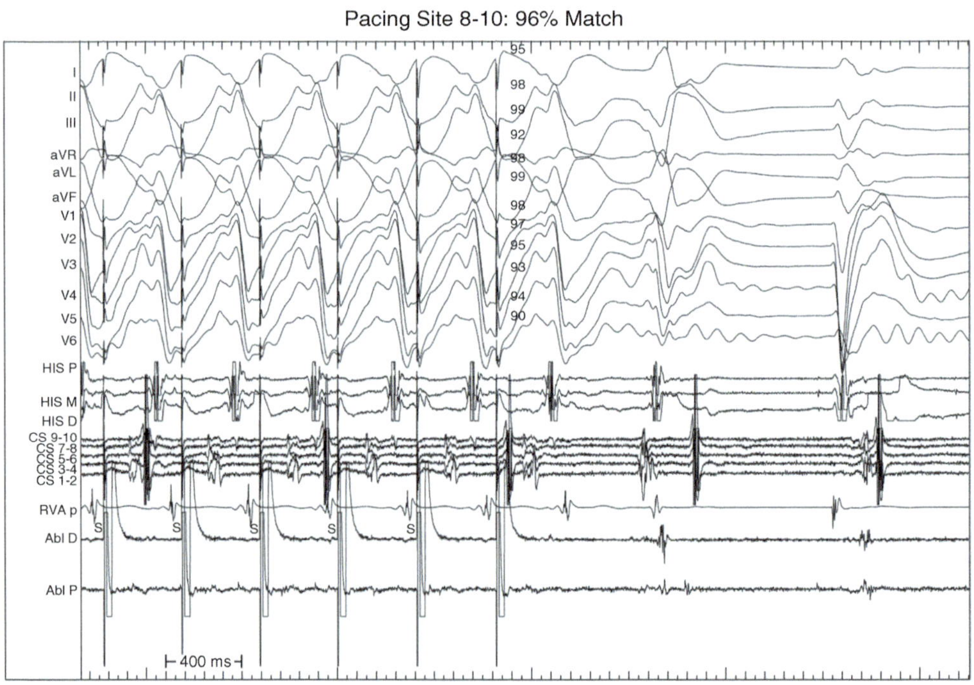

Pacing at a basal lateral side produces a 96% computer match of the morphology of VT-2 (Fig. 27-21).

Critique This Site . . . [Fig. 27-22]

Same Site After VT and Pacing

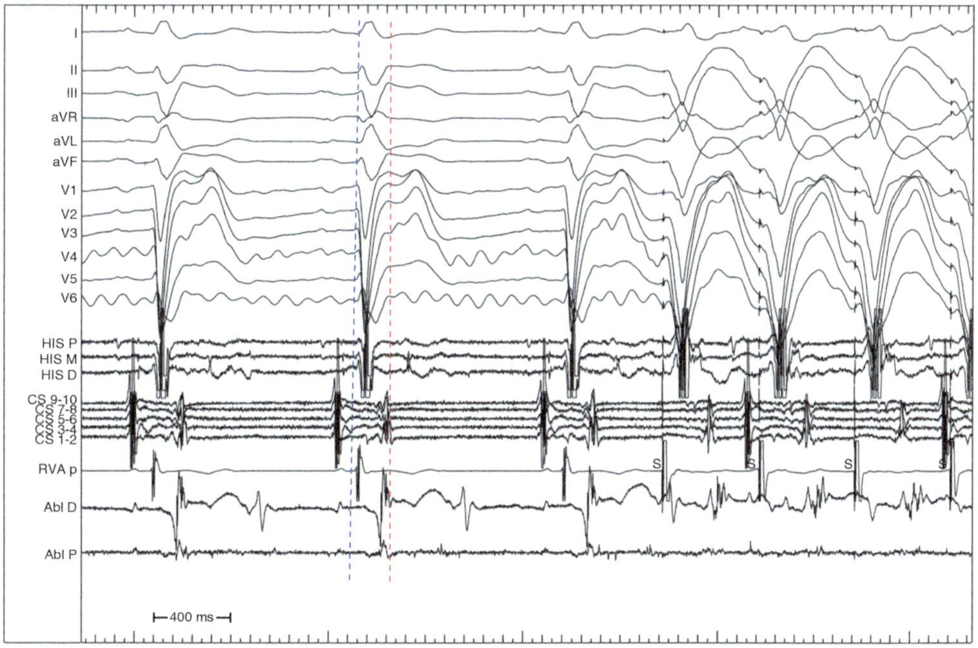

Figure 27-22

Fig. 27-22 shows the sinus rhythm recordings from the site of pace match and diastolic signal during VT-2—not very impressive (no fragmentation or late potential). Pacing the right ventricle, however, unveils a highly fragmented and delayed electrogram. This shows the importance of pacing-induced changes in signal characteristics when looking for local abnormal late activities (LAVA).

Reinitiation of VT-1

VT 1 Reinitiated

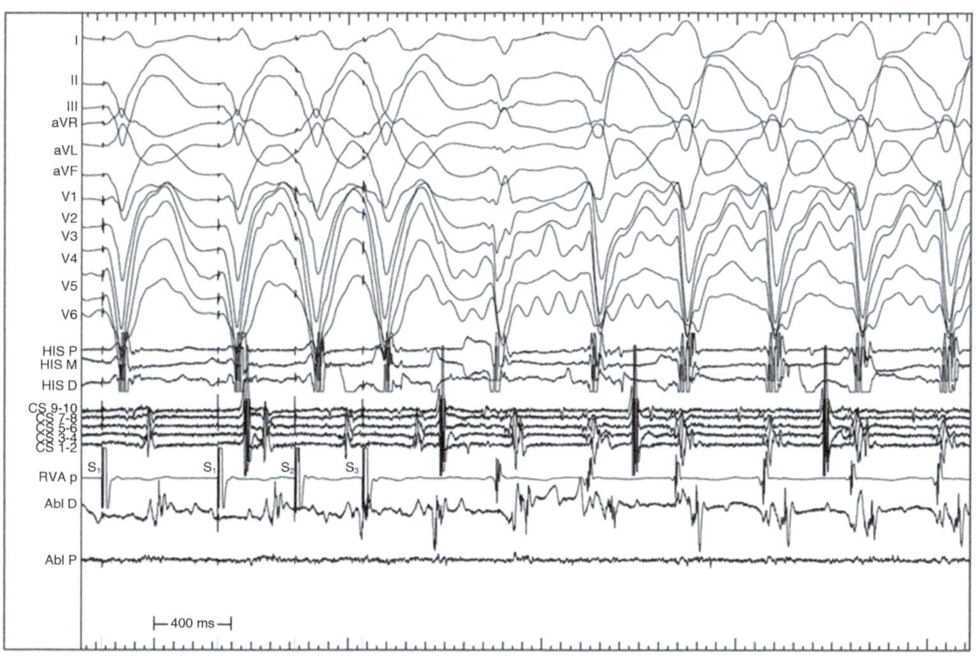

Figure 27-23

In Fig. 27-23, VT was reinitiated to test whether the stimulus that terminated VT without global capture ("nonpropagated termination") was a real phenomenon or chance occurrence (ie, spontaneous change).

Single Extrastimulus Terminates VT-1, Spontaneous Reinitiation, and Further Testing at This Site

What's Going on Here?

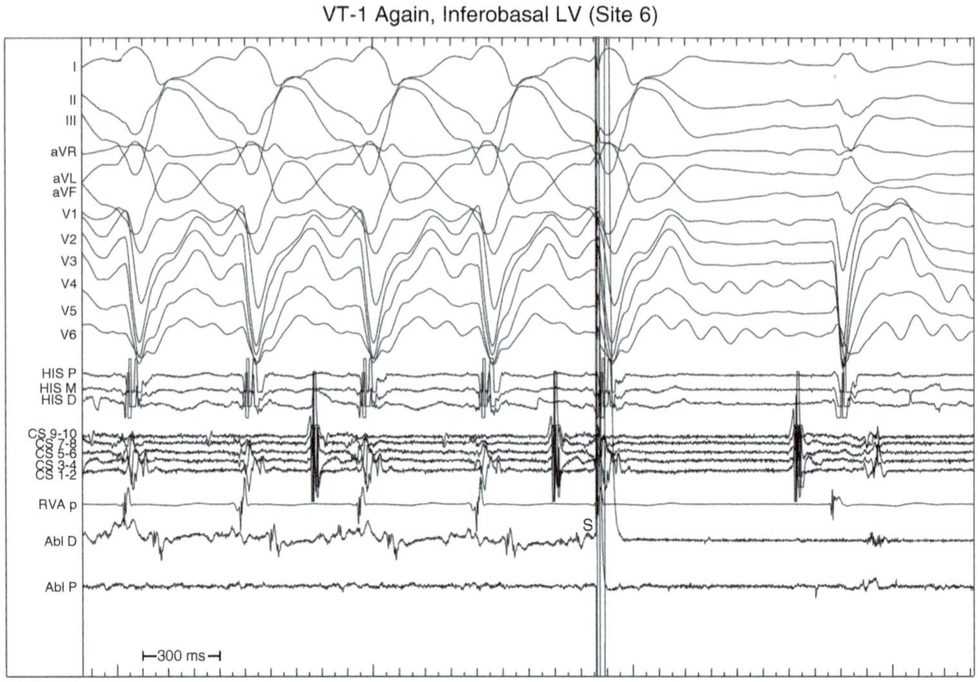

Figure 27-24

At a site very near where an attempt at overdrive pacing terminated VT without propagation, a single extrastimulus terminates VT (Fig. 27-24). This signifies that this is an excellent site for ablation.

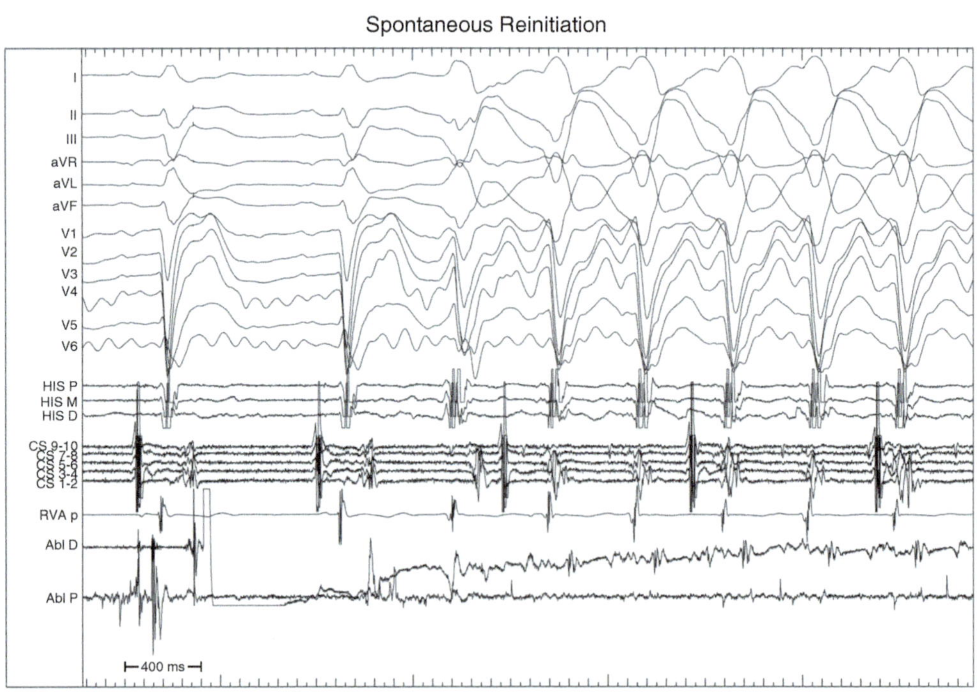

Figure 27-25

Spontaneous initiation of VT occurs when the catheter is at this site, as shown in Fig. 27-25.

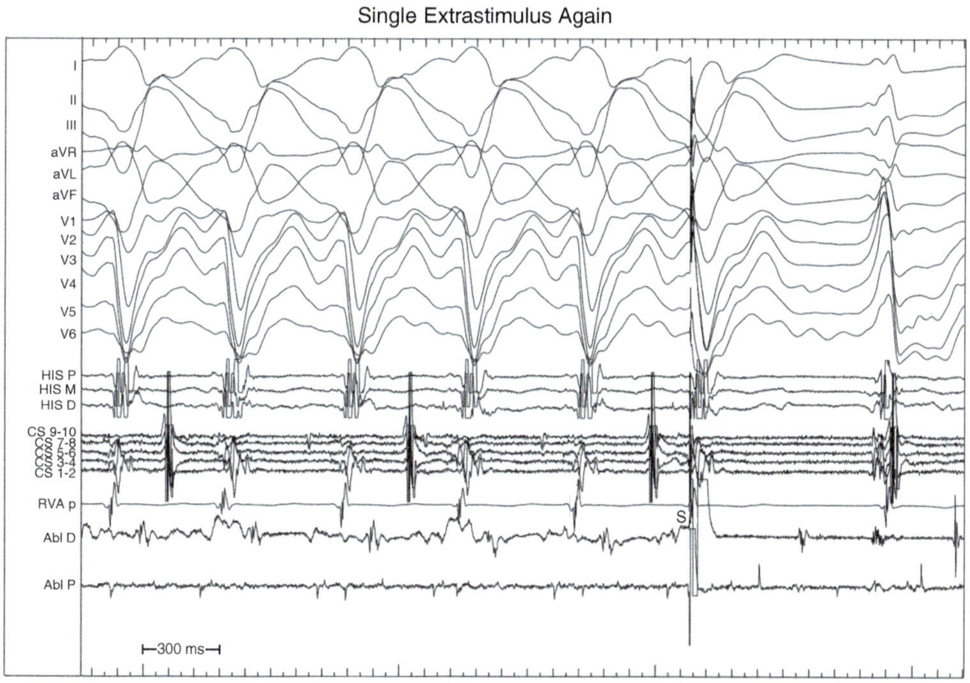

Figure 27-26

Just to prove the point, another single extrastimulus (S) terminates VT without propagation (Fig. 27-26).

Critique This Site . . .

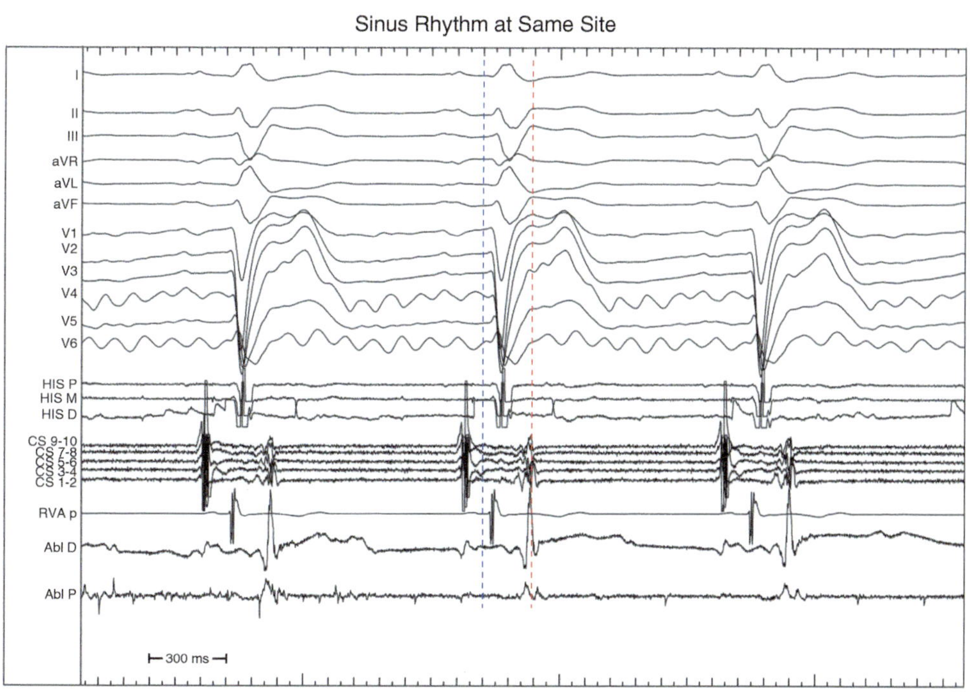

Figure 27-27

A nondescript electrogram is evident during sinus rhythm at the site at which VT was terminated by a single extrastimulus (Fig. 27-27).

Figure 27-28

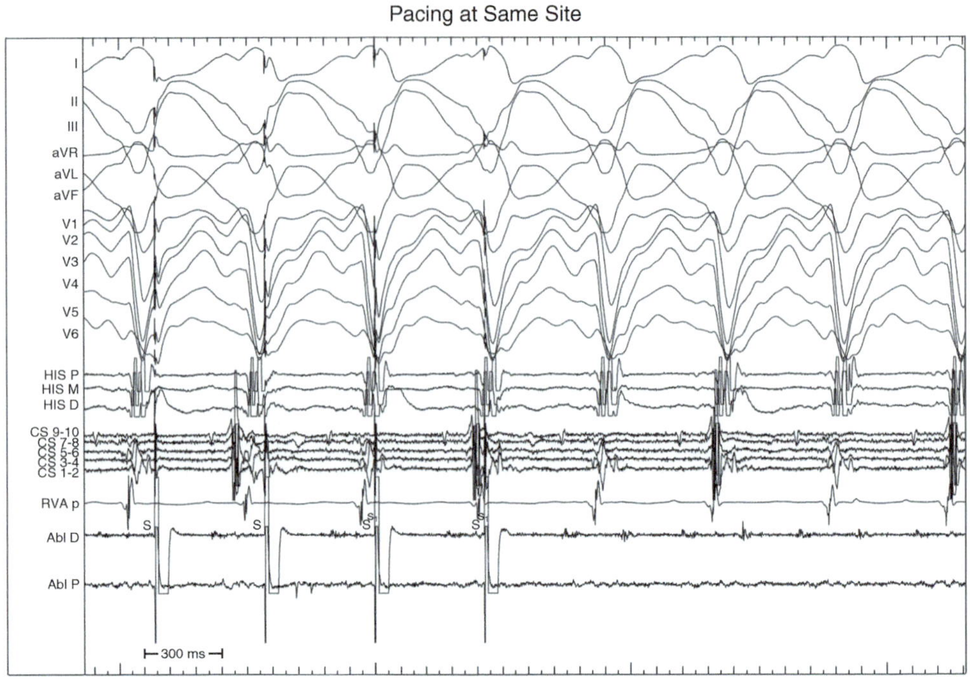

As shown in Fig. 27-28, pacing at this same site reinitiates the same VT.

Ablation and Subsequent Pacing at This Site in VT-1

Figure 27-29

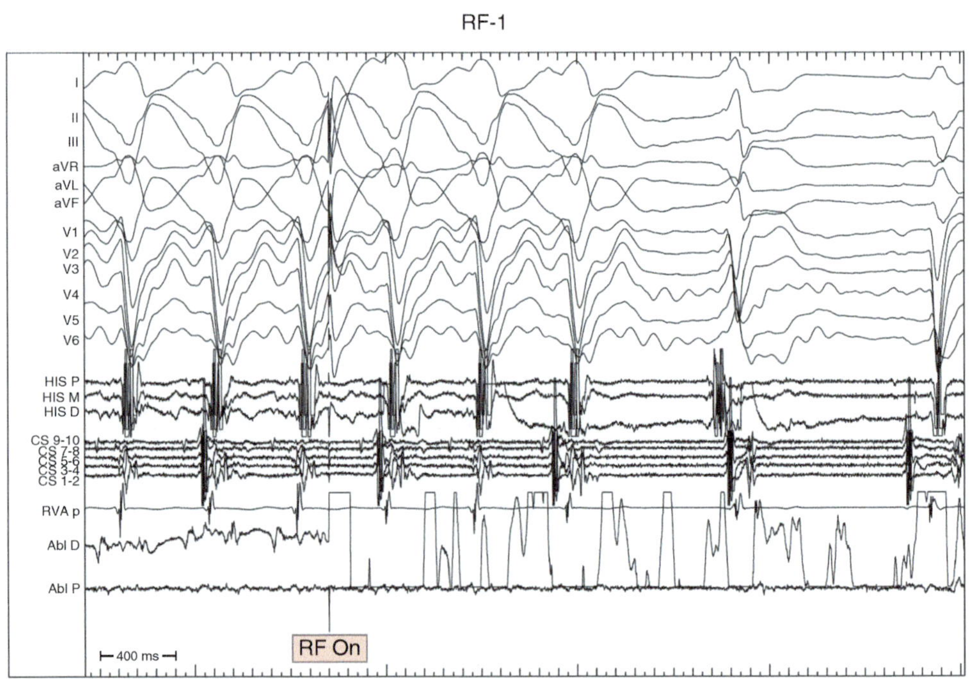

Rewarding our hard work is nearly immediate termination of VT with radiofrequency application at this site (Fig. 27-29).

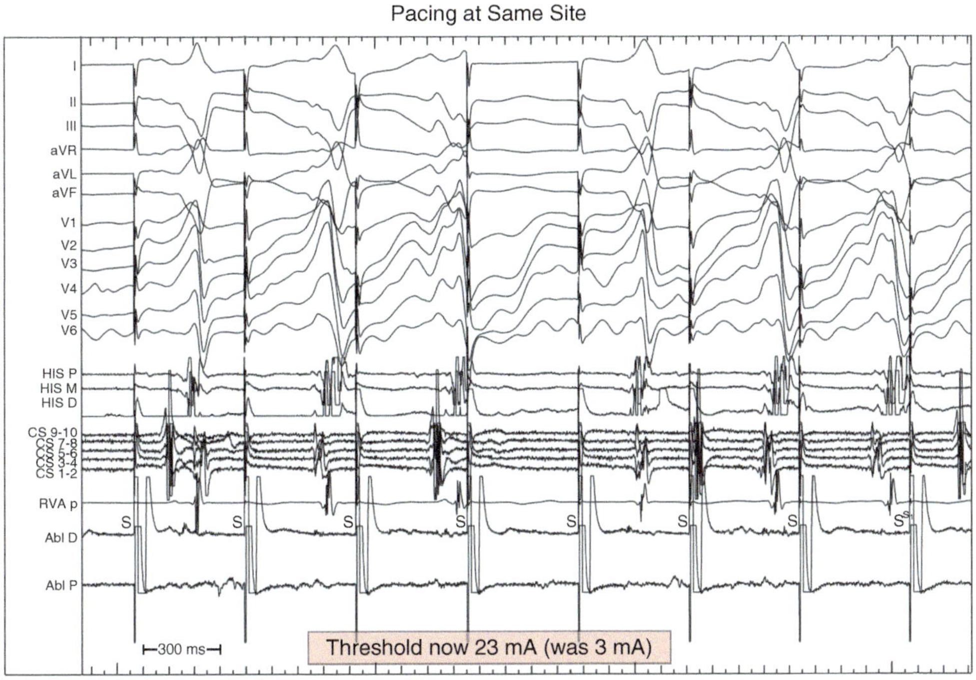

Figure 27-30

VT cannot be reinitiated; a quick check of the pacing threshold at this site after ablation shows it to be markedly elevated (Fig. 27-30).

Initiation and Ablation of VT-3

Critique This Site . . . [Fig. 27-31]

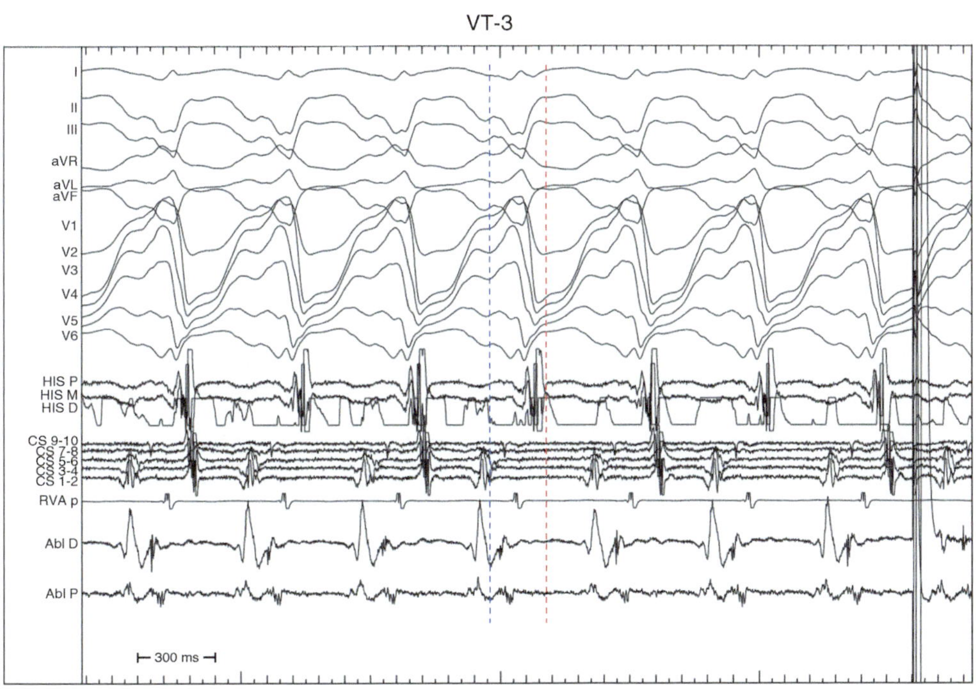

Figure 27-31

However, as can be seen in Fig. 27-31, another VT can be initiated.

Figure 27-32

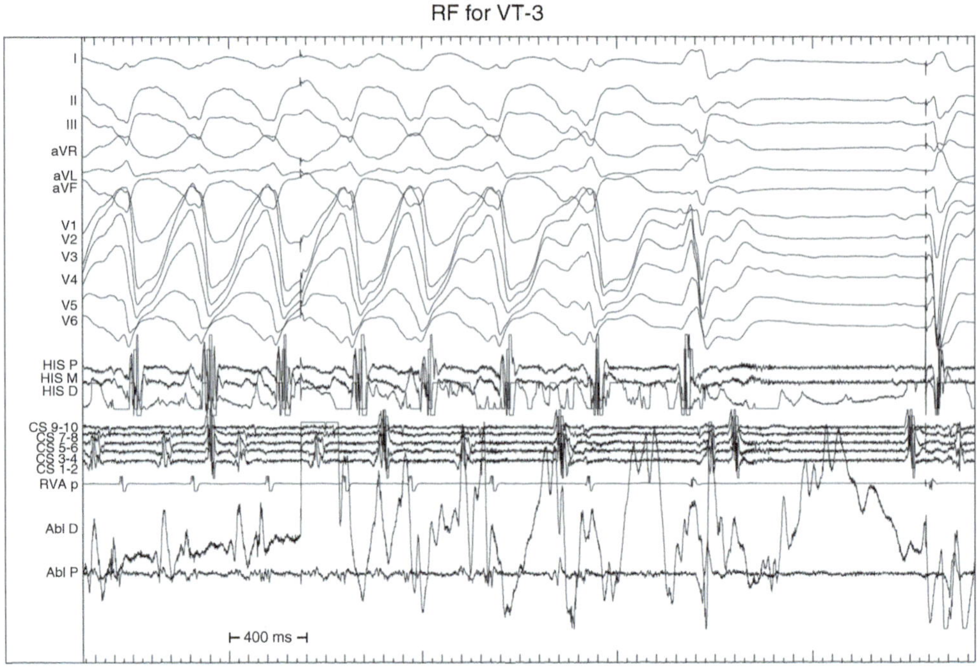

After applying several of the same pacing maneuvers, the VT displayed in Fig. 27-32 is terminated with radiofrequency energy at a site of diastolic activation.

Electroanatomic Mapping Findings

Figure 27-33

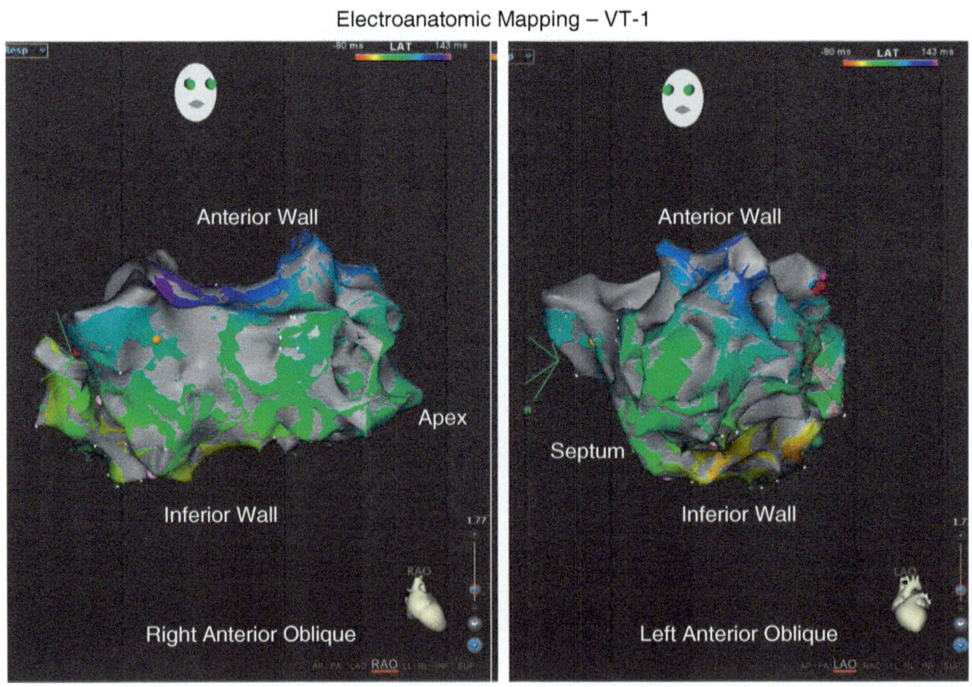

Standard views of the electroanatomic activation map, shown in Fig. 27-33, suggest a region of interest in the inferolateral basal left ventricular free wall (*red* and *orange* areas).

Why So Much Low Voltage? [Fig. 27-34]

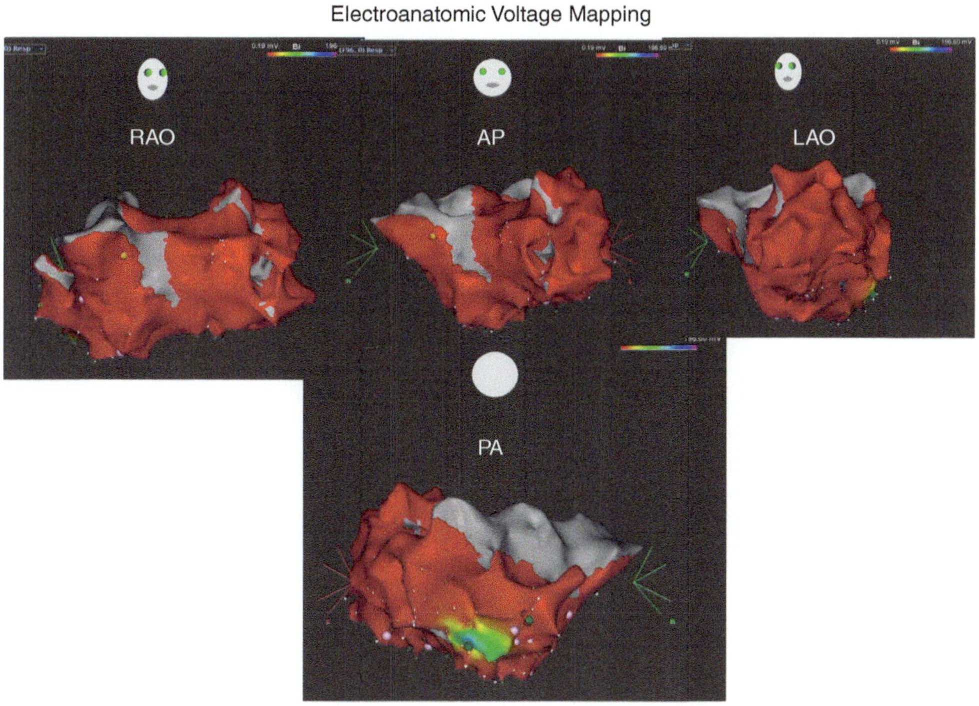

Figure 27-34

In Fig. 27-34, it looks like the entire ventricle, except for a small portion (near where we ablated!), has very low voltage. This does not make sense; the ablated area (diseased) should have low voltage (*red*) while other areas should have more normal voltage (*purple*).

Why Such Different Voltage?

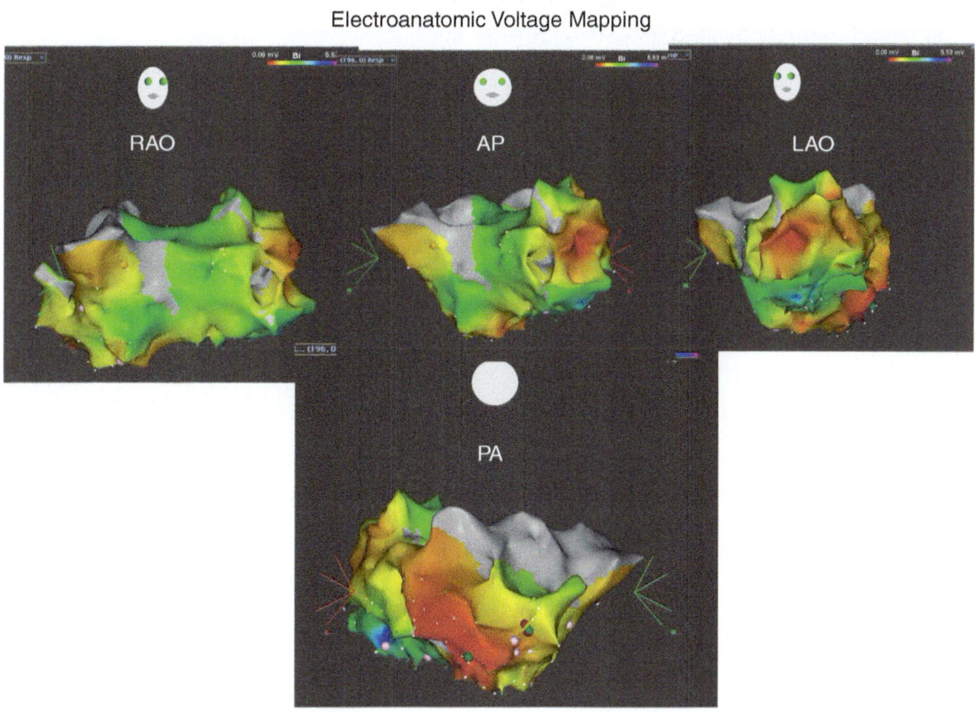

Figure 27-35

The problem is, a single site of the posterior wall had an extremely high voltage, making everything else seem extremely low (Fig. 27-35).

Electroanatomic Mapping

Figure 27-36

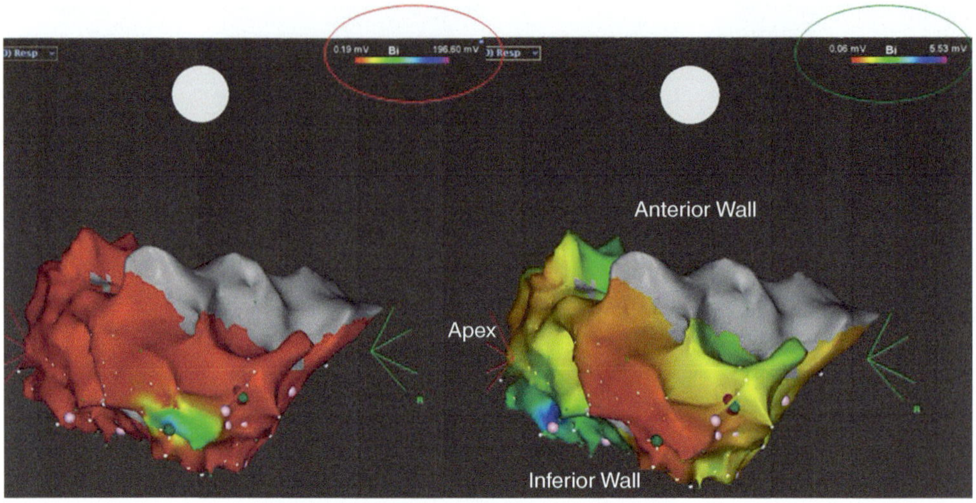

At left of Fig. 27-36 is the original voltage map; at right is the edited voltage map (after adjudicating the computer-designated voltage at one site).

Electroanatomic Mapping

Figure 27-37

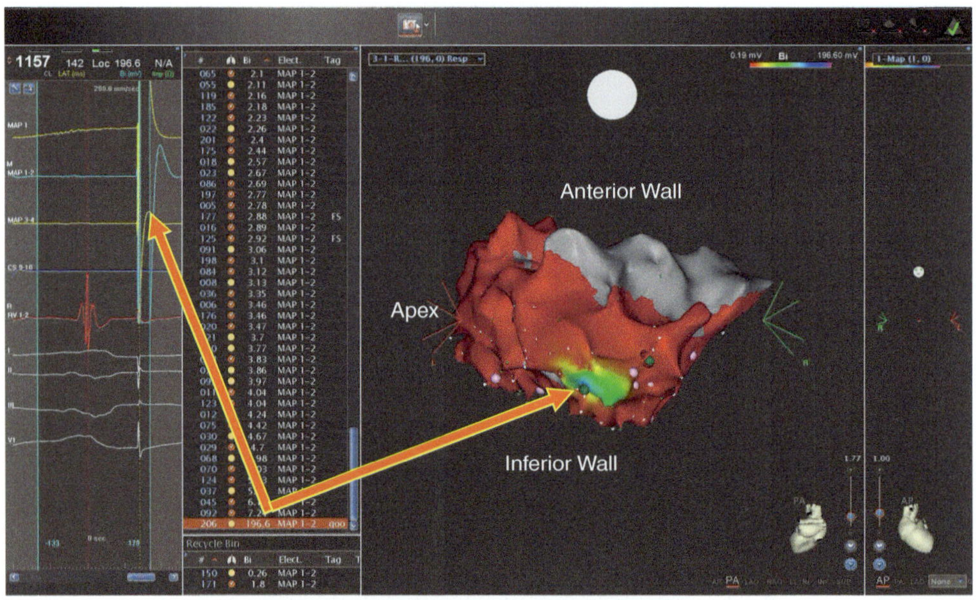

In Fig. 27-37, the point with the falsely high voltage was because of a stimulus artifact.

This *single point* in the voltage map threw everything else off (195 other points that were correct).

Electroanatomic Mapping

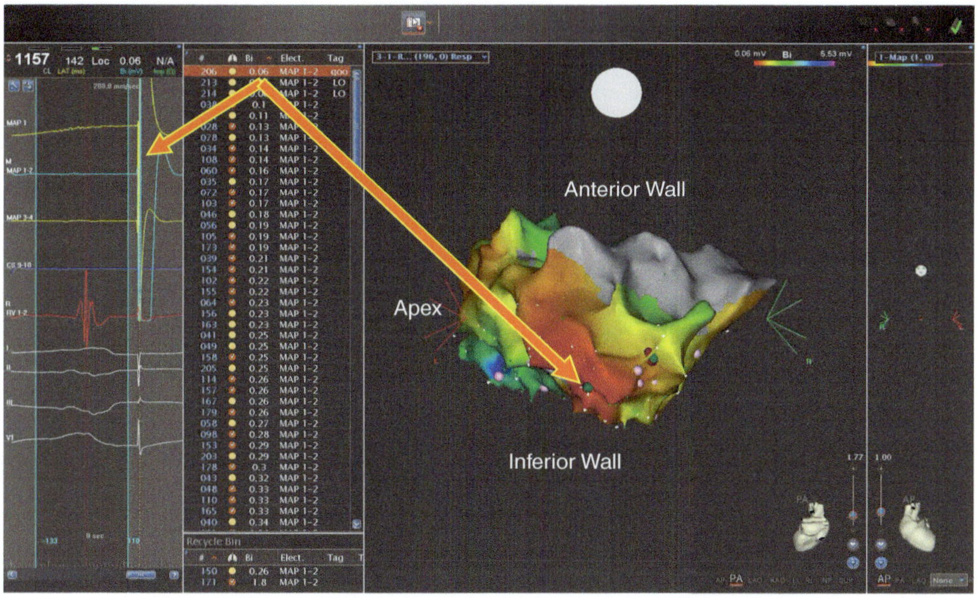

Figure 27-38

In Fig. 27-38 is the correct voltage at that site, obtained by simply sliding the window of interest enough to exclude the stimulus artifact that was causing a problem.

Electroanatomic Mapping

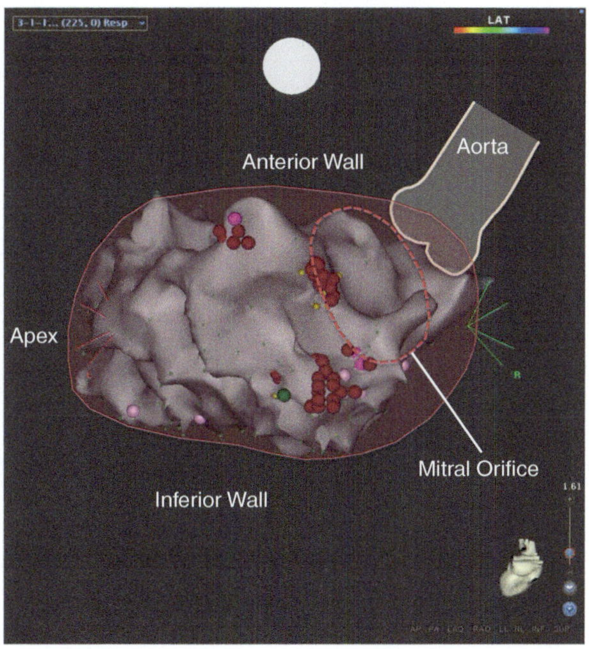

Figure 27-39

In Fig. 27-39, the electroanatomic map as well as ablation sites *(red dots)* are projected on a silhouette of the left ventricle and aorta in a posterior view of the heart.

Summary

- Sometimes it is hard to know what the target area is likely to be (preoperative imaging, ECG in sinus rhythm or VT can help)
- The pathophysiology of VT in dilated cardiomyopathy is fundamentally the same as other scar-based VTs (like post-MI VT); this patient had a small prior MI but LV dysfunction out of proportion to it
- Having *some* information about the spontaneous VT (ICD recordings) can be very useful in deciding what to target
- Serendipitous findings (nonpropagated stimulus terminating VT) are very valuable and should not be ignored
- Voltage mapping can be great but *just one incorrect point* can make interpretation completely wrong

28 Bundle Branch Reentry Ventricular Tachycardia

Case Presentation

A 56-year-old man with inferior wall myocardial infarction (MI) in May 2010 was referred for catheter ablation because of frequent implantable cardioverter-defibrillator (ICD) activity. At the time of his MI, he had percutaneous coronary intervention to the mid-right coronary artery. Left ventricular systolic function was poor at the time and remained so; he underwent biventricular ICD placement for primary prophylaxis of sudden death. Within months, he began experiencing frequent antitachycardia pacing (ATP) and shocks from his ICD because of rapid ventricular tachycardia (VT). Amiodarone was administered; he still received frequent ATP and some shocks, despite additional device reprogramming. He underwent electrophysiology (EP) study and ablation, at which time abnormal electrograms on the left ventricular anterior septum were identified. Only nonsustained VT episodes with multiple left bundle branch block (LBBB) morphologies could be induced. Extensive ablation of anterior septal sites was performed. Unfortunately, even after the procedure, he continued to have episodes of VT requiring ATP or shocks. He was given more amiodarone but still required frequent ATP for treatment of VT. He was referred for repeat ablation.

Baseline ECG (Paced) and Intracardiac Recordings

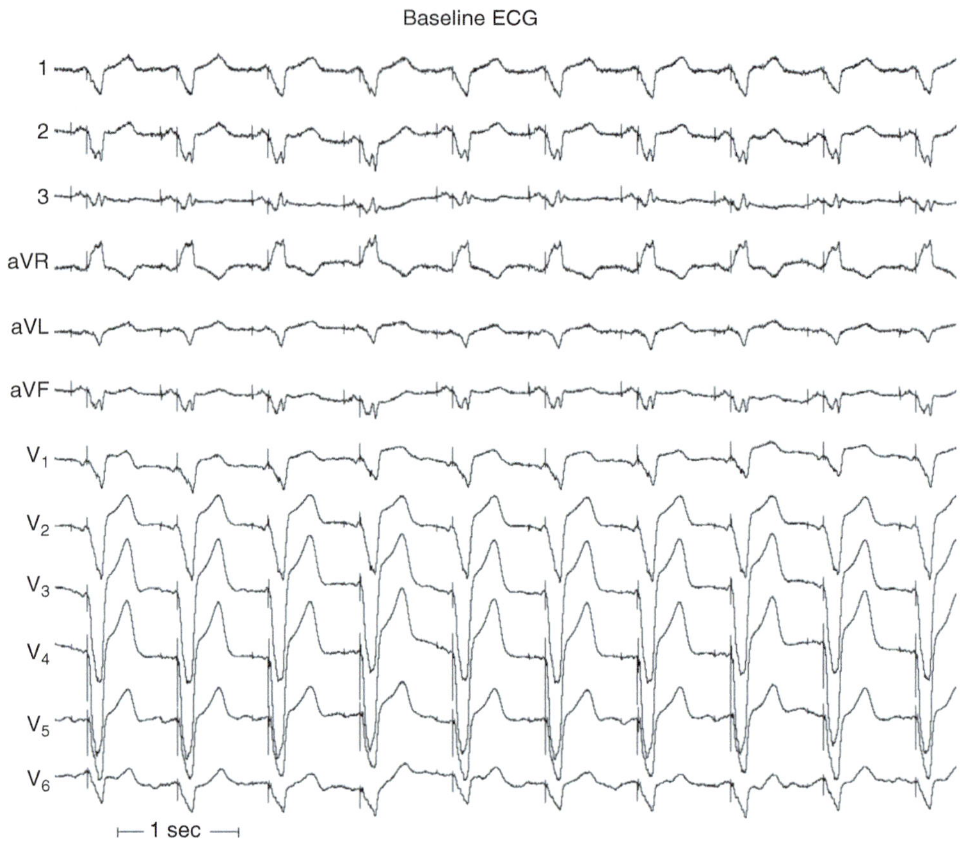

Figure 28-1

The baseline ECG during atrial and biventricular pacing yields few clues as to where mapping attention should be focused (Fig. 28-1).

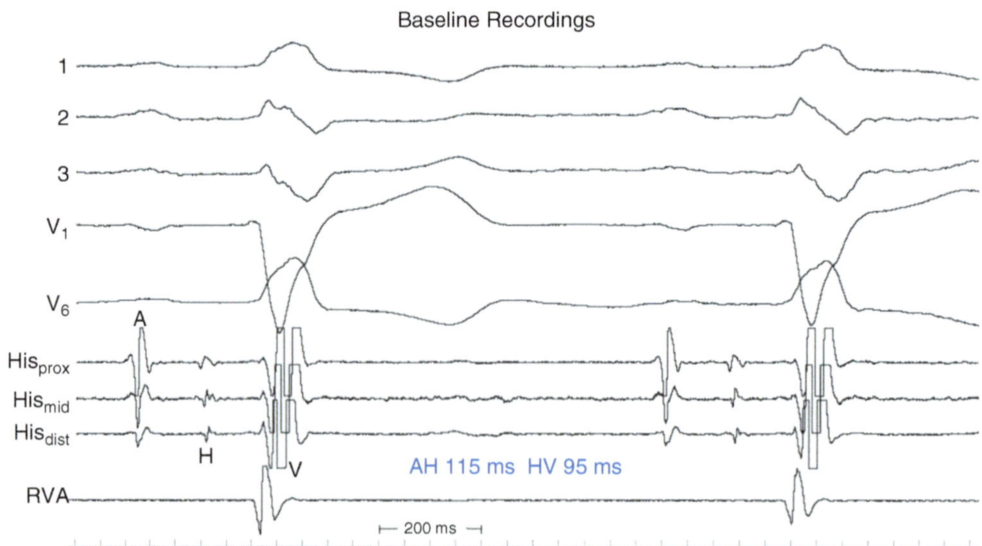

Figure 28-2

When the device was reprogrammed to a backup pacing mode, sinus rhythm with intact AV conduction is revealed. In Fig. 28-2, LBBB is present with intervals as shown.

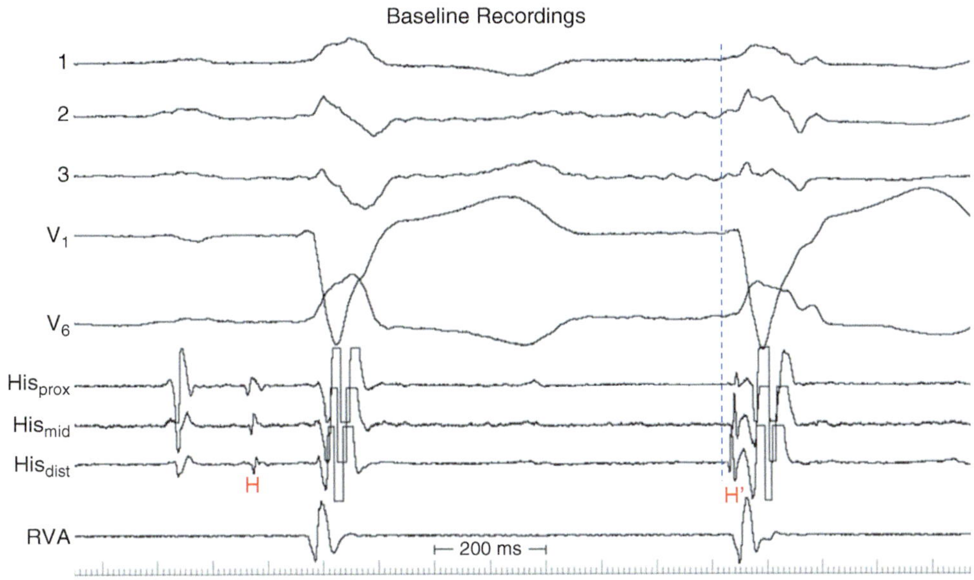

Figure 28-3

In Fig. 28-3, a spontaneous premature ventricular complex occurs that conducts retrogradely over the His bundle (H′, propagated distal to proximal). As early as the retrograde His occurs relative to the QRS onset *(dashed line)*, it must have conducted from the right bundle branch.

Ventricular Stimulation and VT Induction

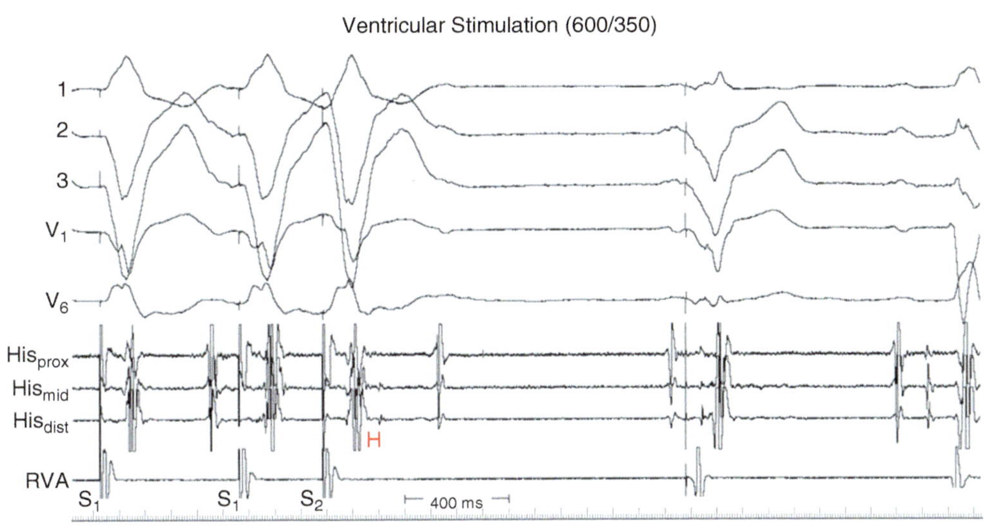

Figure 28-4

With ventricular extrastimulus testing, a His potential (H) is seen "out the back" (retrograde block in RBB with transseptal propagation to the LBB and then to the His bundle) in Fig. 28-4.

Figure 28-5

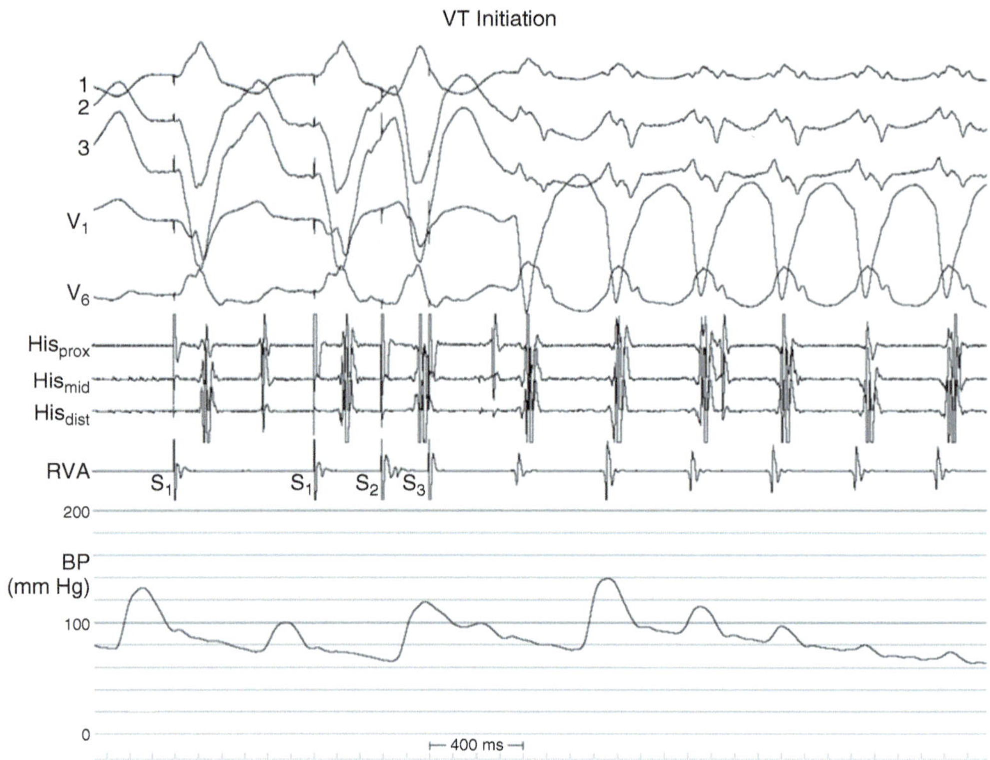

With double ventricular extrastimuli, rapid VT is induced; blood pressure is very poor and pacing termination was necessary within a few seconds after this recording (Fig. 28-5) was made.

Figure 28-6

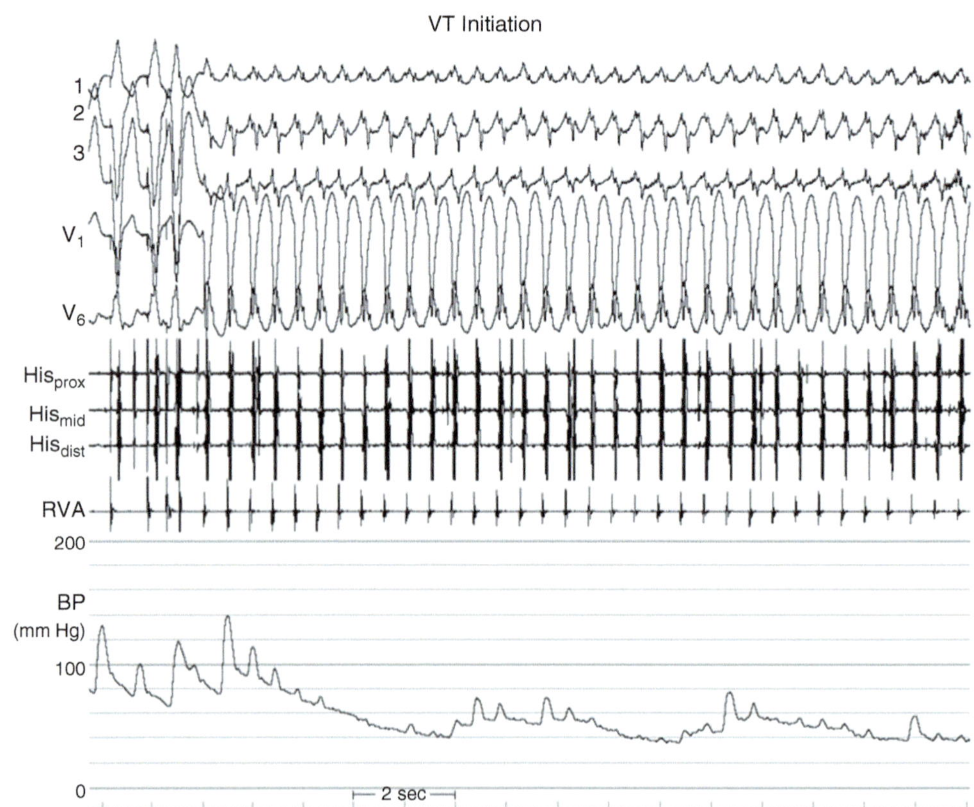

Fig. 28-6 presents the same events at a slower sweep speed and clearly shows the poor blood pressure response during induced VT.

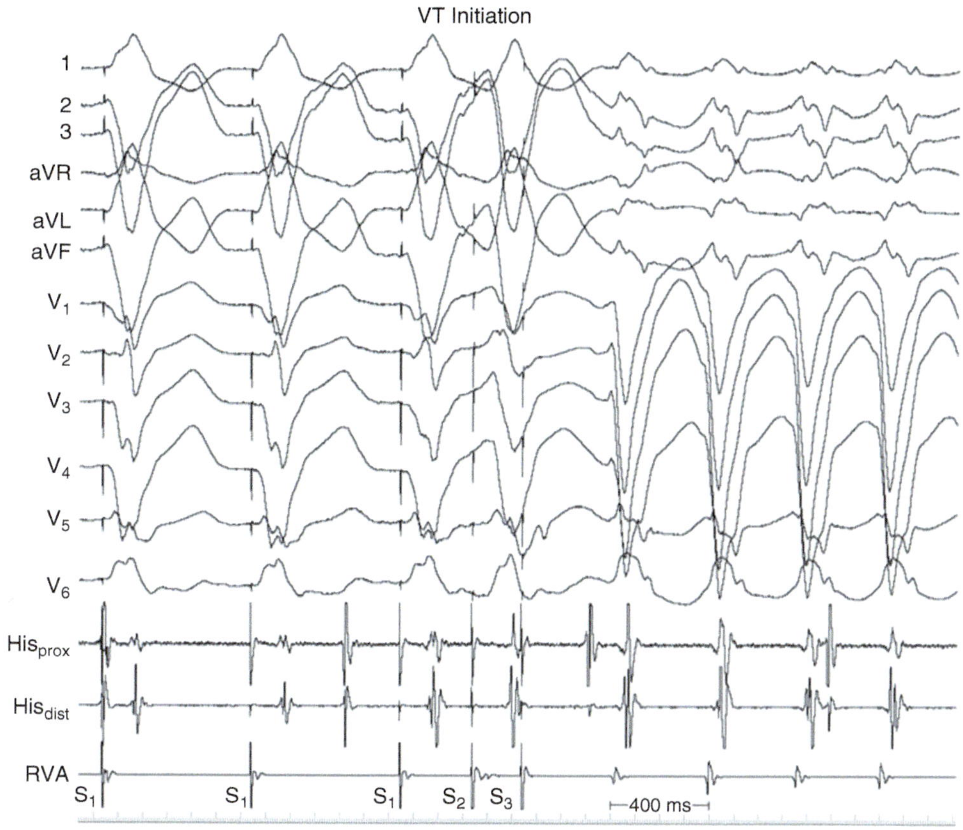

Figure 28-7

In Fig. 28-7, the same events as in the prior figure are shown, but this time displaying all 12 ECG leads. Of note, there is no His potential visible during VT.

VT ECG

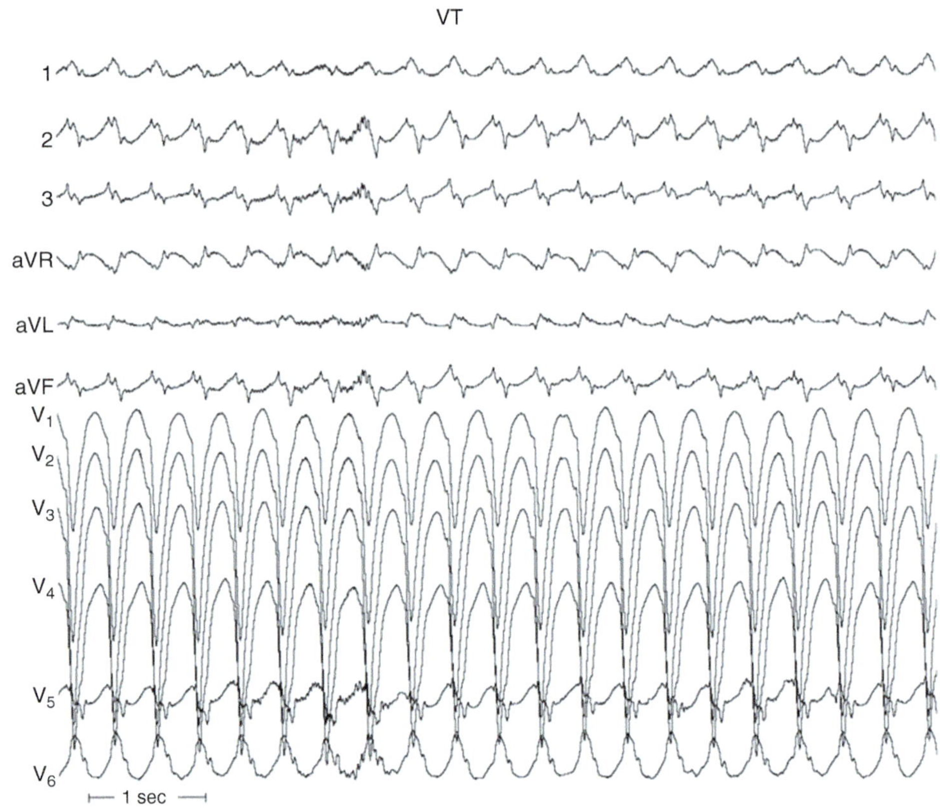

Figure 28-8

The full 12 leads of ECG during this induced VT are shown in Fig. 28-8, having an LBBB morphology (similar to what was described as having been initiated at the previous procedure).

VT Termination

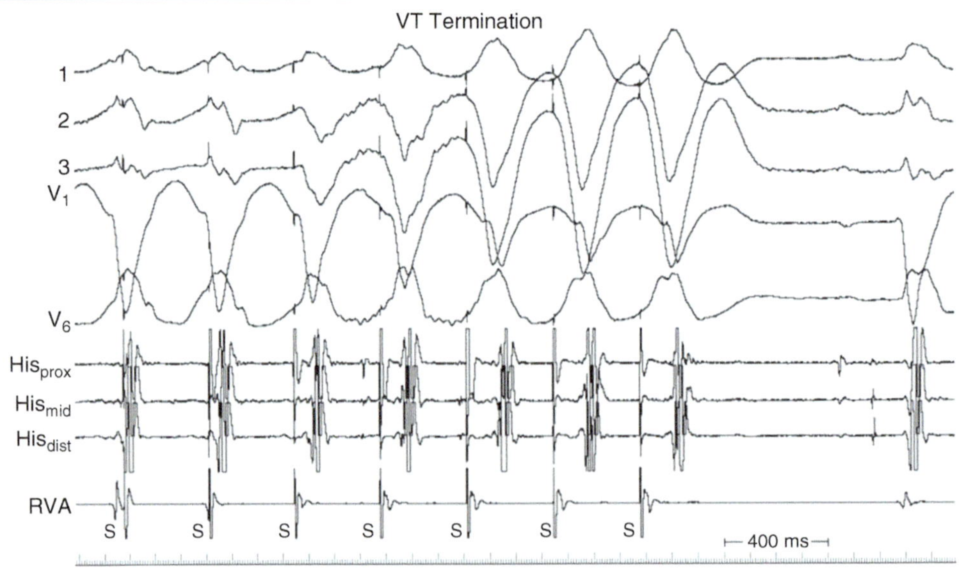

Figure 28-9

Fortunately, a single burst of ventricular pacing was able to terminate VT to sinus rhythm (Fig. 28-9). The situation at this time is as follows: VT is inducible but severe hypotension during VT precludes activation mapping under the current conditions. He had already undergone extensive substrate mapping and ablation, with little beneficial effect. Options at this point include the following: adding an inotropic agent to support blood pressure and reinitiate VT; add procainamide or amiodarone to slow VT rate, hoping for better hemodynamic stability, and attempt activation mapping if VT is tolerated; use pacemapping to guide ablation; repeat substrate mapping and ablation; perform epicardial mapping and ablation; discontinue procedure and come back another day with mechanical hemodynamic support (percutaneous ventricular assist device, etc.)

Baseline ECG (Nonpaced)

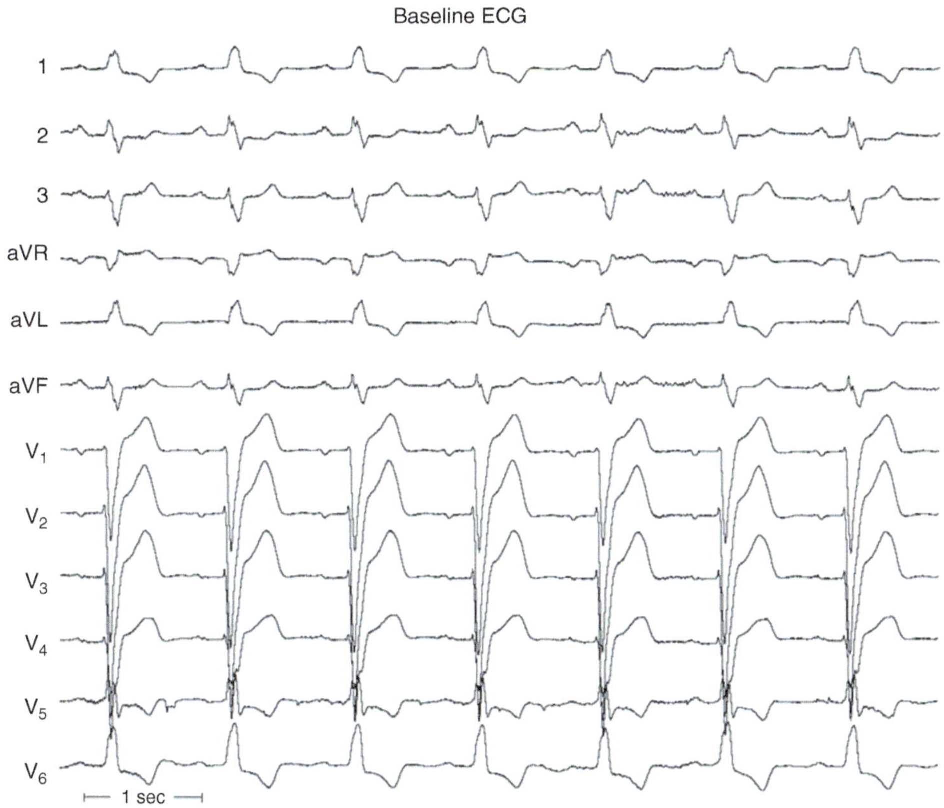

Figure 28-10

Before proceeding, it is worth a look back at what has already been learned in the procedure, starting with the nonpaced ECG at the beginning; this shows a LBBB morphology (Fig. 28-10).

Baseline Intracardiac Recordings Again

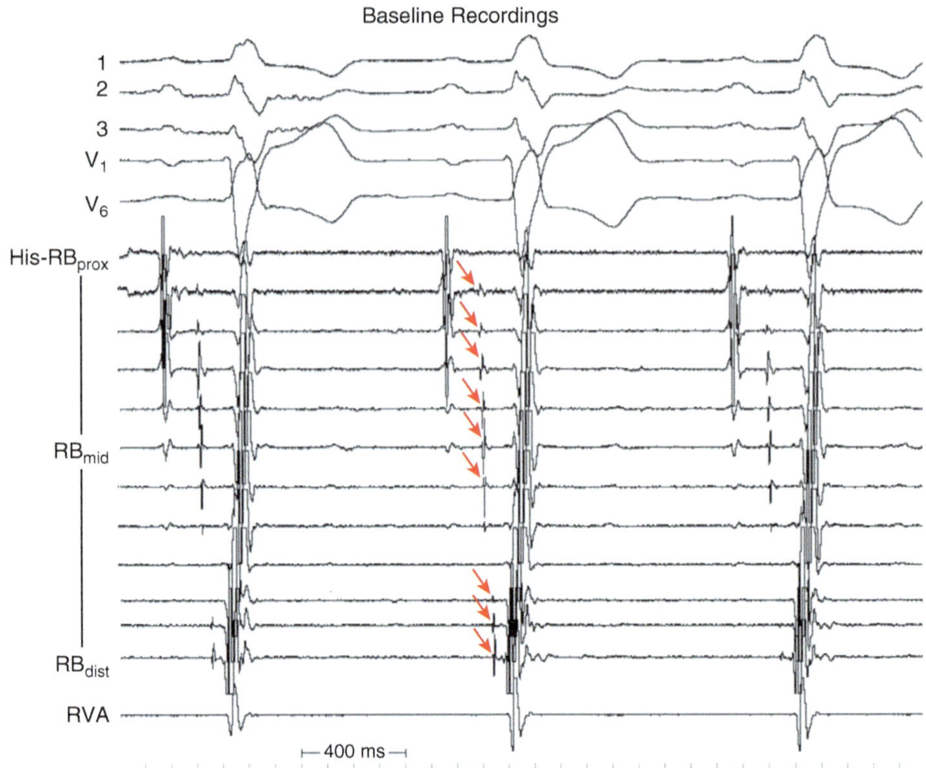

Figure 28-11

Another look back at sinus rhythm before induction of VT shows additional recordings made at the time, but not displayed earlier (Fig. 28-11). A decapolar catheter had been placed roughly in the usual His recording position, extending into the right ventricle along course of the right bundle branch; in addition, the quadripolar catheter usually used for recording the His bundle was placed more distally on the right ventricular aspect of the interventricular septum. Recordings from these two catheters are labeled His-RB_{prox} through RB_{dist}, and show small potentials representing His and RBB recordings *(arrows).*

VT Initiation Again

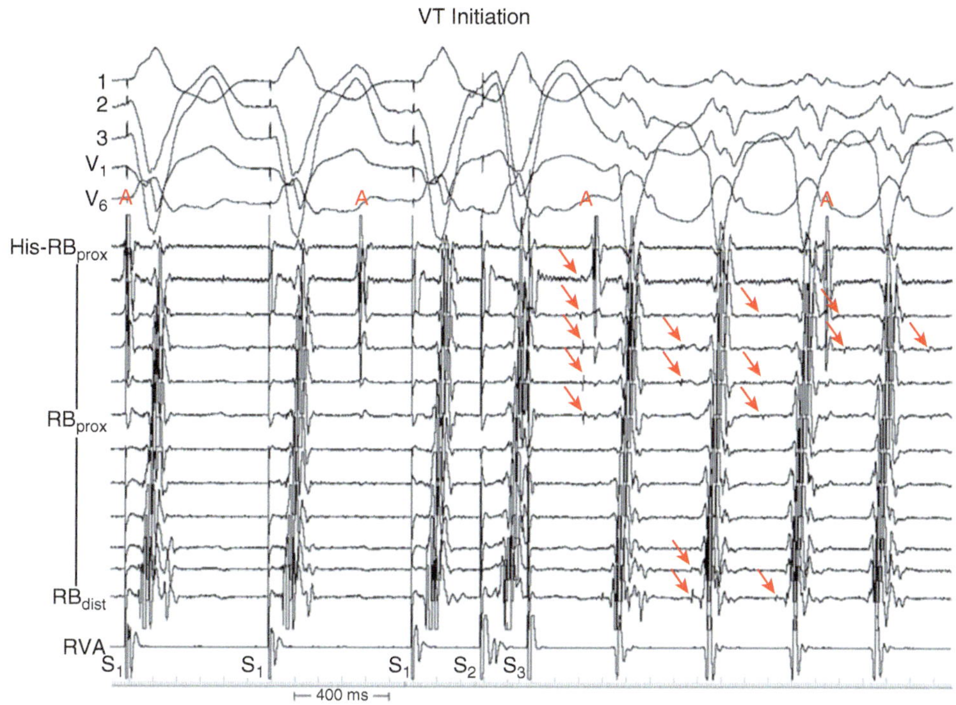

Figure 28-12

Another look back at induction of VT shows the additional recordings described in the prior figure that were made at the time, but not displayed earlier (Fig. 28-12). Recordings from these two catheters show small potentials *(red arrows)* during initiation of VT that are consistent with His and bundle branch potentials; the HV here is about 110 ms (in sinus rhythm, 95 ms). The mere presence of His potentials during VT does not allow a diagnosis of bundle branch reentry (because these are frequently seen in all forms of VT), but is consistent with it. Dissociated atrial electrograms are also seen (*A*).

VT Compared with Sinus Rhythm ECGs

Figure 28-13

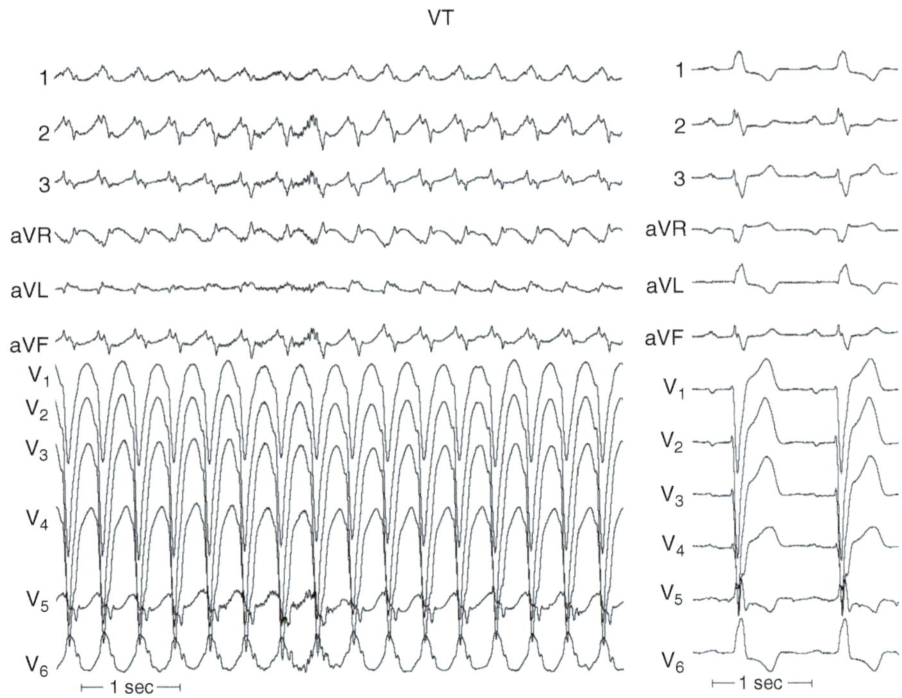

Another look at the 12-lead ECG of VT (in Fig. 28-13) shows similarities to the nonpaced QRS (at right) at the beginning of the procedure.

His Recordings During VT

Figure 28-14

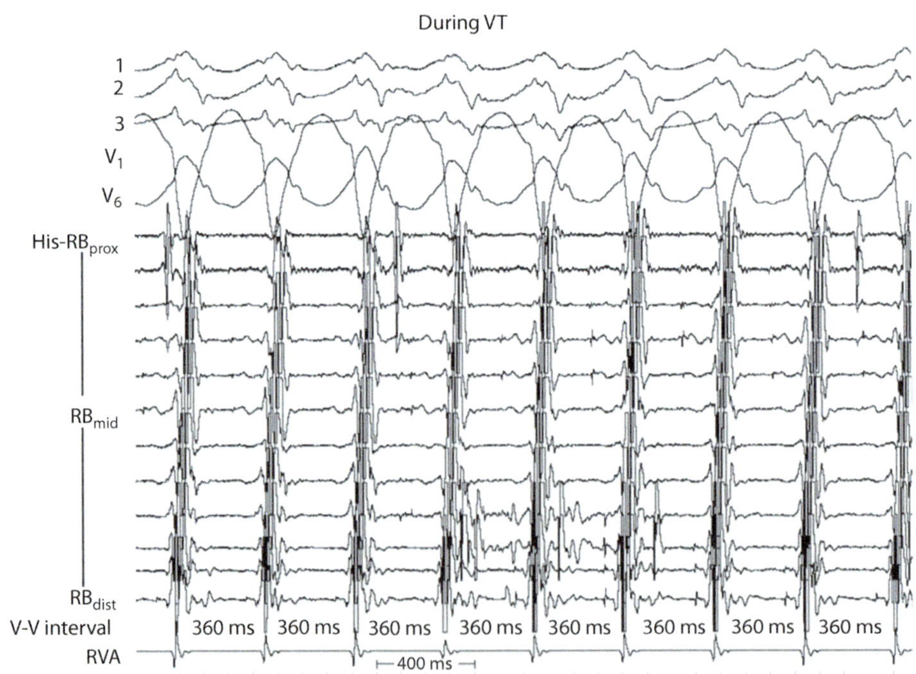

A few seconds after initiation of VT, but before pacing termination, the recordings in Fig. 28-14 were made. All intervals appear constant, affording no opportunity to test which signal leads others.

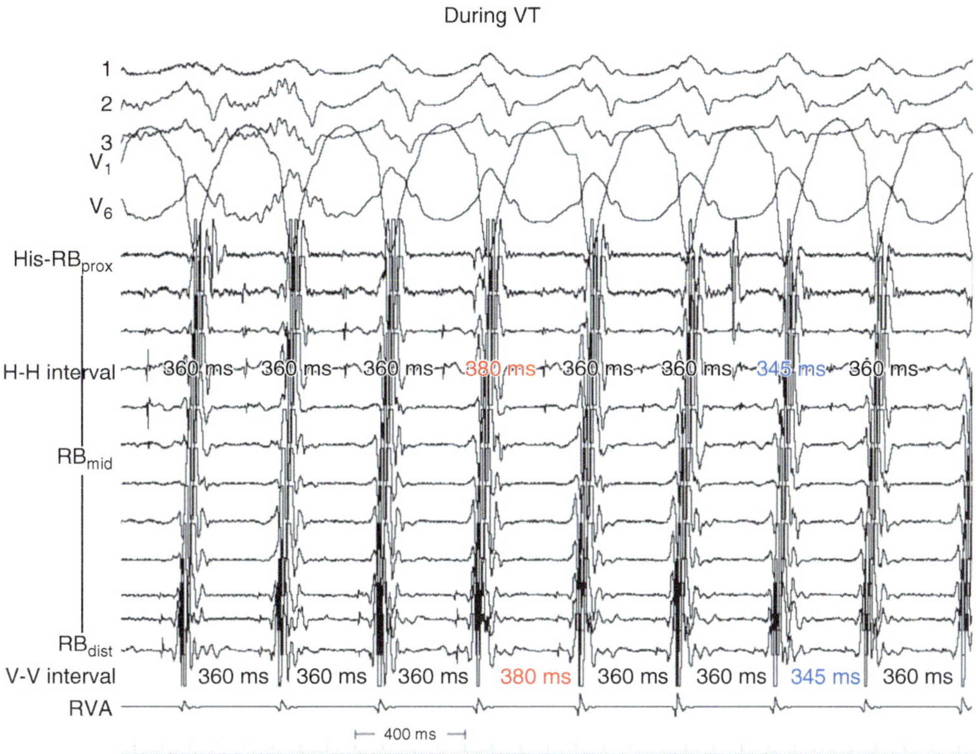

Figure 28-15

A few seconds still later, immediately before pacing termination, some irregularity of VT cycle length is seen (Fig. 28-15); it appears that changes in H-H intervals as shown precede changes in V-V intervals, strongly indicating that His-Purkinje activation drives the VT.

Ablation Site

Figure 28-16

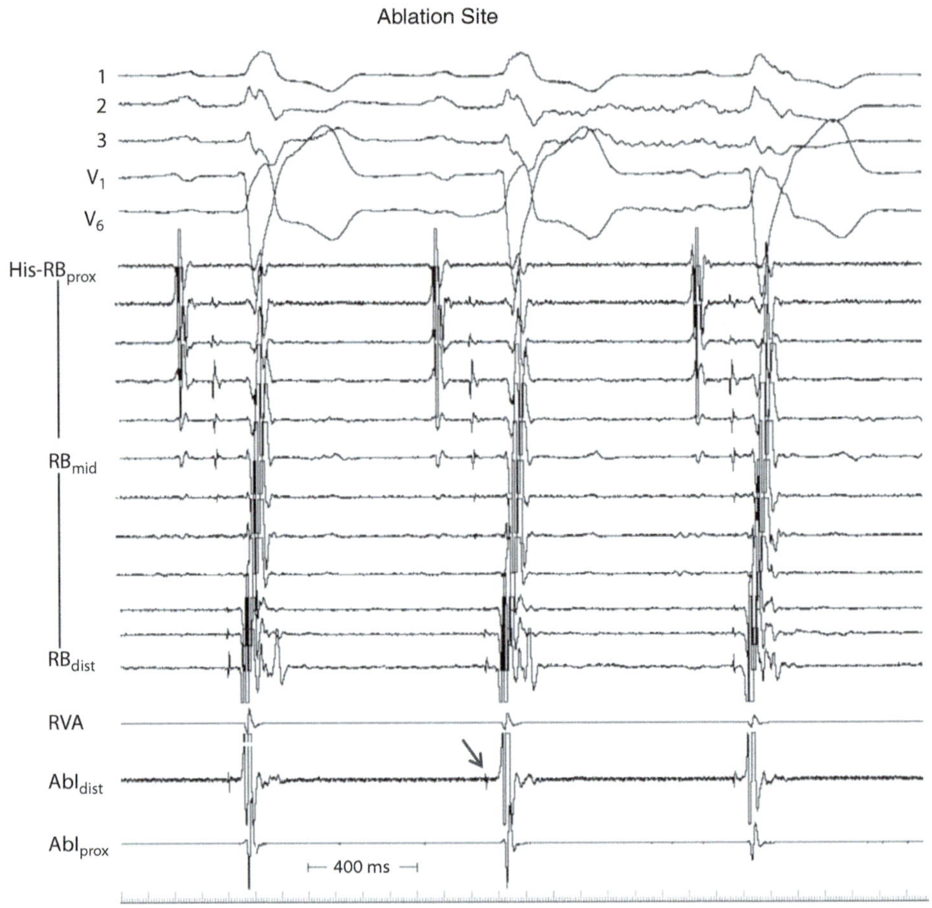

With all the data taken together (LBBB in sinus rhythm and similar morphology in VT; long HV baseline and during VT; H-H changes preceding V-V changes during VT; early activation of the RV apex during VT), a diagnosis of bundle branch reentrant VT was made and the RBB was targeted for ablation. Further maneuvers (attempted entrainment from RV) were not attempted because of hemodynamic instability during VT. In Fig. 28-16, a very small, sharp RBB potential *(arrow)* is evident in the ablation recording. These are often of very low amplitude and may be missed if the signal gain is not adequate.

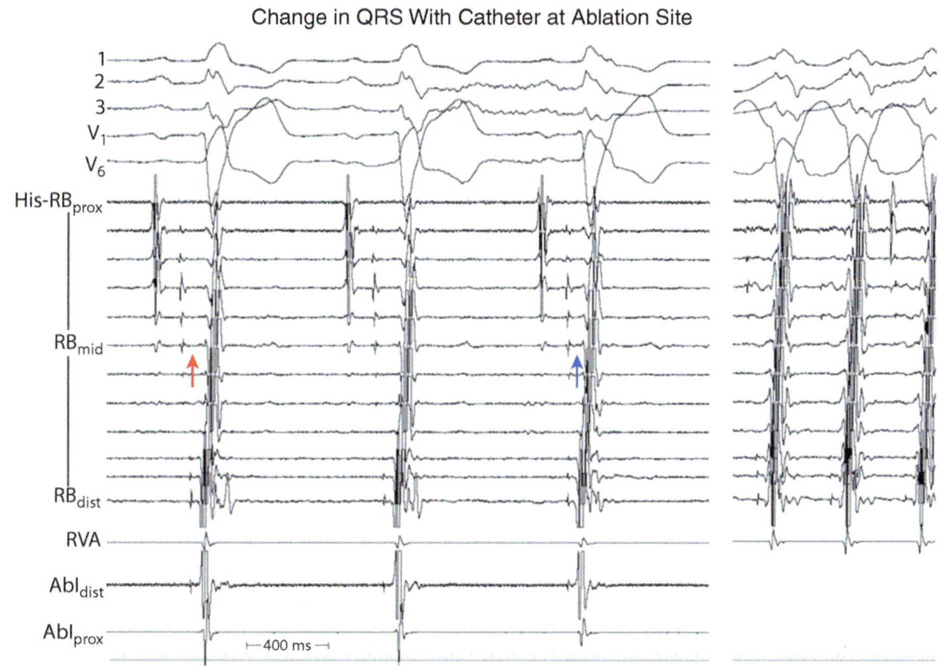

Figure 28-17

Catheter pressure at the ablation site (Fig. 28-17) appeared to cause mild prematurity of the RBB potential (shorter HV interval at *blue arrow* than *red*). Of note, this was accompanied by a slight change in the QRS complex, making it still more like the VT complexes (shown in the right panel). This is likely related to change in the site of breakout from the RBB to initiate ventricular activation.

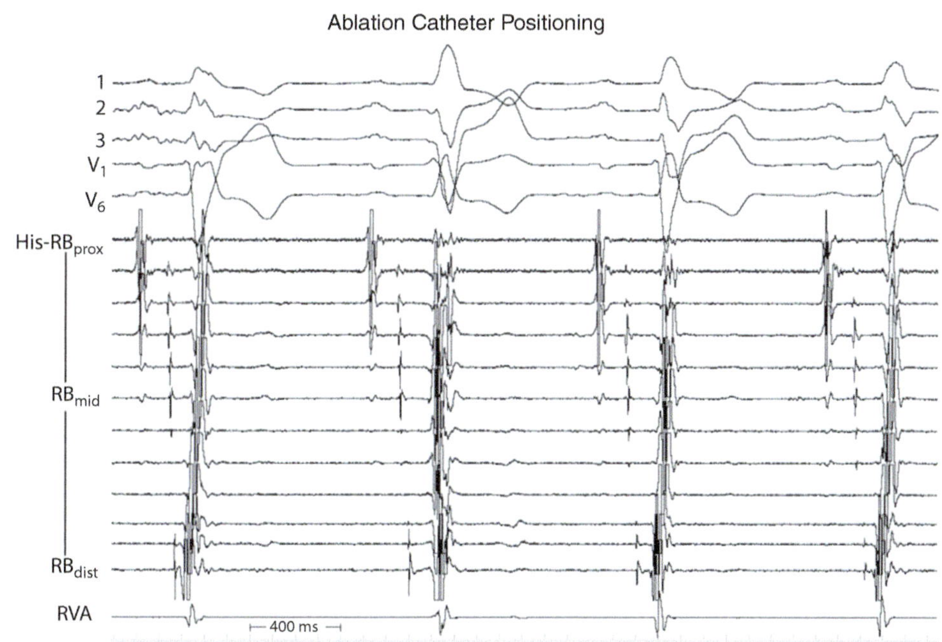

Figure 28-18

Additional catheter manipulation caused further changes in QRS complex and RBB-local ventricular activation times as shown in Fig. 28-18.

RF Ablation

Figure 28-19

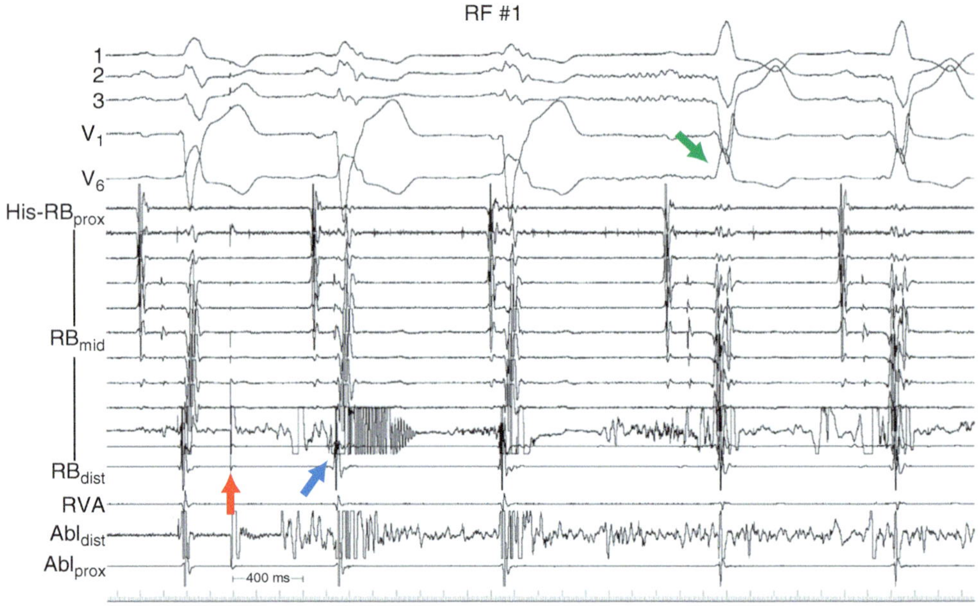

Radiofrequency (RF) energy (Fig. 28-19, delivery starting at *red arrow*) results in an accelerated rhythm *(blue arrows)* from the ablation site followed by elimination of conduction over the RBB *(green arrow)*. As is very often the situation in similar cases, RBBB in the presence of preexisting apparent LBBB does not result in complete heart block, but reveals very slow anterograde conduction over the left bundle branch (showing RBBB with a long HV interval).

Final ECG

Figure 28-20

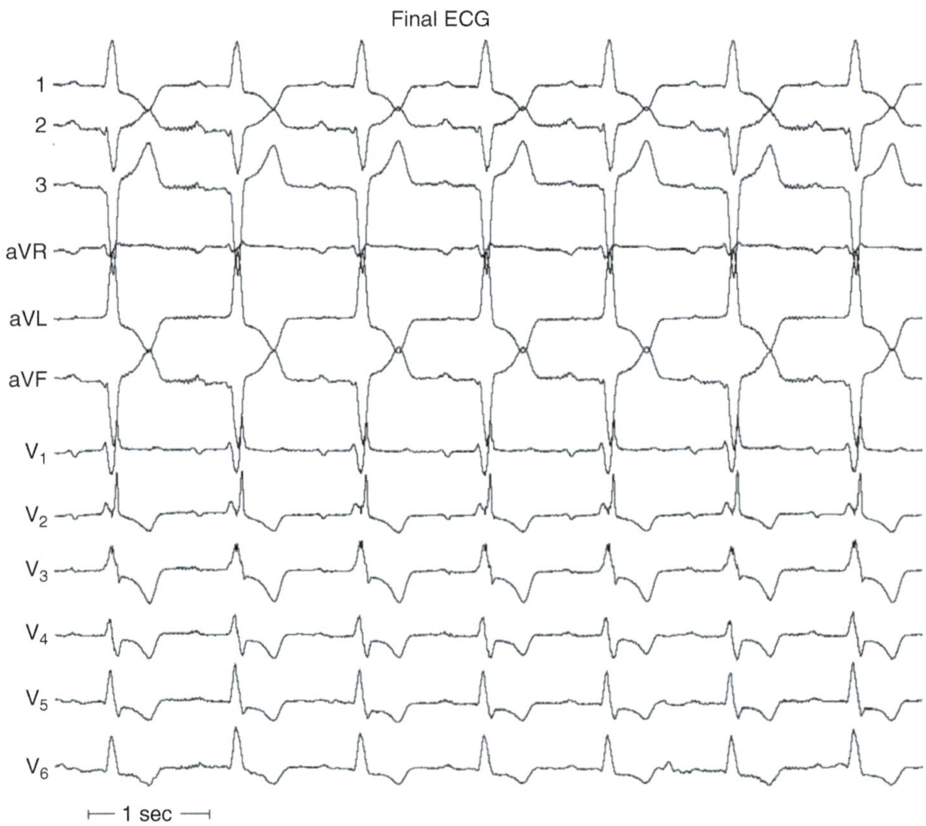

The final 12-lead ECG shows RBBB with left axis deviation.

After ablation, repeat ventricular stimulation showed no inducible ventricular arrhythmias; the patient's ICD was reprogrammed to atrial sensed biventricular pacing. After over 2 years of follow-up, no arrhythmias were detected by the ICD (Fig. 28-20).

Other Examples of Bundle Branch Reentry

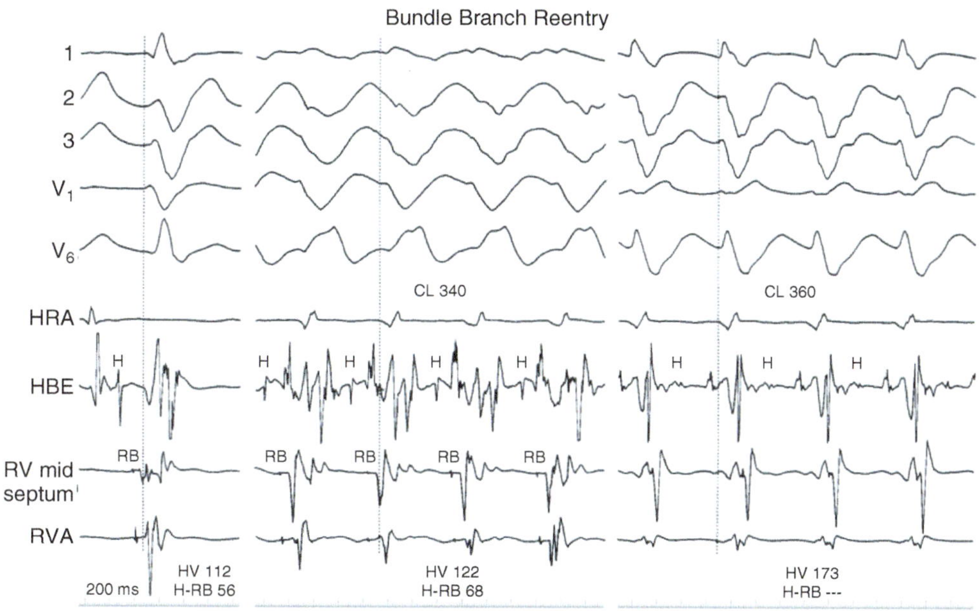

Figure 28-21

In a different patient, two episodes of bundle branch reentry (BBR) with opposite directions of circulation in the His-Purkinje system are illustrated in Fig. 28-21 with sinus rhythm at left, typical LBBB-type BBR in center, and RBBB-type BBR at right. Note relative timing of His and right bundle (RB) branch recordings.

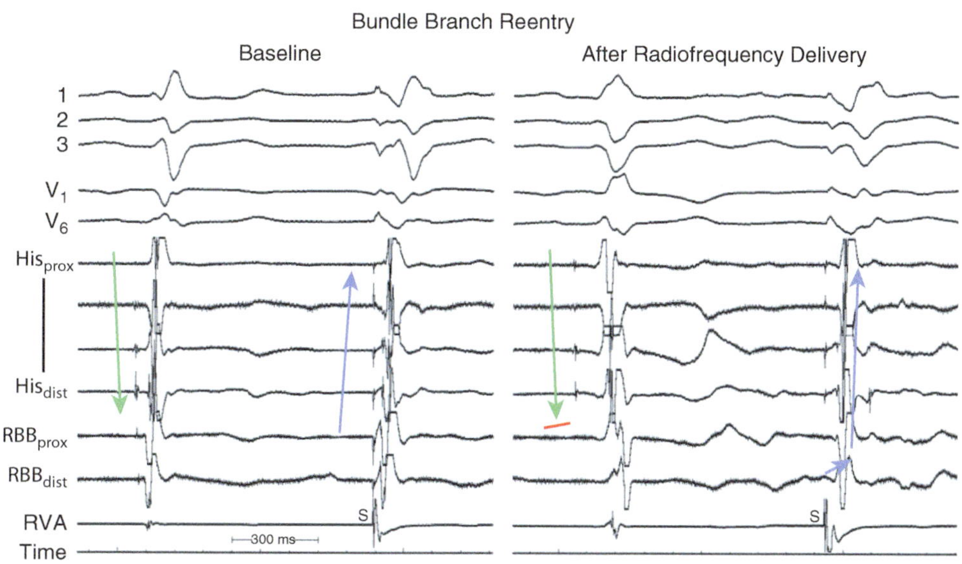

Figure 28-22

In yet another case of BBR, recordings along the RBB are shown in Fig. 28-22 before (baseline) and after RBB ablation, in sinus rhythm (complex at left in each panel) and right ventricular pacing (complex at right in each panel). *Green arrow* indicates anterograde propagation in the RBB during sinus rhythm (blocked after ablation, *red line*), whereas the *blue line* indicates retrograde propagation over the RBB. After ablation, retrograde RBB activation is dramatically delayed (appears after the local ventricular electrogram).

Summary

- Bundle branch reentry is not uncommon in patients with dilated cardiomyopathy
- At least a moderate level of suspicion is necessary for preparing correct recordings to make diagnosis
  - Multiple His + RB recordings are essential (ideally, LB also)
  - Standard catheter setup may easily miss the diagnosis
  - Look for spontaneous variations in VT cycle length (if preceded by H-H changes, BBR is diagnosed)
- Ablation of RB may unmask slow, but present, conduction over the LB with a very long HV interval
- Other myocardial VTs are present in at least 30% of patients, generally necessitating ICD placement (if not already present)

Index

S

T